THE MEASUREMENT OF PERSONAL

THE MEASUREMENT OF PERSONALITY

Readings selected and comments written by

H. J. Eysenck, Ph.D., D.Sc.

Professor of Psychology, University of London

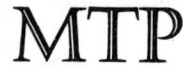

MTP

Published by
MTP Press Limited
St Leonard's House
Lancaster
England

ISBN 0 85200 148 7

Printed in Great Britain at The Spottiswoode Ballantyne Press
by William Clowes and Sons Limited,
London, Colchester and Beccles

CONTENTS

To explain all nature is too difficult a task for any one man or even for any one age. 'Tis much better to do a little with certainty and leave the rest for others that come after you, than to explain all things.

I. NEWTON.

FOREWORD

This book deals with the measurement of personality, in much the same way as an earlier book dealt with the measurement of intelligence (Eysenck, 1973). In each case the major part of the book consists of reprinted articles of particular interest and importance, organized into ten sections, and linked by short commentaries. In each case, the intent is not to produce a textbook, or a survey of all or many of the current approaches to the subject, or an eclectic conglomerate, but rather to try and give a coherent impression of a scientific paradigm. Paradigms, as defined by Kuhn (1962), are "accepted examples of actual scientific practice—examples which include law, theory, application, and instrumentation together—[which] provide models from which spring particular coherent traditions of scientific research". Suppe (1974) has pointed out that, in Kuhn's development of this thesis, the central concept of "paradigm" is not clear; "it is used extremely loosely and becomes bloated to the point of being a philosophical analogue to phlogiston". Masterman (1970) has listed twenty-one different ways in which Kuhn employs "paradigm", not all of which are compatible with each other. In his most recent paper, Kuhn has acknowledged the problem, and suggests two major components of his earlier notion: *exemplars* and *disciplinary matrix*. Exemplars are the accepted applications of symbolic generalizations to various concrete problems one finds in the examples and solutions to the exercises in standard textbooks and laboratory manuals. The disciplinary matrix "is the common possession of a professional discipline", it "contains all those shared elements which make for relative fullness of professional communication and unanimity of professional judgment. These include values for judging the adequacy of scientific work, models, ontological commitments, symbolic generalizations, a language, with meanings specific to that community, for interpreting symbolic generalizations, and so on".

The term "paradigm" is used here roughly in this sense. It would not be appropriate to go into greater detail concerning the philosophical discussions of this concept; the reader must be referred to Suppe's (1974) book for this purpose. Immediately the reader will express a doubt. It is possible to argue that such a paradigm exists in the field of intelligence, although even that statement would be criticized by many psychologists; can it be argued that such a statement can seriously be made in the field of personality? There is indeed a marked difference of status; I would suggest that the paradigm of "intelligence" fashioned by Galton, Spearman, Burt, Thurstone and Binet is not exempt from criticism, but it does constitute a paradigm as defined by Kuhn. As far as personality is concerned, I would say rather that such a paradigm has been developing, and that by now it may be considered to have come of age. The papers assembled in this book are the best evidence for this statement; if the reader is still doubtful after reading through them, then clearly the editor has been over-optimistic!

In trying to present a paradigm, I have had to excise from the enormous literature on personality all those papers which did not deal with the paradigm, directly or indirectly; in doing so I will to many seem to have thrown out the baby with the bath water. The great majority of investigations in the personality field are isolated, one-off pieces of work; at best, we have a series of studies using the same test, but otherwise isolated from general psychology, from theory, and from laboratory studies in experimental psychology. I am not denying that such studies can be of great interest and value; I am suggesting that the prime business of science is the construction of paradigms of the Kuhnian kind, and the failure of psychology in general, and personality theory in particular, to do so has been one of the reasons why many "hard" scientists are reluctant to admit psychology into the charmed circle of science altogether. To many psychologists, this refusal matters not at all; they are quite happy to remain outside the pale, and profess to be uninterested in creating a science which is at all similar to physics, or chemistry, or astronomy. For them, this book will contain nothing of interest; it is written for those who feel that a truly scientific attempt to understand and deal with the concepts of personality research is worth the while—using the term "scientific" here in precisely the same way in which it would be used by a "hard" scientist, or by the philosophers of science who contributed to the Suppe (1974) or the Lakatos and Musgrave (1970) symposia.

The term "measurement" in the title of this book was chosen precisely because it marks the point where science begins, and common sense ends; as Lord Kelvin put it, "One's knowledge of science begins when he can measure what he is speaking about, and express it in numbers". Or, in the words of Clerk Maxwell, "We owe all the great advances in knowledge to those who endeavour to find out how much there is of anything". Measurement, unfortunately, is not as easy and obvious a concept as it is often thought to be; a perusal of the books of Campbell (1920, 1928), Bridgeman (1927), and Ellis (1966) will soon show the complexities which arise. In particular, meaningful scientific measurement is only possible within the confines of some theoretical framework. Consider the simple measurement of length, apparently the most elementary kind of measurement. To measure the distance from London to Edinburgh, simply apply a metal rod, a yard long, so many times; this will give you the answer. Yes, but you would find that the distance apparently was longer in winter than in summer! (Metal rods shrink in the cold, and expand in the heat.) In 1784 when Britain and France co-operated in a project to determine the precise relative positions of the Greenwich and Paris Observatories, William Roy was given the job of measuring a base line for triangulation (which in turn presupposes considerable knowledge of geometry) across Hounslow Heath. He used deal wood rods, and found his results unusable, because the wood shrank and swelled with changing humidity, and he had to remeasure with glass, and finally with steel chain. Thus even in the most elementary type of measurement there is need for a theory—embracing in this case metallurgy, thermodynamics, humidity, and whatnot.

On the other hand, measurement (certainly at the beginning) need not be very precise in order to be called scientific. The basic method involved in measurement in high energy physics was discovered by Ernest Rutherford early in the century. Alpha particles, sent out by some radioactive substance, were used as bullets, and Sidot's Blende, a zinc sulphide with traces of copper, was used to transform into light some of the energy created by an alpha particle striking an atom. The resulting scintillations could be seen with a magnifying glass, and in this way it was possible to spot the occasional sharp deflections suffered by an alpha particle on going through a thin foil. The observer had to wait in pitch darkness for half an hour to get his eyes adapted before starting to count scintillations, and the result was very unreliable with more than fifty and less than one or two scintillations per minute. Weak flashes could be both missed and imagined, and wrong results galore were published, particularly by the Viennese school where students—presumably unbiased because they were not told what they were counting—felt that the more scintillations they saw the better! This early exercise in what we now call *vigilance* (see part IV, page 169) was scientific measurement all the same; the inaccuracy was soon remedied once the theoretical framework was constructed.

This approach to personality via model building and measurement goes counter to the deeper feelings of many psychologists. They would prefer to understand and explain human nature, rather than to measure invariant properties detected in the laboratory. However, as the Nobel Laureate Wigner (1964) has pointed out: "Physics does not endeavour to explain nature. In fact, the great success of physics is due to a restriction of its objectives: it only endeavours to explain the regularities in the behaviour of objects. This renunciation of the broader aims, and the specification of the domain for which an explanation can be sought, now appear to us as an obvious necessity. In fact, the specification of the explainable may have been the greatest discovery of physics so far". I firmly believe that we will only rival the success of physics if we adopt the method described by Wigner in psychology; personality study will forever remain an art, rather than a science, if we do not attempt to construct paradigms, test deductions from the theories belonging to that paradigm, and carry out measurement in line with the theoretical concepts of the paradigm. Even if this belief were correct, it would presumably mean little to those who prefer psychology to be an art rather than a science. The serious problems which we face, nationally and internationally, most of which are psychological problems rather than material ones, may act as a reminder that psychology as an art form has not so far delivered the goods, and does not look like doing so in the future; it might be worth while trying the scientific horse!

As an alternative to Wigner's statement, we may quote Einstein: "The grand aim of all science is to cover the greatest number of empirical facts by logical deduction from the smallest number of hypotheses or axioms". Again, note the absence of terms like "understand" or even "explain", and also the absence of the notion of "cause". Causal connections are difficult concepts to work with, as Hume already demonstrated. The Emperor Justinian thought that sodomy caused earthquakes, a belief no longer shared by many people. However, psychologists, particularly in the personality field, still hold causal beliefs no less quaint than this. Perhaps a return to the simplicity of the aims and methods of science might give us greater control over nature, even though it might destroy the *mystique* of the clinician, whose influence has been very powerful and almost certainly disadvantageous in this field.

If the aim be judged to be a reasonable one (provided that it does not exclude other approaches, having other aims in view), then it may be useful to state explicitly the rules according to which the researcher may proceed. A very brief and necessarily dogmatic statement of the metatheory would encompass the following points.

(1) *There is one set of invariant factors in human behaviour which gives rise to individual differences; these factors can be conceptualized under such headings as abilities, traits, attitudes, etc.* Doubts have often been expressed about the existence and/or importance of such invariant personality factors; thus Thorndike, in an early and typically powerful statement of this position, wrote that "there are no broad, general traits of personality, no general and consistent forms of conduct which, if they existed, would make for consistency of behaviour and stability of personality, but only independent and specific stimulus–response bonds or habits". I have discussed the evidence regarding this elsewhere (Eysenck, 1970), arguing that the weight of the evidence is overwhelmingly against Thorndike's view. Since then, Mischel (1971) and others have revived Thorndike's view, and the emerging doctrine of "situationism" (i.e. the belief that situations contribute more to the variance than does personality) has been much discussed and criticized (e.g. Bowers, 1973; Endler, 1973; Magnusson, 1974). The first section includes a paper on this issue, so that little more needs to be said, other than that this whole book, in a sense, is an answer to Mischel's position; if personality factors were as unimportant compared with the situational ones, then none of the experiments recounted here could have had a successful outcome. Also of course none of the authors taking part in this controversy note the fact that genetic factors are of great importance in the creation of personality differences, as illustrated by another paper in the first section of this book; this too would be impossible unless personality factors possessed the characteristics which Thorndike and Mischel deny. Obviously situations and personality characteristics are both important in determining the outcome of a particular experiment, and their interaction is likely to be of particular relevance. Any view denying the importance of personality invites the criticism which Dr. Johnson made of the plot of Shakespeare's *Cymbeline.*

(2) *Personality factors must be integrated into general psychology by using concepts and theories paradigmatic in that science to explain the observed regularities.* It has always been one of the main criticisms of psychology that it consists essentially of a series of disconnected textbook headings, and that there is no unity whatever linking these chapters together. The truth of this charge becomes obvious when we look at the chapter on personality in any textbook, and search in vain for concepts and theories which we have encountered previously in chapters on perception, learning, memory, conditioning, and so forth. The only person to have tried to forge such links, in a serious attempt to remedy this

situation, was K. Spence; unfortunately he approached personality merely as an extension of the general Hullian system, and his great contribution has suffered from the disfavour into which Hullian learning theory has sunk. As we shall also see, there are other criticisms of his work which make the interpretation of his results problematic; these detailed points will be dealt with in subsequent sections. This, of course, is the fate of all pioneering attempts; here let us merely note that Spence (in the terms of our metatheory) was working along the right lines, and many of his ideas have stood the test of time and are incorporated into the paradigm here offered. It would be a task of supererogation to argue the need for such integration between personality study and general psychology here; if the point is not obvious, then no amount of argument will suffice to convince.

(3) *Personality factors of sufficient width and importance to determine general and invariant patterns of behaviour are likely to be biologically anchored and to be determined strongly by genetic causes.* This statement in particular is likely to make the acceptance of the paradigm here offered difficult, in view of the apparent determination of most psychologists interested in personality study to disregard biological and genetic factors in favour of environmental and social influences. The issue is of course an empirical one, and a whole section of this book is devoted to the discussion of experimental efforts to find a physiological basis for the particular set of invariant factors which we have chosen to use as our example. This third and final statement of our metatheory does not imply any disrespect for, or disregard of, environmental and social factors; these are obviously important for biosocial organisms. What is suggested, rather, is that invariance is more likely to be found in behaviour largely determined by biological causes, including genetic ones. The reader is invited simply to note this third statement of our metatheoretical position, and suspend judgment until he has reviewed the evidence offered.

Substantively, I believe that at the present time there are only three major personality factors outside the cognitive field which present themselves as candidates for the rather searching type of analysis here suggested. These factors have received various names by the different writers who have been concerned with them (usually along descriptive lines); here we shall refer to them as E (extraversion–introversion), N (neuroticism or emotionality, as opposed to stability), and P (psychoticism). Details about the large literature concerning the first two factors can be found in Eysenck and Eysenck (1969), and regarding the third in Eysenck and Eysenck (1976). The work of Cattell (at the higher order end) emerges with very similar factors, and so does that of many other factor analysts. We shall not here enter into a detailed description of the behaviour patterns which are characteristic of persons scoring high and low respectively on these dimensions of personality; let us merely note that they are relatively independent of each other, and of general intelligence, and that scores are distributed in a more or less normal fashion. When the term "type" is used in connection with these dimensions, this is understood to refer to persons at the extremes of these distributions.

All three factors have been linked theoretically and experimentally with biological structures which give rise to the behaviour observed at either extreme of these dimensions (Eysenck, 1967). As we have concentrated in this book on the extraversion–introversion dimension (with only occasional glances at other dimensions), it is the biological theories concerning this variable that we shall be concerned with. The authors of the different papers included in the various sections give sufficient detail of the theory to obviate the need to state it here again, except very briefly. It is suggested that extraverted behaviour is a function of persistently low cortical arousal, while introverted behaviour is a function of persistently high cortical arousal; ambiverts, i.e. persons intermediate with respect to E–I, are on this hypothesis characterized by intermediate degrees of arousal. As arousal (or drive) is a concept which is central to much general theoretical discussion in psychology, it fulfils our second metatheoretical requirement; it remains to be seen, of course, whether or not the empirical evidence does or does not support the theoretical postulation. The introduction to our second section contains some further considerations of the position here adopted.

Crucial to any experimental study of the relevance of arousal to personality is the realization that regressions are likely to be curvilinear rather than linear; if this point is not taken into account, deductions from theory are likely to be erratic. The postulate of a curvilinear relation between arousal or drive and performance was originally made by Yerkes and Dodson (1908); the Yerkes–Dodson Law also contains a second postulate, namely that the inversion of the direct relationship between drive and performance occurs earlier for difficult tasks, later for easy ones (Broadhurst, 1959). Pavlov (1927) enunciated a similar law, or rather, a similar law follows from putting together two of his laws. The first of these is the *law of strength*, which states that the strength of the response is a function of the strength of the stimulus (particularly in respect to conditioned responses); the second is the *law of transmarginal inhibition*, which asserts that with high values of stimulus intensity, the response becomes weaker, rather than stronger (Gray, 1964). (This is also known as "protective inhibition"; Pavlov thought of it as a device for protecting the cortical cells from over-stimulation.) In effect this would produce the same curvilinear regression of drive on performance as the Yerkes–Dodson Law. Third is Hebb (1955), who also postulated an inverted-U relation between drive and "cue function" or cortical efficiency, with an optimum level for response or learning. He also postulated that arousal was the physiological mechanism which underlies motivation, thus effectively substituting a physio-

logical mechanism recognizable by modern physiologists for Pavlov's rather esoteric physiological concepts. In recent years Spence and Broadbent have added important features to this model, the former suggesting that the important distinction was not between easy and difficult tasks, but between prepotent and non-dominant responses, and the latter hypothesizing that greater arousal was linked with special attention to dominant responses. These additional theories are discussed in their place by various authors whose studies are reprinted in later sections.

One advantage of a collection of readings such as this is the fact that by bringing together several examples of the same general law, it can be seen much more clearly than in the case of a single experiment that the law is not invoked *ad hoc*, but that it applies to a wide range of situations and stimuli. The law of transmarginal inhibition, for instance, may appear as a kind of *deus ex machina* when involved to explain a particular finding, such as that a few drops of lemon juice, when placed on the tongue, will increase the salivation rate of introverts drastically, but will leave that of extraverts unaffected; when the lemon juice is swallowed, producing a much stronger stimulation, extraverts show a marked increase in salivation, while introverts show a decrease (Eysenck and Eysenck, 1967). This may be explained in terms of transmarginal inhibition for introverts, but to many readers it will sound rather a doubtful explanation. When it is seen in the light of precisely similar phenomena in relation to evoked potentials as a function of strength of stimulation, eyeblink conditioning as a function of the strength of the UCS, the effect of intersensory stimulation on sensory thresholds, or any other examples included in the studies here reprinted, the explanation assumes quite a different aspect.

The concept of the inverted-U relationship between arousal-drive and performance-learning has been criticized (e.g. Näätänen, 1973), but as the work here presented, and the references contained therein make clear, there is very strong evidence for some such concept, and accordingly it has been retained here. Similarly, there has been much criticism of the concept of arousal, particularly because different methods of measurement have often shown only slight correlations. This point is discussed in the third section, and will not be dealt with here. It is suggested there that the criticism is not well taken, and that the evidence does in fact support the postulation of a physiologically based concept of arousal.

Most of the authors in this book have used the paradigm originally suggested by the writer (Eysenck, 1967), but others have made use of a Pavlovian set of concepts centring on the notion of a "strong" as opposed to a "weak" nervous system. The working out of Pavlovian theories in the personality field has been described well by Gray (1964) and Strelau (1975); necessary details are given in the papers reprinted. There does appear to be good theoretical reason, and also some empirical evidence, to identify the strong nervous system with extraversion, the weak nervous system with introversion, but the evidence is by no means conclusive (Gray, 1967). In addition, there are alternative theories about the physiological basis of extraversion (e.g. Gray, 1970) which implicate other mechanisms, such as the pleasure–pain centres; readers interested in these problems may like to consider how adequate such theories are to account for the majority of the facts contained in this book.

We must now turn to a problem which is endemic in psychology, but which is particularly important in personality research, namely the problem of "failure to replicate", and of failure to verify deductions from a general theory. It will be useful first of all to consider scientific methodology in general, before coming to grips with particular applications of the insights thus gained. This will necessitate a brief look at the present state of thinking among philosophers of science about the nature of science, and the importance of falsification and "falsifiability".

We will not consider old-fashioned and clearly erroneous views, such as inductionism; no science has ever arisen along Baconian principles of random data gathering and subsequent hypothesis formulation. In the early years of the twentieth century, inductive logicians set out to define the probabilities of different theories according to the available total evidence; if the mathematical probability of a theory was high, it qualified as scientific, while if it was low or even zero, it was not scientific. This view has some attractive features, but Popper (1959) destroyed it when he showed that the mathematical probability of all theories, scientific or pseudoscientific, given any amount of evidence, is zero. He showed that scientific theories are not only equally unprovable but also equally improbable; in the long run all our theories will be disproved, so that the "truth" or even the probability criterion has no real relevance.*

Popper (1959, 1963) instead suggested that we should

---

* It is curious and either tragic or comic that practically the only view of the philosophy of science which is at all familiar to psychologists is one which is almost universally rejected by leading philosophers of science. Beginning in the 1920s it became commonplace for philosophers of science to construe scientific theories as axiomatic calculi which are given a partial observational interpretation by means of correspondence rules. This theory was dubbed "the received view on theories", and was of course closely related to the school of logical positivism, although it still flourished after logical positivism had been decisively rejected by the great majority of philosophers. Both logical positivism and the received view became popular among psychologists, due to the efforts of Bergman, Spence and others, just after serious doubts concerning their adequacy had been raised among philosophers, and began to flourish in the kindly but uncritical soil of psychology after they had been coldbloodedly killed by more critical philosophers. The harrowing story is well told by Suppe (1974).

not divide scientific theories from pseudoscientific ones, but rather scientific *method* from pseudoscientific *method*. Scientific method is characterized by the criterion of *falsifiability*; if our theory specifies experimental conditions which could lead to disproof of the theory, then that theory is scientific; if not, not. Thus a proposition may petrify into pseudoscientific dogma or become genuine knowledge, depending on whether we are prepared to state observable conditions which would refute it. On this criterion, Popper decided that Marxism and Freudianism are either pseudosciences, or else they have been refuted; he is never quite clear which of these two outcomes he believes to be the correct one. (This is due to the fact that Marxists and Freudians behave in divergent ways when confronted with "refutations", some trying to change the theory, others trying to argue away the evidence.)

There are difficulties connected with Popper's view which are perhaps not widely enough known. At a conference called to discuss his and Kuhn's views, it became very apparent that the falsification theory itself had serious weaknesses (Lakatos and Musgrave, 1970). Newton's theory of gravitation threw up large numbers of anomalies and contradictions, yet his followers did not give up the theory; they behaved very much like convinced Marxists and Freudians in this respect. As Lakatos once said, "had Popper ever asked a Newtonian scientist under what *experimental* conditions he would abandon Newtonian theory, some Newtonian scientists would have been exactly as nonplussed as are some Marxists and Freudians" (personal communication). Kuhn (1962) not only argued against Popper's falsification criterion, but suggested that historically the accumulation of anomalies to which any theory is subject results in a *revolution* in which new concepts and new problems take over, and in which there is little question of crucial experiments to decide between the theories; these revolutions in some way resemble religious conversions, constituting just an irrational change in commitment. This view also has found many critics; the change from one paradigm to another must have some rational foundation which ought to be identifiable.

Perhaps the most widely accepted view among philosophers of science is that of Lakatos. It may be best to present a brief version of it in his own words; it is important to get the meaning of our terms clear if we are to argue rationally about the relevance of apparently negative evidence. Lakatos's view combines and transcends those of Popper and Kuhn, and while no doubt it too will ultimately be improved upon, it nevertheless at the moment gives us a meaningful and useful standard of scientific propriety.

This is what he says: "In the last few years I have been advocating a methodology of scientific research programmes, which solves some of the problems which both Popper and Kuhn failed to solve. First, I claim that the typical descriptive unit of great scientific achievements is not an isolated hypothesis but rather a research programme. Science is not simply trial and error, a series of conjectures and refutations. 'All swans are white' may be falsified by the discovery of one black swan. But such trivial trial and error does not rank as science. Newtonian science, for instance, is not simply a set of four conjectures—the three laws of motion and the law of gravitation. These four laws constitute only the *hard core* of the Newtonian programme. But this hard core is tenaciously protected from refutation by a vast *protective belt* of auxiliary hypotheses. And, even more importantly, the research programme has also a *heuristic*, that is, a powerful problem-solving machinery, which, with the help of sophisticated mathematical techniques, digests anomalies and even turns them into positive evidence. For instance, if a planet does not move exactly as it should, the Newtonian scientist checks his conjectures concerning atmospheric refraction, concerning propagation of light in magnetic storms, and hundreds of other conjectures which are all part of the programme. He may even invent a hitherto unknown planet and calculate its position, mass and velocity in order to explain the anomaly.

"Now Newton's theory of gravitation, Einstein's relativity theory, quantum mechanics, Marxism, Freudianism, are all research programmes, each with a characteristic hard core stubbornly defended, each with its more flexible protective belt and each with its elaborate problem-solving machinery. Each of them, at any stage of its development, has unsolved problems and undigested anomalies. All theories, in this sense, are born refuted and die refuted. But are they *equally* good? Until now I have been *describing* what research programmes are like. But how can one distinguish a scientific or *progressive* programme from a pseudo-scientific or *degenerating* one?

"Contrary to Popper, the difference cannot be that some are still unrefuted, while others are already refuted. When Newton published his *Principia*, it was common knowledge that it could not properly explain even the motion of the moon; in fact, lunar motion refuted Newton. Kaufmann, a distinguished physicist, refuted Einstein's relativity theory in the very year it was published. But all the research programmes I admire have one characteristic in common. They all predict *novel* facts, facts which had been either undreamt of, or have indeed been contradicted by previous or rival programmes. In 1686, when Newton published his theory of gravitation, there were, for instance, two current theories concerning comets. The more popular one regarded comets as a signal from an angry God warning that He will strike and bring disaster. A little known theory of Kepler's held that comets were celestial bodies moving along straight lines. Now according to Newtonian theory, some of them moved in hyperbolas or parabolas never to return; others moved in ordinary ellipses. Halley, working in Newton's programme, calculated on the basis of observing a brief stretch of a comet's path that it would return in 72 years time; he calculated to the minute when it would be seen again at a well-defined point of the sky. This was incredible. But 72 years later, when both Newton and Halley were long dead, Halley's comet returned exactly as Halley predicted. Similarly, Newtonian scientists predicted the existence and exact motion of small planets which had never been observed before. Or let us take Einstein's programme. This programme made the stunning prediction that if one measures the distance between two stars in the night and if one measures the distance between them during the day (when they are visible during an eclipse of the sun), the two measurements will be different. Nobody had thought to make such an observation before Einstein's programme. Thus in a *progressive* research programme theory leads to the discovery of hitherto unknown novel facts. In degenerating programmes, however, theories are fabricated only in order to accommodate *known* facts. Has, for instance, Marxism ever predicted a stunning novel fact successfully? NEVER. It had some famous *unsuccessful* predictions. It predicted the absolute impoverishment of the working class. It predicted that the first socialist societies would be free of revolutions. It predicted that there will be no conflict of interests between socialist countries. Thus the early predictions of Marxism were bold and stunning but they failed. Marxists explained all their failures: they explained the rising living standards of the working class by devising a theory of imperialism; they explained even why the first socialist revolution occurred in industrially backward Russia. They 'explained' Berlin 1953, Budapest 1956, Prague 1968. They 'explained' the Russian–Chinese conflict. But their auxiliary hypotheses were all cooked up after the event to protect Marxian theory from the facts. The Newtonian programme led to novel facts; the Marxian lagged behind the facts and has been running fast to catch up with them.

"To sum up. The hallmark of empirical progress is not trivial verifications: Popper is right that there are millions of them. It is no success for Newtonian theory that stones, when dropped, fall towards the earth, no matter how often this is repeated. But so-called 'refutations' are not the hallmark of empirical failure, as Popper has preached, since all programmes grow in a permanent ocean of anomalies. What *really* counts are dramatic, unexpected, *stunning* predictions: a few of them are enough to tilt the balance; where theory lags behind the facts, we are dealing with miserable *degenerating* research programmes.

"Now how do scientific *revolutions* come about? If we have two rival research programmes, and one is progressing while the other is degenerating, scientists tend to join the progressive programme. This is the *rationale* of scientific revolutions. But while it is a matter of intellectual honesty to keep the record public, it is not dishonest to stick to a degenerating programme and try to turn it into a progressive one.

"As opposed to Popper the methodology of scientific research programmes does not offer instant rationality. One must treat budding programmes leniently; programmes may take decades before they get off the ground and become empirically progressive. Criticism is not a Popperian quick kill, by refutation. Important criticism is always constructive: there is no refutation without a better theory. Kuhn is wrong in thinking that scientific revolutions are sudden, irrational changes in vision. The history of science refutes both Popper and Kuhn: on close inspection both Popperian crucial experiments and Kuhnian revolutions turn out to be myths: what normally happens is that progressive research programmes replace degenerating ones." (Personal communication.)

On these grounds, the research programme which is implicit in the paradigm discussed in this book must be accepted as strictly in line with the requirement as a progressive programme. It fulfils, as we shall see, the major requirement, namely that it should be productive of novel facts; the reader must be the judge of the degree to which this requirement is in fact fulfilled. The question which arises in relation to failure to replicate, and to failures of deductions to be verified, raises the problem of what Lakatos calls the "protective belt" which surrounds the "hard core" central to every scientific research programme. What sorts of arguments might be part of this protective belt, to take charge of the many anomalies which inevitably surround every research programme? (It is important to emphasize this historical fact, namely the abundance of anomalies in every research programme that ever was; psychologists are apt to abandon a research programme at the first whiff of anomalies, failures of prediction, or lack of replication. A good example is the work of Petrie, discussed in a later section, where a very successful technique, productive of many novel facts, was abruptly abandoned because of a completely irrelevant failure to demonstrate high retest reliabilities, and failure to replicate produced by actual changes in methodology.) Among those that spring to mind are the following.

(1) *Differences in measuring instruments for E–I*. The theory is specifically related to a conception of E–I embodied in the Eysenck Personality Inventory, or its parallel forms, the MPI or the EPQ; many authors have used instead other inventories to measure this dimension, such as the Cattell scales, the Myers–Briggs Type Indicator, the MMPI, the Sensation Seeking scale, the Barratt Impulsiveness scale, the MAS and many more. All these scales correlate with the EPI, sometimes quite highly, but they sample somewhat different portions of the personality factor space, and the differences may be crucial for particular deductions, leading to failure to replicate, or failure to verify deductions which might be verifiable with a proper measure.

(2) *Neglect of experimental parameters*. Deductions from the general theory can and do specify optimal experimental parameters, and if other parameters are chosen then apparent anomalies may be the result. Examples are given in later sections, e.g. in relation to eyeblink conditioning; the prediction of positive correlations between introversion and conditioning, made on the basis of UCS of low or middling intensity, can be upset (predictably) by the choice of UCS of strong intensity; indeed, it is possible to reverse the direction of the correlation in this manner! Similarly, experimental parameters are vital in making predictions regarding the correlation between E–I and EEG arousal; this is discussed in detail in the second section. Neglect of this factor has been responsible for a large number of failures to replicate or verify; it hardly needs saying that these failures are failures of the experimenters involved, not failures of the theory.

(3) *Failure of intermediary theories*. It is acknowledged among philosophers of science that failures to verify predictions from a given theory may be due to faults in the theory *or* to faults in the hypotheses which link the original theory with a particular field. As an example, let us take the writer's prediction that extraverts would show greater reminiscence in pursuit rotor experiments. This prediction was based in part on a linking theory, namely Hull's hypothesis that reminiscence was due to the dissipation of reactive inhibition, an hypothesis which was at the time widely accepted, and indeed almost universal. Later work (summarized in a later section) showed that in fact the dissipation of inhibition hypothesis is wrong, and has to be substituted by a consolidation hypothesis (Eysenck and Frith, 1976). (Actually the prediction from the wrong hypothesis has been verified many times; this demonstrates that wrong theories can generate verifiable predictions! After abandoning the wrong theory, it was necessary to postulate a new link which would join the new, hopefully correct theory with the observed predictions from the old, discredited theory.) Considering that most psychological theories relating to the many diverse phenomena which have been linked with extraversion are themselves of uncertain status, and far from universally agreed, clearly the failure of particular experiments is at least as likely to be due to the postulation of erroneous theories regarding the origin of the specific phenomenon, as to errors in the personality theory itself. If the personality theory is strongly supported in a number of quite dissimilar and divergent deductions, then the probability increases that failure to confirm may be due to erroneous assumptions regarding the new phenomena which form the object of the prediction.

(4) *Neglect of present state*. Trait theories specify, as we shall see later, an average level of arousal, maintained when conditions are mildly arousing; such average levels may be disturbed by many uncontrolled (and usually uncontrollable) external conditions (e.g. smoking or drinking prior to taking part in the experiment, partaking of food or sex, specific arousing properties of the stimuli through conditioning or

cognitive factors, tiredness, etc.). Thus state arousal should routinely be ascertained when testing theories concerning trait theories of arousal; as M. W. Eysenck (1976) has shown, it is often possible for neither state nor trait measures to give significant results, but for the *interaction* to be highly significant. (The same point is made in several of the papers reprinted in later sections.) The testing situation itself may be differentially arousing, and this factor must be taken into account predictively and by actual measurement of state arousal.

(5) *Interaction of different personality factors.* The action of a particular chemical element may be well understood, but chemical elements usually act in combination, and the laws of combination are complex and often difficult to disentangle. Personality factors never act in isolation; this is a simple function of the fact that they are measured in intact persons who must have a position, not only on the personality trait measured, but also on other personality traits (and on intelligence, etc.). Thus we may make predictions about an extravert or an introvert, but we are testing these predictions on extraverts or introverts who are also neurotic or stable, bright or dull, tough- or tender-minded. Such outside differences can sometimes be controlled, e.g. by picking experimental subjects within a narrow band of scores on other traits, but this procedure is essentially limited to consideration of one or at most two such other traits. Usually, other traits are measured but not controlled, and under these circumstances powerful interactions may arise; several examples are given in the papers here reprinted. Thus fluency scores are higher in extraverts than in introverts, as predicted, but only when N is low; when N is high, there are no differences. Sometimes the scoring patterns of extraverts and introverts are reversed when measured in high- and low-N subjects (e.g. Wallach and Gahm, 1960). Prediction and replication may fail when such interactions are not taken into account.

This collection of papers does not contain any which are specifically negative as far as predicted outcome is concerned; however, many papers do contain references to, and discussions of, experiments which failed to confirm the theory; the reader must judge for himself whether these anomalies can be explained along the lines of these five major "protective belts". The existence of such belts should not be taken as evidence of special pleading; they form part of every large-scale theory in the "hard" sciences, and psychology cannot be holier than thou in this respect. Some explanations of failure are in the nature of *post hoc* rationalizations; they are characteristic of degenerating research programmes. It does not seem to the writer that explanations of anomalies arising in the present field are of this character.

In considering philosophical theories concerning the growth of scientific concepts and ideas, it may be useful to remember that specific theories tend to refer, and apply to, certain stages of development of a science. It is usually assumed that such theories have a universal application, but this is almost certainly not so. Scientific concepts develop in the course of history, and different methods of investigation may be appropriate at different stages. Figure 1 may illustrate the kind of relation I have in mind. Usually development starts with ordinary observation and induction; based on these the investigator develops a hunch that certain features of the observation might be invariant—i.e. the sun might rise again tomorrow because in the past it has always risen again after setting. Gradually limited hypotheses are formed, e.g. that the sun is moving around the earth, or vice versa. At this early stage, verification is sought of such hypotheses, and falsification is not very important—there are so many areas of ignorance that apparent falsification may not be as destructive to the hypothesis as it would be at a later stage. (The failure to observe stellar parallax did not render Copernicus' heliocentric hypothesis nugatory.) Gradually hypotheses become more firmly established, and related ones are seen to have certain features in common; out of these related hypotheses a theory is born, such as Newton's theory of gravitation. Such a theory is highly specific in its predictions, and consequently falsification becomes important, although even at this stage simple falsification is not enough to overthrow a theory. Gradually theory develops into law; we tend to refer to theories which have become well established as natural or scientific laws. Falsification of laws is almost anathema; the anomalies in the precession of the perihelion of Mercury were known for centuries, but they were not admitted as disproof of Newton's laws. What is required is a Kuhnian revolution, in the form of an alternative theory; it needed Einstein's theory of relativity to overthrow Newton's theory. Falsification in the simple factual sense was not enough.

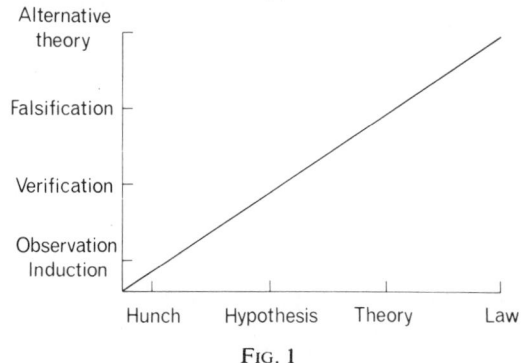

FIG. 1

It may be suggested that the theory discussed in this book is just on the point of moving from the area of being constituted of a set of hypotheses, of varying cogency and support, to that of genuine theory. This would make the search for verification less important, and that for falsification more so. I once labelled the continuum represented on the abscissa in the figure "weak *vs.* strong theories" (Eysenck, 1960); our theory is moving from being "weak" towards a position of greater strength—although of course still far removed from reaching the "strong" extreme. This would only be possible if psychology as a whole were to advance over a wider front; as pointed out before, the testing of personality theories such as this depends for success on supporting theories concerning the particular phenomena under investigation. Without a good theory of reminiscence, predictions from personality theory as to the differential performance of introverts and extraverts rest on insecure foundations; the same is true in the fields of conditioning, learning, memory, perception, motor movement, etc. Nevertheless, the change from even a dozen years ago is noticeable, both in the quality of the work done, and in the convergence of results on a general paradigm. If these trends continue, then a definite step will have been taken to unify the study of personality and that of general and experimental psychology, and to introduce a paradigm which will make possible that accumulation of detailed knowledge which is the routine business of science in its non-revolutionary period.

This introduction has extended to perhaps an undue length, and has covered a number of topics which are not usually dealt with in books on personality. The reason for this is, of course, that the writer's concept of personality, and his suggestions for a proper paradigm in this field, are quite different from the traditional kind of approach, as for instance exhibited in Hall and Lindzey's *Theories of Personality* (1957); few of the views there discussed would coincide with those here presented. Accordingly, it became necessary to outline the reasoning behind an approach which stresses laboratory investigations and theoretical concepts derived from general psychology, biological features and genetic explanations to an extent which is quite unusual in this field. It can be argued that some such paradigm as that presented here is necessary if we are ever to get away from the literary, non-scientific type of personality study which is so current at present; such is the opinion of Brody (1972) who has argued the case at some length. Of course the success of the actual model here investigated is another question; the approach might be right, even though the model turned out a failure. The degree to which our approach differs from the orthodox is perhaps indicated by nothing better than by the fact that the very problems here discussed are not usually raised in typical textbook discussions, or even monograph presentations; answers radically different from those here given are taken for granted.

We must return to a discussion of the concept of measurement, which after all is part of the title of the book. Stevens (1959) defined "measurement [as] the assignment of numerical values to objects or events according to rule—any rule", and proposed that we should classify our scales of measurement according to "their mathematical group structure". Ellis (1966) has shown the untenability of this view, and in any case we would say that it disregards the substantive nature of scientific measurement and concentrates on purely formal properties. True measurement occurs only when the qualitative question of what to measure has been solved, even if only in a preliminary way; to assign numbers to objects or events according to some meaningless or trivial rule is not the scientist's concept of measurement. We would maintain that scientific measurement of a meaningful kind only becomes properly possible once a paradigm has been established, or once a research programme of a progressive kind has begun to be developed. It is for this reason that we believe that studies such as those reprinted here make meaningful the measurement of such personality traits as extraversion–introversion; they are the only way in which we can answer the perennial question posed by students and laymen alike: "How do you know what you are measuring with such scales as the EPI is actually extraversion?" Extraversion is defined in terms of a nomological network, as are all scientific concepts; as Haller put it in 1768: "Natura in reticulum sua genera connexit, non in catenam: homines non possunt nisi catenam sequi, cum non plura simul sermone exponere". We have done our best to explore this network by following each different strand; we believe that in science there is no alternative method.

REFERENCES

BOWERS, K. S. Situationism in psychology: an analysis and a critique. *Psychological Review*, 1973, 80, 307–336.

BRIDGEMAN, P. W. *The logic of modern physics.* London: Macmillan, 1927.

BROADHURST, P. L. The interaction of task difficulty and motivation: the Yerkes–Dodson Law revived. *Acta Psychologica*, 1959, 16, 321–338.

BRODY, N. *Personality: research and theory.* London: Academic Press, 1972.

CAMPBELL, N. R. *Physics, the elements.* Cambridge: Cambridge University Press, 1920.

CAMPBELL, N. R. *An account of the principles of measurement and calculation.* London: Longmans, Green, 1928.

ELLIS, B. *Basic concepts of measurement.* Cambridge: Cambridge University Press, 1966.

ENDLER, N. S. The person versus the situation—a pseudo issue? *Journal of Personality*, 1973, 41, 287–303.

EYSENCK, H. J. *The biological basis of personality.* Springfield: C. C. Thomas, 1967.

EYSENCK, H. J. *The structure of human personality* (3rd Edition). London: Methuen, 1970.

EYSENCK, H. J. *The measurement of intelligence.* Lancaster: Medical and Technical Publishers, 1973.

EYSENCK, H. J. *Experiments: personality* (2 vols). London: Routledge and Kegan Paul, 1960.

EYSENCK, H. J., and EYSENCK, S. B. G. *Personality structure and measurement.* London: Routledge and Kegan Paul, 1969.

EYSENCK, H. J., and EYSENCK S. B. G. *Psychoticism as a dimension of personality.* London: Hodder and Stoughton, 1976.

EYSENCK, H. J., and EYSENCK, S. B. G. Physiological re-activity to necessary stimulation as a measure of personality. *Psychological Reports*, 1967, *20*, 45–46.

EYSENCK, H. J., and FRITH, C. D. *Reminiscence*. London: Academic Press, 1976.

EYSENCK, M. W. Extraversion, activation and the recall of prose. *British Journal of Psychology*, 1976, *67*, 53–62.

GRAY, J. A. *Pavlov's typology*. London: Pergamon Press, 1964.

GRAY, J. A. Strength of the nervous system, introversion–extraversion, conditionability and arousal. *Behaviour Research and Therapy*, 1967, *5*, 151–169.

GRAY, J. A. The psychophysiological basis of introversion–extraversion. *Behaviour Research and Therapy*, 1970, *8*, 249–266.

HALL, C. S., and LINDZEY, G. *Theories of personality*. New York: Wiley, 1957.

HEBB, D. D. Drives and the C.N.S. (conceptual nervous system). *Psychological Review*, 1955, *62*, 243–254.

KUHN, T. S. *The structure of scientific revolutions*. Chicago: University of Chicago Press, 1962.

KUHN, T. S. Second thoughts in paradigms. In: F. S. Suppe (Ed.) *The structure of scientific theories*. London: University of Illinois Press, 1974.

LAKATOS, I., and MUSGRAVE, A. (Eds.). *Criticism and the growth of knowledge*. Cambridge: Cambridge University Press, 1970.

MAGNUSSON, P. The person and the situation in the traditional measurement model. Stockholm: Reports from the Psychological Laboratories, 1974, number 426.

MASTERMAN, M. The nature of a paradigm. In: I. Lakatos and A. Musgrave (Eds.) *Criticisms and the growth of knowledge*. Cambridge: Cambridge University Press, 1970.

MISCHEL, W. *Introduction to personality*. New York: Holt, Rinehart and Winston, 1971.

NÄÄTÄNEN, R. The inverted-U relationship between activational performance: a critical review. *Attention and performance*, Vol. IV. London: Academic Press, 1973.

PAVLOV, I. P. *Conditioned reflexes*. Oxford: Oxford University Press, 1927.

POPPER, K. R. *The logical scientific discovery*. London: Hutchinson, 1959.

POPPER, K. R. *Conjectures and refutations*. London: Routledge and Kegan Paul, 1963.

STEVENS, S. S. Measurement, psychophysics and utility. In: C. W. Churchman and P. Ratoosh (Eds.) *Measurement: definitions and theories*. New York: Wiley, 1959.

STRELAU, J. Pavlov's typology and current investigations in this area. *Nederlands Tijdschrift voor de Psychologie*, 1975, *30*, 171–200.

SUPPE, F. (Ed.) *The structure of scientific theories*. London: University of Illinois Press, 1974.

SUPPE, F. The search for philosophic understanding of scientific theories. In: F. S. Suppe (Ed.) *The structure of scientific theories*. London: University of Illinois Press, 1974.

WALLACH, U. S., and GAHM, R. C. Personality functions of graphic constriction and expansiveness. *Journal of Personality*, 1960, *28*, 73–88.

WIGNER, E. P. Events, laws of nature, and invariance principles. *Science*, 1964, *145*, 995–999.

YERKES, R. M., and DODSON, J. D. The relation of strength of stimulus to rapidity of habit-formation. *Journal of Comparative and Neurological Psychology*, 1908, *18*, 459–482.

PART I

MODELS OF PERSONALITY

This first section of our book covers certain important areas which require discussion before we enter upon the detailed description of work in the specific areas covered in later sections. The first paper reprinted deals with the argument between personality theorists and "situationists"; it demonstrates the obvious, namely that neither personality alone nor situations alone are sufficient to give us much predictive power, and that interaction effects can be very important. The rest of this book will demonstrate amply how powerful personality factors can be provided proper control is exercised over irrelevant and interfering variables; much the same is true of physics, of course. There too the atomistic structure of a metal, and the purpose for which it is being used, determine jointly whether or when it will fracture, or melt; only laboratory investigations can control irrelevant or interfering variables sufficiently to make prediction precise.

Our second paper demonstrates that the three-fold analysis of the major personality variables into P, E and N can be replicated on the animal level; other work has shown that this is possible not only with primates, but that even with the humble rat such a personality factor as neuroticism can be isolated and studied with reference to its heritability, with great precision (Broadhurst, 1975). We then go on to discuss the fact that extraversion is a higher-order concept, i.e. is postulated to account for the intercorrelations between different traits; in particular there appears a major division of the various items in the extraversion–introversion scale into sociability and impulsiveness items. The third paper considers this theme by looking at the heritability of extraversion, and attempts to demonstrate that sociability and impulsiveness are not simply correlated in actual populations, but that it is possible to calculate the degree to which this association is determined by genetic and by environmental factors respectively.

The final two papers deal with alternative models which have attracted a good deal of attention, and which are widely used for experimental purposes. One of these is Cattell's 16 PF battery; the other is the Minnesota Multiphasic Personality Inventory. The two papers here reprinted attempt to show that not only do these models not conflict with that used here, but that they show heartening agreement on essential points. The papers also argue that in so far as the models go beyond that here used, they run into difficulties and may have to be abandoned completely. It would have been useful if a continuation of the Wakefield paper on the MMPI could have been reprinted also, but space did not permit; readers are advised to consult it if they are interested in the relationship between the MMPI system and that here discussed (Wakefield et al., 1975).

It should perhaps be stated here explicitly, even though it may be obvious, that the three dimensions of P, E and N here postulated are not conceived of as the only such dimensions existing, nor that they are believed to account for the whole of human personality. A proper system of description of human personality would resemble the Mendeleeff table of the elements; only a few of the psychological variables have been discovered to date, and it will be a long time before we have sufficient knowledge to even guess at the total number involved. Neither is it suggested that because we have concentrated on the major factors or dimensions, therefore we do not believe in the existence of smaller "group" or "primary" factors. The very conception of higher-order factors, such as extraversion or neuroticism, is based on the orderly correlations between such primary factors, and their isolation and measurement is a task of great importance and relevance. What is being said is simply that (1) higher-order factors are of greater scope and importance, and consequently deserve prior attention, and (2) certain primaries, such as those advocated by Cattell, are subject to criticisms which render their employment hazardous. These are all empirical questions, the evidence regarding which has been reviewed elsewhere (Eysenck and Eysenck, 1969); there seems to be no doubt that higher-order factors have a much better record of replicability than do primaries, and that the range of phenomena related to higher-order factors is much greater than that related to primaries.*

It has been suggested by Guilford (1975) and others that higher-order factors are at a disadvantage as compared with primaries, in that when there is a correlation between an experimental test and a factor score, it is impossible to interpret such a correlation unequivocally in the case of a higher-order factor. Let us assume that the higher-order factor (E in our case) is made up of five primaries (e.g. impulsiveness, sociability, liveliness, activity, carefreeness); then the correlation between an experimental measure (e.g. eyeblink conditioning) and E could be due to any one, or any combination of primaries; the outcome is not definitive. This objection is well taken, and in a later section we shall see that the correlation between E and conditioning is mediated by impulsiveness, rather than by sociability. However, a similar objection can be made in reverse against the use of primaries. A given primary furnishes us with a score which is made up of a general and a specific portion, i.e. it is in part a measure of E, and in part a measure of that primary unalloyed by contamination with other primaries also measuring E. Put more technically, if the primary personality trait we are measuring is impulsiveness, then $V_I = V_E + V_{I(P)} + V_S + V_e$, where V_I denotes the total variance of the impulsiveness scale, V_E that portion of the total variance due to differences in extraversion, i.e. shared with other primaries, $V_{I(P)}$ that portion of the total variance due to impulsiveness as a primary not overlapping with other primaries defining E, V_S the specific variance of the particular test employed and V_e the error variance. Using this score, we are again faced with a measure which is not univocal, because we can now not discriminate between V_E and $V_{I(P)}$; it would not be correct to identify (as Guilford appears to do) V_I and $V_{I(P)}$. Ideally what should be done is to use measures of both primaries and resulting higher-order factors; unfortunately, reliable measures of primaries require long tests, and if several higher-order factors are to be measured, each consisting of many primaries, very long questionnaires are required which may not be filled in with sufficient care and attention by relatively uninterested subjects. There is no solution to this problem which would approximate to the ideal and yet be practically admissible; the best method to be used perhaps is one

which starts out with specific hypotheses, and gears the personality measurement to these hypotheses. An example of this method is given in the Eysenck and Levey paper reprinted in part VII, page 305.

It is interesting to ask why tests such as the MMPI have been so widely used in the U.S.A., and hold such an eminent place in the empirical literature. There can be little doubt that from the scientific point of view the MMPI is based on quicksand; it attempts essentially to replicate to a reasonable degree of similarity the system of diagnosis used by American psychiatrists. This system is the product of committee work, compromise, and guesswork; no-one suggests that it is based on scientific knowledge or experimentation, and even the reliability of the system, when used by experts trained under identical conditions, is very poor (Spitzer and Fleiss, 1974), while the correlation between test and criterion is even poorer (Goldberg, 1965). We thus face the question why anyone should wish to use a test which very poorly mirrors unreliable diagnoses based on a system lacking any scientific foundation (thus it has been shown that identical cases of mental disorder are diagnosed as schizophrenic five times as frequently by American as by British psychiatrists—thus diagnosis becomes a question of the nationality of the psychiatrist, rather than of the disorder of the patient!) The answer presumably lies in the urgent application-directed stance of much of modern psychology; there is little interest in scientific models, experimental investigation of fundamental problems, and gradual approach to better understanding. Immediate application is all, and however worthless the model, and however unreliable and invalid the method, the urgency of the practical problem excuses all. The model here discussed may and probably does have practical applications, but these are quite secondary to its purely scientific features; we are concerned here with a model which must fulfill certain basic scientific requirements before the question of utility is even approached. Thus practical utility, as demonstrated for instance in work with neurotic and criminal groups, would be no excuse for failure to make accurate predictions in laboratory investigations having no purpose but the testing of the model itself. It is important to bring out this feature of our model, in order to prevent misunderstanding; we are concerned with an integral part of general psychology, requiring the same standard of objectivity and concern with experimental details as any other part.

There has been much discussion among philosophers of science about the usefulness and otherwise of models, and the propriety of using such models (Black, 1962; Braithwaite, 1953; Duhem, 1954; Hesse, 1966); such a discussion can best be focused in terms of an example. Consider the theory of heat, where we have two competing theories, namely the thermodynamic and the kinetic theory. Thermodynamics deals with unimaginable concepts of a purely quantitative kind: *temperature*, measured on a thermometer, *pressure*, measured as the

* Even within the range of widely accepted primary personality factors these problems are only too apparent. Thus Howarth (1972) has replicated in a large-scale study using 50 variables and 569 subjects Cattell's findings on factors U.I. 16, 17, 19, 20, 21, 23, 24, and 32, using objective personality tests as originated by Cattell. The results of this replication were very disappointing; of the eight factors for which marker tests were employed, only two gave rise to even approximate replications. Howarth concludes that "contrary to prior expectation what actually emerged from this group of carefully selected Cattell markers were factors which more closely resembled those of Eysenck, especially at second order level" (p. 451).

force exerted per unit area, and *volume*, measured by the size of the container. Nothing is said in the laws of thermodynamics about the *nature* of heat. Bernoulli, in his famous treatise on hydraulics, postulated that all "elastic fluids", such as air, consist of small particles which are in constant irregular motion, and which constantly collide with each other and with the walls of the container. This was the foundation stone of the kinetic theory of heat, which results in a model or picture of events which is eminently "visualizable", and which gives to many people a feeling of greater "understanding", of better and more thorough "explanation", than do the mathematical laws of thermodynamics. Consider for example the "insight" which we seem to gain in looking at Cailletet's famous experiment, which originated cryogenic research, by considering his cooling device as part of a single stroke of an expansion engine! Nevertheless, many phenomena are quite intractible to kinetic interpretations even today, which yield easily to a thermodynamic solution. Models have their own value, but they may in due course be replaced by theories which are not amenable to this approach. It may be said with some confidence that in psychology we have not yet reached this advanced position, and that models are still of great value and utility.

It may be worth while to make a final point about the importance of personality and individual differences research, in both theoretical and applied psychology, and to cast doubt on the logic of those who argue that the contribution of such factors to the variance, in many instances, is rather small. If we can agree that human behaviour is very complex, and that casual factors in any particular situation are probably multiple, then it is obvious that no single factor is likely to account for much of the total variance. Let us assume a total of ten such factors to account for all the non-chance variance of a particular type of behaviour; five of these might be situational and environmental, five genetic and related to personality. Some of these factors might give rise to interaction variance, rather than contribute to the main factors variance, at least in part. We might then find that if every one of our ten factors contributed 10% to the non-chance variance, and if our factors were orthogonal to each other, then we could account for all the non-chance variance of the behaviour in question. To discover, therefore, that any given personality trait might not contribute more than 10% to the variance (and many examples where contributions of much greater size were found are given in the pages that follow) would not be equivalent to stating that this information was not worth having; it is only by repeating the process ten times i.e. by properly specifying and measuring each of the ten contributing variables, that we can obtain a proper understanding and control of the phenomenon in question. To expect that all or most of the variance could be due to a single factor seems unreasonable, particularly in non-laboratory situations; even in laboratory situations it is usually not possible to keep constant important variables such as previous smoking, drinking, eating, sexual intercourse, late nights, boredom, depression, anxiety, and many others, although it may sometimes be possible to get more or less accurate measurements of these.

To take an example, let us imagine that we study 1,000 cars that refuse to start. This could be due to an almost infinite number of causes such as defective starting motor, run-down battery, failure of the ignition system, too thick oil due to cold, etc. An engineer would think it a curious form of criticism to say that none of these multivarious causes were worth studying because none of them accounted for more than 10% of the actual failures observed! What we look for in the first place is a proper understanding of the causal interactions, i.e. the invariances which are involved in the phenomenon we are studying; once this is achieved, we may be able to manipulate one or other of the factors involved. To worry about the contribution of that factor to the variance of a particular, exceedingly complex, phenomenon is not sensible. It seems quite likely that in many situations, particularly of the social kind, chance factors account for a large proportion of the variance, leaving only considerably less than 100% to be explained by systematic sources of variation. Comparisons with the simplest kinds of physical phenomena, studied under extremely well-controlled laboratory conditions, are not very useful here. We must understand the restrictions under which we are working in trying to account for naturally occurring psychological phenomena; even the hard sciences have difficulties in finding factors accounting for 10% of the variance in metereological phenomena! Personality factors have been shown to account for about a third of the extra-chance variance in the field of sexual attitudes and behaviours (Eysenck 1976); it is doubtful if any other factors contribute as much. In laboratory situations even higher values can be achieved, provided the measures used are based on a proper theory. It is the absence of such a theory in all too many cases which is responsible for the failure of personality variables to make as large a contribution in empirical studies as they might.

REFERENCES

BLACK, M. *Models and metaphors*. Ithaca: Cornell University Press, 1962.

BRAITHWAITE, R. B. *Scientific explanations*. Cambridge: Cambridge University Press, 1953.

BROADHURST, P. The Maudsley reactive and nonreactive strains of rats: a survey. *Behaviour Genetics*, 1975, 5, 299–320.

DUHEM, P. *The animal structure of physical theory*. Princeton: University Press, 1954.

EYSENCK, H. J. *Sex and personality*. London: Open Books, 1976.

EYSENCK, H. J. and EYSENCK, S. B. G. *Personality structure and measurement*. London: Routledge and Kegan Paul, 1969.

GOLDBERG, L. R. Diagnosticians *vs.* diagnostic signs. *Psychology Monograph*, 1965, No. 602.

GUILFORD, J. P. Factors and factors of personality. *Psychological Bulletin*, 1975, *82*, 802–814.

HESSE, M. B. *Models and analogies in science*. Notre Dame: University of Notre Dame Press, 1966.

HOWARTH, E. A factor analysis of selected markers for objective personality factors. *Multivariate Behavioural Research*, 1972, *7*, 451–476.

SPITZER, R. L. and FLEISS, J. L. A re-analysis of the reliability of psychiatric diagnosis. *British Journal of Psychiatry*, 1974, *125*, 34–37.

WAKEFIELD, J. A., BRADLEY, P. E., DOUGHTIE, E. R., and KRAFT, I. A. Influence of overlapping and non-overlapping items on the theoretical interrelationships of MMPI scales. *Journal of Consulting and Clinical Psychology*, 1975, *43*, 851–857.

From I. G. Sarason, R. E. Smith and E. Diener (1975). Journal of Personality and Social Psychology, 32, 199–204, *by kind permission of the authors and the American Psychological Association*

Personality Research: Components of Variance Attributable to the Person and the Situation

Irwin G. Sarason, Ronald E. Smith, and Edward Diener
University of Washington

Studies involving personality and situational variables were surveyed. Studies permitting determination of main effects and interactions involving these variables have increased since 1950. In one comparison, situational main effects were significant in 65.5% of the cases, whereas the figure was 31% for individual difference variables and 59.9% for interactions. In another comparison, 35% of situational main effects accounted for more than 10% of the variance, compared with 29% for personality indexes; 19% of the situational variable effects accounted for more than 20% of the variance, compared with 14% of the personality main effects. Low percentages of variance were accounted for by all variables investigated: situational, personality, demographic, and interactions among these variables.

The idea that what a person brings to different situations influences his or her behavior makes intuitive sense. Even the most radical behaviorist readily agrees that the response repertory of the individual is a significant datum for the experimentalist or behavior modifier, although there may be disagreement over the definition and means of measuring elements of the repertory. What has aroused controversy has not been the abstract idea that individual differences by themselves and in interaction with environmental variables influence behavior, but the success with which existing assessment methods provide meaningful measures of individual differences. For example, Mischel (1968, 1969), while recognizing the scientific importance of interrelating individual differences and experimental variables, has expressed disappointment at the low levels of correlation between personality variables and assorted criteria. He cites the high frequency of correlations that account for less than 10% of the variance in the criterion behavior and the infrequent occurrence of significant transsituational consistency in behavior that would support the notion of broad personality traits.

Bowers (1973) has recently presented a

thoughtful analysis of metaphysical, psychological, and methodological aspects of these problems. Eleven studies reviewed by him, all of which involved the transsituational assessment of behaviors of the same subjects, demonstrated that the average amount of variance accounted for by the Personality × Situation interaction exceeds the average amount of variance accounted for by either persons or situations alone. As valuable as they are, studies of this type, in which no attempt is made to assess particular individual difference variables, do not provide information about Personality × Situation interactions. In other words, such designs tell us *what* is the case, but not *why*. The epistemic yield is best regarded as description rather than as understanding of the role of identifiable person variables in behavior. The typical Personality × Situations design employed in contemporary personality research is a factorial one in which groups differing on some individual difference variable are randomly assigned to differing experimental conditions. An analysis of the components of variance attributable to the factors and their interaction in such a design would serve to complement the data reviewed by Bowers, which provide information on the current "state of the phenomenon."

The analysis performed in the present study provides information on the current state of the science of personality in identifying and measuring dispositional variables that

---

Edward Diener is now at the University of Illinois at Champaign–Urbana.

Requests for reprints should be sent to Irwin G. Sarason, Department of Psychology, NI-25, University of Washington, Seattle, Washington 98195.

account for behavior. The study concerns itself with two major considerations. The first involves the question of whether there has been an increase or a decrease in experimental investigations that incorporate personality variables. The second, and of greater relevance to the current controversy regarding situational and dispositional variables, pertains to the relative potencies of individual difference variables and experimentally manipulated variables, and the interaction between these two classes of variables. In the analyses performed, potency was considered from the perspectives of both statistical significance and proportion of behavioral variance accounted for.

METHOD AND RESULTS

The trend over the past two decades of studies that permit estimation of interaction effects was the first topic examined. The journals surveyed were the *Journal of Personality and Social Psychology, Journal of Abnormal and Social Psychology*, and *Journal of Personality*. Table 1 shows that there was an increase in the percentage of studies that permitted determination of interaction effects between individual difference and experimental variables. The increase was from 5% in 1950 to 14% in 1960 to 25% in 1970.

The part of the present survey related to interaction effects included a total of 385

TABLE 1

PERCENTAGE OF EXPERIMENTAL STUDIES
INCLUDING SITUATIONAL AND INDIVIDUAL
DIFFERENCE VARIABLES

1950 ($n = 100$)	1960 ($n = 193$)	1970 ($n = 220$)
Personality and situational or demographic and situational variables		
5%	14%	25%
Personality and situational variables		
5%	9%	11%
Demographic and situational variables		
0%	7%	17%

Note. Journals surveyed were the *Journal of Personality and Social Psychology, Journal of Abnormal and Social Psychology,* and *Journal of Personality. n* = the number of articles surveyed each year.

studies published in the 1971 and 1972 volumes of the *Journal of Personality and Social Psychology,* the *Journal of Personality,* and the *Journal of Consulting and Clinical Psychology*. Many of the journal articles that were reviewed contained more than one dependent variable measure, so that a total of 692 statistical analyses were examined. Also surveyed were studies reported in *Dissertation Abstracts* of 1970.

Two separate analyses of independent samples of published literature were conducted. Analysis 1, based on the 1971 volumes of the *Journal of Personality and Social Psychology* and the *Journal of Personality,* was designed to assess the frequency with which individual difference variables were employed in personality and social psychological research and their likelihood of yielding statistically significant results both alone and in interaction with situational variables. Analysis 2 consisted of an assessment of components of variance accounted for by individual difference and situational variables and their interactions.

Analysis 1 included a total of 254 studies involving 305 separate analyses, which were divided into four classes: (a) those involving only situational independent variables ($n = 147$), (b) those involving only measured personality and attitudinal independent variables ($n = 44$), (c) those involving only demographic (e.g., sex, race, age) independent variables ($n = 12$), and (d) those involving both situational and individual difference variables ($n = 53$). The results of the analysis were tabulated in terms of the percentage of significant ($p < .05$) effects yielded by these classes of independent variables. Studies in which personality scales were correlated with other personality scales were excluded from the analysis so as not to spuriously inflate the percentage of significant results attributable to personality variables. In the case of the group of studies that incorporated both situational and personality-attitudinal variables within factorial designs, it was possible to categorize the magnitude of statistically significant effects (the categories were .05, .025, .01, and .001) and to tabulate the percentage of instances in which the situational main effect, the personality main effect, and the interaction effect yielded the strongest effect in the analysis. As the last column of Table 3 shows, in 77.2% of the analyses, one of the three sources of variance was more highly significant than either of the other two.

The results of Analysis 1 indicated that individual difference variables were incorporated in 42.9% of the studies. As Table 2 indicates, a high percentage of significant results was obtained in studies in which a situational, demographic, or personality variable was the sole independent variable, a fact that is not surprising in light of editorial demands for significant results. Published studies that achieved nonsignificant results generally involved either failures to replicate previous findings or (especially in the case of individual difference variables) failures to demonstrate linkages to behavior that the construct in question would predict.

Of greater interest, however, is the pattern of Analysis 1 results pertaining to studies that incorporated both situational and individual difference variables. These results are presented in Table 3. In these studies, situational variables yielded significant results twice as frequently as did individual difference variables, and were nearly four times as likely to be the most potent variable in the analysis. Also noteworthy, however, is the high frequency with which significant interactions were obtained between situational and individual difference variables, as well as the relatively high percentage of cases in which the interaction was the most potent effect. These results suggest that individual difference variables may be most important in terms of how they interact with situational factors, and that such significant interactions occur nearly as often as do significant main effects for situational variables.

In addition to the evidence of Analysis 1 just presented and that of Analysis 2, to be presented, a set of comparisons was made for reports of empirical research other than those contained in journal articles. We examined PhD theses, summarized in the 1970 issues of *Dissertation Abstracts*, that incorporated individual difference variables and experimentally manipulated variables. It seemed desirable to gauge the trend of results among a group of

TABLE 2

ANALYSIS 1: RESULTS OF STATISTICAL ANALYSES FROM STUDIES EMPLOYING ONLY ONE CLASS OF VARIABLE

Independent variable	No. of analyses	% Significant ($p < .05$)
Situational	147	95.2
Demographic	12	83.3
Personality	59	83.0

research investigations that are typically not reported in journals. Although the emphasis on positive results characterizes dissertations as well as published articles, the emphasis is less in the former than in the latter.

The summaries of studies contained in *Dissertation Abstracts* for 1970 were read and categorized into those in which personality and demographic variables comprised elements in experimental designs in the field of psychology. Because these summaries do not contain many of the details found in journal articles, it was necessary to classify the dissertations not only into those that yielded positive and negative results with regard to main or interaction effects but also into a "cannot say" group. The "cannot say" results typically were too ambiguous to permit conclusions about whether positive or negative results had been obtained. Also in this category were summaries that simply omitted the results of relevance to the present survey. The percentages reported here are restricted to summaries of dissertations that explicitly indicated whether or not the relevant results had attained statistical significance.

At least one personality measure was used in 52 of the 123 dissertations surveyed. Of

TABLE 3

RESULTS OF ANALYSIS 1 OF 53 STUDIES EMPLOYING BOTH SITUATIONAL AND INDIVIDUAL DIFFERENCE VARIABLES

Variables and interaction	% Significant	% Largest effect
Situational (S)	65.5	38.0
Individual differences (I)	31.0	10.4
S × I	59.9	28.8

Note. Results are based on 87 statistical analyses because of multiple dependent variables in several studies. Journals surveyed were the 1971 *Journal of Personality and Social Psychology* and *Journal of Personality*.

the 30 dissertations reporting main effects for personality variables, 53% ($n = 16$) described statistically significant outcomes. Forty-six dissertations reported results relevant to interactions. Of these, 70% ($n = 32$) were statistically significant. There were 48 dissertations dealing with demographic variables whose main effects could be classified unambiguously as being either statistically significant or not significant. Of these, 79% ($n = 38$) were significant. Of the 63 dissertations reporting interactions involving demographic variables, statistical significance was obtained in 71% ($n = 45$) of the cases. Of the 95 dissertations reporting results for situational variables, 63% ($n = 60$) described positive outcomes.

Whereas Analysis 1 was largely concerned with statistical significance, Analysis 2 was concerned with proportions of behavioral variance accounted for by various kinds of independent variables. Hays (1965, p. 382) has described the procedure known as omega squared (ω^2), which may be used to estimate the amount of response variance that can be accounted for by each main and interaction effect in an analysis of variance. The analysis to be described here used the ω^2 procedure to assess components of variance accountable in terms of situational, individual difference, and interaction effects.

Analysis 2 was based on a sample of 102 studies involving 138 analyses of variance published in the 1972 volumes of the *Journal of Personality and Social Psychology* and the *Journal of Personality* and the 1971 and 1972 volumes of the *Journal of Consulting and Clinical Psychology*. The sample was, of necessity, restricted to those studies that presented analysis of variance summary tables from which ω^2 could be computed. Excluded from the ω^2 analysis were trials effects in studies concerned with learning.

The results of Analysis 2 are presented in Table 4. The data summarize the total number of main and interaction effects of each type that were examined in the 138 analyses of variance. It is readily apparent that on the average, individual difference variables account for only a small proportion of variance, either alone or in interaction with other variables. However, it is equally clear that there is little difference between the mean and median proportions of variance accounted for by personality and by situational variables. Interactions involving situational and individual difference variables account for less variance than either of the main effects.

A supplementary analysis was performed on 249 additional analyses from the same journals involving situation, personality, and demographic variables that were analyzed by means of t tests and correlation coefficients. The ω^2 analysis was applied to t test results (Hays, 1965, p. 327), and correlation coefficients were squared in order to provide estimates of accountable variance. Combining these data with the analysis of variance results forms a composite but does not substantially alter the pattern of results. The following mean proportions of variance were accounted for in the composite: situational, $M = 12.8\%$, $SD = 22.6\%$ ($n = 331$); personality, $M = 9.4\%$, $SD = 11.8\%$ ($n = 201$); demographic, $M = 1.5\%$, $SD = 2.6\%$ ($n = 62$).

Table 5 presents a breakdown of the data of Table 4 in terms of the distribution of the variance accounted for by main and interaction effects. The table shows the percentages of results accounting for different proportions of variance. Most striking in the data summarized in this table are the high percentages of results that account for relatively small proportions of the variance within each category of independent variables. Of additional interest is the fact that personality variables are nearly as likely to account for

TABLE 4

RESULTS OF ANALYSIS 2: COMPONENTS OF VARIANCE ACCOUNTED FOR IN TERMS OF SITUATIONAL AND INDIVIDUAL DIFFERENCE VARIABLES AND THEIR INTERACTIONS

Independent variable and interaction	Total number of main and interaction effects analyzed	Mean percentage of variance accounted for	SD	Median percentage of variance accounted for
Situational (S)	247	10.3	13.42	4.5
Personality (P)	53	8.7	11.23	3
Demographic (D)	43	1.8	2.28	1
S × S	118	2.2	7.21	1
S × P	54	4.6	8.77	1
S × D	46	1.2	2.31	0.0
P × D	8	2.0	4.00	0.0
P × P	5	7.3	12.35	2
D × D	4	.2	.002	0.0

PERSONALITY RESEARCH

TABLE 5

DISTRIBUTION OF PERCENTAGES OF THE VARIANCE ATTRIBUTABLE TO MAIN AND INTERACTION EFFECTS

Independent variable	Proportion of variance accounted for									
	≤.01	.01–.05	.05–.09	.10–.14	.15–.19	.20–.29	.30–.39	.40–.49	.50–.59	≥.60
Situational (S)	34	18	13	10	6	9	5	2	2	1
Personality (P)	39	21	11	9	6	6	6	2		
Demographic (D)	65	28	5	2						
S × S	61	18	12	4	2	2		1		
S × P	52	15	22	4		5			2	
S × D	78	20	2							
P × D	78	11		11						
P × P	40	40					20			
D × D	100									

substantial proportions of the variance as are situational variables. For example, 35% of the situational main effects account for more than 10% of the variance, compared with 29% of the personality main effects; 19% of the situational variable effects account for more than 20% of the variance, compared with 14% of the personality variable main effects. The highly skewed nature of the distribution of variance percentages shown in Table 5 suggests that the median might serve as a more suitable measure of central tendency (and as a more accurate reflection of the current state of the science) than does the mean. It can be seen in Table 4 that the median proportion of variance accounted for in no case exceeds 5%.

DISCUSSION

Our survey reveals surprisingly low percentages of variance accounted for by all classes of variables investigated: situational, personality, demographic, and interactions among these variables. If our somewhat negative evaluation of this result is reasonable, then many of the theoretical disputes that permeate the personality literature are explicable in terms of the narrow margin by which results are regarded as psychologically meaningful. Attainment of the .05 level of statistical significance may not provide a sufficiently firm base upon which to erect crisp psychological interpretations and powerful theories. From another perspective, however, by what standard is accounting for, say, only 10% of the variance a poor or disappointing performance? It appears that most current studies are directed toward the investigation of relatively subtle psychological

phenomena, so that we might well expect the present results. If an independent variable is truly powerful (i.e., accounts for a massive proportion of the variance), it is generally also too obvious to be of "theoretical" interest. In any event, no matter how one views the results of the present survey with regard to the potency of individual variables, the state of affairs for situational variables alone is only slightly more favorable.

Although the present variance analysis is to our knowledge the first to be performed on a major segment of the personality–social literature, previous statistical and theoretical analyses of a similar nature have been conducted within specific segments of it (Argyle & Little, 1972; Averill, 1973; Bowers, 1973; Endler, 1973; Endler & Hunt, 1966, 1968, 1969). As mentioned earlier, Bowers (1973), summarizing the results of 11 studies using self-report and observational data, found that Person × Situation interactions accounted for more of the variance (20.77%) than did either main effects for persons (12.71%) or for situations (10.17%). Likewise, Endler (1973) has reported Person × Situation interactions that accounted for higher proportions of the variance than the mean of 4.7% that emerged from the present survey. This seems in no way surprising, since figures presented in this article are a composite representing studies in which the independent variables vary widely along a continuum of theoretical meaningfulness. It seems reasonable to assume that the more theoretically relevant a personality or demographic variable is to the situation to be manipulated and/or the behavior to be studied, the more variance will be accounted for by the Person

I. G. Sarason, R. E. Smith, and E. Diener

× Situation interaction. In addition, as noted here, the figures reported by Endler (1973) and Bowers (1973) are Person × Situation interactions, whereas the present summary is composed of measured Personality × Situational interactions. That is, Bowers' (1973) and Endler's (1973) interactions use individual persons as one variable in their design, and their Person × Situation interaction is therefore a composite of all possible Personality × Situation interactions for the particular situations of interest.

Several considerations that are typically ignored in discussions of the relative merits of dispositional and situational variables are worth noting. One concerns the degree of difference between levels of individual difference variables and experimentally manipulated variables in the factorial Dispositional × Situational experimental design. In most instances, we would expect the dispositional variable to account for more variance if very different groups (such as schizophrenics and normals) were compared than if normal groups differing in locus of control were studied. It may be that in many instances manipulated situational variables, given high degrees of laboratory control, will be more "different" (and less confounded with other variables) than will groups of subjects differing on one imperfectly measured personality variable. On the other hand, unmeasured individual differences may cause subjects to perceive the same rigidly controlled situation in different ways and thereby increase within-cell variance, thus decreasing the proportion of variance accounted for by the situational variable.

The telling points made by Mischel (1968, 1969) and others regarding transsituational consistency of behavior and the low level of predictability of behavior from conventional personality assessment devices have resulted in an increasingly widespread conviction that situational variables are prepotent determinants of behavior and that individual difference variables are, by comparison, of only minor importance. Although limited to a small number of journals over a relatively brief period of time, the present survey suggests that though situational variables do indeed account for a slightly higher proportion of variance, their margin of superiority is by no means striking enough for them to be considered prepotent by comparison.

The results of the present survey are encouraging in one respect. The proportion of studies reported in the literature in which both dispositional and situational variables are incorporated into experimental designs appears to be on the increase. This approach may ultimately result in the greatest epistemic yield for the science of personality. Although a knowledge of situational variables may permit the best prediction of behavior in similar situations, Personality × Situation interactions may contribute greatly to specifying the processes that mediate the situational behavior relationships. Viewed in this light, the issue of the relative potency of situational and dispositional variables becomes secondary in importance to the question of how they might best be concurrently studied to advance our understanding of behavior.

REFERENCES

Argyle, M., & Little, B. R. Do personality traits apply to social behavior? *Journal for the Theory of Social Behavior*, 1972, *2*, 1–35.

Averill, J. R. The disposition of psychological dispositions. *Journal of Experimental Research in Personality*, 1973, *6*, 275–282.

Bowers, K. S. Situationism in psychology: An analysis and a critique. *Psychological Review*, 1973, *80*, 307–336.

Endler, N. S. The person versus the situation—a pseudo issue? *Journal of Personality*, 1973, *41*, 287–303.

Endler, N. S., & Hunt, J. McV. Sources of behavioral variance as measured by the S–R Inventory of Anxiousness. *Psychological Bulletin*, 1966, *65*, 287–303.

Endler, N. S., & Hunt, J. McV. S–R Inventories of hostility and comparisons of the proportions of variance from persons, responses, and situations for hostility and anxiousness. *Journal of Personality and Social Psychology*, 1968, *9*, 309–315.

Endler, N. S., & Hunt, J. McV. Generalizability of contributions from sources of variance in S–R Inventories of Anxiousness. *Journal of Personality*, 1969, *37*, 1–24.

Hays, W. L. *Statistics for psychologists*. New York: Holt, Rinehart & Winston, 1965.

Mischel, W. *Personality and assessment*. New York: Wiley, 1968.

Mischel, W. Continuity and change in personality. *American Psychologist*, 1969, *24*, 1012–1018.

(Received April 1, 1974)

From A. S. Chamove, H. J. Eysenck and H. F. Harlow (1972). Quarterly Journal of Experimental Psychology, *24, 496–504, by kind permission of the authors and the Longman Group Limited*

PERSONALITY IN MONKEYS: FACTOR ANALYSES OF RHESUS SOCIAL BEHAVIOUR

A. S. CHAMOVE,† H. J. EYSENCK,‡ AND H. F. HARLOW

Regional Primate Research Center, University of Wisconsin

Three factor analyses were performed on social interaction data from 168 juvenile macaques. Animals were tested in stable quadrad peer groups; in newly-formed dyads with infant, juvenile, and adult stimulus monkeys; and in similar triads with the stimulus animal plus a familiar cage-mate. Factors emerged, most strongly in the most stable condition, which were interpreted as affiliative, hostile and fearful. These factors were almost entirely independent and resembled the extraversion, psychoticism, and emotionality factors frequently found in humans.

Introduction

Factor analyses of human social behaviour have been undertaken primarily in two areas. The first is upon humans in a solo setting, usually having the subject fill in a questionnaire. The subject is rating his own behaviour in another postulated setting, usually an interacting one. Reliably, factors of introversion–extraversion, emotionality or neuroticism, and psychoticism emerge (reviewed recently by Eysenck and Eysenck, 1968, 1969). Looked at from the point of view of the behaviour patterns on which these factors are based, extraversion is characterized by sociable behaviour, neuroticism by fearful behaviour, and psychoticism by hostile, aggressive behaviour. The second area is upon humans in an interactive setting, usually dyadic. Studies of mother and child (Becker and Krug, 1964; Hatfield, Ferguson and Alpert, 1967), adults (Borgatta, 1964; Schaefer, 1959), children (Borgatta and Sperling, 1963), and infants (Cobb, Grimm, Dawson and Amsterdam, 1967) report factors which can be termed affection or extraversion, emotionality or neuroticism, and assertive reponse to assertiveness. One might expect to find similar patterns of behaviour in the higher subhuman primates. Certainly when primatologists describe behaviour, they often do so using comparable terms.

In subhuman primates two studies have been published, both in the latter category. The first (Locke, Locke, Morgan and Zimmerman, 1964) recorded 10 behaviour categories in 12-year-old rhesus monkeys that had been reared in social isolation (probably not visual or auditory isolation) from soon after birth. The severely restricted repertoire of isolated monkeys, when tested in quadrads, enabled

---

†Present address: Stirling University Psychology Primate Unit, Stirling, FK9 4LA, Scotland.

‡Present address: Institute of Psychiatry, University of London, London, S.E.5., England.

the experimenters to record only the following behaviours: pass, approach, contact, chase, aggression, passive awareness, avoidance, escape, submission, and apparent unawareness. Two factors emerged: dominance, and submission in response to dominance.

Van Hooff (1971) reported a component and cluster analysis of 53 behaviours recorded in a stable group of 25 chimpanzees. Sixty-nine per cent of the variance was accounted for by components termed affinitive or social positive, play, aggressive, and submissive. In addition, contributing a small but significant amount to the results, were factors termed groom, excitement, and "show" or display.

The following is a report of three factor analyses, of 10 behaviours, performed on data from a stable group situation and on data from less stable dyadic and triadic situations.

Method

Subjects

One hundred and sixty eight *Macaca mulatta*, about 85% males, were separated from their mothers at birth and reared in individual mesh cages. They were given daily peer experience starting at between 15 and 90 days of age. For about half the animals this consisted of daily 2-h pairings in the homecage and bi-weekly 1-h group sessions in a playroom or in a large cage. For the rest social experience entailed daily 40-min group sessions in a playroom. All subjects were assigned to a group composed of four age-mates, and all social experience, both pairings and group sessions, involved these group members. All group social interaction was experienced when all four members were present, so that after a few months the group had formed stable social relationships which were retained even when monkey subjects were paired.

Apparatus

The animals were group tested in that particular playroom or large cage to which they had become accustomed through daily group sessions throughout most of their lives. The playrooms used were Wisconsin Playroom II for 44 animals (see Chamove, Waisman and Harlow, 1970, for a description), Wisconsin Playroom III for 36 animals (described by Chamove, 1966), and a standard rectangular mesh cage measuring $3 \times 1.5 \times 1.5$ m for the remaining monkeys. Stimulus testing was carried out in a similar sized cage but fitted with a plexiglas front and a plexiglas partition which could divide the cage in half. It allowed the animals to observe one another in the adaptation interval before testing.

Behaviours were recorded using a bank of 10 Standard Electric Timers activated by 10 microswitches (as described by Chamove, Harlow and Mitchell, 1967). The timers recorded the duration of the following behaviours: *social explore*—any investigation, contact or not, of another animal, primarily looking at another monkey (reliability, $r = 0.88$); *social play*—playing with another monkey, usually a relaxed, complex, and vigorous behaviour ($r = 0.95$); *nonsocial play*—similar behaviour not directed toward another animal ($r = 0.90$); *nonsocial fear*—withdrawal from the environment, scored when no social object could be credited with the instigation of the fear response ($r = 0.96$); *appropriate withdrawal*—avoidance of an animal that is exhibiting hostile behaviour ($r = 0.91$); *inappropriate withdrawal*—withdrawal from an animal exhibiting fear, exploratory, or play behaviour ($r = 0.90$); *hostile contact*—biting or grabbing another animal ($r = 0.96$); *nonhostile contact*—all other behaviours involving physical contact except clinging ($r = 0.95$); *social cling*—clinging to another animal ($r = 0.99$); *noncontact hostile*—($r = 0.91$).

Reliability is given as product-moment inter-observer coefficients.

Procedure

Group Testing was done on all subjects between 9 and 12 months of age, and all monkeys were tested in their group of four a minimum of twice weekly. Testing consisted of at least thirty 60-min sessions during which each animal was observed for three 5-min periods. One experimenter did all the Group Testing. The data were converted to "per cent of total time tested" scores for purposes of analysis.

Stimulus Testing was performed on 63 of the above subjects soon after Group Testing. At 12 months of age the monkeys were housed in groups of four continuously. At approximately 13 months of age the first Stimulus Test was undertaken. The subject was housed in one half of the Stimulus Test cage, separated from the stimulus animal by the plexiglas partition, for a 23-h period. The transparent barrier was then removed and testing immediately begun; it was continued for 15 min unless one of the animals was seriously injured.

Testing involved placing the subject animal with a stimulus animal of relatively constant characteristics in the following 3×2 design. The stimulus monkey was either an infant of approximately 1 month, a juvenile male of approximately 6 months of age and chosen for its playfulness, or an adult male chosen for its docility. The subject was tested with each of these three in the above order in a dyadic social situation. The tests were separated by a period of about 10 days. After the "Alone" Stimulus Test, another three sessions followed. The subject monkey was first paired with an animal from his original four-membered test group. The two animals were quite familiar with one another, having lived together for over a month in a group of four and having interacted with one another from an early age. These two monkeys were then tested *together* with the stimulus animal. Here two experimenters were used. The procedure followed was the same as for the Alone testing except that two animals were adapted for 23 h in half of the test cage, and the test situation was triadic—two subjects and one stimulus monkey. This was called the "Partner" situation.

Analysis of the data was by means of principal components analysis rotated to oblique simple structure (Eysenck and Eysenck, 1969). Interfactor correlations of the promax factors were derived and all factors with eigenvalues less than unity were ignored. Computer limitations forced a division of the Stimulus Test data into two halves, the Alone and the Partner testing situations. As clinging was rarely observed in the Group Test situation, it was deleted from the analysis.

The rationale of the procedure is as follows. The Group Test situation involves a maximum of adaptation to the social test situation. Because of the formation of hierarchies and preferences during their year of social interaction, one would expect a maximum of within-group divergence, the most subordinate subject, e.g. being able to show almost no hostility. Tempered by this very stable structure, personality differences might be expected to emerge.

The Stimulus situation has been shown to demonstrate the effects of early environmental manipulations which the group situation has failed to detect (Mitchell, 1970; Chamove, 1966), but it may be less reflective of habitual modes of social response due to the variability of the various test situations. Dominance position, dyadic alliances, and social response are much more controlled in this stimulus situation. The stimulus infant at 1 month moves about very little and normally elicits very little aggression. The juvenile is very active but always subordinate to the experimental subject, and so aggression is more commonly elicited; play is quite common and fear uncalled for. The docile adult is a test for aggressive-fearful factors. Excessive fear should be rare and aggression rarer, brief submissive gestures being more appropriate with these males. Isolate monkeys, however, suicidally attack all animals (Mitchell, 1970) whereas certain brain damaged monkeys carefully discriminate the objects of their hyper-aggression (Chamove *et al.*, 1970).

The Partner situation is used because it was felt that having a familiar peer present might elicit certain behaviours not elicited in the Alone condition as has been previously found (Chamove, 1966).

Results

The results of the factor analysis of the *Group Test* data are striking. Three clear factors emerge having little intercorrelation: hostile, fearful, and affiliative or sociable (see Table I). These three all show positive intercorrelations. This may be a result of the constrained social situation, for an animal showing play or hostility may induce fear in other animals. Another possible cause of this correlation may be the existence of a kind of monkey which is relatively nonsocial and inactive; he will score low on all behaviours. The factor we have here termed hostility correlates 0·23 with the one we termed fear, 0·34 with affiliation while the affiliation factor correlates 0·21 with fear. These correlations account for only 10% of the variance at most, and we consider them unimportant.

TABLE I

Loading of nine behaviours on three factors resulting from analysis of the quadrad Group Test data and labelled play, fear, and aggression–hostility

	Factors		
Behaviours	I	II	III
Nonsocial play	0·10	0·78	0·02
Social play	−0·07	0·99	0·03
Positive contact	−0·04	0·96	−0·01
Social exploration	0·73	0·39	−0·15
Nonsocial fear	0·99	−0·16	0·04
Inappropriate fear	0·91	0·04	−0·03
Appropriate fear	0·95	0·00	0·14
Noncontact hostility	0·40	−0·10	−0·80
Contact hostility	−0·25	0·04	−0·98

One nonfear variable, noncontact hostility, shows a moderate correlation with the fear factor. This single aberrant score can be explained in terms of the behaviour pattern termed redirected-threats. These are hostile behaviours directed toward a more subordinate animal in an attempt to distract the hostile attentions of a more dominant monkey. The behavioural sequence is initiated by the dominant animal and the redirection is a response to that initiation.

The results of the *Stimulus Test* are less clear, as might be predicted from the unstable nature of the test situation (see Table II). When monkeys are tested in a dyad with the stimulus animal (upper half of Table II), four factors are found. The first loads negatively on infant fear, juvenile fear and hostility, and adult hostility; and positively on infant hostility. The second factor is one of juvenile play versus infant positive contact, probably of an exploratory nature. The third loads on nonsocial fear versus social explore. Both are fairly nonsocial behaviours as they involve little social contact and are seen in nonsocial animals such as long-term isolates. The final factor is social play versus adult hostility.

When monkeys are stimulus tested paired with familiar partners four factors again emerge (lower half of Table II). The first loads positively on play and on cling directed toward the juvenile and adult stimulus animal versus a negative

TABLE II

Loadings on the first four factors resulting from analysis two (upper) and analysis three (lower) of Stimulus Test data when subjects are tested with three types of stimulus monkey

	Behaviours	I			II			III			IV		
		infant	juvenile	adult	infant	juvenile	adult	infant	juvenile	adult	infant	juvenile	adult
"alone" or dyad condition	Nonsocial play	0·04	0·05	0·27	0·16	0·03	0·15	0·22	0·17	0·15	0·02	0·36	0·14
	Social play	0·18	0·23	0·16	−0·06	−0·51	−0·09	0·56	0·22	0·07	0·23	−0·27	0·26
	Positive contact	0·10	−0·24	0·01	0·75	0·48	0·03	0·09	0·00	0·09	−0·13	−0·09	0·21
	Social cling	0·20	−0·36	−0·11	−0·03	−0·26	−0·29	−0·05	0·01	0·04	−0·09	0·05	−0·10
	Social exploration	−0·13	0·01	0·18	0·49	0·35	−0·20	−0·08	−0·21	−0·04	−0·33	0·09	−0·48
	Nonsocial fear	0·28	0·04	0·15	0·03	−0·05	0·12	−0·17	0·06	0·04	0·17	0·52	0·45
	Inappropriate fear	−0·55	−0·64	0·28	0·09	0·12	0·09	0·17	0·21	−0·86	0·15	−0·04	−0·11
	Appropriate fear	0·00	−0·68	−0·37	0·00	0·04	0·07	0·00	0·11	0·08	−0·00	−0·06	−0·34
	Noncontact hostility	−0·02	−0·48	−0·61	−0·01	0·06	−0·08	0·10	−0·23	−0·13	0·17	−0·09	−0·07
	Contact hostility	0·73	−0·33	−0·69	0·06	−0·13	−0·04	0·01	−0·33	−0·19	0·18	0·08	0·12
"partner" or triad condition	Nonsocial play	−0·40	−0·48	0·19	−0·05	0·02	0·31	0·07	0·15	0·48	0·05	0·11	−0·09
	Social play	0·05	0·52	0·24	−0·73	0·16	−0·08	0·37	−0·14	−0·06	0·18	0·44	−0·42
	Positive contact	0·04	0·68	−0·14	0·62	0·11	−0·03	0·04	0·01	−0·13	0·07	0·01	−0·41
	Social cling	0·10	0·50	0·33	−0·06	−0·02	−0·04	0·46	0·21	0·12	0·14	−0·27	−0·08
	Social exploration	0·04	0·44	−0·45	0·70	0·08	0·19	0·01	0·14	−0·01	0·09	−0·25	0·19
	Nonsocial fear	−0·05	−0·05	0·05	0·28	−0·00	−0·22	−0·09	0·15	0·03	−0·38	−0·03	0·12
	Appropriate fear	−0·36	0·05	−0·06	−0·16	−0·16	−0·13	−0·04	−0·42	−0·11	−0·20	0·32	0·15
	Noncontact hostility	−0·10	−0·24	−0·07	−0·65	−0·12	−0·21	−0·35	0·05	−0·65	0·07	−0·11	−0·11
	Contact hostility	−0·14	−0·06	0·18	−0·42	−0·15	0·21	−0·08	−0·05	−0·82	0·02	0·06	−0·20

The column heading "Factors" spans factors I–IV.

loading on nonsocial play and social fear. The second loads on infant hostile and play versus infant explore and nonsocial fear. The third factor loads on adult and infant hostile, juvenile fear versus infant play and cling and adult nonsocial play. The last factor loads positively on juvenile play and inappropriate withdrawal as contrasted with negative loading on adult play, juvenile explore and cling, and infant nonsocial fear. Table III lists the intercorrelations between each of the four factors from both of the Stimulus Test factor analyses. Except for factors I and II, the correlations between pairs of factors is remarkably low suggesting a high degree of independence.

TABLE III

Interfactor correlations of promax factors from Stimulus Testing

Analysis two; dyads			
Factors	II	III	IV
I	0·33	−0·27	0·07
II		−0·18	−0·09
III			0·06
Analysis three; triads			
Factors	II	III	IV
I	0·61	−0·12	−0·08
II		−0·17	−0·04
III			−0·03

The complexity of the Stimulus Test data is what one might expect if for no other reason than that different behaviours are elicited in the six situations. For example, in the Partner or triad situation the subjects exhibit less juvenile-directed hostility, less inappropriate fear toward the adult, more adult hostility, and less nonsocial fear, substituting partner-directed clinging in many cases for nonsocial fear. Factors III and IV, found in the Alone condition, are represented in factor I of the Partnered situation; factors II and III of the Partner test are found in IV and I respectively of the Alone condition.

The first factor of the Alone condition and second factor of the Partner test are clearly a social fear and hostile category. The second factor of the dyadic test appears comparable to an affectional category, showing play toward the juvenile and restrained positive and exploratory behaviour toward the infant, the first infant these monkeys had ever seen. The first factor of the triad or Partner test, like factors III and IV on the dyad test, seem also to reflect an affectional character, perhaps more comparable to the meaning of extraversion. We see here an animal exhibiting play toward the juvenile and other monkeys, showing some avoidance of other animals, considerable nonsocial play, and some hostility toward the playful juvenile stimulus monkey. The last triad factor dichotomizes between adult play and juvenile play.

Discussion

The factor analysis of the Group Test has resulted in three clear behaviour factors: fearful, hostile, and affectionate. These patterns of behaviour are not dissimilar to those which gave rise to the three major factors in research on human personality; neuroticism-stability, extraversion–introversion, and psychoticism. It would be premature to seek to prove the identity of the factors in these different species; no acceptable method exists at the moment for any such proof. What would be required to make the identification reasonable would be the incorporation of these factors in a nomological network, rather in the fashion adopted by Eysenck and Broadhurst (1964) with reference to emotionality in rats. Thus it should not prove impossible to test whether affectionate (extraverted) monkeys have lower cortical arousal patterns than do non-affectionate ones; similarly, it should be possible to test for differences in conditioning between the two groups. A programme for testing the suitability of the "neuroticism" tag for the fearful animals could with advantage follow that adopted for emotionality in rats. Psychoticism might be the most difficult factor to investigate, for the simple reason that least is known about it in the human population. However, even here such behaviours as lack of co-operation or inappropriate aggression should be susceptible to observation and quantification.

It might at first seem surprising that similar factors emerge from two different species, but there are good reasons for expecting such agreement. The first reason is linked with the simple fact that monkeys and men (and rats also) have similar anatomico-physiological structures to subserve emotional/fearful behaviour, i.e. an autonomic system and a visceral brain, and arousal behaviour, i.e. a cortex linked with an ascending reticular formation; one would expect individual differences in behaviour to be linked with differences in the functioning of both these systems, and these behavioural differences would be expected to be the more similar to those observed in humans, the closer the species under investigation was to *Homo sapiens*. As regards psychoticism, it is much more difficult at this moment to suggest a biological locus for this trait, but a close relation has been observed with masculinity. The possibility of a link with some hormonal secretion related to the sex glands would be supported by recent investigations of rhesus monkeys (Rose, Holady and Bernstein, 1971).

The second reason is that we are here concerned with social behaviour, i.e. how one animal behaves towards another, and the major possibilities of such behaviour seem to be limited to the three patterns we noted; an animal can be friendly-sociable-affectionate, it can be hostile-aggressive-cruel, or it can be fearful-emotional-withdrawing. Most if not all social behaviour can be grouped under these three main headings, and it is perhaps not too surprising that these patterns should emerge as factors in our investigation. Nor is it surprising that the picture is somewhat more complex (and confused) when we turn from the Group Test data to those collected in the Stimulus Test. This would be expected if for no other reason than that different behaviours are inevitably elicited in the six situations by the different "stimulus" patterns.

This observational study demonstrates marked individual differences between monkeys in their social behaviour. These differences are apparently highly reliable, and characteristic of the animals concerned, and may thus be regarded as aspects of the "personality". Yet experimental work with monkeys, and other animals as well, seldom pays attention to their "personality". We would argue that this omission is a serious one, just as experimentation in human subjects can be very misleading if it leaves out of account personality factors like extraversion-introversion (Eysenck, 1967). In rats a whole host of experimental studies can be shown to be influenced profoundly by differences in emotionality, and quite different theoretical conclusions can be drawn from identical experiments depending on the strain of animals used (Eysenck and Broadhurst, 1964; Eysenck, 1967). The usual process of "averaging" serves simply to relegate such "personality" factors to the error term, which thus becomes unduly swollen and often far exceeds in importance the main effects looked for. Personality factors usually emerge as "interaction" factors, and may serve materially to reduce the size of the error term. It is in this function that we see the main importance of our findings; work with monkeys too should bear in mind the importance of individual differences and use scores on these factors to keep the error term as small as possible. In addition there is of course the possibility that continued work along these lines will increase our knowledge about "personality" factors in animals, and humans as well. In view of the lack of knowledge in this field, such increases would be more than welcome.

This research was supported by United States Public Health Service Grants FR-00167 and MH-11894 from the National Institutes of Health to the University of Wisconsin Regional Primate Research Center and Department of Psychology Primate Laboratory, respectively. The authors would also like to thank Roberta Sprengel for testing assistance.

References

BECKER, W. C. and KRUG, R. S. (1964). A circumplex model for social behavior in children. *Child Development*, **35**, 371–96.

BORGATTA, E. F. (1964). The structure of personality characteristics. *Behavioural Science*, **9**, 8–17.

BORGATTA, E. F. and SPERLING, B. C. (1963). A note on the stability of peer judgements in independent situations. *Journal of Psychological Studies*, **14**, 45–8.

CHAMOVE, A. S. (1966). The effects of varying infant peer experience on social behavior in the rhesus monkey. Unpublished M.A. thesis, University of Wisconsin.

CHAMOVE, A. S., HARLOW, H. F. and MITCHELL, G. A. (1967). Sex differences in the infant-directed behavior of preadolescent rhesus monkeys. *Child Development*, **38**, 329–35.

CHAMOVE, A. S., WAISMAN, H. A. and HARLOW, H. F. (1970). Abnormal social behavior in phenylketonuric monkeys. *Journal of Abnormal Psychology*, **76**, 62–8.

COBB, K., GRIMM, E. R., DAWSON, B. and AMSTERDAM, B. (1967). Reliability of global observations of newborn infants. *Journal of Genetic Psychology*, **110**, 253–67.

EYSENCK, H. J. (1967). *The Biological Basis of Personality*. Springfield: C. C. Thomas.

EYSENCK, H. J. and BROADHURST, P. L. (1963). Experiments with animals. In EYSENCK, H. J. (Ed.), *Experiments in Motivation*. Oxford: Pergamon.

EYSENCK, H. J. and EYSENCK, S. B. G. (1969). *The Structure and Measurement of Personality*. London: Routledge & Kegan Paul.

EYSENCK, S. B. G. and EYSENCK, H. J. (1968). The measurement of psychoticism: a study of factor stability and reliability. *British Journal of Social and Clinical Psychology*, **7**, 286–94.

HATFIELD, J. S., FERGUSON, L. R. and ALPERT, R. (1967). Mother-child interaction and the socialization process. *Child Development*, **38**, 365–414.

LOCKE, K. D., LOCKE, E. A., MORGAN, G. A. and ZIMMERMAN, R. R. (1964). Dimensions of social interactions among infant rhesus monkeys. *Psychological Reports*, **15**, 339–49.

MITCHELL, G. A. (1970). Abnormal behavior in primates. In ROSENBLUM, L. (Ed.), *Primate Behavior: Developments in Field and Laboratory Research*. London: Academic Press.

ROSE, R. M., HOLADAY, J. W. and BERNSTEIN, I. S. (1971). Plasma testosterone, dominance rank and aggressive behaviour in male rhesus monkeys. *Nature*, **231**, 366–8.

SCHAEFER, E. S. A. (1959). A circumplex model for maternal behavior. *Journal of Abnormal and Social Psychology*, **59**, 226–35.

VAN HOOFF, J. A. R. A. M. (1971). *Aspects of the Social Behaviour and Communication in Human and Higher Non-Human Primates*. Rotterdam: Bronder.

Received 13 *March* 1972

Eratum: Table 2, triad condition: Appropriate fear should read Inappropriate fear, and the loadings for Appropriate fear are—0·00, −0·48, −0·50, 0·00, −0·10, −0·01, 0·01, 0·06, −0·10, 0·00, −0·06, 0·13.

From L. Eaves and H. J. Eysenck (1975). Journal of Personality and Social Psychology, *32*, 102–112, *by kind permission of the authors and to the American Psychological Association*

The Nature of Extraversion: A Genetical Analysis

Lindon Eaves
Department of Genetics,
University of Birmingham,
Birmingham, England

Hans Eysenck
Institute of Psychiatry,
University of London,
London, England

A biometrical–genetical analysis of twin data to elucidate the determinants of variation in extraversion and its components, sociability and impulsiveness, revealed that both genetical and environmental factors contributed to variation in extraversion, to the variation and covariation of its component scales, and to the interaction between subjects and scales. A large environmental correlation between the scales suggested that environmental factors may predominate in determining the unitary nature of extraversion. The interaction between subjects and scales depended more on genetical factors, which suggests that the dual nature of extraversion has a strong genetical basis. A model assuming random mating, additive gene action, and specific environmental effects adequately describes the observed variation and covariation of sociability and impulsiveness. Possible evolutionary implications are discussed.

One of the central problems in personality research has been the question of whether such higher order factors as extraversion can be regarded in any meaningful sense as *unitary* or whether there are several independent factors, such as "sociability" and "impulsiveness," which should not be thrown together artificially. Carrigan (1960) concluded her survey of the literature by saying that "the unidimensionality of extraversion/introversion has not been conclusively demonstrated" (p. 355); she further pointed out that several joint analyses of the Guildford and Cattell questionnaires show that at least *two* independent factors are required to account for the intercorrelations between the extraversion–impulsiveness variables. These two factors, she suggested, may correspond to the European conception of extraversion, with its emphasis on impulsiveness and weak superego controls, and the American conception, with its emphasis on sociability and ease in interpersonal relations. Eysenck and Eysenck (1963) have reported quite sizable correlations between sociability and impulsiveness, a conclusion replicated by

We are indebted to the Colonial Research Fund and the British Medical Research Council for their support of the investigation. We are grateful to J. Kasriel for the collection of data and to the twins for their continued cooperation.

Requests for reprints should be sent to Lindon Eaves, Department of Genetics, University of Birmingham, Birmingham, B15 2TT, England.

Sparrow and Ross (1964); this would suggest that there is a close connection between the two conceptions (Eysenck & Eysenck, 1969). Furthermore, Eysenck and Eysenck (1967) have shown that the correlations of extraversion items (whether sociability or impulsiveness) with subjects' reactions on a physiological test devised on theoretical grounds were proportional to their loadings on the extraversion factor. The recognition that extraversion is a unitary factor in behavior is thus vindicated by prediction from a psychological theory as much as by a correlation between primary factors (Eysenck, 1967).

We now develop a model for the genetical and environmental determinants of extraversion and of its primary components, sociability and impulsiveness. Our intention is to analyze the phenotypic variation and covariation of sociability and impulsiveness into their genetical and environmental components in order to determine, as far as our data permit: (a) the simplest model for the genetical and environmental variation of extraversion considered as a unitary trait and (b) the simplest model for the genetical and environmental determination of the interaction between subjects and the component tests of extraversion, sociability and impulsiveness.

In fulfilling these aims, we are led to compare the unitary and dual models of extraversion with regard to their relative contri-

LINDON EAVES AND HANS EYSENCK

butions to the representation of both genotypic and environmental determinants of variation among the responses of subjects to a personality inventory.

Earlier research from the standpoint of the psychological theory underlying this work has mainly been concerned with the analysis of extraversion as a unitary trait (Shields, 1962). Claridge, Canter and Hume (1973) reported analyses of extraversion, sociability, and impulsiveness, but these authors themselves admitted that their samples were too small to justify the kind of analysis we attempt here. Our model will be derived from an analysis of twin data and will, therefore, inevitably reflect the limitations of twin studies as sources of genetical information (Jinks & Fulker, 1970). Even twin studies, however, have seldom been used to best advantage. We hope that our particular analysis will have the additional virtue of demonstrating how twin data in general may be manipulated to test simple hypotheses about the causes of variation. We have adopted the methods and notation of biometrical genetics (Mather & Jinks, 1971) because we believe them to be the most precise and general, while embodying a defined procedure for the analysis of continuous variation which may be extended readily to the analysis of human behavior (Jinks and Fulker, 1970).

DATA

The analysis is based on the responses of 837 pairs of adult volunteer twins to an 80-item personality inventory. Of these items, 13 formed a scale of sociability, and 9 items were scored to provide a measure of impulsiveness. The relevant items are given in Table 1. On the basis of a short questionnaire concerning similarity during childhood, the twins were classified as monozygotic or dizygotic.[1] Such a procedure is surprisingly reliable (Cederlöf, Friberg, Jonsonn, & Kaij, 1961). A sample of

[1] The twins were asked: (a) "Do you differ markedly in physical appearance and coloring?" and (b) "In childhood were you frequently mistaken by people who knew you?" If consistent replies were not given, reference was made to previous questionnaires, twins' letters, and additional information in an attempt to assess zygosity. Many of the twins have been blood-typed subsequently, and the original diagnoses have generally been confirmed (Kasriel, J., personal communication, December 1974).

TABLE 1

PERSONALITY INVENTORY ITEMS INCLUDED IN THE ANALYSIS

Item	Key
18. Do you suddenly feel shy when you want to talk to an attractive stranger?	−S
23. Generally, do you prefer reading to meeting people?	−S
27. Do you like going out a lot?	+S
30. Do you prefer to have few but special friends?	−S
36. Can you usually let yourself go and enjoy yourself a lot at a gay party?	+S
40. Do other people think of you as being very lively?	+S
44. Are you mostly quiet when you are with other people?	−S
48. If there is something you want to know about, would you rather look it up in a book than talk to someone about it?	−S
56. Do you hate being with a crowd who play jokes on one another?	−S
66. Do you like talking to people so much that you never miss a chance of talking to a stranger?	+S
69. Would you be unhappy if you could not see lots of people most of the time?	+S
75. Do you find it hard to really enjoy yourself at a lively party?	−S
77. Can you easily get some life into a rather dull party?	+S
1. Do you often long for excitement?	+I
4. Are you usually carefree?	+I
8. Do you stop and think things over before doing anything?	−I
12. Do you generally say things quickly without stopping to think?	+I
16. Would you do almost anything for a dare?	+I
20. Do you often do things on the spur of the moment?	+I
33. When people shout at you, do you shout back?	+I
59. Do you like doing things in which you have to act quickly?	+I
62. Are you slow and unhurried in the way you move?	−I

Note. S denotes an item scored for sociability, I for impulsiveness; + indicates that "yes" scored 1, and − indicates that "no" scored 1 for scale under consideration.

digzygotic twins of unlike sex has been included in our study because these provide a critical diagnostic test of sex limitation. The composition of the sample by sex and zygosity is given in Table 2.

The mean sociability and impulsiveness scores of the five groups are given in Table 3. An analysis of the variation between and within groups revealed highly significant (but substantively fairly small) differences between groups with respect to the sociability scores. The groups did not differ with respect to their mean impulsiveness scores. We shall regard

TABLE 2

STRUCTURE OF TWIN SAMPLE

Twin type	No. pairs
Monozygotic female	331
Monozygotic male	120
Dizygotic female	198
Dizygotic male	59
Unlike-sex dizygotic	129

the groups as representative of the same population as far as their means are concerned. The groups are homogeneous with respect to their dispersion, as will become clear from the subsequent genetical analysis. The pooled standard deviations within groups were 3.0015 and 1.7586 for sociability and impulsiveness, respectively.

Since we wished to minimize the possibility of spurious interaction between subjects and tests, we standardized the raw scores of the twins on both sociability and impulsiveness by dividing the scores by the corresponding average within-groups standard errors. For each group of twins separately, the mean squares within pairs and between pairs were calculated for each of the standardized scales. The analogous within-pairs and between-pairs mean products were also calculated. The mean squares and mean products form the basic statistical summary for the analysis to follow (see Table 4).

We studied the inheritance of extraversion by analyzing the mean squares derived from the subjects' total scores of the two standardized tests. The mean squares for the twins on the measure of extraversion (E) may be

TABLE 3

MEAN SOCIABILITY AND IMPULSIVENESS
SCORES OF TWIN GROUPS

Twin type	N	M	
		Sociability	Impulsiveness
MZf	662	6.5045	3.7039
MZm	240	5.7875	3.8125
DZf	396	6.6869	3.7525
DZm	118	6.6441	4.0678
DZos	258	6.4884	3.7054

Note. Abbreviations are as follows: MZf = monozygotic female, MZm = monozygotic male, DZf = dizygotic female, DZm = dizygotic male, and DZos = unlike-sex dizygotic.

TABLE 4

MEAN SQUARES AND MEAN PRODUCTS WITHIN AND
BETWEEN TWIN PAIRS FOR STANDARDIZED
SOCIABILITY AND IMPULSIVENESS SCORES

Item	df	MS (S)	MS (Imp)	MP (S–I)
Between MZf pairs	330	1.5339	1.3777	.6517
Within MZf pairs	331	.5394	.6403	.1762
Between MZm pairs	119	1.5595	1.2904	.3126
Within MZm pairs	120	.4817	.6630	.1497
Between DZf pairs	197	1.0855	1.1804	.3069
Within DZf pairs	198	.8380	.8408	.2918
Between DZm pairs	58	1.3919	.9799	.6309
Within DZm pairs	59	.6693	.8441	.1516
Between DZos pairs	128	.9457	1.2839	.3638
WIthin DZos pairs	129	.9290	.7697	.3581

Note. Abbreviations are as follows: MZf = monozygotic female, MZm = monozygotic males, DZf = dizygotic female, DZm = dizygotic male, and DZos = unlike-sex dizygotic. MS = mean square, MP = mean product; S = Sociability and I = impulsiveness. No correction for the main effect of sex was necessary for the DZos.

derived directly from the mean squares and mean products (MP) of Table 4, since $MS_E = MS_{(S+I)} = MS_S + MS_I + 2MP_{S,I}$, where S and I refer to sociability and impulsiveness.

Just as we obtained an E score for each subject by summing over tests, so we may obtain a difference (D) score for each subject by taking the difference between his scores on the standardized tests. The MS derived from these differences summarizes the variation arising because subjects do not perform consistently on the two tests. We may obtain the MS for the D scores directly from the raw MS and mean products of Table 4, since

$$MS_D = MS_{(S-I)} = MS_S + MS_I - 2MP_{(S,I)}.$$

The mean squares for E and D are found in Table 5. Clearly, since the mean products are all positive, the MS_E's are larger than the corresponding MS_D's. Since we are only concerned with these particular tests, the mean squares between subjects for E contain none of the interaction variation. Thus the fact that the MS_E's are approximately twice as large as the MS_D's is an indication that E accounts for more of the total variation of the two tests than D.

We analyze the MS_E to provide a genetical model for variation in extraversion, and we analyze the MS_D to determine the extent to

LINDON EAVES AND HANS EYSENCK

which genetical or environmental factors contribute to the resolution of E into sociability and impulsiveness. Finally, we show that the covariation of sociability and impulsiveness reflects both genetical and environmental factors by an analysis of the raw mean squares and mean products of Table 5.

METHODS

Formulation of the Model

Most analyses of classical twin studies have merely demonstrated the existence of a genetical component of variation by showing that monozygotic twins are more alike than are dizygotic twins. Such an intuitive approach is imprecise and does not lead to any exact predictions about the similarity between other degrees of relatives. For this reason the classical approach is not very helpful in guiding the design of future research. In adopting the methods of biometrical genetics we are able to specify, for a given set of assumptions about the kinds of gene action and environmental effects, precise expectations for the components of variance (and consequently for the mean squares) derived from the analysis of variance of any group of relatives. Furthermore, having specified our assumptions and the consequent expectations of mean squares, we are able to provide a statistical test of the agreement between observations and expectations and, consequently, to test the validity of the assumptions we made at the outset.

Clearly, twin data of the kind we have summarized in this article do not allow us to test any but the simplest set of assumptions about the causes of variation. We also recognize that failure of particular assumptions in principle may not lead to failure of the model in practice, either because sample sizes are too small for the test to be sufficiently powerful (see, e.g., Eaves & Jinks, 1972) or because failure of certain assumptions may contribute more to a bias in estimation than to departures of what is observed from what is expected.

We now consider individually the assumptions we make in the analyses which follow. Some of these are an undesirable necessity of the limited data we have available and may not be tested very powerfully by our analysis. Other assumptions are quite likely to be disproved in practice, even with the data available, if they are unjustified. We emphasize that these limitations apply not to the method, which is the most explicit and flexible available, but to the particular data upon which we seek to build our model. Other experimental designs would enable us to test with greater conviction the assumptions which we now make tentatively, (Eaves, 1972; Jinks & Fulker, 1970).

1: Alleles and loci act additively and independently. We assume that there is no dominance, epistasis, or linkage for the loci contributing to variation of the traits under consideration. If our other assumptions are justified, nonadditive variation may be detected in principle with our data, but in practice the necessary sample sizes are likely to be too large (Eaves, 1972). Failure of either of the two following assumptions may make the de-

TABLE 5

MEAN SQUARES FOR EXTRAVERSION AND INTERACTION OF SUBJECTS AND COMPONENT TESTS

Item	df	MS	
		E = S + I	D = S − I
Between MZf pairs	330	4.2150	1.6082
Within MZf pairs	331	1.5321	.8273
Between MZm pairs	119	3.4751	2.2247
Within MZm pairs	120	1.4441	.8453
Between DZf pairs	197	2.8797	1.6521
Within DZf pairs	198	2.2624	1.0952
Between DZm pairs	58	3.6336	1.1100
Within DZm pairs	59	1.8166	1.2102
Between DZos pairs	128	2.9572	1.5020
Within DZos pairs	129	2.4749	.9825

Note. Abbreviations are as follows: MZf = monozygotic female, MZm = monozygotic male, DZf = dizygotic female, DZm = dizygotic male, and DZos = unlike-sex dizygotic. E refers to extraversion, and D refers to the interaction of subjects and component tests. S and I refer to sociability and impulsiveness, respectively.

tection of nonadditive variation virtually impossible with the data of our study.

2: Mating is random. There is little evidence of assortative mating for extraversion. We might expect to detect the genetical consequences of assortative mating provided there is substantial genetical variation and a fairly high correlation between spouses (Eaves, 1973a). The design of the present study, however, since it involves twins reared together, makes it impossible to distinguish the effects of assortative mating from those of environmental influences shared by members of the same twin pair. Eysenck (1974) reports a nonsignificant correlation for the extraversion scores of husbands and wives. This suggests that assortative mating can safely be discounted as a factor contributing to the genetical variability of extraversion.

3: All environmental effects are specific to individuals within families. Most of the twins in our study lived together, especially when they were young. The fact that both individuals in a pair have the same biological mother and grew up in the same family may make both monozygotic and dizygotic twins more alike than we would expect on the basis of our simple genetical and environmental model. For twins reared together, such effects are formally indistinguishable from those of assortative mating and, if they are substantial, may contribute to failure of our simple model, which assumes that assortative mating and common environmental influences make a negligible contribution to the observed variation. We have some independent test of the contribution of postnatal shared environmental influences for extraversion because we would expect the intrapair differences of twins to increase with the period of separation. Although age and duration of separation are, of course, highly correlated, we can detect no relationship between the intrapair difference for extraversion scores

TABLE 6

A GENETICAL AND ENVIRONMENTAL MODEL FOR A SET OF OBSERVED MEAN SQUARES

MS	Coefficient of parameter	
	D_R	E_1
Between MZf pairs	1	1
Within MZf pairs	·	1
Between MZm pairs	1	1
Within MZm pairs	·	1
Between DZf pairs	$\frac{3}{4}$	1
Within DZf pairs	$\frac{1}{4}$	1
Between DZm pairs	$\frac{3}{4}$	1
Within DZm pairs	$\frac{1}{4}$	1
Between DZos pairs	$\frac{3}{4}$	1
Within DZos pairs	$\frac{1}{4}$	1

Note. Abbreviations are as follows: MZf = monozygotic female, MZm = monozygotic male, DZf = dizygotic female, DZm = dizygotic male, and DZos = unlike-sex dizygotic. D_R refers to an additive genetical component, and E_1 refers to a within-family environmental component.

and the age or duration of adult and juvenile separation of these twins. We hope to make a detailed consideration of this issue the subject of a future publication. We assume, until we have evidence to the contrary, that any environmental variation for the traits in question is the result of influences which are unique to particular individuals rather than shared by members of the same family. If such an assumption were clearly unjustified, then we would find our observations quite obviously did not coincide with our expectations and we would be forced to reject our simple model.

Jinks and Fulker (1970) showed in their biometrical genetical reanalysis of Shields's (1962) extraversion data that common environmental influences must be fairly unimportant. This adds some weight to our assumption that common environmental influences can be ignored, but we should first indicate the likely sensitivity of our experiment for detecting such effects if they still contribute to the variation between pairs.

Power calculations, familiar in the context of biometrical genetics, (e.g., Eaves, 1972; Eaves & Jinks, 1972; Kearsey, 1970) reveal that a sample of approximately 220 pairs of monozygotic and the same number of dizygotic pairs would allow us to be roughly 50% certain of detecting common environmental influences which accounted for 20% of the total variation against the background of an additive genetical component which accounted for about 40% of the total variation. This gives some indication of the power of the present study to detect common environmental influences (and the confounded consequences of assortative mating), provided there is no nonadditive genetical variation. To be 95% certain of detecting a common environmental component of this magnitude, sample sizes would have to be about four times as great.

4. *Sex linkage and sex limitation are absent.* If we were to adopt the usual practice of analyzing correlations rather than mean squares, we would have only poor tests of sex linkage and sex limitation. We would, however, expect the numerical values of comparable mean squares to vary significantly between sexes in the presence of sex linkage or sex limitation except under very restrictive assumptions about the magnitudes and types of gene effects (see Mather & Jinks, 1971). In applying our model to the mean squares rather than to the correlations, we may expect any gross distortion due to either of these causes to result in significant failure of the model.

5. *Genotypic and environmental deviations are uncorrelated.* Under some circumstances we might expect genotype–environmental covariation to contribute to failure of our simple genetical model for monozygotic and dizygotic twins. These circumstances, however, are rather restricting for a study of this type, and we should be cautious about assuming that the adequacy of the model for twin data means that we can ignore this source of variation. As a consequence of the covariation of genotype and environmental effects we could, in principle, find that the environmental components for dizygotic and monozygotic twins are no longer comparable. In practice we are unlikely to detect such differences with these data.

6. *Any variation due to the interaction of genotype and environment is confounded with the environmental variation within families.* It is inevitable that any interaction between genotypic effects and those environmental influences specific to individuals will be confounded with variation due to specific environmental factors in human studies (Jinks & Fulker 1970). We hope that an analysis of such interactions for personality variables will be the subject of a future article. If we are justified in our assumption that there are no common environmental influences, then we are also justified in our assumption that these do not interact with the genotype. Should our model fail because of common environments, we would find that our estimate of the additive genetical component was biased by the variation due to any interaction of these influences with genotypic factors.

We represent the six assumptions by writing a model for the *mean squares* for pairs of monozygotic and dizygotic twins in terms of an additive genetical component (D_R) and a within-family environmental component (E_1). Mather and Jinks (1971) showed how D_R may be defined in terms of the frequencies and effects of many loci. The coefficient chosen for D_R will depend on the mating system. Since we are assuming mating to be random, the coefficients involve no further unknown parameter and may be written for monozygotic and dizygotic twins as they are shown in Table 6. The expectation for a *within-pair mean square* is simply the expectation for the corresponding *within-family component of variance*, σ_w^2, and the expectation for a *between-pair mean square* is σ_w^2 plus twice the expectation for the corresponding *between-families component of variance*, σ_b^2. Full tables of expectations of mean squares and variance components for different kinds of relatives may be found elsewhere (e.g., Eaves, 1973a; Jinks & Fulker, 1970; Mather & Jinks, 1971).

LINDON EAVES AND HANS EYSENCK

Estimating Parameters and Testing the Model

If we consider only one trait we have, in this study, 10 observed mean squares. Let these be written as the column vector $\mathbf{x}$. Our model (see Table 6) involves two parameters whose coefficients in the expectations of $\mathbf{x}$ may be represented by the 10×2 design matrix $\mathbf{A}$. We may obtain our estimates of the two parameters, denoted by the two-element vector $\hat{\boldsymbol{\theta}}$, by solving the simultaneous equations:

$$\hat{\boldsymbol{\theta}} = (\mathbf{A'WA})^{-1}\mathbf{A'Wx},$$

where $\mathbf{W}$ is the (10×10) matrix of information about the observed statistics. When the $\mathbf{x}$ are mean squares, the amount of information about mean square $\mathbf{x}_i$ is $n_i/2(\varepsilon\mathbf{x}_i)^2$, where n_i is the degrees of freedom corresponding to $\mathbf{x}_i$. Clearly we do not know $\varepsilon\mathbf{x}$ until the model has been fitted so we have to use the observed $\mathbf{x}$ to provide trial values for the amounts of information and proceed iteratively until our $\varepsilon\mathbf{x}$ are stable. In practice, however, it is often unnecessary to go beyond the first cycle provided the model is adequate, since $\mathbf{x}$ will then be a close approximation to $\varepsilon\mathbf{x}$. For the case in which we are considering a single trait and our mean-squares are all independent, $\mathbf{W}$ is diagonal and the computations for simple models are not tedious. Providing that our observed statistics are normally distributed, our estimates of $\boldsymbol{\theta}$ are the maximum-likelihood estimates and the scalar

$$S = (\mathbf{x} - \varepsilon\mathbf{x})'\mathbf{W}(\mathbf{x} - \varepsilon\mathbf{x})$$

is distributed as a chi-square with degrees of freedom equal to the number of statistics less the number of parameters estimated from the data. The assumption of normality is probably not far from the truth with the sample sizes available. Should this chi-square be significant, we would be compelled to reject our model as inappropriate for the description of the variation for the trait under consideration.

Although the preceding statistical considerations are not new, they have not been generally applied to the genetical analysis of human behavior, with the result that data have been used inefficiently, standard errors of estimates rarely quoted, and assumptions rarely tested. The usual analyses of twin data either concentrate on the variation within pairs or on a comparison of monozygotic and dizygotic correlations. The method we employ combines both approaches in a single test of a simple model. In effect, our test of the D_R, E_1 model is not merely testing whether the within-pair variances differ for the two types of twins but whether the estimates derived from within-pair comparisons can be used to predict the variation between pairs. We expect the prediction to be poor if certain of our assumptions fail. These and other considerations, such as that of sex limitation, are all combined in our weighted least-squares analysis of the full set of raw mean squares.

RESULTS

Genetical Analysis of Extraversion

The estimates of the parameters and the elements of their covariance matrix, $(\mathbf{A'WA})^{-1}$,

TABLE 7

GENETICAL ANALYSIS OF EXTRAVERSION

Parameter	Estimate	χ^2	df	P
D_R	2.2487	98.50	1	<.001
E_1	1.5280	276.04	1	<.001
Residual		7.05	8	.50
V D_R	.051336	—	—	
V E_1	.008458	—	—	
Cov $D_R E_1$	−.011814	—	—	

Note. D_R refers to an additive genetical component, and E_1 refers to a within-family environmental component. V and Cov refer to variance and covariance, respectively.

are given for extraversion in Table 7. We see from the nonsignificant residual χ^2 that our model is clearly adequate so that the data give no reason to suppose that our assumptions are unjustified. We divide the square of each estimate by the corresponding variance term to give, for each estimate, a $\chi^2(1)$ which tests the significance of that parameter. Clearly both D_R and E_1 are highly significant components of the variation in extraversion.

On the basis of our tests of the model we tentatively adopt the view that most of the genetical variation is additive and most of the environmental variation can be attributed to E_1. We may use our estimates to estimate the proportion of the population variance for extraversion which can be attributed to genetical causes. Since all of the variation is additive, we have no need of the distinction between "broad" and "narrow" heritability in the present context; we just estimate:

$$\hat{h}^2 = \tfrac{1}{2}\hat{D}_R/(\tfrac{1}{2}\hat{D}_R + \hat{E}_1)$$

$$= .424 \text{ for extraversion.}$$

This means that 42% of the variation in extraversion may be attributed to genetical causes. In the present case E_1 includes variation due both to "unreliability" and "real" specific environmental influences. There seems little point in correcting for unreliability if all predictions are to be made on the basis of one administration of a test such as that analyzed here. If our genetical model is in fact appropriate, we may predict the correlations between other degrees of relatives for extraversion as measured by this test. For parents and offspring, for example, we would expect a correlation of $\tfrac{1}{2}h^2 = .21$. Such data as we have suggest that the observed correlation is

TABLE 8

GENETICAL ANALYSIS OF INTERACTION BETWEEN SUBJECTS AND TESTS OF SOCIABILITY AND IMPULSIVENESS

Parameter	Estimate	χ^2	df	P
D_R	.8591	62.94	1	<.001
E_1	.8359	288.95	1	<.001
Residual	—	8.76	8	>.30
$V\,D_R$	.011727	—	—	—
$V\,E_1$	.002418	—	—	—
$Cov\,D_R E_1$	−.003277	—	—	—

Note. D_R refers to an additive genetical component, and E_1 refers to a within-family environmental component. V and Cov refer to variance and covariance, respectively.

somewhat lower but not significantly so. Such a difference, if it turned out to be significant, might be attributed to the interaction of the genotypic difference between individuals with an overall differences between the environments of parents and offspring or to the fact that our estimate of the heritability is somewhat biased by undetected common environmental effects. A common environmental effect which accounted for about 10%–15% of the total variance might explain the disparity and is more likely than not be to undetected in our study.

We obtained estimates of the internal consistency of the scales. For sociability the reliability was about .75 and for impulsiveness, .60. We may correct our heritability estimate for unreliability provided we can assume the Subjects × Items interactions estimate experimental error only. Using the estimates of genetical and environmental variance and covariance obtained below, we found the heritability of extraversion, after correction, to be .57. By correcting for unreliability, we have attempted to partition the environmental variation for extraversion into that part which may reflect stable environmental influences on the development of the trait and that part due to experimental error. If subjects and items interact, the contribution of experimental error to E_1 will be overestimated. Such interactions may have a genetical component which we could analyze using the methods adopted in this article. Confounded with our "true" environmental variation will remain variation reflecting day-to-day changes in behavior whose contribution can only be assessed by repeated measurement.

Genetical Analysis of Subject × Tests Interaction

The results of the analysis of the mean squares for the D scores appear in Table 8. Broadly speaking the results for the interaction are very similar to those for E. The main difference is the reduction by half, in this case, of the estimates of D_R and E_1. This reflects the greater discriminating power of E resulting from the positive covariation of sociability and impulsiveness. However, the simple model is again adequate, since the residual $\chi^2(8)$ is not significant. D_R and E_1 are, once more, highly significant. This means that the discrimination between sociability and impulsiveness is justified in genetical terms. We have to conclude that not all the genetical factors contributing to variation in sociability and impulsiveness contribute equally and consistently to both. We estimate the heritability of the interaction to be .339. Although this value is somewhat lower than that for E, the difference is not large and we must notice that the *relative* contribution of unreliability variation will be greater for the interaction than for E. Using the reliabilities given above, and the estimates of the genetical and environmental variance and covariance components from a later analysis (see below), we estimate the heritability of the interaction of subjects and tests to be .72. The marked change reflects the relatively large positive environmental correlation between sociability and impulsiveness, particularly when the environmental variances are corrected for unreliability.

Table 9 summarizes the results of both analyses in terms of the proportions of the total variation of sociability and impulsiveness

TABLE 9

THE RELATIVE CONTRIBUTIONS OF GENOTYPIC AND ENVIRONMENTAL FACTORS OF EXTRAVERSION AND SUBJECTS × TESTS INTERACTION TO THE VARIATION BETWEEN SUBJECTS FOR SOCIABILITY AND IMPULSIVENESS

Causal factor	Psychological factor		Total
	Extraversion	Interaction	
Genetical	.2870(.3402)	.1096(.2631)	.3966(.6035)
Environmental	.3900(.2156)	.2134(.1807)	.6034(.3963)
Total	.6770(.5558)	.3230(.4440)	1.0000(.9998)

Note. Proportions of estimated reliable variation are given in parenthesis.

LINDON EAVES AND HANS EYSENCK

TABLE 10

RESULT OF FITTING SIMPLE MODEL TO VARIATION AND COVARIATION
OF SOCIABILITY AND IMPULSIVENESS

Parameter	Estimate	Covariance ($\times 10^4$) of estimate with estimate of						$\chi^2(1)$
		D_{RS}	D_{RI}	D_{RSI}	E_{IS}	E_{II}	E_{ISI}	
D_{RS}	.9214	67.05	8.54	23.89	−14.80	−1.61	−4.92	126.63*
D_{RI}	.7132		68.38	24.01	− 1.62	−19.34	−1.93	74.33*
D_{RSI}	.3419			38.08	− 4.92	− 5.64	−9.30	30.70*
E_{IS}	.5410				10.42	1.11	3.41	280.77*
E_{II}	.6441					14.32	9.92	290.45*
E_{ISI}	.1758						6.68	46.27*

Note. The parameters D_{RS}, D_{RI}, D_{RSI}, E_{IS}, E_{II}, and E_{ISI} correspond to the components of the mean squares of sociability, impulsiveness, and the mean products of the two traits, respectively.
* $P < .001$.

scores which may be attributed to the genetical and environmental components of extraversion and the interaction of subjects and tests. Approximately three fifths of the total variation is environmental (from the row totals of Table 9) and two thirds of the total variation is attributable to the extraversion factor (from the column totals of Table 9). The proportion of environmental variation is fairly consistent over columns, and the proportion of variation accounted for by extraversion is fairly consistent over rows. In Table 9 we also present a summary for the scales after the environmental components have been corrected for unreliability. So far we have shown that genetical factors probably contribute to individual differences in both E and D scores. A qualitative consideration of the conclusion suggests that E is more discriminating than D genetically and environmentally and leads us to the view that the positive covariation of sociability and impulsiveness has a basis which is both genetical and environmental. We could verify this directly by a statistical comparison of our estimates to test whether the estimates of D_R and E_1 are significantly greater than the corresponding estimates for D. We prefer, however, to estimate separately the genetical and environmental components of the variation and covariation of sociability and impulsiveness scores, since this will allow us to estimate the genetical and environmental correlations between the traits.

Analysis of Variation and Covariation of Sociability and Impulsiveness

The weighted least-squares procedure described above may be extended without undue complication to the simultaneous analysis of the variances and covariances of multiple variables (Eaves & Gale, 1974). In this case, however, separate D_R's and E_1's are fitted for the variance and covariance terms. The information matrix, **W**, is no longer diagonal, since the model is fitted to mean squares and mean products which are no longer independent because each subject yields measurements on every trait.

In this instance the model is fitted to the 30 statistics of Table 5. Now six parameters are specified, D_{RS}, D_{RI}, $D_{RS,I}$, E_{IS}, E_{II}, and $E_{IS,I}$. These correspond to the components of the mean squares of sociability, impulsiveness, and the mean products of the two traits, respectively. The method and the definition of the parameters is discussed in more detail by Eaves and Gale (1974).

There are thus 30 statistics. Six parameters are estimated from the data, so the residual chi-square for testing the goodness of fit of the model has 24 degrees of freedom. This chi-square changed by less than .2% between the first and second cycle of the weighted least-squares analysis, when $\chi^2(24) = 29.41$, $p \simeq .20$. Thus the adequacy of the D_R, E_1 model for the variation and covariation of sociability and impulsiveness was confirmed.

The estimates of the six parameters and their covariance matrix are given in Table 10. Clearly all the estimates differ significantly from zero. We estimate the heritability of sociability to be .460 and that of impulsiveness to be .356. Using, once more, our estimates of reliability, we infer that about 54% of the environmental variation for sociability is "reliable" variation, assuming that we have accounted for all the unreliability. For impulsiveness the comparable figure is 38%. We may now obtain estimates of the proportion of *reliable* variance which is due to genetical causes. Our estimates are .61 for sociability and .60 for impulsiveness. There is, therefore, convincing evidence that both traits are under some degree of genetical control. This finding is not new. Claridge, Canter, and Hume (1973) reported an apparent genetical component of variation for both scales. Our model-fitting approach, however, leads us to suggest that there is no evidence of nonadditive genetical variation and no evidence of common environmental effects. Furthermore, we have demonstrated that the covariance of sociability and impulsiveness probably has a genetical basis but that environmental factors also contribute significantly to the covariation of the two scales. The extent to which the two traits may be regarded as sharing common genetical and environmental factors is represented by the genetic and environmental correlations r_{D_R} and r_{E_1}, respectively:

$$r_{D_R} = D_{RS,I}/(D_{RS} \cdot D_{RI})^{\frac{1}{2}}$$
$$= .42$$
$$r_{E_1} = E_{1S,I}/(E_{1S} \cdot E_{1I})^{\frac{1}{2}}$$
$$= .32.$$

Variation due to unreliability contributes to E_1 but not to D_R so we might expect the observed environmental correlation to be less than the genetic correlation. These correlations are a little less, though not considerably less, than the phenotypic correlation of .468 reported for sociability and impulsiveness by Eysenck and Eysenck (1969).

Providing we are justified in assuming the unreliability components of sociability and impulsiveness to be uncorrelated, we may correct our estimate of r_{E_1} for unreliability using the estimates of reliability given above. We now find that r_{E_1} is .66. This indicates that the unitary nature of extraversion is clearly evident in the environmental determinants of the trait, even though the genetical correlation between sociability and impulsiveness is rather less. Eaves (1973b) suggested, on the basis of a multivariate genetical analysis of monozygotic twins, that "the apparently unitary nature of extraversion at the phenotypic level could be due to environmental rather than to genetical

influences." The different analysis we have presented here confirms this conclusion.

We should perhaps clarify what this finding means. It does not necessarily support the view that extraversion is an "environmental mold" trait, to use the conception of Cattell, that is, a trait which reflects the structure of environmental influences inherent in the environment itself. We may obtain exactly the same picture because the organism, by virtue of the integration of its nervous system, *imposes* a unitary structure on externally unstructured environmental influences contributing to the development of behavior.

CONCLUSIONS

The analyses presented above suggest the following principal conclusions.

1. Genetical factors contribute both to the variation and covariation of sociability and impulsiveness.

2. Environmental factors also contribute to the covariation of sociability and impulsiveness.

3. The genetical correlation between the two factors is estimated to be .42, the environmental correlation to be .66 after correction for unreliability.

4. Combining sociability and impulsiveness scores by addition to provide a measure of extraversion provides the most powerful single means of discriminating between individuals with respect to the genetical and environmental determinants of their responses to the sociability and impulsiveness items of the questionnaire.

5. The interaction between subjects and tests has a significant genetical component, so there is some justification for regarding sociability and impulsiveness as distinguishable genetically.

Furthermore we conclude:

6. About 40% of the variation in sociability, impulsiveness, and their combinations, as measured by this questionnaire, can be attributed to genetical factors.

7. Our data are consistent with the view that the genetical variation is mainly additive.

8. We find no evidence for a large effect of the family environment on any of the traits studied, but the environmental influences

specific to individuals (including unreliability of measurement) account for about 60% of the variation.

9. Mating is effectively random for the traits in question.

10. The genetical and environmental determinants of variation are homogeneous over sexes, suggesting that the effects of sex linkage and sex limitation are negligible.

DISCUSSION

Our analysis is necessarily tentative because it is based only on monozygotic and dizygotic twins. We would be particularly cautious about discounting genotype–environment correlations as an additional source of variation. It must also be emphasized that genotype–environment interaction may well be confounded with E_1 so that variation which we have ascribed to environmental factors may itself have a genetical component. We hope to clarify this matter in the future.

Between 30% and 40% of the variation in components of extraversion may be due to environmental factors that cannot be attributed to the inconsistency of the test. All of the detectable environmental variation is specific to individuals rather than common to families. This suggests that attempts to relate extraversion to aspects of the individual's "family background" are unlikely to be productive unless the family background has a direct genetical association with extraversion. Even though we might be able to measure social and domestic factors shared by members of the same sibship, we would not expect these to be very highly correlated (say, not more than $r = .2$) with the mean extraversion score of the sibship. Consistently larger correlations between such shared environmental factors and the mean raw E scores of sibship would lead us to suspect our simple model.

Since a considerable proportion of the variation in extraversion and its components is clearly due to environmental influences specific to individuals, we could expect, in principle, to relate the intrapair differences of monozygotic twins to differences in their environmental experiences. That this is feasible in principle, however, does not aid our efforts to specify or detect such likely influences. Attempts to predict the variation in extraversion for a random sample of individuals by measuring concomitant social or other variables, however, may be misleading, because any association we find could reflect either genetical or environmental communality of the traits in question. Merely attaching the label "social" to a trait does not constitute a prior case for environmental causation. Analyses of the kind we have conducted for the covariation of components of extraversion would have to be employed for the other variables if we were to discriminate between environmental and genetical association between extraversion and other variables in the social "environment."

The fact that between 60% and 70% of the "reliable" variation is genetically determined does not, of course, suggest which genes are involved nor what may or may not be done to modify the trait. It does, however, suggest that the segregation and recombination of alleles may be a primary cause of variation in the dimension of personality we have studied here. At the level of population biology it means that extraversion, like most other traits, reflects genetical polymorphism and as such is exposed to the directional, stabilizing or disruptive influence of natural selection. As far as we can judge from studies on other organisms (Kearsey & Kojima, 1967; Mather, 1966; 1967), we find that directional selection has been characteristically associated with the evolution of a genetical system demonstrating a large amount of directional dominance and duplicate gene interactions. When natural selection has favored intermediate phenotypes, the genetical system involves predominately additive effects, and dominance, if any, is ambidirectional. It would be too early to say whether our failure to detect nonadditive variation merely reflects the design of our study, the (relatively) low heritability, or the small amount of dominance relative to the additive variation. It may be difficult to obtain a definite answer to such questions for this trait because of the large samples required and because of the formal inability to disentangle completely the additive, dominance, and epistatic components of gene action for natural populations even when these can be raised in strictly experimental situations (Mather, 1974). We suggest very tentatively that the polymorphism we detect for extraversion and its components may be subject to stabilizing selection because, as far as we can tell at the moment, the genetical variation is additive. That is, we should conclude that neither extreme introversion nor extraversion has been favored systematically during human evolution. It is possible that without either extreme the fitness of a human population would have suffered at sometime or other. We can at least conceive of situations in which individuals of more impulsive or sociable temperament may well have promoted the survival of themselves and their close relatives. Similarly, we can imagine that there are times or situations in which it would be advantageous to have the persistent, attentive behavior characteristic of introverts. In contrast to this, we may consider a trait such as high intelligence for which there is as uggestion of directional dominance (Jinks & Eaves, 1974; Jinks & Fulker, 1970) and for which, therefore, we suspect a history of directional selection. In the case of intelligence, it is difficult to conceive of as many plausible situations in which relatively high intelligence could not confer upon an individual greater reproductive fitness than average. Such speculations about the evolutionary significance of personality are less well founded at this stage because we cannot infer the genetical system with any great degree of confidence. We believe, however, that such speculations are legitimate if they engender a more systematic and thoughtful approach to the collection and analysis of data on human behavioral traits.

REFERENCES

Carrigan, P. M. Extraversion-introversion as a dimension of personality: A reappraisal. *Psychological Bulletin*, 1960, *57*, 329–360.

Cattell, R. B. The description and measurement of personality. New York: World Book, 1946.

Cederlöf, R., Friberg, L., Jonsonn, E., & Kaij, L. Studies in similarity of diagnosis in twins with the aid of mailed questionnaires. *Acta Genetica (Basel)*, 1961, *11*, 338–362.

Claridge, G., Canter, S., & Hume, W. I. *Personality differences and biological variations: A study of twins.* New York: Pergamon Press, 1973.

Eaves, L. J. Computer simulation of sample size and experimental design in human psychogenetics. *Psychological Bulletin*, 1972, *77*, 144–152.

Eaves, L. J. Assortative mating and intelligence: An analysis of pedigree data. *Heredity*, 1973, *30*, 199–210. (a)

Eaves, L. J. The structure of genotypic and environmental covariation of personality measurements: An analysis of the PEN. *British Journal of Social and Clinical Psychology*, 1973, *12*, 275–282. (b)

Eaves, L. J., & Gale, J. S. A method for analysing the genetical basis of covariation. *Behavior Genetics*, 1974, *4*, 253–267.

Eaves, L. J., & Jinks, J. L. Insignificance of evidence for differences in heritability of I.Q. between races and social classes. *Nature*, 1972, *240*, 84–88.

Eysenck, H. J. *The biological basis of personality.* Springfield, Ill.: Charles C Thomas, 1967.

Eysenck, H. J. Personality, premarital sexual permissiveness and assortative mating. *Journal of Sex Research*, 1974, *10*, 47–51.

Eysenck, H. J., & Eysenck, S. B. G. On the unitary nature of extraversion. *Acta Psychologica*, 1967, *26*, 383–390.

Eysenck, H. J., & Eysenck, S. B. G. *Personality structure and measurement.* London: Routledge & Kegan Paul, 1969.

Eysenck, S. B. G., & Eysenck, H. J. On the dual nature of extraversion. *British Journal of Social and Clinical Psychology*. 1963, *2*, 46–55.

Jinks, J. L., & Eaves, L. J. I.Q. and inequality. *Nature*, 1974, *248*, 287–289.

Jinks, J. L., & Fulker, D. W. A comparison of the biometrical genetical, MAVA and cassical approaches to the analysis of human behavior. *Psychological Bulletin*, 1970, *73*, 311–349.

Kearsey, M. J. Experimental sizes for detecting dominance variation. *Heredity*, 1970, *25*, 529–542.

Kearsey, M. J., & Kojima, K. The genetic architecture of body weight and egg hatchability in *Drosophila melangaster. Genetics*, 1967, *56*, 23–37.

Mather, K. Variability and selection. *Proceedings of the Royal Society of London, Series B*, 1966, *164*, 328–340.

Mather, K. Complementary and duplicate gene interactions in biometrical genetics. *Heredity*, 1967, *22*, 97–103.

Mather, K. Non-allelic interaction in continuous variation of randomly breeding populations. *Heredity*, 1974, *32*, 414–419.

Mather, K., & Jinks, J. L. *Biometrical Genetics.* London: Chapman Hall, 1971.

Shields, J. *Monozygotic twins.* Oxford: University Press, 1962.

Sparrow, N. H., & Ross, J. The dual nature of extraversion: A replication. *Australian Journal of Psychology*, 1964, *16*, 214–218.

(Received March 11, 1974)

From H. J. Eysenck (1972). British Journal of Social and Clinical Psychology, *11*, 265–269, *by kind permission of the author and the Avenue Publishing Company*

Primaries or Second-order Factors: A Critical Consideration of Cattell's 16 PF Battery

By H. J. EYSENCK

University of London

Intercorrelations between certain Cattell 16 PF scales contributing to the second-order factors exvia–invia and adjustment–anxiety were corrected for attenuation, in order to test Cattell's views about the relative importance of primary and second-order factors. It was found that when the contribution of second-order factors was extracted from the battery, very little was left over for primaries to measure, and it was concluded that in Cattell's own data there is no good evidence to suggest that primaries make any independent contribution to measurement apart from the higher-order factors.

There are considerable similarities between the personality descriptions given by the factor-analysis based systems of Cattell, Guilford and Eysenck; these similarities, however, appear only in the higher-order factors called extraversion–introversion and neuroticism–stability by Eysenck, and exvia–invia and adjustment–anxiety by Cattell (Eysenck & Eysenck, 1969). While the factors extracted at this level from sets of questions contributed by these three authors are virtually identical, there is little agreement on primary (first-order) factors; furthermore, Eysenck was unable to replicate Cattell's or Guilford's factors on his samples (Eysenck & Eysenck, 1969). As far as Cattell's primaries are concerned, this failure seems common; Peterson (1960) in the U.S.A. and Greif (1970) in Germany similarly failed to provide any kind of replication. It could be argued, in the case of the Eysenck & Eysenck studies, that the method of rotation used was dissimilar to that used by Cattell; however, Promax (Hendrickson & White, 1966) was devised in our laboratories by two former collaborators of Cattell's with intent to capture the principles underlying his own methods, and a study carried out in Cattell's own laboratory has shown Promax to be equivalent to Cattell's own methods (personal communication).

Even if Cattell's factors were replicable, there would still be disagreement on the relative importance and value of primary factors and of second-order factors. Cattell is quite specific in his claims: 'The primary factors give one most information, and we would advocate higher strata contributors only as supplementary concepts.... It is a mistake, generally, to work at the secondary level only, for one certainly loses a lot of valuable information present initially at the primary level' (Cattell *et al.*, 1970, pp. 111–12). Eysenck's position is equally clear; he would maintain that second-order factors are far more meaningful psychologically (Eysenck, 1967*a*), and that little if any information is lost by disregarding the primaries in such personality studies as those reported by Cattell. It is not suggested that this would always and inevitably be so; in the field of intelligence testing Eysenck would still regard *g* as the most important single factor, but would certainly agree that half a dozen or so

H. J. EYSENCK

of primaries make a definite contribution to prediction in many cases (Eysenck, 1967*b*; Vernon, 1965; McNemar, 1964).

Such an argument should be amenable to factual settlement, and the present paper constitutes an attempt to provide some information which may be considered relevant. Cattell *et al.* (1970) have published a table (p. 113) of intercorrelations between the 16 PF scale scores of 423 male and 535 female college students, separately; they used the sum of scores on forms A and B for this purpose. Many of these are quite high, but for our purposes these raw correlations are not very useful as they are of course very much lower than the 'true' correlations between scales by virtue of the rather low reliabilities. Our argument will be that if the correlations between scales contributing to a particular factor (exvia, or anxiety) at the second-order level are at or near unity, then clearly the individual scales (primaries) make no contribution over and above that made by the second-order factor. To test this hypothesis we must correct the existing correlations for attenuation; without this correction the failure of the observed correlations to reach unity may be due entirely to random error rather than to factor-specific contributions. For this purpose, reliability coefficients are required for the scales used; fortunately correlations between scales A and B (which Cattell *et al.* consider 'parallel forms' on p. 32) are given in their Table 5.3 for 6476 subjects, and have been used for our calculations. It would have been more suitable if these reliabilities had been calculated on the actual sample studied, but the requisite data are not available; this may introduce some minor errors into the computations. On the other hand, the reliabilities of the figures may be considerably improved because they are based on much larger numbers; it is possible that advantages and disadvantages balance out in this case. This correlation between parallel forms, Cattell calls 'equivalence coefficient'; as he points out, there are many different 'reliability' coefficients in the literature, all having quite different properties, and it is necessary to be quite specific about one's use of the term.*

Table 1 gives the corrected correlations for men (upper half) and women (lower half) between the five scales which, according to Cattell, contribute to his anxiety second-order factor. Scale H, which is also included by him, has been omitted because it also contributes to exvia–invia, the other main second-order factor, and correlates more highly with this. Out of 20 coefficients, 12 are above unity, and another three are only just below unity; this leaves five coefficients in the 0·8's (three in all) and below (two). Coefficients above unity are, of course, evidence of

---

* It might be argued that 'equivalence coefficients' are not the proper reliabilities to use in correction for attenuation, and that some form of split-half reliability ought to have been used. Such would not be Cattell's own view, and to give his theory the optimum opportunity to prove itself we have followed his own reasoning in our procedure. It should also be noted that there are gross differences in the empirical literature about the split-half reliabilities to be expected in relation to Cattell's 16 scales; Greif (1970) gives an interesting comparison (Table 2 in his paper) of his own findings and Cattell's. For scale A, Cattell reports a correlation of 0·82, Greif of 0·28; for scale M, the values are 0·79 and 0·21; for scale N, 0·65 and −0·04. The average reliability in Greif's study is only 0·37. Had we used these reliabilities, conclusions about the intercorrelations between scales corrected for attenuation would have been much more adverse than those actually recorded.

Primaries or Second-order Factors

Table 1. *Intercorrelations between Cattell's five 'anxiety' scales,*
corrected for attenuation

		C(−)	L	O	Q$_3$(−)	Q$_4$
C(−)	(Low ego strength)	—	1·14	1·22	1·04	1·19
L	(Suspiciousness)	0·98	—	0·86	0·78	1·15
O	(Guilt proneness)	1·24	0·66	—	0·95	1·24
Q$_3$(−)	(Low self-sentiment)	1·02	0·80	0·87	—	0·97
Q$_4$	(High ergic tension)	1·23	1·04	1·11	1·14	—

overcorrection, and may be due to the fact that the reliabilities were calculated on groups other than the ones furnishing the actual correlations between scales; similarly, the lower coefficients may be evidence of undercorrection. However we look at these figures, they do not justify Cattell's claim that work with the second-order factors would cause one to 'lose a lot of valuable information present initially at the primary level'. As far as one can see, practically all the information contained unreliably in the primaries is contained reliably in the second-order factor; very little information indeed is left over for contribution by the primaries.

The position is not quite as clear in Table 2, which presents the intercorrelations

Table 2. *Intercorrelations between Cattell's five 'exvia' scales,*
corrected for attenuation

		A	E	F	Q$_2$(−)	H
A	(Affecto-thymia)	—	0·44	0·66	0·91	0·69
E	(Dominance)	0·28	—	0·94	0·18	0·89
F	(Surgency)	0·61	0·85	—	1·07	1·00
Q$_2$(−)	(Group adherence)	0·93	0·04	0·78	—	0·86
H	(Venturesomeness)	0·50	0·72	0·87	0·76	—

between the five scales which according to Cattell contribute to the second-order factor exvia–invia. Only two out of 20 correlations exceed unity, and another six could be rounded up to 0·9; this leaves 12 correlations below this level. Of these, three belong to scale H (Venturesomeness) which, as already noted, also loads on the anxiety factor; as its contribution is spread over two second-order factors, its correlations for either must of course be considerably lower than unity. Of the remaining coefficients, two are very low, viz. those referring to the correlations between E (Dominance) and Q$_2$ (Group adherence) in the male and female samples respectively. This would appear to be a good example of what Frenkel-Brunswik (1942) has called the principle of alternative manifestation; 'different classes of behavioral expressions were often related to one drive as alternative manifestations of that drive…. One drive variable may circumscribe a family of alternative manifestations unrelated to each other: the meaning of the drive concept emerges in terms of families of divergent manifestations held together dynamically or genotypically, though often not phenotypically'.

Other correlations which are well below unity are those involving A and E, and A and F. A and E are both noted by Cattell as being involved in second-order factor 3 (Pathemia); E is also involved in factor 4 (Independence), and A in factor 5 (Naturalness). F is involved in factor 8 (Superego strength). We thus find that primaries whose intercorrelations do not come up to unity when second-order factors 1 and 2 are concerned are also involved in other second-order factors; this would be impossible if all their variance were taken up by one second-order factor.

If it is permissible to draw any conclusions from these figures, it must be that they fail to support Cattell's statement quoted at the beginning of this paper; primary factors add little to the contribution made by second-order factors, with the possible exception of the 'alternative manifestations' factors contrasting extraverted attitudes leading to either leadership or group adherence. The figures given are not incompatible with a general view which would regard the primaries advocated by Cattell as random groupings of items either measuring extraversion or neuroticism, or occasionally both (i.e. the items making up his factor H). Such a view would also be compatible with the fact that several writers have found it impossible to replicate Cattell's factors in independent analyses, using both his items and his methods of analysis and rotation. The figures upon which this tentative conclusion is based are of course not very precise, for reasons already given, and the fact that several of the corrected correlations exceed unity bears witness to this. In this lack of accuracy, of course, psychology is an exact replica of physics; as Taylor *et al.* (1970) point out, 'contrary to popular opinion, physics is usually not a very exact science.... In some cases finding agreement to within an order of magnitude (a factor of 10) is a considerable achievement'. And the reason for this lack of exactitude is the same in both sciences: 'First, most experiments deal with a complex system in which a variety of interrelated and often poorly understood phenomena are involved. Second, the pertinent theory usually provides only an approximation based on a simplified conceptual model of the system' (p. 62). In spite of the obvious inaccuracies in our calculations, the data do seem to support reasonably well the writer's conception of the relation between primary and second-order factors, and to contradict that advocated by Cattell. At the very least, the data and analyses presented seem to require some form of proof from Cattell to substantiate his contention that 'one certainly loses a lot of valuable information present initially at the primary level' in working with second-order factors only. Even restricting ourselves to two only of the eight second-order factors Cattell claims to have isolated, this just does not seem to be so.

It is interesting to speculate on the reasons for this rather strange phenomenon. Eysenck & Eysenck (1969) have drawn attention to a continuum ranging from factors which are essentially tautological (T factors) to factors which are made up of many complex and divergent items (C factors); Guilford and Eysenck, in so far as they deal with primaries, are concerned more with the former, whereas Cattell is concerned with the latter. This difference emerges also in the stress laid by these different authors on high factor loadings, leading to simple structure defined by clusters of similar items (Guilford and Eysenck), or rather on high hyperplane counts (Cattell), which are compatible with much lower factor loadings, and particularly with much lower item correlations within a given primary factor. The resulting factors are called by Cattell 'surface' (T factors) and 'source' (C factors) traits, but these terms are question begging; there is no independent evidence to show that Cattell's factors come any closer to some truly fundamental 'source' of human behaviour, and there is some evidence that Eysenck's E and N factors do

Primaries or Second-order Factors

(Eysenck, 1967*a*). As far as our analysis goes, it seems to suggest that far from being 'source' traits, Cattell's primaries are chance aggregations of items measuring E, or N, or both, as well as possibly some other second-order factors. This conclusion fits in well with the argument presented by Eysenck & Eysenck (1969) that replicable primaries are of the 'T' type, and that replicable 'C' type factors are always of the second-order kind, at least in the non-cognitive personality field.

There is now considerable international agreement regarding the vulnerability of Cattell's system to these criticisms (Becker, 1961; Borgatta, 1962; Greif, 1970; Levonian, 1961*a, b*; Peterson, 1960; Timm, 1968). Greif, for instance, points out that, in his detailed analysis, out of 170 items only 28 correlate more highly with the scale they are supposed to measure than with some other scale; out of 15 scales there are six without a single item which correlated more highly with the scale it is supposed to measure than with some other scale. He also concludes, as we have done, that 'the 16 scales cannot by any means be regarded as functionally independent, but are relatively highly correlated' (p. 211). Clearly, Cattell's hypothesis of 16 functionally independent factors being measured by his test requires considerable support if it is to continue being accepted by test users.

REFERENCES

BECKER, W. C. (1961). A comparison of the factor structure and other properties of the 16 PF and the Guilford-Martin personality inventories. *Educ. psychol. Measur.* **21**, 393–404.

BORGATTA, E. F. (1962). The coincidence of subtests in four personality inventories. *J. soc. Psychol.* **56**, 227–244.

CATTELL, R. B., EBER, H. W. & TATSUOKA, M. G. (1970). *Handbook for the Sixteen Personality Questionnaire (16 PF)*. Champaign, Ill.: Institute for Personality and Ability Testing.

EYSENCK, H. J. (1967*a*). *The Biological Basis of Personality*. Springfield, Ill.: Thomas.

EYSENCK, H. J. (1967*b*). Intelligence assessment: a theoretical and experimental approach. *Br. J. educ. Psychol.* **37**, 81–98.

EYSENCK, H. J. & EYSENCK, S. B. G. (1969). *Personality Structure and Measurement*. San Diego: Knapp.

FRENKEL-BRUNSWIK, E. (1942). Motivation and behaviour. *Genet. Psychol. Monogr.* **26**, 121–265.

GREIF, S. (1970). Untersuchungen zur deutschen Übersetzung des 16 PF Fragebogens. *Psychol. Beitr.* **12**, 186–213.

HENDRICKSON, A. E. & WHITE, P. O. (1966). A method for the rotation of higher-order factors. *Br. J. math. statist. Psychol.* **19**, 97–103.

LEVONIAN, E. (1961*a*). A statistical analysis of the 16 Personality Factor Questionnaire. *Educ. psychol. Measur.* **21**, 589–596.

LEVONIAN, E. (1961*b*). Personality measurement with items selected from the 16 PF Questionnaire. *Educ. psychol. Measur.* **21**, 937–946.

McNEMAR, Q. (1964). Lost: our intelligence? Why? *Am. Psychol.* **19**, 871–882.

PETERSON, D. R. (1960). The age generality of personality factors derived from ratings. *Educ. psychol. Measur.* **20**, 461–474.

TAYLOR, B. N., LAUGHENBERG, D. N. & PARKER, W. H. (1970). The fundamental physical constants. *Scient. Am.* **223** (4), 62–78.

TIMM, U. (1968). Reliabilität und Faktorenstruktur von Cattells 16 PF Test bei einer deutschen Stichprobe. *Z. exp. angew. Psychol.* **15**, 354–373.

VERNON, P. E. (1965). Ability factors and environmental influences. *Am. Psychol.* **20**, 723–733.

Manuscript received 15 *March* 1971

From J. A. Wakefield, Jr., B.-H. L. Yom, P. E. Bradley, E. B. Doughtie, J. A. Cox and I. A. Kraft (1974). British Journal of Social and Clinical Psychology, *13*, 413–420, *by kind permission of the authors and the Avenue Publishing Company*

Eysenck's Personality Dimensions: a Model for the MMPI

By JAMES A. WAKEFIELD JR, BYONG-HEE LEE YOM,
PEGGY E. BRADLEY, EUGENE B. DOUGHTIE
AND JOHN A. COX

University of Houston

AND IRVIN A. KRAFT

Baylor College of Medicine

Nine of the ten clinical scales of the MMPI were considered as measures of the neuroticism, psychoticism and extraversion personality dimensions of Eysenck. The correspondence between the conceptual placement of the subtests in Eysenck's three-dimensional space and their empirical placement in factor space was tested for 205 married males and again for 205 married females. The correspondence was significant for both sexes but considerably stronger for the females than for the males.

Eysenck (1970*a*; H. Eysenck & S. Eysenck, 1969) has proposed a dimensional system of personality consisting of psychoticism (P), neuroticism (N) and extraversion (E) dimensions. These three dimensions have been shown to be reliably and orthogonally measurable with adults (Eysenck, 1971, 1970*b*; H. Eysenck & S. Eysenck, 1971) and with children (S. Eysenck & H. Eysenck, 1969).

Scales for measuring two of the dimensions, N and E, were developed early (Eysenck, 1956), and several attempts have been made to equate these dimensions with factors obtained from the Minnesota Multiphasic Personality Inventory (MMPI) (Goorney, 1970; Hundleby & Connor, 1968; Corah, 1964). A method for measuring the third dimension, P, was more recently developed (S. Eysenck & H. Eysenck, 1968) and is still regarded more as a research tool than as a practical measure of psychosis (cf. Claridge & Chappa, 1973).

The present study attempts to show further the relationship between the three dimensions of Eysenck's personality theory and the empirically developed MMPI. In order to demonstrate the relationship, nine of the ten clinical scales are considered as measures of points in Eysenck's three-dimensional framework. (The Mf scale is not so considered.) MMPI scales that are commonly held to measure neuroticism are Hs, D and Hy (Meehl, 1956; Gough, 1946). Indicators of psychoticism are Pa, Pt and Sc (Winter & Stortroen, 1963; Ruesch & Bowman, 1945). The Si scale (Drake, 1946) was originated as a measure of the non-clinical introversion–extraversion dimension of personality.

The Ma scale has been considered an indicator of neurosis (e.g. Rousell & Edwards, 1971). Also, persons who score high on this scale tend to be outgoing and energetic (Carson, 1969). For these reasons the Ma scale is considered to measure both the neuroticism and extraversion dimensions of Eysenck's theory.

The Pd scale is associated with psychoticism. The Pd scale supposedly measures psychopathic character disorders (Carson, 1969). However, the failure of the MMPI to discriminate between such character disorders and psychosis has been noted (Affleck & Garfield, 1960). High scores on this scale also indicate a tendency to 'act out' (Carson, 1969). This scale is considered to measure both psychoticism and extraversion.

In Eysenck's theory the placement of the nine scales is as shown in Fig. 1. The three neurotic scales correspond to positive values on the N dimension. The three psychotic scales correspond to positive values on the P dimension. The Si scale corresponds to a negative value on the E dimension. Ma should have positive values on both the E and N dimensions. Pd should have positive values on both the P and E dimensions.

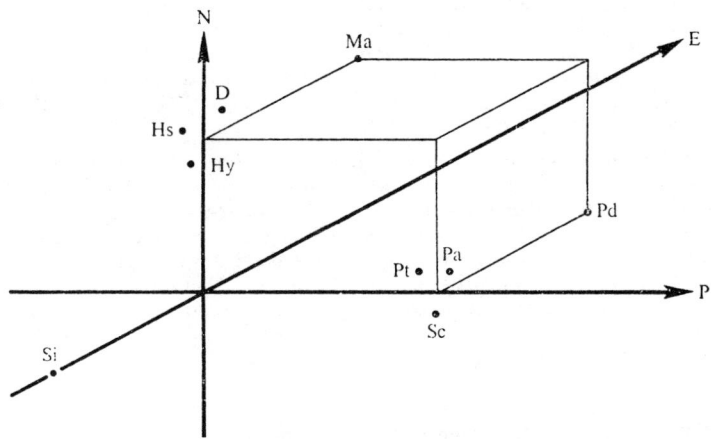

Fig. 1. Conceptual placement of nine MMPI scales in
Eysenck's three-dimensional personality theory

The correspondence between the empirical relationships among the MMPI scales and their theoretical placement in Eysenck's system is tested by a procedure presented by Wakefield & Doughtie (1973). The procedure involves specifying the relative lengths of interpoint distances from the theory and comparing each theoretically ordered pair of distances with the empirically ordered magnitudes of the distances in factor space.

METHOD

Theoretical interpoint distances

Among the three neurotic scales there are three distances. Since the scales measure variations of the same construct, neuroticism, the distances among them should be relatively short. The three interpoint distances among the psychotic scales should likewise be short. These six distances are called *short* distances.

There are nine interpoint distances from the three neurotic scales to the three psychotic scales, three distances from the neurotic scales to Si, three from the psychotic scales to Pd, and one interpoint distance from Ma to Pd. These 22 distances should be longer than the short distances; they are called *middle* distances.

Eysenck's Personality Dimensions

The two remaining interpoint distances are from Si to Ma and from Si to Pd. These should be the longest distances and are called *long* distances.

Theoretical distance relations

Each of the six *short* distances should be shorter than each of the 22 *middle* distances. This yields 132 ordered pairs of distances. Further, both of the *long* distances should be longer than each of the 22 *middle* distances. This yields 44 more ordered pairs of distances. From the theoretical structure presented in Fig. 1, there is a total of 176 ordered pairs of distances.

Subjects

The subjects were 205 married couples who took the MMPI in the course of obtaining psychiatric services for their children.

Factor analysis

The three validity scales and ten clinical scales of the MMPI were scored for each person. In the analysis, each couple was considered as a single case, thus giving 26 variables. A 26×26 matrix of product-moment correlations was obtained, analysed by the principal components method, and rotated to simple structure by the varimax method (Harman, 1970).

Empirical distances in factor space

Principal component analysis was used to place the MMPI scales in multidimensional space. The dimensionality of the space was defined by the number of orthogonal components obtained with eigenvalues greater than $1 \cdot 0$. Each scale could then be located as a single point in the space by considering its loadings on the resulting components as coordinates on a set of orthogonal axes. Euclidean distances, in the space defined by the principal component analysis, between every pair of MMPI scales for the males and between every pair of MMPI scales for the females were computed (Coombs *et al.*, 1970, p. 61; Harman, 1970, chap. 4) using the formula:

$$d(XY) = \left[\underset{i=1}{N} \Sigma (a_{xi} - a_{yi})^2 \right]^{\frac{1}{2}},$$

where $d(XY)$ is the distance from point X to point Y and a_{xi} is the loading of variable X on component i.

Test of the correspondence between the theoretical structure and the empirical placement of points in factor space

Shepard (1962 *a*, *b*) has shown that any rank order of N points is free to occur in a space of at least $(N-1)$ dimensions. In order to test the geometric model of nine points representing the nine MMPI scales, eight or more dimensions were necessary. (Eight dimensions were obtained, making the test possible.)

Each ordered pair of distances derived from the geometric representation in Fig. 1 was compared with the empirical order of magnitude of the corresponding pair of distances in factor space for males. The comparisons were repeated for the females. The number of correctly ordered pairs of distances was obtained for each sex.

If the points were arranged randomly in factor space, any distance would be equally likely to be greater than or less than another distance. At random, one-half of the 176 distance pairs would be expected to be ordered in the correct direction (i.e. 88). Using the normal approximation to a binomial test for goodness of fit (Siegel, 1956, pp. 36–42):

$$z = [(r \pm 0 \cdot 5) - Np]/\sqrt{(Npq)},$$

where z is a standard normal score, r is the number of theoretical and empirical distance pairs with the same order, N is the total number of observations (176), and p is the probability of the occurrence of a correct order at random ($0 \cdot 5$), it was found that 100 distance orders must occur in the correct direction to reject the null hypothesis of no relation between the empirical placement of the points and the theoretical structure at the $0 \cdot 05$ level. To reject

JAMES A. WAKEFIELD JR AND OTHERS

at the 0·01 level requires 104 correct orders. Rejection of the null hypothesis supports the contention that the MMPI scales are interrelated in the fashion prescribed in Fig. 1.

RESULTS

Further information (Table A*) has been deposited with the British Library at Boston Spa, Yorkshire LS23 7BQ, U.K., as Supplementary Publication No. SUP 90007 (eight pages). It contains the intercorrelations of the 26 MMPI scales

Table 1. *Rotated components of married couples' MMPI scales*
($n = 205$)

Variables	Components							
	1	2	3	4	5	6	7	8
Husband								
L	−0·34	0·09	−0·04	−0·18	0·51	0·23	−0·25	0·15
F	0·78	0·11	−0·02	−0·09	0·05	0·03	0·02	0·03
K	−0·59	0·03	−0·03	−0·02	0·62	−0·12	0·16	0·04
Hs	0·74	−0·11	−0·01	0·14	0·25	0·13	−0·27	−0·21
D	0·59	0·02	−0·02	0·02	0·31	0·54	0·15	−0·04
Hy	0·31	−0·02	0·04	0·11	0·79	−0·15	0·06	−0·18
Pd	0·79	0·19	0·04	−0·06	0·12	−0·11	0·09	0·06
Mf	0·23	0·04	0·01	−0·09	0·03	0·25	0·72	−0·07
Pa	0·47	0·12	−0·08	0·01	0·42	0·05	0·34	0·29
Pt	0·87	0·01	0·08	0·05	−0·17	0·24	0·11	−0·06
Sc	0·88	0·13	0·03	−0·00	−0·13	0·13	0·12	0·04
Ma	0·63	0·07	0·10	−0·10	−0·13	−0·55	0·03	0·04
Si	0·39	0·06	0·09	−0·00	−0·29	0·76	−0·01	0·03
Wife								
L	−0·00	−0·14	−0·04	0·04	−0·02	0·01	−0·15	0·81
F	0·00	0·70	0·33	−0·07	−0·08	0·10	−0·16	0·21
K	−0·00	−0·46	−0·53	0·29	0·00	−0·08	0·20	0·36
Hs	−0·11	0·43	0·38	0·61	0·02	0·13	−0·19	−0·14
D	0·09	0·28	0·71	0·46	0·01	−0·03	0·13	0·09
Hy	−0·04	0·17	−0·11	0·92	0·01	−0·02	0·11	0·10
Pd	0·18	0·73	0·21	0·32	−0·07	−0·02	0·05	−0·08
Mf	−0·13	−0·09	0·04	0·22	0·03	−0·31	0·61	−0·13
Pa	0·09	0·69	0·08	0·21	0·07	−0·02	0·72	0·08
Pt	0·09	0·65	0·64	0·09	0·08	0·00	0·07	−0·23
Sc	0·10	0·81	0·44	0·10	0·04	0·01	−0·05	−0·14
Ma	0·09	0·73	−0·28	−0·04	0·11	−0·00	−0·12	−0·37
Si	0·02	0·17	0·92	−0·10	−0·05	−0·00	0·01	0·03

(13 for the husbands and 13 for the wives). The eight rotated components are presented in Table 1. The eight components accounted for 75·2 per cent of the total variance of husbands' and wives' MMPI scores.

The interpoint distances between the males' scales in the eight-dimensional space defined by the components in Table 1 are included in Table A. Table A also contains the interpoint distances between the females' scales.

* Available from the Library's Photocopying Services at a prepaid flat rate of 25p including postage. (Outside U.K. the price is 30p for Europe and 42½p elsewhere.) Please quote the Supplementary Publication No. when ordering.

Eysenck's Personality Dimensions

Also included in Table A are lists of the empirical distance pairs that correspond
(= 1) and fail to correspond (= 0) to the theoretical structure of Fig. 1 for males
and for females. For the males, 111 of the 176 distance pairs were in the correct
order, indicating a significant ($P < 0.01$) correspondence between the empirical
placement of the MMPI scales in factor space and the conceptual placement of the
scales in Eysenck's three-dimensional personality framework. For the females, 134
of the 176 distance pairs were in the correct order, supporting ($P < 0.01$) the
correspondence of the females' inventory scores to the theoretical model.

Although unexpected, it should be noted that the difference in the degrees to
which the males and the females corresponded to the model was large – 23 distance
pairs. The standard deviation of the random binomial distribution of correct
distance orders used to test the correspondence between the data and the theory
was 6·63. The difference of 23 between the number of correct observations for the
males and the number of correct observations for the females was more than three
standard deviations in this distribution.

The correlations between the corresponding scales of the married couples are
generally small. The largest was 0·31 between the Pd scales of the two sexes. While
those correlations are small, they contain some reliable information about selective
mating. As this information is not relevant to the theoretical model suggested here,
it is presented elsewhere (Yom *et al.*, 1974).

DISCUSSION

The components

The first component was a general male personality dimension. Almost all of the
male MMPI scales loaded highly on this component. K was negatively loaded on
this component. None of the females' scales loaded on it.

The second component was associated with the females' personalities. The
paranoid scales (Sc, Pt, Pa) and F, Hs, Pd and Ma contributed to the variance of
this component. K was negatively associated with this component, as it was with the
general personality component for males.

The third component is a female introversion component. High loadings for Si
and D lead to this interpretation. K is negatively loaded and two of the psychotic
scales (Pt and Sc) are strongly loaded on this component.

The fourth component is female neuroticism. Strong loadings occur for the
'neurotic triad' for the females. No other scales load heavily on this component.

The fifth component is composed of variance from the males' MMPI scales.
Two of the validity scales (L and K) and Hy and Pa contributed to this component.

The sixth component represents introversion for the husbands. Si and D load
positively, and Ma, which was considered to measure extraversion, loads strongly
in the negative direction.

The seventh component is the only one that includes variance from both the
husbands and the wives. The component is composed of variance from the Mf
scales of both sexes. This component measures variance of husbands and wives
on the MMPI in similar manners. The Spearman rank-order correlation (Siegel,

1956, pp. 202–13) between the husbands' loadings from the 13 MMPI scales on this component and the wives' loadings is 0·86 ($P < $ 0·01).

The only large loading on the eighth component is the L scale for the females.

Of the eight components extracted from the 26 MMPI scales obtained from both members of 205 married couples, there were three primarily from the husbands' scales, four from the wives' scales, and one from both the husbands' and the wives' scales.

The relationship between Eysenck's dimensions and the placement of
MMPI scales in eight-dimensional space

The investigators (Goorney, 1970; Hundleby & Connor, 1968) who have previously been concerned with using the MMPI within Eysenck's theoretical framework have accepted Eysenck's tests as measures of his constructs. They have been concerned to show that the MMPI and certain scales of Eysenck's tests share variance. That certain MMPI scales have variance in common with Eysenck's E and N dimensions has been shown (Corah, 1964).

To the established empirical correspondence between the MMPI and measures of two of Eysenck's constructs, the present study added support for the relationship on a conceptual level. If the terms neuroticism, psychoticism, and extraversion-introversion were conceptualized similarly by the developers of the MMPI and by Eysenck, and if both Eysenck's theory and the MMPI are valid, the MMPI scales should be expected to be interrelated in a manner consistent with the theory. The MMPI scales are shown to be geometrically placed in such a manner. The scales approach an arrangement consisting of a cluster of neurotic scales, a cluster of psychotic scales, a measure of introversion, and two scales each of which measures extraversion and one of the other constructs.

Use of the MMPI to measure the constructs of Eysenck's personality theory was supported for both married males and married females. Data of the present study indicate that correspondence between the theory and the personality inventory is stronger for females than for males. This observation was not expected, and no attempt will be made to explain it. This apparent difference in the degrees to which the two sexes produce personality inventory scores in correspondence with the neuroticism, psychoticism and extraversion dimensions of personality should be replicated in different populations of males and females and using different personality measures.

The correspondence between Eysenck's theory and the MMPI scales is interesting in two ways. First, it gives a unified theoretical framework within which to use the MMPI. While the MMPI was developed to function as a simple predictor of certain clinical categories, the literature about this inventory contains a great many statements that deviate from simple empiricism. These statements, however, are typically partial and unintegrated, and thus fall short of being theoretically satisfying. The present attempt to view the MMPI within a theoretical framework related nine of the ten clinical scales of the MMPI to all three of Eysenck's personality dimensions.

A second aspect of the correspondence between the MMPI and the three

42

personality dimensions is the support it gives Eysenck's dimensional conception of personality. The MMPI was not developed to correspond to Eysenck's personality theory. The actual geometric correspondence between the inventory and the theory suggests that the theory has a reality apart from the test construction skills of the theorist.

REFERENCES

AFFLECK, D. C. & GARFIELD, S. L. (1960). The prediction of psychosis with the MMPI. *J. clin. Psychol.* **16**, 14–26.

CARSON, R. C. (1969). Interpretive manual to the MMPI. In J. N. Butcher (ed.), *MMPI: Research Developments and Clinical Applications*. New York: McGraw-Hill.

CLARIDGE, G. S. & CHAPPA, H. J. (1973). Psychoticism: a study of its biological basis in normal subjects. *Br. J. soc. clin. Psychol.* **12**, 175–187.

COOMBS, C. H., DAWES, R. M. & TVERSKY, A. (1970). *Mathematical Psychology*. Englewood Cliffs, N.J.: Prentice-Hall.

CORAH, N. L. (1964). Neuroticism and extraversion in the MMPI: empirical validation and exploration. *Br. J. soc. clin. Psychol.* **3**, 168–174.

DRAKE, L. E. (1946). A social IE scale for the MMPI. *J. appl. Psychol.* **30**, 51–54.

EYSENCK, H. J. (1956). The questionnaire measurement of neuroticism and extraversion. *Riv. Psicol.* **50**, 113–140.

EYSENCK, H. J. (1970a). A dimensional system of psychodiagnostics. In A. R. Mahrer (ed.), *New Approaches to Personality Classification*. New York: Columbia University Press.

EYSENCK, H. J. (1970b). Personality and attitudes to sex: a factorial study. *Personality* **1**, 355–376.

EYSENCK, H. J. (1971). Personality and sexual adjustment. *Br. J. Psychiat.* **118**, 593–608.

EYSENCK, H. J. & EYSENCK, S. B. G. (1969). *Personality Structure and Measurement*. San Diego: Knapp.

EYSENCK, H. J. & EYSENCK, S. B. G. (1971). The orthogonality of psychoticism and neuroticism: a factorial study. *Percept. mot. Skills* **33**, 461–462.

EYSENCK, S. B. G. & EYSENCK, H. J. (1968). The measurement of psychoticism: a study of factor stability and reliability. *Br. J. soc. clin. Psychol.* **7**, 286–294.

EYSENCK, S. B. G. & EYSENCK, H. J. (1969). 'Psychoticism' in children: a new personality variable. *Res. Educ.* **1**, 21–37.

GOORNEY, A. B. (1970). MPI and MMPI scores, correlations and analysis for a military aircrew population. *Br. J. soc. clin. Psychol.* **9**, 164–170.

GOUGH, H. G. (1946). Diagnostic patterns on the Minnesota Multiphasic Personality Inventory. *J. clin. Psychol.* **2**, 23–27.

HARMAN, H. H. (1970). *Modern Factor Analysis*. Chicago: University of Chicago Press.

HUNDLEBY, J. D. & CONNOR, W. H. (1968). Interrelationships between personality inventories: the 16 PF, the MMPI and the MPI. *J. consult. clin. Psychol.* **32**, 152–157.

MEEHL, P. E. (1956). Profile analysis of the MMPI in differential diagnosis. In G. S. Welsh & W. G. Dahlstrom (eds.), *Basic Readings on the MMPI in Psychology and Medicine*. Minneapolis: University of Minnesota Press.

ROUSELL, C. H. & EDWARDS, C. N. (1971). Some developmental antecedents of psychopathology. *J. Personality* **39**, 362–377.

RUESCH, J. & BOWMAN, K. (1945). Prolonged post-traumatic syndromes following head injury. *Am. J. Psychiat.* **102**, 145–163.

SHEPARD, R. N. (1962a). The analysis of proximities: multidimensional scaling with an unknown distance function. I. *Psychometrika* **27**, 125–140.

SHEPARD, R. N. (1962b). The analysis of proximities: multidimensional scaling with an unknown distance function. II. *Psychometrika* **27**, 219–246.

SIEGEL, S. (1956). *Nonparametric Statistics*. New York: McGraw-Hill.

WAKEFIELD, J. A. Jr. & DOUGHTIE, E. B. (1973). The geometric relationship between Holland's personality model and the Vocational Preference Inventory. *J. counsel. Psychol.* **20**, 513–518.

JAMES A. WAKEFIELD JR AND OTHERS

WINTER, W. D. & STORTROEN, M. A. (1963). A comparison of several MMPI indices to differentiate psychotics from normals. *J. clin. Psychol.* **19**, 220–223.

YOM, B. L., BRADLEY, P. E., WAKEFIELD, J. A. Jr., KRAFT, I. A., DOUGHTIE, E. B. & COX, J. A. (1974). A common factor in the MMPI scales of married couples. *J. pers. Assess.* (in the Press).

Manuscript received 31 August 1973

Revised manuscript received 2 March 1974

PART II

THE PHYSIOLOGICAL BASIS OF PERSONALITY

The general theory of extraversion with which we are here concerned states that differential states of arousal are responsible ultimately for a given person's position on the E–I continuum, such that persons innately predisposed to have resting patterns of high arousal will tend to develop introverted behaviour patterns. Persons with intermediate resting patterns of arousal will tend to develop intermediate or ambivert behaviour patterns. It is also part of this theory that the differential states of arousal are the result, in part at least, of the activity of the ascending reticular activating system, but this is not an essential part of the theory (alternative sources of arousal could be imagined), and as this part of the theory is not directly testable in human subjects we will not be concerned with it specifically in this chapter; the involvement of the ARAS in human states of arousal is entirely dependent on, and deduced from, animal experimentation (Eysenck, 1967).

As far as the association of cortical arousal and E–I is concerned, two major points must be remembered. In the first place, the theory refers to the resting state; it is not suggested that differences in arousal would be manifested under all conditions. Clearly an extravert writing an important examination, or viewing a burlesque show, or playing in a tennis tournament, would probably show higher arousal than an introvert sitting at home, tired, watching a boring TV play. But in the second place, a "resting" state may be difficult to define; what is restful for one person may be boring to another, and excessive boredom may produce either sleep or high arousal! This point will be discussed in detail presently.

The very concept of arousal may of course produce doubt and criticism; it is often suggested that (1) there are many different meanings of the term, and that these do not refer to the same basic phenomenon, and (2) that as different measures (physiological) of arousal do not correlate together at all highly, therefore no central concept of arousal can be postulated. Some of these difficulties are discussed by Andrew (1974). As he

points out, arousal may mean: 1. *Responsiveness*—the likelihood at a particular moment that any one of a number of different stimuli will evoke the response appropriate to it if presented. 2. *Behavioural intensity*—the vigour and completeness of whichever response is elicited. 3. *Activation*—determination of the kind of response which is possible (e.g. grooming, or copulation). 4. *Drive*—the association together in time of a group of responses, which may be held to include alert responses, cardiac acceleration, increase in postural tonus and a variety of "emotional" responses. 5. *Sensory input*—regulation of the level of sensory input, possibly including mechanisms of selective attention. 6. *Physiological system*—syndrome resulting from increased activity in the ascending activating system. As Andrews goes on to say, "some or all of these meanings are commonly confused together, which greatly reduces their value in description and analysis". This is true in part, but only in part. It is feasible to hypothesize that meaning (6) above is causally related to certain other meanings, linking them together to form a proper definition of arousal; such a hypothesis is testable, and in the body of this work we shall encounter several papers which have done precisely this. Whether arousal is defined in terms of Hebb's "conceptual nervous system", or is really related to the central nervous system (and how) is not a question which can be answered *a priori*.

The fact that different psychophysiological measures of arousal correlate poorly together cannot be gainsaid, but this is a far cry from denying the existence of meaningfulness of the concept itself. The correct answer to this objection has probably been given by Thayer (1967, 1970), who postulated self-report systems of arousal which "can be considered the result of phenomenological awareness of total bodily functioning", and that as such they might be more representative of general bodily activation than any single peripheral physiological system. He constructed a questionnaire of arousal (the Activation-Deactivation Adjective Check

List) which, when factor analysed, gave rise to four factors, one of which (General Activation) seems to come closest to our concept of arousal. Correlations with different physiological measures, under varied conditions, and with different groups of subjects, demonstrated the usual lack of high correlations among the physiological measures, but also quite strong correlations between the questionnaire measure and the individual and summed physiological measures (correlations running into the 0·6 to 0·7 range). As he points out, "it seemed apparent that self-report measures correlated better with physiological measures than the physiological measures correlated among themselves". When it is realized that his physiological measures included such variables as skin conductance, heart rate, muscle action potential, and finger blood volume, but did not include others, such as EEG, which have often been regarded as more relevant (Otto and Weber, 1974), it will be clear that by having an even larger choice of physiological measures we could probably obtain even higher correlations with verbal report measures of experienced arousal.

The Thayer list, or that of Bohlin and Kjellberg (1975) is of course a measure of state, rather than of trait arousal; this is an important distinction first made by Cicero (45 B.C.). As he points out, it is one thing to be prone to colds, another to be actually suffering from one at a given time, just as it is one thing to be irascible (i.e. prone to anger), and another to be actually angry at a particular instant of time. "Estque aliud iracondum esse, aliud iratum, ut differt *anxietas* ab *angore*; neque enim omnes anxii qui angerentur aliquando nec qui anxii semper angentur." (IV, XII 27). (As irascibility differs from anger, so differs anxious temperament from a feeling of anxiety; for not all men who are at times anxious possess an anxious temperament, nor are those who possess an anxious temperament always feeling anxious.) Similarly, not all men who are aroused upon occasion possess a high state of arousal, nor are those who possess a high general arousal level always highly aroused. We integrate (introspectively) the incoming signals from our arousal-mediating physiological systems to produce a feeling of arousal at a given time; this is *state arousal*. Integrating these states over time (provided circumstances are sufficiently equal) would produce an estimate of trait arousal, or E–I.

One particular danger to which the concept of arousal is prone is confusion with another concept which I have termed activation (Eysenck, 1967), although these terms are used synonymously by many people, and although Thayer, for instance, uses activation for what I would prefer to call arousal. Arousal, in my terminology, refers to cortical activity mediated by the ARAS; activation refers to autonomic activity mediated by the limbic system, and coordinated by the visceral brain. The introspective correlate to arousal

is alertness; that of activation is emotion. A complication arises because strong activation (emotion) inevitably produces strong arousal as well; thus while the two systems are independent most of the time (i.e. under conditions of low emotional activation), they become interdependent under conditions of high emotional activation. This point is not likely to prove bothersome under conditions of laboratory testing of deductions from the general theory, where experimenters attempt to put subjects into a state of low emotional activation; but where there is a suspicion that this effort may not have been made, or may not have succeeded, caution may be needed in interpreting the results. As there are individual differences in level of arousal, and arousability, so there are individual differences in level of activation, and emotionality; this gives rise to the personality dimension N (neuroticism). When the influence of N is not ruled out in laboratory investigations, this dimension of personality may interact with E–I, and several papers included in this book demonstrate this effect. Strictly speaking all tests produce a minimum of emotional activation, and thus individual differences in N must always be looked at and their possible influence investigated; tasks which do not seem to involve stress to the experimenter may nevertheless produce strain in some at least of his (high N) subjects.

When we look at the literature on physiological measures of personality, with particular reference to the E–I dimension, it is the EEG which claims prior attention. Excellent reviews of the literature have been published by Gale (1973, 1974). Gale points out that of the possible outcomes (extraverts show less arousal, extraverts show more arousal, and extraverts are not differentiated from introverts), all have in fact been reported by some workers; this would seem to suggest that the search may be fruitless. However, Gale suggests two major reasons why such a conclusion would be premature. In the first place, he points out a large number of faults in the published papers, mostly stemming from poor techniques of measurement. These can and should be corrected. But he also points out that parameter differences in the different studies would lead one to predict differential outcomes. As he says: "Eysenck's theory of the neurophysiological basis of extraversion–introversion . . . allows us to demonstrate that *differences in testing conditions* and *differences in experimental procedures* will lead to the three different outcomes. Different types of task make different demands upon Ss. Extraverts are 'stimulus hungry' and introverts are 'stimulus aversive'. Therefore extraverts and introverts will respond differently to different experimental treatments, depending upon how much stimulation they provide."

Essentially, Gale's hypothesis is that the predicted higher arousal of introverts is most (or only) likely to be found under experimental conditions which are neither too boring nor too stimulating, i.e. under conditions producing medium degrees of arousal. (This is an extension of the argument concerning the optimum "resting state" briefly alluded to above.) "If experimental conditions are boring and monotonous, the extraverted subjects will arouse themselves and actively seek stimulation from themselves or from the laboratory, while introverted subjects exposed to the same conditions will find those conditions soothing and conducive to obedience of the experimental instructions to relax. If on the other hand the task is challenging and interesting, then it provides a ready source of varied stimulation for the stimulus-hungry extravert. Such intensely arousing conditions might oblige the introvert to cut off all input and by this drastic step, reduce local arousal." In this manner, extraverts would raise their arousal level in response to minimally stimulating conditions, and introverts would lower theirs in response to maximally stimulating conditions, in either case producing an apparent failure of the prediction. This is but one example of the fact that control of experimental parameters is absolutely essential in testing deductions from theories such as that dealt with in this book, and that a proper theory should predict the effects of differences in parameter conditions.

Gale gives a list of published studies, grouping them into those where conditions were highly arousing, moderately arousing, and very little arousing; admittedly the grouping is *post hoc*, and information is not always sufficient in the published papers to make decisions completely reliable. Nevertheless, he finds that of the studies involving moderate arousal, seven out of seven show the predicted greater arousal in introverts; in the other two groups, nine out of nine fail to show this effect, very much as we would expect. To these studies we can add three more which have been published since Gale completed his survey (Montgomery, 1975; Rösler, 1975; Strelau and Terelak, 1974); all three are in line with prediction. Thus in ten cases where introverts can be expected to show greater EEG arousal, they have been found to do so, while in nine cases out of nine where we would expect no difference, or a greater show of arousal in extraverts, this effect has been found. Not too much should be made of this apparent 100% success in the 19 studies surveyed; there is inevitably much subjectivity entering into the grouping of the experimental conditions. Nevertheless, it does seem that direct proof of the general hypothesis linking EEG arousal with extraversion–introversion is not entirely missing. The study reprinted below has been chosen to exemplify the sort of work that is being done, and the sort of result that may be expected when great care is taken over the experimental details. For a complete picture, Gale's survey papers and particularly his extensive critical comments should be consulted.

Because of the difficulties in direct tests of the theory,

Gale has suggested an interesting alternative method, and has indeed already carried out a whole series of experimental tests following this paradigm. As he puts it, "what we have tried to do is to select experimental paradigms which Eysenck and others have shown to yield personality effects, and to translate these paradigms into a form which allows us to examine EEG correlates of behaviour". In other words, our theory predicts that introverts would do better than extraverts on tests of vigilance, and as we shall see this is indeed so. Provided that our theory is correct which ascribes this difference to differences in arousal, then it should follow that good and poor performance on a vigilance task would be characterized by high and low EEG arousal respectively. Clearly this approach can be extended to a large number of different experimental tasks. Consider one example: Bartol and Martin (1974) have predicted and shown that extraverts prefer complex to simple material, on the hypothesis that such material would be more arousing. Gale *et al.* (1975) have shown that inspection of 27 projected patterns produced differences in occipital EEG arousal which were associated in the predicted direction with the number and variety of elements in the patterns. This type of approach is promising, and will no doubt be continued.

The remaining papers in this section need little discussion as they each introduce the particular field, and the theories involved. They also contain discussions of previous research, so that no detailed introduction would seem to be necessary. All six papers in this section cover quite different ground, and yet they are all clearly tied together by the concept of "arousal". Critics who seek to abolish this concept would still be faced with this set of empirical findings, and would be required to account for it in theoretical terms; in the absence of any hint of such alternative theories it may be advisable to retain the concept, at least for the time being. It is easier to improve useful concepts, than to invent new ones.

One point may be worth drawing attention to. The hypothesis formulated by Gale to explain the occasional arousal of extraverts in EEG experiments essentially reproduces Pavlov's Law of Transmarginal Inhibition (at least as far as strongly arousing stimuli are concerned); when stimulation reaches a degree which is considered possibly injurious, inhibitory forces reduce the intensity of stimulation. Two of the studies reproduced in this section provide evidence for the applicability of this law in psychophysiological studies of human subjects, and also demonstrate that it applies with particular force to introverts—as of course it should, given their higher degree of arousability. The first is the study by Zuckerman, Murtaugh and Siegel, which deals with evoked potentials as a response to light flashes of different intensity; the other is the study by Eysenck and Eysenck on increase in rate of salivation as a function of strength of acidity of the stimulus. In both cases there is a break in the increase in response as a function of strength of stimulation for the introverts, and these two examples will be replicated many more times in papers reprinted in later sections. There is thus good evidence for the applicability of this law, and its particular relationship with personality.

These studies also raise a problem. Pavlov was thinking of very high intensities of stimulation, while the intensities here involved in laboratory investigations are rather low; even the most intense stimulation is still well within the limits of tolerance which most subjects would accept. This means that Pavlov's notion of defining intensity in terms of what might actually be physically injurious to the organism cannot be reconciled with the facts; we must search for another definition. Possibly "unpleasant" rather than injurious; there is some evidence (to be reviewed later) to indicate that introverts avoid, and extraverts search out, somewhat more intense stimuli which are well below the level of possible injury to the nervous system. With this exception, Pavlov's Law of Transmarginal Inhibition seems to account very well for some otherwise inexplicable findings, and links up with the general arousal theory of extraversion–introversion very neatly to predict effects which are spectacular and on any other grounds rather unexpected. These are the characteristics of a good theory.

One set of studies has not been included in this section, although perhaps they ought to have been so included.* Studies of the sedation threshold are certainly psychophysiological in nature, and they provide strong evidence for a theory linking arousal with introversion. Eysenck (1963) has reviewed the early evidence in favour of his drug postulate, according to which stimulant drugs (e.g. amphetamine, caffeine) shift an individual towards greater arousal (greater introversion), while depressant drugs (alcohol, sodium amytal) shift an individual towards lesser arousal (greater extraversion). Given a *terminus ad quem* (the sedation threshold, defined in terms of EEG changes, or behaviour on experimental tasks, or even life behaviour), extraverts should require lesser amounts of depressant drugs to reach this threshold, on the grounds that they start out nearer the terminus. Shagass and Kerenyi (1958) have demonstrated this quite clearly, and Sloane, Davidson and Payne (1965) have provided a good replication study. (There are many more such studies in the literature which confirm the general outcome.) The relation is in fact unexpectedly close; Sloane *et al.*, in the study just mentioned, find a correlation of 0·57, which, when corrected for attenuation for unreliability in

the two measures which enter into the correlation, is raised to almost 0·80! Such statistical corrections always make assumptions which may not be entirely justified, but on the whole there is no doubt that sedation thresholds and extraversion are in fact closely related. It is unfortunate that psychologists have not often included measures of the sedation threshold in their experiments; of all the physiological tests described it is perhaps the simplest, the most reliable, and the most valid (in terms of correlation with E). Perhaps the need for medical coverage in using a drug has been a deterrent; in spite of this drawback it may be hoped that in the future this test will be more widely used. On theoretical grounds it provides perhaps the best evidence for the link between arousal and introversion, as well as being experimental in the strictest sense, i.e. working through the manipulation of conditions, rather than just relying on correlations using static tests.

REFERENCES

ANDREW, R. J. Arousal and the causation of behaviour. *Behaviour*, 1974, *51*, 135–165.

BARTOL, C. R. and MARTIN, R. B. Preference of complexity as a function of neuroticism, extraversion, and amplitude of orienting responses. *Perceptual and Motor Skills*, 1974, *38*, 1155–1160.

BOHLIN, G. and KJELLBERG, A. Self-reported arousal. *Scandinavian Journal of Psychology*, 1975, *16*, 203–208.

CICERO, N. T. *Tuscularum disputationum*. London: Heinemann, 1927 (original: 45 B.C.).

EYSENCK, H. J. (Ed.) *Experiments with drugs*. London: Pergamon Press, 1963.

EYSENCK, H. J. *The biological basis of personality*. Springfield: C. C. Thomas, 1967.

EYSENCK, H. J. (Ed.), *Readings in extraversion–introversion*. London: Staples, 1971.

GALE, A. The psychophysiology of individual differences; studies of extraversion and the EEG. In: P. Kline (Ed.), *New approaches in psychological measurement*. London: John Wiley and Sons, 1973.

GALE, A. EEG studies of extraversion–introversion: sources of experimental error. Paper presented at the International Conference on Temperament and Personality, Warsaw 21st–24th October, 1974.

GALE, A., SPRATT, G., CHRISTIE, B. and SMALLBONE, A. Stimulus complexity, EEG abundance gradients, and detector efficiency in a visual recognition task. *British Journal of Psychology*, 1975, *66*, 289–298.

MONTGOMERY, P. S. EEG alpha as an index of hysteroid and obsessoid personalities. *Psychological Reports*, 1975, *36*, 431–436.

OTTO, E. and WEBER, H. EEG—Aktivitätsmuster, Augenbeuegungen, Lidschlag rate und Herzschlag frequenz bei visueller Informationsverarbeitung. *Zeitschrift für Psychologie*, 1974, *182*, 284–306.

RÖSLER, F. Die Abhängigkeit des Elektro-encephalogramms von den Persönlichkeitsdimensionen E und N sensu Eysenck und unterschiedlich aktivierenden Situationen. *Zeitschrift für experimentelle und angewandte Psychologie*, 1975, *22*, 630–667.

---

* The topic has been covered adequately in Eysenck's *Readings in Extraversion–Introversion* (1971), and it was decided not to include in this volume any articles reprinted in that three-volume presentation. No new studies have appeared since the appearance of these volumes.

SHAGASS, C. and KERENYI, A. B. Neurophysiological studies of personality. *Journal of Nervous and Mental Diseases*, 1958, *126*, 141–147.

SLOANE, R. B., DAVIDSON, P. O. and PAYNE, R. W. Anxiety and arousal in psychoneurotic patients. *Archives of General Psychiatry*, 1965, *13*, 19–23.

STRELAU, J. and TERELAK, J. The alpha-index in relation to temperamental traits. *Studia Psychologica*, 1974, *16*, 40–50.

THAYER, R. E. Measurement of activation through self report. *Psychological Reports*, 1967, *20*, 663–678.

THAYER, R. E. Activation states as assessed by verbal report and four psychophysiological variables. *Psychophysiology*, 1970, *7*, 86–94.

From A. Gale, M. Coles and J. Blaydon (1969). British Journal of Psychology, *60*, 209–223, *by kind permission of the authors and Cambridge University Press*

EXTRAVERSION–INTROVERSION AND THE EEG

By ANTHONY GALE, MICHAEL COLES AND JENNIFER BLAYDON

Department of Psychology, University of Exeter

Studies relating measures of the EEG to extraversion–introversion are reviewed and criteria set up for their evaluation. A new measure of mean dominant frequency is proposed. Extravert and introvert EEGs are compared, firstly across the whole frequency range (with eyes closed) and secondly across theta, alpha and beta ranges under alternating conditions of eyes closed/ eyes open. With the eyes closed, the extravert EEG is higher in integrated output than the introvert EEG across the whole measured range, the differences in output being greater in the lower alpha range. Such differences in alpha are not so readily apparent with eyes closed when recording with a gross filter which fails to discriminate among within-alpha frequencies. However, with eyes open, and given monotonous visual stimulation, even a gross filter shows differential output. Prolonged recording also reveals differences in theta and beta; these differences are stronger when the eyes are shut.

According to Sisson & Ellingson (1955, p. 357) 'no study has been done conclusively showing a relationship between any feature of the normal adult EEG recorded under standard conditions and any personality trait or variable'. This statement is no longer true. However, a number of recent studies suffer from series defects and much of the earlier work is still referred to with bland inattention to its inadequacies (Eysenck, 1967).

Studies relating the EEG to personality must satisfy three requirements: (i) adequate quantification of the EEG, (ii) adequate measurement of personality, and (iii) a theoretical rationale for predicting what relation holds between these two variables. This paper is concerned with attempts to relate the EEG to extraversion–introversion (Eysenck, 1957) and presents some new evidence. Table 1 gives a summary of earlier work. It will be observed that virtually all the effort in this field has been directed at the alpha frequencies (8–13 c/sec.). But the methods used to quantify the alpha band vary considerably ('high–low', dominant frequency, percentage, amplitude, abundance, correlogram, rate of change of potential). Comparison of the available studies is therefore difficult.

PREVIOUS WORK

Only one study satisfies all the requirements set out above. Savage (1964) selected four groups on the basis of MPI (Eysenck, 1959) score (high E high N, high E low N, low E high N and low E low N). Savage showed: (i) that extraverts have significantly higher amplitude than introverts ($P < 0.01$), (ii) that there is no correlation between alpha amplitude and neuroticism, but (iii) that there *is* a significant interaction between extraversion and neuroticism, the high E high N group having lower alpha amplitude than high E low N ($P < 0.05$). The first finding supports predictions based on Eysenck's distinction between extraverts and introverts in terms of generation of cortical inhibition (Eysenck, 1957). Savage takes alpha amplitude as an operational definition of cortical inhibition. (His justification for failing to include measures of alpha index and frequency is that 'investigations using the latter have been incon-

ANTHONY GALE, MICHAEL COLES AND JENNIFER BLAYDON

clusive' (Savage, 1964, p. 99).) Since extraverts generate cortical inhibition more readily, their alpha amplitude is higher. The failure to find a correlation between *neuroticism* and the EEG supports Eysenck's view only to the extent that he predicts that individual differences in alpha activity are due to differences in extraversion–introversion. In Eysenck's most recent review of the field, he makes no specific prediction concerning the relation of EEG and *neuroticism as such*. However, he does predict how the two dimensions will *interact*: 'introverted neurotics (low E high N) tend to have fast EEG activity, whereas extraverted neurotics (high E high N) tend to have exceptionally slow EEG activity' (Eysenck, 1967, p. 68). Within the alpha range, amplitude and frequency are negatively correlated (Knott & Travis, 1937). Moreover, all arousal studies of the EEG associate low frequency with high voltage (HVS) and high frequency with low voltage (LVF) (Thompson, 1967). Thus Savage's third finding (which Eysenck omits to mention) clearly contradicts Eysenck's statement. This contradiction is unfortunate, since Savage's study avoids Eysenck's major criticism of work in this field. Eysenck points to a basic methodological flaw in two types of investigation; firstly, those studies which have claimed a relation between arousal measures and neuroticism and, secondly, those studies which have failed to reveal differences on arousal measures between extraverts and introverts. Eyzenck's criticism is a sound one and is based on the *orthogonality* of neuroticism to extraversion–introversion. He points out that such studies typically employ clinical groups. Since anxiety state patients are likely to be both introverted and neurotic, extraversion–introversion and neuroticism are confounded. Even where non-clinical groups are employed, studies comparing extraverts with introverts fail to control for neuroticism, and vice versa (Eysenck, 1967). It is therefore unfortunate that the one EEG study which makes use of a dimensional framework fails in part to support Eysenck's predictions.

Earlier studies were inconclusive. Gottlober (1938) found extraverts to have a high alpha index, but Henry & Knott (1941) failed to replicate Gottlober's results. They found extraversion to be *negatively* but insignificantly correlated with alpha index. Apart from pointing out that Gottlober's population is strongly weighted in favour of his conclusions, they present a reworking of his data and show his results to be equivocal, the more objective of his techniques of personality assessment leading to a less significant result. More recently, Marton & Urban (1966) report significant differences in mean alpha frequency (extraverts 9·15 c/sec., introverts 11·1 c/sec.; $P < 0.01$). However, nine of the introverted group of 20 subjects 'were without alpha rhythm' (p. 107). They do not report whether these nine subjects were included in the calculation of the means; their exclusion would be difficult to justify on statistical grounds. Moreover, in view of the fact that only a small number of people have little or no alpha (Glaser, 1963), the absence of alpha activity in 22·5 per cent of Marton & Urban's sample remains a mystery. They also fail to report on what basis their subjects were designated extravert or introvert. Glass & Broadhurst's (1966) results appear to be in direct contradiction to those of Gottlober, Savage and Marton & Urban. Glass & Broadhurst find extraversion to be negatively and significantly correlated with per cent alpha and with rates of change of potential (r.c.p.), high r.c.p. being equated to 'increased alpha amplitude'. They claim that the low-frequency analysis used by Savage fails to distinguish between *change in prevalence* and

Table 1. *Studies relating the EEG to extraversion–introversion*

Author	Personality measure	EEG measures	Results
Gottlober (1938)	Subjective rating and Nebraska Personality Inventory	30 sec.; eyes closed; per cent time alpha (index); manual scoring	Extraverts have higher alpha index
Henry & Knott (1941)	NPI	300 sec.; eyes closed; alpha index, i.e. 50 per cent alpha = 'high' alpha; 8–12 c/sec. and 7 μV; manual scoring	Introverts have higher index (not significant)
Mundy-Castle (1955)	Primary–secondary function (as measured by a number of tasks)	20 min.; eyes closed; mean alpha frequency	Alpha frequency correlated with primary function (equated by Eysenck (1953) with extraversion)
Nebylitsyn (1963)	Predominance of excitation or inhibition in dynamism (as measured by a number of tasks)	Derivation unknown; alpha, beta and theta; index, amplitude and frequency	Subjects with predominance of inhibition in dynamism have high alpha index and amplitude but low frequency; high beta (amplitude, index and frequency) and high theta frequency. This group could be equated with extraverts (Gray, 1967)
Savage (1964)	Maudsley Personality Inventory (1959)	240 sec.; eyes closed; low-frequency analysis of 8–13 c/sec. filter; alpha 'amplitude'	Extraverts have higher amplitude. Interaction with neuroticism
Glass & Broadhurst (1966)	Either MPI or Eysenck Personality Inventory (1964)?	Unknown duration; derived between tasks (arithmetic calculations; Glass, 1964); alpha index and rate of change of potential (r.c.p.); opisometric scoring	Extraversion negatively correlated with both r.c.p. and alpha index
Marton & Urban (1966)	Unknown	Alpha index and frequency; manner of derivation unknown	Extraverts have higher index and lower frequency
Fenton & Scotton (1967)	MPI	30 sec.; eyes closed; alpha index: mean amplitude; 8–13 c/sec. and 15 μV; manual scoring	Negative (but not significant) correlation between extraversion and both index and amplitude
Hume (1968)	EPI	Duration unknown; manual scoring of output of alpha band filter	Alpha index and extraversion have positive loadings on the same factor
Gale, Coles & Blaydon	EPI	(i) 110 sec.; eyes closed; 2–20 c/sec. divided into nine frequencies; low-frequency analysis giving mean integrated output and mean dominant frequency (m.d.f.) (ii) 10 min. eyes open; 10 min. eyes closed; theta, alpha and beta	(i) Extraverts have higher integrated output on all measured frequencies and lower m.d.f. (ii) Extraverts have higher theta, alpha and beta integrated output with eyes open and eyes closed

ANTHONY GALE, MICHAEL COLES AND JENNIFER BLAYDON

change in amplitude, whereas their own opisometric technique (Glass, 1964) enables them to make this distinction. Thus Savage's findings might be due to short bursts of high voltage (but infrequent) alpha. Had Savage included an alpha percentage or index measure, this issue could be resolved. It is not clear, however, how Glass & Broadhurst sample their 'resting' EEG. It appears (Glass, 1964) to be a within-task sample rather than one derived from continuous rest. To justify their sampling technique they must predict how extraverts and introverts would be *differentially* affected by the task in question. Moreover, their study (like those of Gottlober and Henry & Knott) is open to Eysenck's criticism of confounding extraversion–introversion with neuroticism, since no correlation measure is given for extraversion–introversion and neuroticism within their sample. (Clearly, earlier studies cannot be criticized for failing to acknowledge theoretical considerations which are only recent in origin. However, Eysenck's current views on personality structure impose limitations on the interpretation of the earlier work.) Fenton & Scotton (1967) also find a negative (but insignificant) correlation between both alpha amplitude and index, and extraversion. However, they employ a manual method of scoring. The absence of automatic scoring techniques transforms the quantification of the EEG into a sort of projective test, not unlike the Rorschach inkblots. The difficulties of non-automated scoring have been well summarized by Walter (1963). Fenton & Scotton acknowledge this difficulty and present a scorer reliability study, which shows that the same scorer has a good chance of giving the same score to the same record on two occasions. A reliability study employing at least two scorers on the same material would have raised the credibility of their technique. Hume (1968), in an elaborate factor analytic study (of which only a preliminary report is available), finds high loadings on the EPI to be linked with high alpha index. However, Hume's results are obtained from manual scoring of the instantaneous (non-integrated) output of a single (7·5–13·5 c/sec.) filter.

Gray (1967) argues for an identification of extraversion–introversion with either the strong–weak dimension of Pavlov–Teplov (Gray, 1964) or the equilibrium in dynamism of Nebylitsyn. Nebylitsyn (1963) employs EEG indices (among others) to distinguish subjects with predominance of excitation in dynamism from those with predominance of inhibition in dynamism. The latter group have low frequency, high amplitude and high alpha index and also high beta (frequency, index and amplitude) and high theta frequency. But indices of basal EEG do *not* distinguish strong from weak nervous systems. Thus, if any identification is to be made between Russian and Western personality dimensions, then extraversion and predominance of inhibition in dynamism are clearly good candidates on the basis of EEG data. However, evidence derived from behavioural and other measures is by no means as clear-cut (Gray, 1967).

Mundy-Castle (1955) reports a high positive correlation between *primary function* and alpha frequency. Savage (1964) claims that Mundy-Castle's findings are positively related to his own; in fact, the converse is the case. Because Eysenck (1953, 1957) equates primary function with extraversion, Mundy-Castle's results are in direct contradiction to those of Savage, since higher frequency is associated with *lower* voltage (Knott & Travis, 1937). It may be that Savage is confused by Eysenck's earlier (1953) adoption of Mundy-Castle's findings. In 1953 Eysenck says that

Extraversion–introversion and the EEG

extraversion (equated with primary function) is linked with *higher frequency* alpha. However, in 1967 Eysenck no longer identifies extraversion with primary function and, in accepting Savage's first finding, claims by implication that extraverts have *low frequency* alpha. It is therefore not clear whether Mundy-Castle's findings would now be considered by Eysenck to have any bearing on the present discussion. In order to rule them out of court, Eysenck must either show Mundy-Castle's work to be methodologically unsound or reject his own very convincing arguments concerning the identification of primary function with extraversion.

In summary, studies relating the EEG to extraversion–introversion leave much to be desired. The earlier studies are deficient in the light of Eysenck's current theory of personality structure and therefore fail to recognize the possible interacting effects of extraversion–introversion and neuroticism. None of the studies appear to have an adequate theoretical rationale for predicting the outcome of their procedures, or more important, for accounting for failure to replicate the results of other studies. In terms of the quantification of the EEG also, descriptors are variable and confusing and often indicate a failure to appreciate the basic properties of EEG waveforms. In this respect, our own study, which employs low-frequency analysis (and thereby confounds amplitude with prevalence), is also deficient. To avoid begging a number of questions, the term 'integrated output' is employed throughout this paper.

The present study

We have recently completed a study relating extraversion–introversion and neuroticism to basal and habituation data derived from a number of physiological measures (EEG, heart rate, skin conductance, finger-pulse volume and respiration) (Gale, Coles & Kline, in preparation). The present investigation was conducted as a pilot to that larger study. Our aim was to replicate Savage's first finding (that extraversion is positively correlated with alpha amplitude) and in addition to extend his work in three ways: (i) to extend the basal EEG data over a wider range of frequencies (see Fig. 1); (ii) to examine, in particular, differences in theta and beta frequencies, as well as alpha; and (iii) to measure the effect of the EEG of an eyes open condition.

This third aim represents a departure from previous personality studies, which, without exception, measure resting EEG with eyes closed. We predicted that, given monotonous visual stimulation during an eyes open condition, the differences obtained by Savage for an eyes closed condition would be replicated or even amplified. This prediction is based on a number of assumptions. (*a*) Eyes open is a more 'arousing' condition than eyes closed. This assumption is of course generally accepted and has been examined experimentally in great detail by Daniel (1966). But (*a*) only holds when the available visual stimulation contains some of the 'arousing' qualities outlined by Berlyne (1960). Thus (*b*) prolonged and monotonous visual stimulation is 'de-arousing' (Berlyne, 1960) even when the eyes remain open. The repetitive and monotonous nature of the stimulation will induce cortical inhibition (Eysenck, 1967), which will be characterized by an augmentation of alpha activity which will increase in amplitude over time. Theoretically speaking, there is nothing to prevent such activity reaching its eyes closed level. Since extraverts develop cortical inhibition more readily, they will exhibit this effect earlier. A similar prediction is made on

ANTHONY GALE, MICHAEL COLES AND JENNIFER BLAYDON

alternative grounds (c) that extraverts, being 'stimulus hungry' (Eysenck, 1967; Howarth, 1964), will in the presence of unavoidable monotonous stimulation, undergo a reduction of cortical excitation. In EEG terms, this also should lead to increased alpha amplitude, the effect occurring more readily in the extravert group. But since the notion of 'stimulus hunger' has been devised for the typical 'stimulus-seeking' behaviour of extraverts, assumptions (b) and (c) above appear to lead to contradictory predictions. First, that extraverts, in generating cortical inhibition, will become less responsive and show greater alpha amplitude. Secondly, that extraverts, being stimulus hungry, become less and less tolerant of sensory deprivation and *more responsive* in their search for extra stimulation, leading to reduction in alpha amplitude.

However, the outcome depends very much on the experimental situation. When given the opportunity to obtain stimulation, extraverts will do so (Bakan, 1959; Claridge, 1960; Howarth, 1964; Weisen, 1965). But when no opportunity to search for stimulation is given, extraverts become less responsive (Bakan *et al.* 1963; Claridge, 1960; Colquhoun & Corcoran, 1964; Hogan, 1966). It is of course possible that a third state of affairs may be brought about, where extraverts develop reactive inhibition even to responses necessary to the secondary task or source of additional stimulation (Jensen, 1966).

In the present study, every attempt was made to reduce sources of additional stimulation. It was therefore predicted that subjects would become less responsive and that alpha amplitude (with eyes open) would tend, with prolonged monotony, to reach its eyes shut level. Thus this study not only examines basal differences in EEG but attempts to induce change.

METHOD

Subjects. Subjects were assigned to two equal groups of 12 on the basis of EPI score (Eysenck & Eysenck, 1964); mean E score for extraverts 17·3, mean E score for introverts 8·1; S.D. 1·52 in both cases. No subject had an N score of more than 11, giving two groups similar in composition to Savage's high E low N and low E low N. Subjects were five male and 19 female undergraduate students at the University of Exeter (mean age 21 yr. 4 mth.).

Apparatus. The subject reclined on a bed in a soundproof cubicle (Industrial Acoustics Corp., Type 4024) with a constant room temperature of 65° F. The head of the bed was surrounded by a screen of black card, so that the subject lay with his head facing upward from the lower inner surface of a black cube (3 ft. square), the nearest surface to the face not being less than 2 ft. Constant moderate illumination (8·5 LM ft.²) was provided by a hidden bulb, giving light through a small window (3 ft. × 6 in.), set above the subject's line of regard, in the upper edge of the front face of the screen. Instructions were given to the subject through an intercom system. SLE pad electrodes (silver/silver chloride) were placed transoccipitally for bipolar recording, interelectrode resistance being below 5 kohms. The EEG was recorded on a Sanei' Type PG 802 Polygraph calibrated to give a 34 mm write-out (peak to trough) for 100 μV, time constant 0·3 sec. Continued write-out of the voltage output of 10 separate filters, integrated over an epoch of 5 sec., was provided by a Sanei' Type EA 201 Low Frequency Analyser, calibrated to give a resolution of 60 × 1 mm intervals. The following filters were used. For trial 1: filter numbers 1 (2–4·5 c/sec.), 2 (4·5–6·5 c/sec.), 3 (6·5–7·5 c/sec.), 4 (7·5–8·5 c/sec.), 5 (8·5–9·5 c/sec.), 6 (9·5–10·5 c/sec.), 7 (10·5–11·5 c/sec.), 8 (11·5–14·5 c/sec.), 9 (14·5–20 c/sec.); and for trials 1–10: filter numbers 2, 9 and 10 (8–13 c/sec.), Recording of both traces was on continuous millimetre graph paper (Recorder Chart No. PR 38012), run at 5 mm/sec.

Extraversion–introversion and the EEG

Procedure and statistical treatment

Experimental schedule (C, eyes closed; O, eyes open)

Trials (2 min. each)	1	2	3	4	5	6	7	8	9	10
Extraverts	C	O	C	O	C	O	C	O	C	O
Introverts	C	O	C	O	C	O	C	O	C	O

(i) *Baseline differences over nine filters.* For the first 2 min. eyes closed trial all integrated output values were extracted for all analyser filters 1–9. Since it was not possible to sychronize the analyser with the onset and termination of trials, first and final epoch values were eliminated. This gave a total continuous sample of 110 sec. per filter, represented by the means of 22×5-sec. epochs per filter. The nine filter means per subject were fed into an analysis of variance whose main treatments were personality (extraversion-introversion) and filters (1–9). (Fig. 1; Myers, 1966.)

(ii) *Mean dominant frequency* (m.d.f.). The analysis of baseline differences in (i) is designed

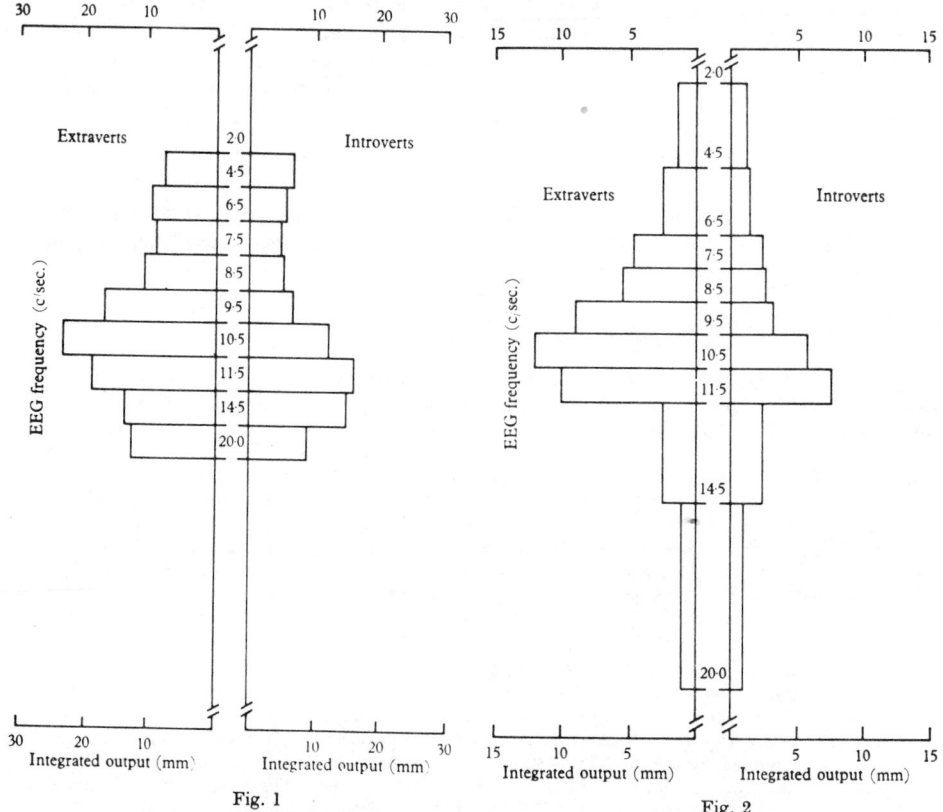

Fig. 1.

Fig. 2.

Fig. 1. Baseline differences between extraverts and introverts with eyes closed. Mean integrated output per filter per group derived from 110 sec. continuous recording.

Fig. 2. Baseline differences between extraverts and introverts with eyes closed. Distributions of integrated output (as shown in Fig. 1) when filter frequency ranges are divided into 0·5 c/sec. steps.

14-2

Anthony Gale, Michael Coles and Jennifer Blaydon

to show whether there is any difference between the two groups in total integrated output or in terms of concentration of integrated output within the available filters. An alternative, more sensitive analysis was performed on the same data, first for the whole frequency range (2–20 c/sec.) and secondly for the within-alpha range (7·5–14·5 c/sec.). *The analysis employed assumes a normal distribution across the EEG frequency range, the mean value for that distribution being the m.d.f.* Division of the EEG frequency range between 2·0 and 20 c/sec. into 0·5 c/sec. intervals yielded a total of 38 derived intervals. The mean energy per derived interval was calculated by dividing the mean energy of its original filter by the number of derived intervals within the filter. Mean energy per derived filter for the two groups is shown in Fig. 2. Means (m.d.f.) and standard deviations were derived from the frequency distributions for each individual subject. For this calculation the amount of energy in each original filter was taken to represent the frequency of occurrence of activity within that filter. This activity was regarded as occurring at the mid-point of that filter. The personality group distributions of m.d.f.s and S.D.s were then compared (*t* test).

(iii) *Effect of eyes open and eyes closed conditions on theta (4·5–6·5 c/sec.), alpha (8–13 c/sec.) and beta (14·5–20 c/sec.).* An identical testing procedure was employed for all subjects; a sequence of 10 alternated 2-min., eyes closed, eyes open trials, commencing with eyes closed. Onset and conclusion of each trial was recorded on the polygraph. Twelve alternate 5-sec. integrated epoch values were extracted for each 2-min. period for the three frequency bands. (In this case, a single filter—8–13 c/sec.—was employed for the alpha frequencies.) First and final epoch values were eliminated because they contained energy from adjacent trials. Mean integrated output (in mm) was calculated for the remaining 10 epochs, representing a total sample of 50 sec. (10 × 5-sec.) per trial. Thus the filter scores for each subject were reduced to 10 mean values, representing 5 × 50 sec. eyes closed and 5 × 50 sec. eyes open. This technique of sampling provided a total sample of 500 sec. for each of the three filters, representing an overall recording time of 20 min. These 10 mean values for each of the theta, alpha and beta bands were fed into three separate analyses of variance (one per filter), whose main treatments were personality (extraversion–introversion), viewing (eyes closed–eyes open) and trials (1–5 for each of the viewing treatments).

Results

(i) *Baseline differences over nine filters.* (Table 2.) Mean integrated output is differentially distributed for both filters and personality groups. The total output (over the whole frequency range) is greater for extraverts. When the whole frequency range is considered, the interaction effect may be largely attributed to the differences on filter numbers 4, 5 and 6 (as opposed to the differences in the other filters) ($P < 0.05$);

Table 2. *Baseline differences: analysis of variance on integrated output, varying personality (P) and filters (F)*

Source	D.F.	S.S.	M.S.	F	P
Total	215	16972·54	—	—	—
Between subjects	23	7428·99	—	—	—
P	1	1506·28	1506·28	5·60	< 0·05
S/P	22	5922·71	269·21	—	—
Within subjects	192	9543·55	—	—	—
F	8	3525·55	440·69	14·86	< 0·005
PF	8	801·41	100·18	3·38	< 0·05
SF/P	176	5217·59	29·65	—	—

when the within-alpha filters alone are considered the interaction effect may similarly be accounted for by comparison of the differences on the lower filters (numbers 4, 5, 6) with those on the higher (numbers 7, 8) ($P < 0.05$; Scheffé test of multiple comparisons).

Extraversion–introversion and the EEG

(ii) *Mean dominant frequency.* When all filters are considered (2–20 c/sec.), neither the m.d.f. nor the standard deviation values are significantly different. However, they are both significantly different (*t* test) when the within-alpha range alone is considered (7·5–14·5 c/sec.).

(iii) *Effect of eyes closed and eyes open conditions (viewing effect) on theta, alpha and beta frequencies.* (Tables 4–6; Fig. 3.) Mean integrated output is higher with eyes

Table 3. *Baseline differences: comparison of extravert and introvert m.d.f.s and S.D.s (t test)*

	Extravert	Introvert	t	P
For the whole measured range (2–20 c/sec.)				
M.D.F.	9·99	10·23	0·98	n.s.
S.D.	3·43	3·70	1·53	n.s.
For the alpha range (7·5–14·5 c/sec.)				
M.D.F.	10·25	10·80	3·25	< 0·005
S.D.	1·50	1·68	1·99	< 0·05

Table 4. *Analysis of variance on integrated output for the theta filter (4·5–6·5 c/sec.), varying personality (P), trials (T) and viewing (V)*

Source	D.F.	S.S.	M.S.	F	P
Total	239	3549·49	—	—	—
Between subjects	23	3035·75	—	—	—
P	1	494·79	494·79	4·28	< 0·05
S/P	22	2540·96	115·50	—	—
Within subjects	216	513·74	—	—	—
T	4	4·22	1·05	n.s.	—
PT	4	8·03	2·01	n.s.	—
ST/P	88	120·50	1·37	—	—
V	1	126·73	126·73	19·68	< 0·005
PV	1	13·44	13·44	n.s.	—
SV/P	22	141·59	6·44	—	—
TV	4	0·93	0·23	n.s.	—
PTV	4	2·03	0·51	n.s.	—
STV/P	88	96·27	1·09	—	—

Table 5. *Analysis of variance on integrated output for the alpha filter (8–13 c/sec.), varying personality (P), trials (T) and viewing (V)*

Source	D.F.	S.S.	M.S.	F	P
Total	239	.41095·56	—	—	—
Between subjects	23	21640·97	—	—	—
P	1	3743·81	3743·81	4·60	< 0·05
S/P	22	17897·16	813·51	—	—
Within subjects	216	19454·59	—	—	—
T	4	71·39	17·85	n.s.	—
PT	4	61·28	15·32	n.s.	—
ST/P	88	928·95	10·56	—	—
V	1	13188·32	13188·32	76·12	< 0·005
PV	1	58·71	58·71	n.s.	—
SV/P	22	3811·58	173·25	—	—
TV	4	23·03	5·76	n.s.	—
PTV	4	145·56	36·39	2·75	< 0·05
STV/P	88	1165·77	13·25	—	—

ANTHONY GALE, MICHAEL COLES AND JENNIFER BLAYDON

closed for all three filters. Extraverts have higher mean integrated output for all three filters. However, the extent of the difference between personality groups is not consistent over the viewing treatment. For theta and beta, the difference obtains at

Table 6. *Analysis of variance on integrated output for the beta filter (14·5–20 c/sec.), varying personality (P), trials (T) and viewing (V)*

Source	D.F.	S.S.	M.S.	F	P
Total	239	7717·96	—	—	—
Between subjects	23	6223·82	—	—	—
P	1	1086·30	1086·30	4·65	< 0·05
S/P	22	5137·52	233·52	—	—
Within subjects	216	1494·14	—	—	—
T	4	2·51	0·63	n.s.	—
PT	4	1·14	0·29	n.s.	—
ST/P	88	116·57	1·32	—	—
V	1	639·61	639·61	26·51	< 0·005
PV	1	106·67	106·67	4·42	< 0·05
SV/P	22	530·93	24·13	—	—
TV	4	2·50	0·63	n.s.	—
PTV	4	3·33	0·83	n.s.	—
STV/P	88	90·88	1·03	—	—

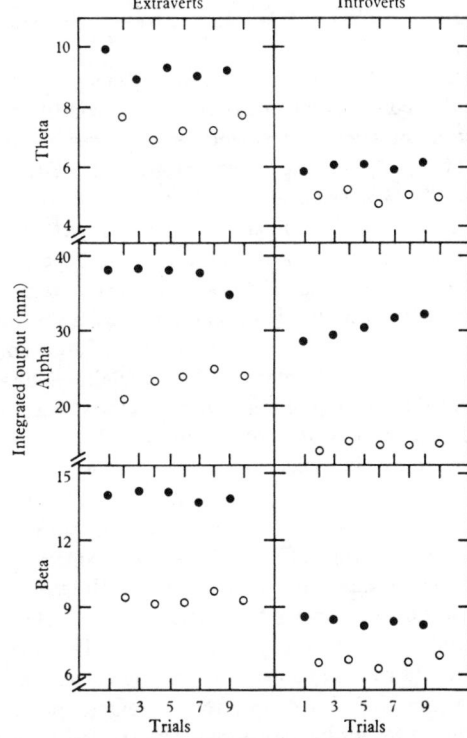

Fog. 3. The EEG of extraverts and introverts. Effect of eyes closed (●) and eyes open (○) on the integrated output of theta (4·5–6·5 c/sec.), alpha (8–13 c/sec.) and beta (14·5–20 c/sec.) frequencies over trials.

Extraversion–introversion and the EEG

the 5 per cent level for the eyes closed condition only, and for alpha, at 5 per cent for the eyes open only (*t* test, two-tailed). (If a lower level of confidence is accepted— *t* test, one-tailed—none of the within-viewing personality differences fall short of the 5 per cent level.) The interaction effect for beta may be expressed in terms of the differential effect of viewing on the personality groups, the difference within viewing for extraverts being greater. There is no main trials effect.

DISCUSSION

This study confirms the view that there are differences in the EEG characteristics of introverts and extraverts. With eyes closed the extravert EEG is higher in integrated output across the whole measured range, the divergence in output being greater in the lower alpha range. Differences in alpha activity are not so readily apparent with eyes closed when recording with a gross filter which fails to discriminate frequencies within alpha: however, with eyes open even a gross filter discriminates between extraverts and introverts. Prolonged recording also reveals differences in theta and beta; these differences are stronger when the eyes are shut.

We have therefore provided additional corroboration for the work of Savage (1964), Marton & Urban (1966) and Hume (1968) and further support for Gray's (1967) view that extraverts have similar EEG characteristics to subjects showing predominance of inhibition in dynamism.

In addition, this study is less open to criticism. Savage extracts his data from a continuous eyes closed record. Given ideal recording conditions, our technique of alternating short periods of viewing treatments is preferable. When all sources of distraction are eliminated, subjects lapse very rapidly into EEG signs of drowsiness. Thus Savage's result might be attributable to the typical waxing and waning of alpha against a background of increased amplitude, associated with drowsiness or the onset of stage A sleep (Oswald, 1962). It is presumably this type of variation to which Glass & Broadhurst (1966) refer. Given the prediction that extraverts fall asleep more readily in a sensory deprivation situation, then Savage's findings are not, strictly speaking, related to basal EEG but rather to a measure of speed of onset of light sleep under conditions of low levels of stimulation. This variable is likely to confound any study involving prolonged recording of inactive eyes closed periods. Moreover, such a procedure must involve a high degree of unpredictable experimental error; there must be few testing procedures in experimental psychology which include an instruction to the subject to 'lie quietly, do nothing, and keep your eyes shut'. The introduction of even a simple task imposes a modicum of constraint on the behaviour of the subject. The absence of a trials effect (Tables 4–6) confirms the authenticity of the present study in terms of baseline measurement with eyes closed; subjects were no more drowsy at the end of testing than they were at the beginning. A triple interaction between trials, viewing and personality would confirm one of our experimental hypotheses, namely that both groups, but more particularly the extravert group, would show progressive de-arousal to prolonged monotonous stimulation. Scrutiny of the trial means for alpha shows that the triple interaction (Table 5) does not lend itself to this interpretation. However, progressive de-arousal might involve a slight shift in frequency *within* the alpha range. The single 8–13 c/sec. filter employed in this part of the study would not reveal such changes. This problem requires further investigation.

The introduction of an eyes open condition has enabled us to demonstrate that visual monotony induces differences in alpha activity between extraverts and introverts which are not so readily apparent when the eyes are shut. Thus our results are compatible with earlier negative or equivocal results.

The source of the differences in the EEG between extraverts and introverts is unclear. Savage attributes the higher voltage output of the extravert group to 'cortical inhibition, be it "basal", reactive or conditioned'. But the 'cortical inhibition' construct, devised largely for the description of response characteristics, begs several questions. It is a neurophysiological construct linked by Eysenck to reactive inhibition, which in turn, was employed by Hull to explain variability in response. Indeed, Savage uses the terms reactive inhibition and cortical inhibition interchangeably. But are terms devised to describe responses appropriate to the measurement of EEG? Are resting measures, or even induced changes, to be treated as responses, analogous, say, to responses of subjects in a pursuit rotor task? And how much of the theoretical framework erected around the construct of reactive inhibition is transferable to the EEG or indeed to any other physiological measure? In the interest of parsimony, it is more reasonable in the present study to identify EEG activity measured from the occiput with some construct related to visual input. In this context, Eysenck's constructs of 'cortical excitation' and 'sensory hunger' are more appropriate. They allow for a correlation of measures of stimulus complexity with measures of EEG arousal, while avoiding the difficult problem of the definition of units of response.

The 'arousal' construct has been employed to explain differences between extraverts and introverts on a number of tasks (Eysenck, 1967) and in many animal studies the EEG is taken as an operational measure of the level of arousal. The higher voltage and lower frequency alpha and the higher voltage theta would appear to support the view that extraverts are less aroused than introverts. An inverse relation between alpha amplitude and arousal (within the waking stage) is generally accepted. However, Daniel (1967) fails to correlate any measure of alpha activity with performance on a vigilance task. Since there have been very few studies correlating alpha activity with adequate measures of performance, the issue is unresolved. Sleep research has identified increased theta with the onset of drowsiness (Oswald, 1962), but Daniel finds errors of omission in his vigilance task to be associated with *decrease* in theta amplitude. Animal studies implicate hippocampal theta (recorded direct from deep brain areas) in the acquisition of conditioned responses (Grastyan et al., 1959) and in other alerted states (Green & Arduini, 1954). However, the functional role of hippocampal theta is open to a number of interpretations (Routtenberg, 1966).

According to Walter (1959, p. 297) augmentation of theta is associated with 'feelings of disappointment and frustration...evoked by the termination...of an agreeable stimulus'. Thus the possibility arises that theta occurs as a measure of *absence* of stimulation and that theta output is inversely proportional to complexity of stimulation. Gale, Dunkin & Coles (in preparation) demonstrate reduced theta to patterned as opposed to plain visual displays, but this is true of *all* frequencies below 13 c/sec.

Extraversion–introversion and the EEG

The position is no less clear with beta. The difficulty lies in the interpretation of the low-frequency analysis data; does a high beta value represent more or less beta? Since low-frequency analysis confounds prevalence with abundance and textbooks normally refer to beta as 'very low voltage activity' (Thompson, 1967), it is difficult to know what 'high voltage beta' implies. Furthermore, the commonly held assumption that alpha blocking involves the replacement of alpha waves by beta waves (Calvet *et al.*, 1965) is unsubstantiated. Gengerelli & Parker (1966, p. 70) report that 'when the eyes are opened and the subject is in a state of perceptual alertness, the amplitude in this range (8–12 c/sec.) clearly diminishes; but there is *no corresponding enhancement of the amplitude in the higher frequencies*'.

The presence of both high alpha *and* high beta voltages in extraverts explains in part the failure of Fenton & Scotton (1967) to obtain differences in habituation rates. Since extraverts have higher alpha and higher beta, visual analysis is *more likely* to detect 'blocking responses', i.e. a reduction in alpha and the 'presence' of beta. Because it is easier to detect a response in extraverts, the scales are weighted against the prediction that they will habituate before introverts. (It is not at all clear how Marton & Urban (1966) detected alpha blockade and desynchronization in subjects without alpha rhythm.)

According to Mundy-Castle (1951) high beta is positively correlated with the M type alpha rhythm found 'predominantly in subjects habitually using vivid visual imagery' (Golla *et al.*, 1943). It is tempting to speculate that extraverts are driven to vivid visual imagery in order to stave off the monotony of our experimental set-up. Unfortunately, the M type alpha rhythm is typically of *low* voltage, whereas we have shown extraverts to have high voltage alpha.

Conclusion

One major difficulty in the correlation of personality measures with the EEG is the problem of the meaningful description of the EEG waveform spectra. Daniel's (1964) correlogram techniques, which combine measures of amplitude, frequency and rhythmicity, are the most adequate descriptors of EEG arousal (Van Olst & Orlebeke, 1967). When a number of conditions are set up which may be ranked (on an intuitive basis) along an arousal continuum, the correlogram ratios are shown to be more satisfactory correlates of behavioural arousal than any single parameter (Daniel, 1966). Unfortunately, their use involves considerable capital outlay on electronic processing devices. Nevertheless, it is still possible to work with old fashioned low-frequency analysis techniques, provided that care is taken in interpretation.

However, many of the measures currently in use are arbitrary, if derived from primary recordings alone, without the assistance of electronic analysis (see Table 1). The notion of 'alpha index' or 'per cent time alpha' must be dependent upon the capacity of the scorer to detect the presence or absence of alpha on the record. In fact, alpha activity is rarely absent from normal records; the continuous write-out of the instantaneous value of alpha filters is typically continuously active (though to a greater or lesser degree) at all points of the arousal continuum. Therefore, measures of alpha index can only be based upon cut-off points dependent upon scorer reliability. One advantage of measured integrated value is that it does provide a con-

ANTHONY GALE, MICHAEL COLES AND JENNIFER BLAYDON

tinuous scale, thus avoiding the problem of the definition of 'high' or 'low' alpha. The general relation between frequency and amplitude (Knott & Travis, 1937) should be recognized and studies reporting measures of the one should acknowledge studies including measures of the other. 'Dominant frequency' measures must take account of fluctuations in alpha frequency as behavioural arousal varies (Oswald, 1962). When the testing procedures employed are conducive to drowsiness and light sleep, different sections of the record are not strictly comparable. When one considers the sorts of attentional tasks on which extraverts are shown to be inferior (Eysenck, 1967) it is apparent that the most fruitful work in this area might well lie in the examination of moment-to-moment frequency fluctuations and their relation to performance, rather than of the gross evaluation of long-term measures, which tends to mask them.

The authors wish to thank Dr. L. H. Shaffer for assistance with the statistical treatment of the results. Michael Coles is an S.S.R.C. research student.

REFERENCES

BAKAN, P. (1959). Extraversion–introversion and improvement in an auditory vigilance task. *Br. J. Psychol.* **50**, 325–332.

BAKAN, P., BELTON, J. A., & TOTH, J. C. (1963). Extraversion–introversion and decrement in an auditory vigilance task. In D. N. Buckner & J. J. McGrath (eds.), *Vigilance: a Symposium*, pp. 22–23. New York: McGraw-Hill.

BERLYNE, D. E. (1960). *Conflict, Arousal and Curiosity.* New York: McGraw-Hill.

CALVET, J., CALVET, M. C. & LANGLOIS, J. M. (1965). Diffuse cortical activation waves during so-called desynchronized EEG patterns. *J. Neurophysiol.* **28**, 893–907.

CLARIDGE, G. S. (1960). The excitation–inhibition balance in neurotics. In H. J. Eysenck (ed.), *Experiments in Personality*, vol. 2. New York: Prager.

COLQUHOUN, W. P. & CORCORAN, D. W. J. (1964). The effects of time of day and social isolation on the relationship between temperament and performance. *Br. J. soc. clin. Psychol.* **3**, 226–231.

DANIEL, R. S. (1964). Electroencephalographic correlogram ratios and their stability. *Science, N.Y.* **145**, 721–723.

DANIEL, R. S. (1966). Electroencephalographic pattern quantification and the arousal continuum. *Psychophysiol.* **2**, 146–160.

DANIEL, R. S. (1967). Alpha and theta EEG in vigilance. *Percept. mot. Skills* **25**, 697–703.

EYSENCK, H. J. (1953). *The Structure of Human Personality.* London: Methuen.

EYSENCK, H. J. (1957). *The Dynamics of Anxiety and Hysteria.* London: Routledge & Kegan Paul.

EYSENCK, H. J. (1959). *Maudsley Personality Inventory.* London: University of London Press.

EYSENCK, H. J. (1967). *The Biological Basis of Personality.* Springfield, Ill.: Thomas.

EYSENCK, H. J. & EYSENCK, S. B. G. (1964). *Eysenck Personality Inventory.* London: University of London Press.

FENTON, G. W. & SCOTTON, L. (1967). Personality and the alpha rhythm. *Br. J. Psychiat.* **113**, 1283–1289.

GALE, M. A., COLES, M. G. H. & KLINE, P. Extraversion–introversion, neuroticism, and habituation of the orientation reaction. (In preparation.)

GALE, M. A., DUNKIN, E. N. & COLES, M. G. H. Visual input and the EEG. (In preparation.)

GENGERELLI, J. A. & PARKER, C. E. (1966). Spectrographic analysis of electroencephalograms under conditions of alertness and relaxation. *J. Psychol.* **63**, 67–72.

GLASER, G. H. (1963). The normal electroencephalogram and its reactivity. In G. H. Glaser (ed.), *EEG and Behaviour*, pp. 3–23. New York: Basic Books.

GLASS, A. (1964). Mental arithmetic and blocking of the occipital alpha rhythm. *Electroenceph. clin. Neurophysiol.* **16**, 595–603.

GLASS, A. & BROADHURST, A. (1966). Relationship between EEG as a measure of cortical activity and personality variables. *Electroenceph. clin. Neurophysiol.* **21**, 309.

Extraversion–introversion and the EEG

GOLLA, F. L., HUTTON, E. L. & WALTER, W. G. (1943). The objective study of mental imagery. *J. ment. Sci.* **89**, 216–223.

GOTTLOBER, A. B. (1938). The relationship between brain potentials and personality. *J. exp. Psychol.* **22**, 67–74.

GRASTYAN, E., LISSAK, K., MADARASZ, I. & DONHOFFER, H. (1959). Hippocampal electrical activity during the development of conditioned reflexes. *Electroenceph. clin. Neurophysiol.* **11**, 409–430.

GRAY, J. A. (1964). Strength of the nervous system as a dimension of personality in man: a review of work from the laboratory of B. M. Teplov. In J. A. Gray (ed.), *Pavlov's Typology*, pp. 157–287. Oxford: Pergamon Press.

GRAY, J. A. (1967). Strength of the nervous system, introversion–extraversion, conditionability and arousal. *Behav. Res. Ther.* **5**, 151–169.

GREEN, J. D. & ARDUINI, A. A. (1954). Hippocampal electrical activity in arousal. *J. Neurophysiol.* **17**, 533–557.

HENRY, C. E. & KNOTT, J. R. (1941). A note on the relationship between 'personality' and the alpha rhythm of the electroencephalogram. *J. exp. Psychol.* **28**, 362–366.

HOGAN, M. J. (1966). Influence of motivation on reactive inhibition in extraversion–introversion. *Percept. mot. Skills* **22**, 187–192.

HOWARTH, E. (1964). Differences between extraverts and introverts on a button-pressing task. *Psychol. Rep.* **14**, 949–950.

HUME, W. I. (1968). The dimensions of central nervous arousal. *Bull. Br. psychol. Soc.* **21**, 111. (Abstract.)

JENSEN, A. R. (1966). The measurement of reactive inhibition in humans. *J. gen. Psychol.* **75**, 85–94.

KNOTT, J. R. & TRAVIS, L. E. (1937). A note on the relationship between duration and amplitude of cortical potentials. *J. Psychol.* **3**, 169–172.

MARTON, M. & URBAN, Ya. (1966). An electroencephalographic investigation of individual differences in the processes of conditioning. *Proc. 18th Int. Congr. Exp. Psychol., Moscow*, pp. 106–109.

MUNDY-CASTLE, A. C. (1951). Theta and beta rhythm in the electroencephalograms of normal adults. *Electroenceph. clin. Neurophysiol.* **3**, 477–486.

MUNDY-CASTLE, A. C. (1955). The relationship between primary–secondary function and the alpha rhythm of the electroencephalogram. *J. nat. Inst. Personnel Res.* **6**, 95–102.

MYERS, J. L. (1966). *Fundamentals of experimental Design*. Boston: Allyn & Bacon.

NEBYLITSYN, V. D. (1963). An electroencephalographic investigation of the properties of strength of the nervous system and equilibrium of the nervous processes in man using factor analysis. In B. M. Teplov (ed.), *Typological Features of Higher Nervous Activity in Man*, vol. 3, pp. 47–80. Moscow: Acad. Pedagog. Nauk RSFSR.

OSWALD, I. (1962). *Sleeping and Waking*. Amsterdam: Elsevier.

ROUTTENBERG, A. (1966). Neural mechanisms of sleep: changing view of reticular formation function. *Psychol. Rev.* **73**, 481–499.

SAVAGE, R. D. (1964). Electro-cerebral activity, extraversion and neuroticism. *Br. J. Psychiat.* **110**, 98–100.

SCHEFFÉ, H. (1959). *The Analysis of Variance*. New York: Wiley.

SISSON, B. D. & ELLINGSON, R. J. (1955). On the relationship between 'normal' EEG patterns and personality variables. *J. nerv. ment. Dis.* **121**, 353–358.

THOMPSON, R. F. (1967). *Foundations of Physiological Psychology*. New York: Harper & Row.

VAN OLST, E. H. & ORLEBEKE, J. F. (1967). An analysis of the concept of arousal. *Nederl. Tijdschr. Psychol.* **22**, 9, 583–603.

WALTER, W. G. (1959). Intrinsic rhythms of the brain. In J. Field (ed.), *Handbook of Physiology*. Sec. 1: *Neurophysiology*, vol. 1, pp. 279–298. Washington, D.C.: American Physiological Society.

WALTER, W. G. (1963). Technique—interpretation. In D. Hill & D. Parr (eds.), *Electroencephalography*, pp. 65–98. London: Macdonald.

WEISEN, A. (1965). Differential reinforcing effects of onset and offset of stimulation on the operant behavior of normals, neurotics and psychopaths. (Unpublished Ph.D. thesis, University of Florida.)

(*Manuscript received* 9 *December* 1968)

From A. Crider and R. Lunn (1971). Journal of Experimental Research in Personality, *5,* 145–150, *by kind permission of the authors and Academic Press*

Electrodermal Lability as a Personality Dimension[1]

ANDREW CRIDER AND ROBERT LUNN

Williams College

Spontaneous fluctuation rate and speed of orienting response habituation of the palmar skin potential were measured in 22 subjects on two occasions 7 days apart. While spontaneous fluctuation rate showed moderate reliability, habituation speed proved to be a highly stable individual difference characteristic. Both measures were highly intercorrelated, suggesting their use as alternate indices of an underlying electrodermal lability dimension. An analysis of the relationship of the two measures with scales loading on major self-report test factors was also performed. Both were randomly related to neuroticism but negatively correlated with extraversion and impulsivity. These validities were of somewhat greater magnitude for habituation speed than for fluctuation rate.

Following an innovative study by Lacey and Lacey (1958), a good deal of interest has been focused on the use of frequency measures of electrodermal activity as individual difference variables. Lacey and Lacey distinguished between electrodermal "labiles" and "stabiles" in terms of the frequency of spontaneous bursts of activity in skin resistance recordings, a measure which has since been shown to be inversely related to the speed of habituation of the electrodermal orienting response to serially presented stimuli. Studies examining both spontaneous fluctuation rate, at rest or during stimulation, and resistance to habituation of the elicited orienting response have without exception found a positive relationship, the reported correlations ranging from .40 to .74 in various investigations (Corah & Stern, 1963; Johnson, 1963; Katkin & McCubbin, 1969; Koepke & Pribram, 1966; Lader & Wing, 1966; Mundy-Castle & McKiever, 1953; Purohit, 1966; Stern, Stewart, & Winokur, 1961; Stern, Winokur, Stewart, & Leonard, 1963). The two measures can thus be thought of as alternate indices of a more basic individual difference dimension, which in general usage is labeled "electrodermal lability."

[1] Supported in part by PHS Grant MH 18558. Address reprint requests to Dr. Andrew Crider, Department of Psychology, Williams College, Williamstown, Mass. 01267.

Electrodermal lability appears to be a relatively stable psychophysiological trait. Reports of test–retest reliabilities of resting fluctuation rate range from .54 to .89 over 24- to 48-hr periods in various populations (Corah & Stern, 1963; Docter & Friedman, 1966; Johnson, 1963; Lacey & Lacey, 1958). Over the longer run, 1-month and 1-year reliabilities of .62 and .50 have been reported by Docter and Friedman (1966) and Dykman, Ackerman, Galbrecht, and Reese (1963). In the case of habituation speed, Bernstein (1967) found a 6- to 10-week stability of .65 in a mixed population of normals and psychotics.

It is noteworthy that neither fluctuation rate nor habituation speed is appreciably correlated with widely employed amplitude measures of electrodermal activity. For example, the correlation between resting fluctuation rate and skin conductance across Ss is typically reported in the range, $.30 \pm .10$ (Corah & Stern, 1963; Johnson, 1963; Koepke & Pribram, 1966; Lacey & Lacey, 1958; Stern, Winokur, Stewart, & Leonard, 1963). Although Johnson (1963) found a positive relationship between fluctuation rate and the amplitude of the skin resistance response (GSR) elicited by the initial stimulus in an habituation series, this has not been confirmed in other investigations (Galbrecht, Dykman, Reese, & Suzuki, 1965; Koepke & Pribram, 1966;

Lader & Wing, 1966; Purohit, 1966; Wilson & Dykman, 1960). Lader and Wing (1966) likewise failed to find any significant correlations between habituation speed and either skin conductance level or GSR amplitude. The concept of electrodermal lability therefore appears to be independent of allied concepts such as orienting reflexiveness (Maltzman, 1967), defined by individual differences in electrodermal amplitude measures.

Little is known of the psychological correlates of electrodermal lability. A favored hypothesis relating lability differences to trait anxiety no longer seems tenable in light of a number of reports of a random relationship between fluctuation rate and self-report measures of neuroticism (Burdick, 1966; Lader & Wing, 1966; Purohit, 1966) or manifest anxiety (Johnson, 1963; Katkin & McCubbin, 1969; Koepke & Pribram, 1966). Two studies have similarly failed to find any relationship between habituation speed and neuroticism (Lader & Wing, 1966; Mangan & O'Gorman, 1969).

Studies of patient groups suggest, on the other hand, that electrodermal lability may reflect individual differences in extraversion. Lader and Wing (1966) reported that anxiety neurotics showed both higher fluctuation rates and slower habituation than normal controls, while others have found lower fluctuation rates in psychopaths as compared with both normal and neurotic controls (Fox & Lippert, 1963; Hare, 1968; Lippert & Senter, 1966). Since anxiety neurotics and psychopaths show similarly elevated scores on neuroticism scales but differ in degree of extraversion (Corah, 1964; Eysenck, 1967), these data suggest a negative relationship between lability measures and psychometric extraversion in the normal population.

Support for this notion comes from studies by Jones (1950) and Block (1957), both of whom reported negative correlations between judges' ratings of extraverted behavior and gross indices of electrodermal lability. Jones partitioned a group of adolescents into "high reactives" and "low reactives" on the basis of the average magnitude of the GSR elicited by a series of verbal stimuli, a measure most likely related to habituation speed. The low reactives were rated as more assertive, animated, talkative, and attention-seeking than the high reactives, who in turn were judged as calmer, more deliberative, cooperative, and responsible. Similarly, Block separated a group of students into "reactors" and "nonreactors" in terms of the number of GSRs observed during an interview situation, a gross measure probably reflecting both spontaneous fluctuation rate and habituation speed. The nonreactors were judged as more hostile, independent, and rebellious than the reactors, who were seen as relatively more submissive, introspective, and responsible.

In addition to supporting the hypothesis of a negative relationship between electrodermal lability and extraversion, both of the above reports are consistent with descriptions of extreme scorers on the psychometric dimension of impulsivity, as discussed by Gough (1957), Heist and Yonge (1968), and Sanford, Webster, and Freedman (1957). Impulsivity appears in factor analytic studies of self-report devices as an oblique factor correlated positively with both extraversion and neuroticism (Kassebaum, Couch, & Slater, 1959). High impulsives are thus extraverted-neurotic and low impulsives introverted-stable. Kassebaum et al. characterize the positive and negative poles of this dimension as impulsive, erratic, and delinquent vs controlled, intraceptive, and responsible.

Based on the foregoing considerations, then, the present study was designed to test the following hypotheses: (1) both the rate of spontaneous skin potential fluctuation and the speed of habituation of the skin potential orienting response are reliable characteristics of the individual; (2) the two measures are sufficiently intercorrelated to justify regarding them as alternate indices of a more general trait of electrodermal lability; (3) both indices are more highly, and negatively, correlated with psychometric extraversion than with neuroticism, and (4) both indices will show their highest correlations with psychometric indices of impulsivity.

ELECTRODERMAL LABILITY AND PERSONALITY

METHOD

Subjects. Twenty-two male undergraduate volunteers served as subjects.

Procedure. Each subject was tested on two separate occasions spaced 7 days apart. The same procedure was followed in both sessions: the subject was seated in a lounge chair in a sound-attenuated cubicle, which was temperature controlled at 70°F and separated from the recording and programming equipment in an adjacent cubicle. Following electrode placement, the subject was instructed to remain alert, to refrain from undue movement, and to anticipate sporadic sounds over a loudspeaker placed on the wall above and to the right of the chair. A 5-min rest period followed adjustment of the recording equipment. The experiment proper began with the introduction of a moderate-intensity masking white noise rated at 72 dB at the position of the subject. Five minutes later, a series of 90 dB, 1300 Hz tones of 2-sec duration were delivered over the loudspeaker. The tones, which interrupted the white noise, were programmed randomly at 40- to 80-sec intervals around a mean of 60 sec. The stimuli continued for 20 trials or until an habituation criterion of three successive nonresponse trials occurred.

The MMPI was administered to each subject prior to the first recording session.

Apparatus. Palmar skin potential activity was recorded on two channels of a Grass Model 7 polygraph via nonpolarizing Ag–AgCl sponge electrodes placed approximately 20 cm apart on the right palm and forearm. Skin surfaces were cleaned with rubbing alcohol. One polygraph channel was used to measure the dc potential difference between the two electrodes via a chopper-stabilized Model 7P1 preamplifier having a gain setting of 10 mV/cm. This signal was also passed through a Model 7P5 ac preamplifier set at the maximum time constant of .45 sec and at a gain of 0.2 mV/cm. This combination of ac recording and increased sensitivity made it possible to recognize rapid electrodermal changes from the base line as small as .1 mV. Since ac coupling at a .45-sec time constant introduces some distortion and attenuation of the true response, the dc channel served primarily as a monitor of the fidelity of the high gain ac signal.

A conventional white noise generator and a Hewlett–Packard Model 200 AB oscillator served as stimulus sources. Experimental events were programmed with a tape programmer and solid-state logic.

Measures. Fluctuation rate scores were taken as the simple frequency of negative-going skin potential responses occurring during the last 4 min of white noise preceding the habituation series. A criterion response was defined as a change of at least .1 mV on the ac channel. Two or more successive fluctuations occurring within 6 sec were tallied as one response. Habituation speed scores were taken as the trial number at which three successive tone presentations failed to elicit a response of at least .1 mV within 3 sec of tone offset.

MMPI protocols were commercially scored, yielding standard scores on 25 clinical and research scales. Scales were chosen for correlation with the electrodermal measures on the basis of their loading on the factors isolated in the Kassebaum *et al.* (1959) study of MMPI and MMPI-derived scales. According to this analysis, the best estimators of the first two orthogonal factors of neuroticism and extraversion are, respectively, Welsh's (1956) anxiety (A) and reflected repression-denial ($-R$) scales. Similarly, the three scales loading most clearly on the oblique impulsivity factor are Gough's (1957) impulsivity (Im) and reflected social responsibility ($-Re$) scales and the MMPI hypomania (Ma) scale. In addition, the MMPI psychopathic deviate (Pd) scale was included with this triad in light of its strong correlation with each of them. Neither Ma nor Pd were K corrected.

RESULTS

The means and standard deviations for the first session lability measures were: habituation speed, 10.86 and 5.93; spontaneous fluctuation rate, 6.36 and 5.42. For the second session they were: habituation speed, 10.54 and 6.77; spontaneous fluctuation rate, 8.41 and 6.53. Table 1 presents the test–retest reliabilities (r) of the two measures, as well as their intercorrelation based on each subject's sum on each measure across the two sessions. Spontaneous fluctuation rate stablility was of moderate

TABLE 1

RELIABILITIES AND INTERCORRELATION OF HABITUATION SPEED AND SPONTANEOUS FLUCTUATION RATE[a]

	Habituation	Fluctuations
Habituation	.70**	
Fluctuations	.75**	·54*

[a] Habituation–fluctuation intercorrelation based on two-session sums.

* $p < .01$.

** $p < .001$.

magnitude, the $r = .54$ consistent with the 1-month and 1-year values previously reported (Docter & Friedman, 1966; Dykman *et al.*, 1963). In contrast, habituation speed proved to be quite stable ($r = .70$), which suggests its use as the more efficient index of electrodermal lability.

That the two measures seem to be reflecting the same underlying phenomenon is seen in their highly significant intercorrelation ($r = .75$). This value is nearly equivalent to the intercorrelation of the two measures in the second session alone ($r = .73$), but a good deal higher than their intercorrelation for the first session ($r = .51$). In general, the correlations of the electrodermal measures with the self-report scales showed similar reductions in magnitude from total to second to first sessions. Both sets of data thus point to the dubious validity of single-session determinations of lability and correspondingly emphasize the importance of repeated testings for achieving stable individual difference estimates.

Table 2 presents the validities of the two-session habituation and fluctuation scores with the test dimensions. As hypothesized, both measures were uncorrelated with neuroticism but significantly negatively related to extraversion. A systematic relationship with scales loading on impulsivity also appeared, with six of the eight coefficients attaining significance. Given the somewhat greater reliability of habituation speed over spontaneous fluctua-

tion rate, the generally higher validities of the former would be anticipated. That the correlations with impulsivity were not notably higher than those with extraversion, as hypothesized, may be due to the somewhat atypical nature of the sample with regard to the impulsivity measures. Although standard scores were not available for *Im*, the means for *Ma*, *Pd*, and *Re* were all significantly different from 50 ($p < .05$). Further correlations were run with the remaining MMPI clinical scales, but none attained significance.

DISCUSSION

The results by and large supported the initial hypotheses. Skin potential measures of spontaneous fluctuation rate and speed of orienting response habituation are sufficiently stable for individual difference analyses. Their high degree of intercorrelation argues for their use as alternate indices of a trait of electrodermal lability, although the somewhat more reliable habituation speed measure is *ipso facto* the better candidate for validity determinations. This latter point is borne out by a consideration of the magnitudes of the correlations between the two measures and the various MMPI scales. While both showed similar patterns of relationship, the size of the correlations were generally greater for habituation speed. The results also confirmed the anticipated random relationship of electrodermal lability with neuroticism and the negative

TABLE 2
CORRELATIONS OF HABITUATION SPEED AND SPONTANEOUS FLUCTUATION RATE
WITH MMPI FACTOR ESTIMATORS

Factor Scale	Neuroticism A	Extraversion (−)R	Impulsivity				Mean[a]	Standard Deviation
			Im	*Ma*	(−)*Re*	*Pd*		
Habituation	−.02	−.48*	−.42*	−.40*	−.57**	−.42*	21.41	11.71
Fluctuations	−.06	−.38*	−.32	−.41*	−.24	−.46*	14.77	10.91
Mean	52.73	50.41	9.09[b]	58.91	53.18	56.27		
Standard Deviation	10.96	8.02	3.00[b]	9.71	6.10	9.55		

[a] Sum of two sessions.
[b] Raw scores.
* $p < .05$, one-tailed.
** $p < .01$, one-tailed.

relationships of lability with extraversion and impulsivity, although the magnitude of the correlations with impulsivity were not notably greater than those with extraversion, as had been anticipated.

It should be noted that previous attempts to isolate significant covariations between Maudsley Personality Inventory extraversion and electrodermal lability measures have yielded inconclusive or negative results (Burdick, 1966; Lader & Wing, 1966; Martin, 1960; Purohit, 1966). The present study differed from former investigations in at least two important respects. The first was the use of repeated testings in order to arrive at stable estimates of individual differences in lability. The second was the use of Welsh's A and R scales to measure neuroticism and extraversion. Not only are these two scales known to be factorily pure and orthogonal (Kassebaum et al., 1959), but they have also been shown to discriminate between normals, dysthymics, and hysterics in the manner specified by Eysenck's (1967) two-factor personality typology (Corah, 1964). Thus these MMPI scales may be more sensitive measures of neuroticism and extraversion in unselected samples than the Maudsley test.

A recent study by Mangan and O'Gorman (1969) suggests, however, that the present results are replicable when subjects are preselected for extreme scores on the Eysenck Personality Inventory, a revision of the Maudsley test. In two separate experiments, measures of skin resistance habituation speed were taken from groups defined by the extremes of neuroticism and extraversion on this scale. No significant difference in habituation speed appeared between high and low neuroticism groups in either experiment. However, introverts were found to habituate significantly more slowly than extroverts in one experiment, while in the second an interaction between neuroticism and extraversion appeared, with stable introverts (nonimpulsives) showing the slowest habituation.

The results are also in substantial agreement with the findings of Jones (1950) and Block (1957), whose data were based on trait ratings by independent observers. That the same sorts of validities were obtained in the present study with self-report devices suggests a degree of multi-method measurement consistency. The extent to which these electrodermal-personality trait covariations are stable across measurement situations deserves to be further investigated as a first step in isolating underlying mechanisms.

REFERENCES

BERNSTEIN, A. S. The orienting reflex as a research tool in the study of psychotic populations. In I. Ruttkay-Nedecky, L. Ciganek, V. Zikmund, & E. Kellerova (Eds.), *Mechanisms of orienting reaction in man.* Bratislava: Slovak Academy of Sciences, 1967.

BLOCK, J. A study of affective responsiveness in a lie-detection situation. *Journal of Abnormal and Social Psychology,* 1957, **55**, 11–15.

BURDICK. J. A. Autonomic lability and neuroticism. *Journal of Psychosomatic Research,* 1966. **9**, 339–342.

CORAH. N. L. Neuroticism and extraversion in the MMPI: Empirical validation and exploration. *British Journal of Social and Clinical Psychology,* 1964, **3**, 168–174.

CORAH, N. L., & STERN, J. A. Stability and adaptation of some measures of electrodermal activity in children. *Journal of Experimental Psychology,* 1963, **65**, 80–85.

DOCTER. R. F., & FRIEDMAN. L. F. Thirty-day stability of spontaneous galvanic skin responses in man. *Psychophysiology,* 1966, **2**, 311–315.

DYKMAN, R. A.. ACKERMAN, P. T.. GALBRECHT, C. R., & REESE. W. G. Physiological reactivity to different stressors and methods of evaluation. *Psychosomatic Medicine,* 1963. **25**, 37–59.

EYSENCK, H. J. *The biological basis of personality.* Springfield: Charles C Thomas, 1967.

FOX, R., & LIPPERT, W. Spontaneous GSR and anxiety level in sociopathic delinquents. *Journal of Consulting Psychology,* 1963, **27**, 368.

GALBRECHT, C. R., DYKMAN, R. A., REESE, W. G., & SUZUKI. T. Intrasession adaptation and intersession extinction of the components of the orienting response. *Journal of Experimental Psychology,* 1965, **70**, 585–597.

GOUGH. H. G. *California Psychological Inventory Manual.* Palo Alto: Consulting Psychologists Press, 1957.

HARE. R. D. Psychopathy, autonomic functioning, and the orienting response. *Journal of Abnormal Psychology,* 1968. **73**, 1–24.

HEIST, P.. & YONGE. G. *Omnibus Personality*

Inventory Manual. New York: Psychological Corporation, 1968.

JOHNSON, L. C. Some attributes of spontaneous autonomic activity. *Journal of Comparative and Physiological Psychology,* 1963, **56,** 415–422.

JONES, H. E. The study of patterns of emotional expression. In M. L. Reymert (Ed.). *Feelings and Emotions.* New York: McGraw-Hill, 1950.

KASSEBAUM, G. G., COUCH, A. S., & SLATER. P. E. The factorial dimensions of the MMPI. *Journal of Consulting Psychology,* 1959, **23,** 226–236.

KATKIN, E. S., & McCUBBIN, R. J. Habituation of the orienting response as a function of individual differences in anxiety and autonomic lability. *Journal of Abnormal Psychology,* 1969, **74,** 54–60.

KOEPKE, J. E., & PRIBRAM, K. H. Habituation of GSR as a function of stimulus duration and spontaneous activity. *Journal of Comparative and Physiological Psychology,* 1966, **61,** 442–448.

LACEY, J. I., & LACEY, B. C. The relationship of resting autonomic activity to motor impulsivity. *Research Publications, Association for Research in Nervous and Mental Disease,* 1958. **36,** 144–209.

LADER, M. H., & WING, L. *Physiological measures, sedative drugs, and morbid anxiety.* New York: Oxford University Press, 1966.

LIPPERT, W. W., & SENTER, R. J. Electrodermal responses in the sociopath. *Psychonomic Science,* 1966, **4,** 25–26.

MALTZMAN, I. Individual differences in "attention": The orienting reflex. In R. M. Gagne (Ed.), *Learning and individual differences.* Columbus: Merrill. 1967.

MANGAN, G. L., & O'GORMAN, J. G. Initial amplitude and rate of habituation of orienting reaction in relation to extraversion and neuroticism. *Journal of Experimental Research in Personality,* 1969, **3,** 275–282.

MARTIN, I. Variations in skin resistance and their relationship to GSR conditioning. *Journal of Mental Science,* 1960, **106,** 281–287.

MUNDY-CASTLE, A. C., & McKIEVER, B. L. The psychophysiological significance of the galvanic skin response. *Journal of Experimental Psychology,* 1953, **46,** 15–24.

PUROHIT, A. P. Personality variables, sex-difference, GSR responsiveness and GSR conditioning. *Journal of Experimental Research in Personality,* 1966, **1,** 166–173.

SANFORD, N., WEBSTER. H., & FREEDMAN, M. Impulse expression as a variable of personality. *Psychological Monographs,* 1957. **71** (11 Whole No. 440).

STERN, J., STEWART, M., & WINOKUR, G. An investigation of some relationships between various measures of galvanic skin response. *Journal of Psychosomatic Research,* 1961, **5,** 215–223.

STERN, J. A., WINOKUR. G., STEWART. M. A., & LEONARD, C. Electrodermal conditioning: Some further correlates. *The Journal of Nervous and Mental Disease,* 1963, **137,** 479–486.

WELSH, G. S. Factor dimensions A and R. In G. S. Welsh and W. G. Dahlstrom (Eds.). *Basic readings on the MMPI in psychology and medicine.* Minneapolis: University of Minnesota Press. 1956.

WILSON, J. W. D., & DYKMAN, R. A. Background autonomic activity in medical students. *Journal of Comparative and Physiological Psychology,* 1960. **53,** 405–411.

From G. L. Mangan and J. G. O'Gorman (1969). Journal of Experimental Research in Personality, *3*, 275–282, *by kind permission of the authors and Academic Press*

Initial Amplitude and Rate of Habituation of Orienting Reaction in Relation to Extraversion and Neuroticism[1]

GORDON L. MANGAN AND JOHN G. O'GORMAN

The University of Queensland

Received May 16, 1968; Revised October 16, 1968

Initial amplitude and rate of habituation of the GSR component of the orienting reaction (OR) to an auditory stimulus of moderate intensity, which within the neo-Pavlovian system are indices of the properties of dynamism of excitation and of inhibition were related to measures of neuroticism and extraversion. It was found that neuroticism relates primarily to initial amplitude and extraversion to habituation rate.

Pavlov (1951–1952) claimed that the processes underlying extinction or habituation of the orienting reaction (OR) and the conditioned response (CR) were similar, both being dependent on the generation of internal inhibition. Vinogradova (1961), Sokolov (1963), and Stein (1966) have proposed that OR extinction is a gradually elaborated negative conditioned reflex process in which the conditioned stimulus (CS) is the onset of the stimulus to be habituated. According to Nebylitsyn (1966) extinction of the OR leads to the formation of a functional inhibitory structure.

Although no systematic investigation of the basic parameters and characteristics of the OR were attempted in the Pavlovian laboratories, it was generally accepted that the weak nervous system is characterized by an almost inextinguishable OR to any stimulus. OR was usually measured by galvanic skin response (GSR), which is considered to be one of the most satisfactory indices (Voronin, Sokolov, and Bao-Khua, 1959). Rapid extinction of OR was interpreted as indicating a predominance of inhibitory processes, and slow extinction a predominance of excitatory processes. Thus, rate of extinction of OR was assumed to

reflect the balance of inhibitory and excitatory processes, according to strength.

In a recent statement, Nebylitsyn (1966) identifies rate of extinction, initial amplitude and duration as basic OR parameters. He reports a significant correlation ($r = +.68$, $N = 24$) between OR extinction rate and speed of formation of differentiations. From this evidence, he claims that rate of OR extinction depends largely on the property, dynamism of inhibition, i.e., the speed of generation of inhibition, usually measured by the ease of development of inhibitory CRs. The dynamism dimension, in Nebylitsyn's system, is assumed to be orthogonal to the strength-sensitivity dimension.

Initial magnitude of OR, however, appears to be dependent on a complex set of relationships. Both Yermolayeva-Tomina (1963), using a GSR measure, and Rozhdestvenskaya, Nebylitsyn, Borisova and Yermolayeva-Tomina (1960), using a vascular measure, report significant positive correlations between initial OR magnitude and rate of OR extinction. To this extent, initial OR magnitude is related to dynamism of inhibition.

Although Rozhdestvenskaya (1963) found little evidence of a relationship between dynamism of excitation, measured by speed of elaboration of positive CRs, and initial OR magnitude, Nebylitsyn

[1] Contribution to a program of studies of the relationship between neo-Pavlovian properties of higher nervous activity and western personality dimensions.

(1966), in a re-analysis of Yermolayeva-Tomina's (1963) GSR data, reports that Ss with a predominance of dynamism of excitation showed slower OR extinction and greater initial magnitude of response than those Ss exhibiting predominance of dynamism of inhibition. The correlations, however, were suggestive rather than significant.

Nebylitsyn (1966) also maintains that initial OR amplitude cannot be completely independent of the strength of the nervous system with regard to excitation. Since the strong nervous system is less sensitive, there should be an inverse relationship between strength of nervous system and initial OR magnitude, i.e., Ss with weak nervous systems should have more expressive ORs, especially to stimuli of weak or average intensity. Although there is little evidence of such dependence, Nebylitsyn suggests that the influence of sensitivity may be concealed by dynamism factors.

Thus it seems likely that while rate of OR extinction is due primarily to dynamism (i.e., speed of generation) of inhibition, initial OR amplitude is related to both dynamism of inhibition and dynamism of excitation, or the balance between these two properties, while at the same time, strength-sensitivity of the nervous system with regard to excitation might be marginally involved.

Western studies relating these OR parameters to personality measures are few and equivocal. A sex difference in GSR habituation rate has been reported (Berry and Martin, 1957; Kimmel and Kimmel, 1965). Although a number of investigators report no significant correlation between GSR habituation rate and manifest anxiety (Galbrecht, Dykman, Reese, and Suzuki, 1965; Koepke and Pribram, 1966), or MPI neuroticism (Martin, 1960), Lader and Wing (1966) reported that anxiety neurotics habituated GSR at a significantly slower rate than normals. And although GSR habituation rate has been shown to be unrelated to extraversion, or "secondary function" (Martin, 1960; Mundy-Castle and McKiever, 1953), Marton and Urban (1966) showed that extraverts developed EEG and GSR habituation in significantly fewer trials than introverts.

Conflicting findings from these studies might be attributable to different criteria used in selecting samples, to procedural variations, or to differences in habituation criteria employed. Lader and Wing's (1966) criterion of clinically diagnosed anxiety appears to be unrelated to manifest anxiety (Sampson and Bindra, 1954); the auditory stimulus used by Marton and Urban (1966) was characterized by them as "weak," compared with the 100-db stimuli used by Martin (1960) and Lader and Wing (1966), the 94-db stimulus employed by Koepke and Pribram (1966), and the "harsh" auditory stimulus used by Mundy-Castle and McKiever (1953), all of which might be expected to elicit a defensive, rather than an orienting reaction (Sokolov, 1963).

Results from studies relating magnitude of OR on the first presentation of the stimulus to personality measures are highly contradictory. Dykman, Reese, Galbrecht, and Thomasson (1959) report that Ss high on self-rated anxiety gave larger GSRs to the first presentation of an auditory stimulus; Galbrecht et al. (1965), however, state that throughout the habituation series, Ss with the highest scores on the anxiety test (MAS) actually gave the smallest GSRs, a finding which accords with Lader and Wing's (1966) conclusion that anxiety, clinically defined, results in smaller GSRs both on initial presentation of the stimulus, and throughout the habituation series. On the other hand, a number of studies disclose no evidence of relationship between initial OR magnitude to an auditory stimulus, and manifest anxiety scores (Dykman et al., 1959; Koepke and Pribram, 1966; Maltzman and Raskin, 1965) and between initial OR magnitude to a visual stimulus and MPI defined neuroticism and extraversion (Lovibond, 1963).

The present study was planned to investigate the relationship between the Eysenck and Eysenck (1964) Personality Inventory (EPI) variables of extraversion (E) and neuroticism (N) and initial amplitude and rate of GSR habituation to an auditory stimulus of moderate intensity.

METHOD

There are two series in the present experiment. In both series, GSR amplitude to the first presentation of the stimulus, and GSR habituation rate, were measured with Ss selected on the basis of their E and N scores on the EPI. In Series 1, both E and N scores were varied to give four combinations of high and low scorers on the two dimensions. In Series 2, N was held constant for all Ss, and the method of stimulus presentation was changed.

Series 1

Subjects. Twenty male Ss within the age range 19–23 years were selected from an undergraduate class in Psychology at the University of Queensland on the basis of their E and N scores on Form B of the EPI. The mean for the class on the E scale was 12.12 with a standard deviation of 3.91, and the mean on the N scale was 7.76 with a standard deviation of 4.44. Depending on whether their scores fell one standard deviation above or below the class mean on both scales, five Ss were allocated to each of four groups–high N: high E, high N:low E, low N:high E, and low N: low E.

Material. A tone of 1000-cps frequency was recorded on magnetic tape from a Levell Decade Oscillator and amplified to an intensity of 60 db through a loudspeaker. The duration of the tone was 3 sec and the inter-tone interval varied on a random schedule from 16 to 24 sec with a series mean of 20 sec. A three channel Halliburton Deceptograph with pen write-out was used to obtain the GSR record. One of the channels recorded GSR, a second was used as an event marker driven through a relay from the loudspeaker.

Procedure. The experiment was conducted in a sound attenuated room. Subject was seated at a table with the loud-speaker in front of him some 3 feet away. Silver-nickel electrodes were attached to the palmar surface of the first and third fingers of S's right hand above the whorls of the finger tips. No electrolyte was used and the only site preparation consisted in wiping the fingers dry.

The subject was asked to rest his right forearm on the table in front of him. He was informed that the experiment would take approximately 10 minutes, that no response was required from him, and that no shock would be used at any time. He was asked to relax and to move as little as possible during the experiment.

When it appeared that the GSR record had stabilized, the tape recorder was switched on and the experiment commenced. All Ss received 30 presentations of the tone.

Series 2

Subjects. Twenty-four male Ss within the age range 18–25 years were selected from an undergraduate class in Psychology at the University of Queensland on the basis of their E and N scores on Form B of the EPI. The mean for the class on the E scale was 12.56 with a standard deviation of 5.25 and the mean on the N scale was 7.26 with a standard deviation of 4.40. Twelve Ss whose scores fell one standard deviation above the class mean on the E scale and within one standard deviation of the class mean on the N scale were allocated to the extravert group; and twelve Ss whose scores fell one standard deviation below the class mean on the E scale and within one standard deviation of the class mean on the N scale were allocated to the introvert group.

Material. A tone of 380-cps frequency was recorded on magnetic tape from a Levell Decade Oscillator and presented to S at an intensity of 57 db through high fidelity headphones. The duration of the tone was 400 msec and the inter-tone interval varied on a random schedule from 16 to 24 sec with a series mean of 20 sec. The method of GSR recording was the same as that employed in Series 1.

Procedure. In the present experiment Ss received only 16 presentations of the auditory stimulus. In all other respects the procedure was the same as that followed in Series 1.

RESULTS

In analyzing Ss' records a pen deflection was scored as a GSR to the tone stimulus if it occurred within 1.5–3.5 sec after stimulus onset (Stewart, Stern, Winokur, and Freedman, 1961). The GSR was measured in millimeters (mm) as the length of the perpendicular from the smallest post-stimulus level to an extension of the basal prestimulus level. No transformation of the units of mms deflection was performed and no attempt was made to remove the dependence in these difference scores on the prestimulus level. The problems of transformation of units and dependence of change scores on basal level are continuing issues in studies with the GSR (Venables and Martin, 1967). In the present investigation the simplest unit available was used. Dependence in the measure was not controlled as Galbrecht et al. (1965) reported little difference between change scores and scores in which dependence had been removed using a technique similar to the regression technique suggested by Lacey (1956). Furthermore, Montague and Coles (1966) have argued that removal of dependence on basal level in GSR scores may work against demonstration of differences in Ss hypothesized to differ in arousal.

Two measures were taken from each record for analysis, an initial amplitude measure and a rate of habituation index. The initial amplitude measure was the magnitude of the GSR in arbitrary units of millimeter deflection to the first presentation of the auditory stimulus in the series. Rate of habituation was determined as the number of tone presentations required for three presentations of the tone to elicit zero response, i.e., a pen deflection of less than 1 mm (Sokolov, 1963).

Initial Amplitude Data

Series 1. The mean size of initial GSR for the four groups, high N:high E, high N:low E, low N:high E and low N:low E was analyzed using a 2×2 Analysis of Variance which is summarized in Table 1.

TABLE 1
ANALYSIS OF VARIANCE OF INITIAL GSR SIZE FOR SERIES 1 Ss

Source	df	MS	F
Neuroticism	1	1513.8	34.80[a]
Extraversion	1	64.8	1.41
N × E	1	115.2	2.42
Error	16	43.5	

[a] $p < .01$.

In view of the significant main effect for N, a comparison of individual means for this factor was made following Winer (1962). It was found that, for introverts, the mean size of the initial OR for low N Ss (20.6 mm) was significantly greater than that (8.0 mm) for high N Ss ($t = 4.27$, $p < .01$).

For the group of extraverts, it was found that the mean size of initial GSR for the low N Ss (29.0 mm) was significantly greater than that (6.8 mm) for the high N Ss ($t = 3.93$, $p < .01$). Thus for both the extravert and introvert groups, low N Ss

showed a reliably greater GSR to the first presentation of the auditory stimulus.

Although the overall analysis showed no significant main effect for the E factor, comparisons of individual means were performed. It was found that, for the low N group, extraverts showed a significantly larger GSR than introverts ($t = 2.97$, $p < .01$), but for the high N group, there was no reliable difference between extraverts and introverts on this measure.

Series 2. In analyzing results in this series, data available from 12 Ss who had been selected and tested using the same procedure as that employed in Series 2 were incorporated in the analysis, giving a total sample of 36 Ss. As these additional Ss received eight presentations only of the auditory stimulus, however, their records could not be assessed for rate of habituation using the index of number of trials to zero response.

The mean size of initial GSR for the group of 18 extraverts was 19.0 mm and for the group of 18 introverts was 13.2 mm A t test revealed a significant difference in these means at less than the .05 level ($t = 1.81$, df 34; two tailed). It was concluded that extraverts show a larger GSR to the first presentations of an auditory stimulus than do introverts.

Habituation Data

Series 1. A 2×2 Analysis of Variance was performed on the rate of habituation scores for the Ss in each of the four groups in Series 1. This analysis is summarized below in Table 2.

Although no significant effects for N or E were found, there was a significant in-

TABLE 2
ANALYSIS OF VARIANCE OF HABITUATION RATE FOR SERIES 1 Ss

Source	df	MS	F
Neuroticism	1	96.80	0.72
Extraversion	1	20.00	0.15
N × E	1	924.80	6.85[a]
Error	16	135.16	

[a] $p < .05$.

teraction between the effects of these variables on rate of habituation. Tests on the simple effects of the variables were, therefore, performed (Winer, 1962). The analysis showed that for low N Ss, the difference between the mean number of trials (13.8) to the criterion of habituation for extraverts was significantly different from the mean number of trials (29.2) to the criterion for introverts ($F = 4.50$, $p < .05$), and that for introvert Ss, the mean number of trials (11.2) to the habituation criterion for high N Ss was significantly different from the mean number of trials (29.2) to the criterion for low N Ss ($F = 5.99$, $p < .05$). No other tests of simple effects proved statistically reliable.

The results of this series thus indicate that low N extraverts and high N introverts habituate GSR at a significantly faster rate than low N introverts.

Series 2. In this series, it was found that the mean number of trials to habituation for the extravert group was 4.75, while the mean for the introvert group was 14.76. A t test of the difference between means gave a significant value ($t = 6.47$, df 22, $p < .001$, one tailed). Thus the finding in Series 1 of a significantly faster rate of habituation for low N extraverts than for low N introverts is in part replicated in this Series.

DISCUSSION

The results of the present study indicate conclusively that both extraversion and neuroticism, as measured by the EPI, are related both to rate of OR habituation and to amplitude of response to the first presentation of the stimulus, the OR index being GSR to an auditory stimulus of moderate intensity. The interrelationships of these variables, however, are exceedingly complex. This is indicated in the following summary table, in which the four experimental groups are characterized as being fast or slow in habituation rate, and as showing large or small amplitude of initial response.

Nebylitsyn (1966), in his theorizing, maintains that OR extinction rate, whether the response be vascular, cortical or vaso-

TABLE 3
INITIAL AMPLITUDE AND HABITUATION RATE OF GSR FOR THE FOUR EXPERIMENTAL GROUPS

	High N: High E	High N: Low E	Low N: High E	Low N: Low E
Initial amplitude	Small	Small	Large	Large
Habituation rate	Slow	Fast	Fast	Slow

motor, whether in the auditory or visual modality, is the prime index of dynamism of inhibition, or the speed of generation of inhibition. On this assumption, both the low-anxious extraverts and the high-anxious introverts display greater dynamism of inhibition than the other two groups. And if, in fact, dynamism of inhibition involves both extraversion and neuroticism, it is not surprising that studies in which one dimension only is varied have shown no significant relationship between rate of OR habituation and either extraversion or neuroticism.

GSR amplitude to the presentation of the first stimulus in the series appears to be primarily a function of level of neuroticism, in that low-anxious Ss—particularly the low N:high E group—gave a significantly larger GSR than high-anxious Ss. This provides some confirmation of the observation of Galbrecht et al. (1965) that Ss scoring high on MAS expressed the smallest GSRs, and the similar conclusion reached by Lader and Wing (1966) in their study. Initial amplitude appears also to be related to level of extraversion, in that, under the constraint of low N scores (Series 2), extraverts show significantly larger initial ORs than introverts.

Nebylitsyn (1966) suggests that initial OR amplitude is largely a measure of the predominance of dynamism of excitation over dynamism of inhibition. If there are grounds for assuming such a relationship, the present data assert that Ss low on neuroticism possess relatively greater dynamism of excitation.

These findings do not seem explicable in terms of the greater sensitivity, i.e., lower LATs, of Ss low on the neuroticism scale.

What evidence there is suggests a moderate relationship between sensitivity and extraversion (Siddle, Morrish, White, and Mangan, 1969), none between neuroticism and sensitivity (Granger, 1957).

One final point might be worth mentioning. Eysenck (1957) originally suggested that extraverts, due to a predominance of inhibition, might be expected to condition slowly and extinguish rapidly, while introverts might be expected to condition quickly and extinguish slowly. The evidence he adduces in support of this proposition, however, is unimpressive. Eysenck has suggested recently (1966) that extraversion might be equated with the Russian dimension of strength-sensitivity, with the introverts being weak or sensitive. The diffiiculty of this new approach has been discussed elsewhere (White, Mangan, Morrish, and Siddle, 1969).

Nebylitsyn's recent statement (1966) however, that ease of elaborating positive and negative CRs is a function of the dynamism of excitation and inhibition, rather than of strength-sensitivity of nervous processes has sharply refocussed the problem of the relationship of certain personality dimensions to conditioning behavior. Eysenck and Eysenck (1964) have assumed near-zero correlation between EPI neuroticism and extraversion, the latter being related to conditioning behavior. Spence (1964), on the other hand, has offered evidence of a relationship between manifest anxiety, which correlates around $+0.8$ with MPI neuroticism (Jensen, 1958), and conditioning performance.

Some basis for reconciliation between the opposing views of Eysenck and Spence can be detected in Frank's (1956, 1957) argument that, assuming a negative correlation between extraversion and neuroticism, selection of extraverted Ss should be biased in favor of low-anxious Ss, and selection of low-anxious Ss in favor of highly extraverted Ss. Selection in terms of one dimension would thus result in a disproportionately large number of high E:low N Ss in both the high E and low N groups, each of which is assumed, by Eysenck and Spence, respectively, to condition poorly.

Since Sokolov (1963) claims that OR maintenance is critical during the establishment of the CR, it is at least a possibility that the poor conditioning performance from both high extraverts and Ss low on the MAS is due to rapid OR habituation from the high E:low N Ss.

This, of course, is speculative. The present findings simply confirm that EPI extraversion and, to a lesser extent, neuroticism, relate to OR habituation rate, which is a prime index of the neo-Pavlovian property of higher nervous activity, dynamism of inhibition, and that neuroticism, and to a lesser degree, extraversion, relate to initial OR amplitude, which appears to involve dynamism of excitation, in its relation to dynamism of inhibition.

REFERENCES

BERRY, J. L., AND MARTIN, B. GSR reactivity as a function of anxiety, sex and instructions. *Journal Abnormal and Social Psychology*, 1957, **54**, 9-12.

DYKMAN, R. A., REESE, W. G., GALBRECHT, C. R., AND THOMASSON, P. J. Psychophysiological reactions to novel stimuli: measurement, adaptation, and relationship of psychological and physiological variables in the normal human. *Annals of the New York Academy Sciences*, 1959, **79**, 43-107.

EYSENCK, H. J. *The dynamics of anxiety and hysteria*. London: Routledge and Kegan Paul, 1957.

EYSENCK, H. J. Conditioning, introversion, extraversion and the strength of the nervous system. In V. D. Nebylitsyn (Organizer), Sympos. 9, *Physiological bases of individual psychological differences*. 18th Int. Congr. Psychol., Moscow: 1966. Pp. 33-44.

EYSENCK, H. J., AND EYSENCK, S. B. G. *Manual of the Eysenck Personality Inventory*. London: University of London Press, 1964.

FRANKS, C. M. Conditioning and personality: A study of normal and neurotic subjects. *Journal Abnormal and Social Psychology* 1956, **2**, 143-150.

FRANKS, C. M. Personality factors and the rate of conditioning. *British Journal of Psychology*, 1957, **48**, 119-126.

GALBRECHT, C. R., DYKMAN, R. A., REESE, W. G., AND SUZUKI, T. Intrasession adaptation and intersession extinction of the components of the orienting response. *Journal of Experimental Psychology*, 1965, **70**, 585-597.

GRANGER, G. W. Night vision and psychiatric disorders. Cited by J. A. Gray, Strength of the nervous system, introversion-extraversion, conditionability and arousal. *Behaviour Research and Therapy*, 1967, **5**, 151–169.

JENSEN, A. R. The Maudsley Personality Inventory. *Acta Psychologica*, 1958, **14**, 314–325.

KIMMEL, H. D., AND KIMMEL, E. Sex differences in adaptation of the GSR under repeated applications of a visual stimulus. *Journal of Experimental Psychology*, 1965, **70**, 536–537.

KOEPKE, J. E., AND PRIBRAM, K. H. Habituation of GSR as a function of stimulus duration and spontaneous activity. *Journal of Comparative and Physiological Psychology*, 1966, **61**, 442–443.

LACEY, J. I. The evaluation of autonomic responses: Toward a general solution. *Annals of New York Academy Sciences*, 1956, **67**, 123–164.

LADER, M. H., AND WING, L. Physiological measures, sedative drugs, and morbid anxiety. *Maudsley Monographs*, 1966, No. 14, London: Oxford University Press.

LOVIBOND, J. H. Conceptual thinking, personality and conditioning. *British Journal of Social and Clinical Psychology*, 1963, **2**, 100–111.

MALTZMAN, I., AND RASKIN, D. C. Effects of individual differences in the orienting reflex on conditioning and complex processes. *Journal of Experimental Research in Personality*, 1965, **1**, 1–16.

MARTIN, I. The effects of drugs on palmar skin resistance and adaptation. In H. J. Eysenck (Ed.), *Experiments in personality*. Vol. 1, Psychogenetics and psychopharmacology. London: Routledge and Kegan Paul, 1960.

MARTON, M., AND URBAN, IA. An electroencephalographic investigation of individual differences in the processes of conditioning. In V. D. Nebylitsyn (Organizer), Sympos. 9, *Physiological bases of individual psychological differences*. 18th Int. Congr. Psychol., Moscow: 1966. Pp. 106–109.

MONTAGUE, J. D., AND COLES, E. M. Mechanism and measurement of the galvanic skin response. *Psychology Bulletin*, 1966, **65**, 261–279.

MUNDY-CASTLE, A. C., AND McKIEVER, B. Z. The psychophysiological significance of the GSR. *Journal of Experimental Psychology*, 1953, **46**, 15–24.

NEBYLITSYN, V. D. *Osnovniye svoistva nervnoi systemi cheloveka*. (Basic properties of the human nervous system.) Moscow: Akademiya Pedagogicheskikh Nauk RSFSR, 1966. Unpublished English translation by M. Kravchenko, University of Queensland, 1968.

PAVLOV, I. P. *Polnoye sobraniye sochinyenii*. (Complete selected works.) Moscow: 1951–1952. Akademi Nauk SSSR. Cited by V. D. Nebylitsyn,

Osnovniye svoistva nervnoi systemi cheloveka. (Basic properties of the human nervous system.) Moscow: Akademiya Pedagogicheskikh Nauk RSFSR, 1966. Unpublished English translation by M. Kravchenko, University of Queensland, 1968.

ROZHDESTVENSKAYA, V. I. Determining the equilibrium of the fundamental nervous processes by the plethysmograph method. *In* B. M. Teplov (Ed.), *Tipologicheskiye osobennosti vysshei deyatelnosti cheloveka*, Vol. 3, 1963. Cited by V. D. Nebylitsyn, *Osnovniye svoistva nervnoi systemi cheloveka*. (Basic properties of the human nervous system.) Moscow: Akademiya Pedagogicheskikh Nauk RSFSR, 1966. Unpublished English translation by M. Kravchenko, University of Queensland, 1968.

ROZHDESTVENSKAYA, V. I., NEBYLITSYN, V. D., BORISOVA, M. N., AND YERMOLAYEVA-TOMINA, L. B. A comparative study of a number of indices of the strength of the nervous system in man. *Voprosy psikhologii*, 1960, **5**, 41–56. Cited by V. D. Nebylitsyn, *Osnovniye svoistva nervnoi systemi cheloveka*. (Basic properties of the human nervous system.) Moscow: Akademiya Pedagogicheskikh Nauk RSFSR, 1966. Unpublished English translation by M. Kravchenko, University of Queensland, 1968.

SAMPSON, H., AND BINDRA, D. "Manifest" anxiety, neurotic anxiety and rate of conditioning. *Journal Abnormal and Social Psychology*, 1954, **49**, 256–259.

SIDDLE, D. A. T., MORRISH, R. B., WHITE, K. D., AND MANGAN, G. L. The relationship of sensitivity and reactivity of the nervous system to extraversion. *Journal of Experimental Research in Personality*, 1969, **3**, 264–267.

SOKOLOV, E. N. *Perception and the conditioned reflex*. Translated by S. W. Waydenfeld. Oxford: Pergamon, 1963.

SPENCE, K. W. Anxiety (drive) level and performance in eyelid conditioning. *Psychological Bulletin*, 1964, **61**, 129–139.

STEIN, L. Habituation and stimulus novelty: a model based on classical conditioning. *Psychological Review*, 1966, **73**, 352–356.

STEWART, M. A., STERN, J. S., WINOKUR, S., AND FREEDMAN, S. An analysis of GSR conditioning. *Psychological Review*, 1961, **68**, 60–67.

VENABLES, P. H., AND MARTIN, I. *A manual of psychophysiological methods*. Amsterdam: North Holland, 1967.

VINOGRADOVA, O. S. *Orientirovochny refleks i ego neirofisiologicheskie mekhanizmy*. (The orientation reflex and its neurophysiological mechanisms.) Moscow: Akademiya Pedagogicheskikh Nauk RSFSR, 1961. Cited by V. D. Nebylitsyn,

Osnovniye svoistva nervnoi systemi cheloveka. (Basic properties of the human nervous system.) Moscow: Akademiya Pedagogicheskikh Nauk RSFSR, 1966. Unpublished English translation by M. Kravchenko, University of Queensland, 1968.

VORONIN, L. G., SOKOLOV, E. N., AND BAO-KHUA, U. Type features of the orientation reflex in man. *Voprosy psikhologii,* 1959, **5,** 73–88. Cited by V. D. Nebylitsyn, *Osnovniye svoistva nervnoi systemi cheloveka.* (Basic properties of the human nervous system.) Moscow: Akademiya Pedagogicheskikh Nauk RSFSR, 1966. Unpublished English translation by M. Kravchenko, University of Queensland, 1968.

WHITE, K. D., MANGAN, G. L., MORRISH, R. B., AND SIDDLE, D. A. T. The relation of transmarginal inhibition to extraversion and neuroticism. *Journal of Experimental Research in Personality,* 1969, 3, 268–274.

WINER, B. J. *Statistical principles in experimental design.* New York: McGraw-Hill, 1962.

YERMOLAYEVA-TOMINA, L. B. On the question of the use of the psychogalvanic response index for determining nervous system type in man. *In* B. M. Teplov (Ed.), *Tipologicheskiye osobennosti vysshei nervnoi deyatelnosti cheloveka,* Vol. 3, 1963. Cited by V. D. Nebylitsyn, *Osnovniye svoistva nervnoi systemi cheloveka.* (Basic properties of the human nervous system.) Moscow: Akademiya Pedagogicheskikh Nauk RSFSR, 1966. Unpublished English translation by M. Kravchenko, University of Queensland, 1968.

From M. Zuckerman, T. Murtaugh and J. Siegel (1974). Psychophysiology, *11*, 535–542, *by kind permission of the authors and the Society for Psychophysiological Research*

Sensation Seeking and Cortical Augmenting-Reducing

Marvin Zuckerman, Thomas Murtaugh, and Jerome Siegel

University of Delaware

ABSTRACT

The experiment was designed to establish the relationship between the Sensation Seeking Scales (SSS) and cortical augmenting-reducing. Forty-nine male undergraduate Ss were used. Ss were presented with five intensities of light flashes in randomly presented blocks of trials at each intensity. Averaged evoked response (AER) amplitudes were measured at each intensity of light. Augmenting-reducing was measured for each S as the slope of the relationship between stimulus intensity and amplitude of response. This slope measure correlated very significantly ($r = .59$) with the Disinhibition subscale of the SSS and positively, but not significantly, with other subscales. Comparing the low and high scorers on the Disinhibition scale, a significant interaction between groups and stimulus intensities was found but no main effects of stimulus intensity or groups were found. The high Disinhibitors did not differ from the lows at the low stimulus intensities but did differ significantly at the highest intensity where the lows showed a marked reducing tendency. The results show an interesting convergence between the Disinhibition type of sensation seeking, manic tendencies, and the AER.

DESCRIPTORS: Sensation Seeking Scales, Augmenting-reducing, Average evoked response, EEG.

The original Sensation Seeking Scale (SSS; Zuckerman, Kolin, Price, & Zoob, 1964) was developed as an attempt to measure individual differences in a hypothetical (Zuckerman, 1969) "optimal level of stimulation" and "optimal level of arousal." This first scale (called the "General" scale) of sensation seeking showed promising construct validity, and indicated that sensation seeking might be a trait underlying other traits such as changeableness, autonomy, exhibitionism, and field independence (Zuckerman & Link, 1968). Since the latter study indicated that sensation seeking might be multidimensional, factor analyses were done on an expanded questionnaire, and four new factor scales added to the General SSS (Zuckerman, 1971). The scales of the new form (IV) of the SSS have been related to personality traits measured by the Minnesota Multiphasic Personality Inventory (MMPI) and 16 Personality Factor (PF) tests, variety of sex and drug experience, use of alcohol, preferences for complexity in designs, and openness to experience (Zuckerman, Bone, Neary, Mangelsdorff, & Brustman, 1972). A summary of research on the SSS can be obtained in a mimeographed manual.[1]

Several years ago the senior author's research focused on a search for a

This research was supported by a grant from the University of Delaware Research Foundation.

The authors are indebted to Dr. Monte Buchsbaum for his freely given and generous assistance in advising us on the methods and procedures of the basic experiment.

Address requests for reprints to: Dr. Marvin Zuckerman, Department of Psychology, University of Delaware, Newark, Delaware 19711.

[1]The manual may be obtained by writing to the senior author, same address as for reprints.

possible biological basis for the sensation seeking motive. A study was done on habituation of the electrodermal orienting reflex (OR) (Zuckerman, 1972). High scoring Ss on the General SSS had greater ORs than lows on initial stimulus presentations, but habituated to the level of the lows by the second stimulus presentations. Recently Neary and Zuckerman (1973) extended these findings from visual to auditory stimulation. These results suggested that high sensation seekers are hyperarousable in response to novel stimulation and suggested that sensation seekers have a high balance of excitatory over inhibitory processes in the CNS.

In 1971 Buchsbaum published a note in *Science* suggesting a relationship between sensation seeking and cortical augmenting-reducing as measured by the amplitude of the average evoked response (AER) to increasing intensities of visual stimulation. Buchsbaum had tested college students on the SSS and found tendencies for high scorers to be augmenters (increasing amplitude of AER with increasing stimulus intensity) while low scorers tended to be reducers (decreasing amplitudes with increasing intensities). The basic AER intensity experiment is described in Buchsbaum and Pfefferbaum (1971). Buchsbaum, Goodwin, Murphy, & Borge (1971) have also reported that manic patients are generally augmenters while depressed patients are reducers. Lithium, a drug which tends to reduce manic episodes, also reduces the augmenting pattern in manics.

These results were of great interest because they suggested a more direct test, than the OR provided, of the hypothesis of an excitable CNS underlying sensation seeking. Buchsbaum's findings on manic patients were also interesting because the Hypomania scale of the MMPI has been the one most consistently correlated with the SSS in college students (Zuckerman et al., 1972), psychiatric offenders (Blackburn, 1969), and male felons and female delinquents (Thorne, 1971). The behavior of manics typically looks like sensation seeking out of control; their optimal levels of stimulation are extraordinarily high.

The present study was an attempt to: (1) test the relationship between sensation seeking and cortical augmenting-reducing with a new sample of college students and slightly changed procedures, (2) compare the SS scales in the magnitudes of their relationship with augmenting-reducing, (3) to test the relationship between other personality variables (extraversion and neuroticism, and state anxiety) and augmenting-reducing. Extraversion was used because Eysenck (1967) has suggested that central neural excitation-inhibition characteristics may underlie this dimension of personality. State anxiety was used because prior work on the OR (Neary & Zuckerman, 1973) showed that state anxiety (but not trait anxiety) was related to the magnitude of the initial OR.

Method

Subjects

Sixty-five male undergraduate students in an introductory psychology course were selected from a subject pool pretested on the SSS. The subjects (Ss) were selected and processed in two groups. In the first group of 21 Ss, all males in the pool at that time were employed. With the second group of 44 Ss, some initial attempt was made to select them from the extremes of the distribution of the Disinhibition subscale. However, this attempt was abandoned due to scheduling priorities, and the distribution of Ss finally drawn was essentially normal and did not differ in mean or variance from the normative group.

Of the 65 Ss selected, 2 declined to participate when informed of the nature of the experiment; 2 Ss were eliminated when questioning revealed a history of epilepsy; 2 Ss were terminated prematurely after experiencing adverse effects during the recording session; 6 Ss did not yield adequate records as a function of equipment malfunction; and 4 Ss were subsequently discarded when their records did not meet scoring criteria. The remaining 49 Ss provided the data for statistical analysis. The ages of these Ss ranged from 17 to 35, with a median age of 19.

Pre-Recording Procedure

Upon keeping his appointment, each S was shown the experimental apparatus and told that an attempt would be made to record his brain waves while being shown flashing lights. He was then asked a series of questions to detect any use of drugs or medications, as well as any history of epilepsy. The S was brought into an isolation chamber (Industrial Acoustics Corporation) and seated in a comfortable chair which had been fitted with a headrest designed to both restrict head movement after electrode placement, and maintain a distance of 50 cm between the head and the stimulus screen. Prior to electrode placement, each S was given the "Today" form of the Multiple Affect Adjective Check List (MAACL, Zuckerman & Lubin, 1965). Electrodes were attached and the polygraph recording was calibrated. Ss were then asked to blink and grimace in order to obtain a standard for detection of these artifacts in the recording period. Each S was asked to relax, fixate at a midpoint on the stimulus screen, and refrain from blinking.

Recording Procedure

The S's EEG was recorded, using silver disk electrodes, between vertex and left ear with forehead as ground. A Grass Model 7 polygraph with P5 amplifiers was used. The amplifier filters were set for a low frequency cut off at 0.3 Hz and a high frequency cut off at 500 Hz. The manufacturer's specifications give a 50% roll off at 0.3 Hz (the low end) and 500 Hz (the high end). The amplifier response is flat between 1 Hz and 125 Hz. Data were recorded on a 7 channel Sanborn FM tape recorder, Model 3917B, and averaged by a Nuclear Chicago Data Retrieval Computer, Model 7100, using 400 data points over a 500 msec analysis interval. A Moseley, Model 7590, X-Y point plotter recorded the curves for measurement.

Flash stimuli of 10 μsec duration were generated by a Grass PS2 Photostimulator. Five intensities of light flashes were randomly presented to the S in blocks containing 30 flashes of the same intensity. The interstimulus interval was 1 sec and the interblock interval was 6 sec. Each intensity of Grass photostimulator settings, 1, 2, 4, 8, and 16, was presented 120 times. Light intensity measured through the use of a photomultiplier yielded the following light intensity values at 52 cm from the screen: Joules/cm² per pulse at stimulus intensity settings, $1 = .08, 2 = .12, 4 = .17, 8 = .20, 16 = .25$.

Flashes were presented to open-eyed Ss through a transilluminated diffusion screen. The screen consisted of ⅛ in. window glass, 61 cm high by 102 cm wide, which had been frosted by four coats of silica spray. The flash tube and housing were sound attenuated within a cardboard enclosure packed with fiberglass and sealed in front with a 6 mm thick sheet of plexiglass, but some

click sound was audible. However, in recordings obtained under the same
conditions with the light stimulus masked, no time locked potentials were
recorded. During the recording session, the isolation chamber was darkened.
Immediately following the session, the S was given an Eysenck Extraversion-Introversion scale, an open-ended questionnaire, and subsequently
debriefed.

Scoring Procedure

AER amplitudes were measured, as described by Buchsbaum and
Pfefferbaum (1971), generally from a positive peak at 70–100 msec (P1) to a
negative peak at 90–150 msec (N1). An attempt was made to maintain the
criteria for both P1 and N1 within a range of 5 msec for each S across
intensities. Additionally, all records were required to demonstrate the P1–N1
phenomena through at least four of the five intensity levels. The location of the
positive peak varied somewhat between Ss. The mean locus of peaks was 88
msec; the peaks fell between 75 and 100 msec for 76% of the Ss, between 80
and 95 msec for 53% of the Ss, and between 85 and 89 msec for 27% (the
mode). A blind scoring procedure was employed (the SSS scores were unknown
while the AER records were being scored). A measure of the relative rate of
AER amplitude increase with increasing stimulus intensity was obtained for
each S by fitting a straight line to amplitude measurements at each of the
intensity levels, using least square techniques. Slopes were calculated through 4
of the 5 points if a peak could not be identified at one of the intensity levels.

Results

Table 1 gives the mean standard scores and standard deviations of the
sample of 49 Ss on the SS scales. None of these differ significantly from the
normative sample of 686 males, also drawn from Introductory Psychology
classes at the University of Delaware.

Table 1 shows the correlations between the personality and state anxiety
variables and the individual slopes of the amplitude-intensity relationships.
Only one of these 8 correlations was significant. However the magnitude of the
correlation between the Disinhibition scale and augmenting ($r = .59$, $p < .00005$,
one-tailed) argues against this being a chance relationship.

Table 1 also shows previously obtained correlations (study II a, Zuckerman
et al., 1972) between the SSS subscales and the Hypomania scale of the MMPI
in 60 male college students. Although the differences between most of the
correlations are small it is interesting to observe that the SSS subscales correlate
(rho = 1.0) with augmenting in direct order of their correlation with the MMPI
Hypomania scale; Disinhibition being most highly correlated with both augmenting and Hypomania, and Thrill and Adventure Seeking being least correlated with either augmenting or Hypomania.

In order to compare the amplitudes of high and low Disinhibition in interaction with stimulus intensities it was necessary to exclude Ss with peaks
absent at one of the stimulus intensities. The group was divided in half on the
basis of Disinhibition scores. Eight Ss fell at the median (48) of the distribution
on Disinhibition so these Ss were also discarded for this analysis; 4 of the 8 had
already been discarded because of a missing peak at one stimulus intensity.
This left 14 lows (Dis scores 33–45) and 14 highs (Dis scores 51–69).

Fig. 1 shows the mean AER amplitudes for low and high Disinhibitors at
each level of stimulus intensity. The augmenting pattern of the highs is appar-

ent in their increasing amplitude of response, with only a slight reversal at intensity 8. The lows began reducing after 2 with a sharp reduction going from 8 to 16.

An analysis of variance (Winer, 1962, p. 302) was done on these data with high vs low Disinhibition as the between groups source of variance, and stimulus intensities and the groups by intensities as the within Ss sources of variance. The results are presented in Table 2. The interaction between Disinhibition groups and stimulus intensities was significant, the main effects were not significant. Further analyses were done to analyze the interaction.

T tests were performed between low and high Disinhibitors at each stimulus

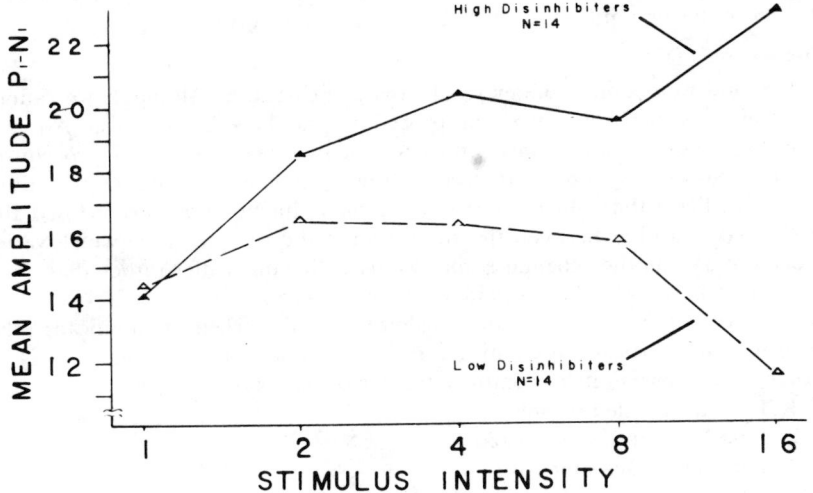

Fig. 1. Mean AER amplitudes* for low and high Disinhibition scorers at each level of stimulus intensity.

*Amplitudes are in arbitrary mm deflection units. Each mm unit =.42 μV.

TABLE 1

Augmenting-reducing and hypomania vs SS scales, EPI scales, and MAACL anxiety scale

Scales	$\bar{X}^a$	SD	r with slope (Aug.-Red.)	r with MMPI Hypomania[b]
General	50.5	10.1	.23	.30*
Thrill & Adventure Seeking	49.6	11.0	.08	.04
Experience Seeking	50.2	9.8	.23	.26*
Disinhibition	48.3	9.3	.59***	.43**
Boredom Susceptibility	49.8	11.5	.16	.18
EPI:Extraversion	50.5	8.9	.10	—
EPI:Neuroticism	48.4	8.1	.10	—
MAACL State Anxiety	52.3	10.0	.16	—

[a]Standard T scores of this sample, Normative Group means = 50, SDs = 10.
[b]From Zuckerman et al., 1972, Ss = 60 undergraduate males.
*$p < .05$, **$p < .001$, ***$p < .0001$.

TABLE 2

Analysis of variance on amplitudes of response

Source	df	MS	F
Groups (Disinhibition)	1	568	< 1
Within Groups	26	713	
Stimulus Intensities (SI)	4	71	1.79
Interaction (Dis × SI)	4	112	2.83*
SI × Ss Within Groups	104	40	

*$p < .05$.

intensity. The difference between groups was significant only at the highest stimulus intensity (16). Analyses of variance were performed between stimulus intensities within each of the groups. The differences between intensities were significant within the high Disinhibitor group (F (5/14) = 2.63, $p < .05$) but not significant within the low group.

A possibility existed that the marked difference between high and low Disinhibitors at the highest stimulus intensity was due to excessive blinking or squinting by the lows, in contrast to the highs. The EEG records of lows and highs were checked for indications of these phenomena. The incidence was almost exactly the same in both groups, and statistically insignificant. It would therefore appear that these types of reactions cannot account for the augmenting and reducing tendencies which differentiated the groups.

Discussion

Why did we obtain stronger results than Buchsbaum? Although we cannot be positive, certain changes in the procedure may have been crucial. An eyes open procedure was used in contrast to Buchsbaum's eyes closed procedure. Since reducing is most likely to occur at the highest intensities, our procedure was more likely than Buchsbaum's to reveal reducing. With eyes closed the eyelid acts as a filter between the stimulus and the receptor (one which varies from S to S). Another change is that we used five intensities rather than four which may have yielded more reliable slope measures.

Since Disinhibition was the only scale to show a marked or significant relationship with cortical augmenting-reducing a description of this scale is in order. The following items comprise this factor scale[2]:

1. I like to gamble for money.
2. I like "wild" uninhibited parties.
3. I enjoy the companies of real "swingers."
4. I often like to get high (drinking liquor or smoking marijuana).
5. It's normal to get bored after a time with the same sexual partner.
6. Most adultery happens because of sheer boredom.
7. I like to date members of the opposite sex who are physically exciting.
8. Keeping the drinks full is the key to a good party.
9. A person should have considerable sexual experience before marriage.
10. I could conceive of myself seeking pleasures around the world with the "jet set."
11. I like people who are sharp and witty even if they do sometimes insult others.
12. Almost everything enjoyable is illegal or immoral.
13. I enjoy watching many of the "sexy" scenes in movies.
14. I feel best after taking a couple of drinks.

A perusal of these items indicates why the scale was called "Disinhibition." In males its highest correlations with the MMPI are with the Hypomania and Psychopathic Deviate scales (Zuckerman et al., 1972). It correlates highly ($r = .60$) with the Surgency scale of the 16 PF test and negatively with the Super-Ego and Controlled scales of that test. It correlates significantly with alcohol use in both males and females but does not correlate with drug use in males. It correlates with variety of sexual experience in both males and females.

[2]The SSS uses a forced choice item with a choice between a sensation seeking and a sensation reducing response. Only the sensation seeking options are reproduced here.

The Disinhibitor seems to be a person who uses alcohol as a disinhibitor of sexual and social inhibitions rather than as a tranquilizer. He pursues a hedonistic philosophy, and shows psychopathic tendencies in his lack of guilt or control. He enjoys others for their stimulating qualities rather than for their reliability or stability.

Like Buchsbaum and Pfefferbaum (1971) the present study shows that reducing occurs at the highest stimulus intensities and probably reflects some kind of central inhibitory mechanism. The absence of such a protective function in the high Disinhibitors corresponds to an absence of effective inhibition in their behavior. The reduction of inhibition may be a threatening state to some, but it is a desirable state for Disinhibitors. The data suggest that the behavior tendency may rest on a characteristic of the nervous system. This characteristic may be what Pavlov, in an early classification, called the "Equilibrium" of the CNS (Gray, 1964). Equilibrium was considered as the balance between the excitatory and inhibitory processes of the CNS. Another possibility is that the phenomena may correspond to what Teplov (1964) called the "Strength" dimension. This dimension is defined as the capacity of the cortical cells to endure stimulation which is extreme in duration or intensity. A strong nervous system can endure intense stimulation; a weak one generates what Pavlov termed "transmarginal inhibition." The concept of equilibrium suggests that the reducing tendency stems from inhibition from some other area of the nervous system than the one being stimulated. The concept of strength seems to assume that the dampening of response stems from some kind of neural exhaustion in the cortical areas stimulated.

An explanation of the data in more conventional Western neurophysiological terms is based on findings of cortical-subcortical homeostatic relationships. Subcortical structures involved in regulating the levels of arousal have been shown to modulate cortical neural activity (Moruzzi & Magoun, 1949; Knispel & Siegel, 1972, 1973). In addition, evidence is accumulating that corticofugal descending influences serve to regulate brainstem arousal systems. Koella and Ferry (1963) and Dell, Bonvallet, and Hugelin (1961), using different procedures, have demonstrated that the cortex can exert both phasic and tonic inhibitory influences upon the arousal system. These studies support the position that a reticulo-cortico-reticular negative feedback loop regulates and maintains the level of arousal at an optimal set point or range. An additional inference about the significance of such a mechanism is that it also serves to prevent a cortical overload to excessive stimulation.

This feedback mechanism may in fact be the neuronal basis for the Pavlovian concept of an equilibrium between excitatory and inhibitory processes. Comparable empirical support at the neural level for the Russian hypothetical concept of strong and weak nervous systems is much more tenuous. The data that do exist on this are summarized by Nebylitsyn (1972, pp. 131–142).

In terms of the findings reported here, it is hypothesized that individuals lie along a dimension of excitatory-inhibitory equilibrium set-points; i.e., people differ as to the level of reticulo-cortical (excitatory) activation which will trigger the corticofugal (inhibitory) feedback necessary to dampen and control further reticular arousal. Subjects who show decreasing evoked potential amplitudes with increasing flash intensities (the reducers), according to this view, possess a low threshold for initiation of the corticofugal inhibitory process. Thus, at stimulation intensities above this point, increasing levels of stimulation produce increasing cortical inhibitory influences which regulate the arousal level to a given set point and insulate the individual from sensory overload. The augmenters are individuals who possess a neural set point which permits them to accept and process higher levels of stimulation before their cortico-reticular inhibitory threshold is reached.

This set point or threshold level may be a basic property of the nervous system and thus determine the dimension of personality which is measured by the SSS. Individuals who score low on the Disinhibition scale of SS may possess a neural process which effectively buffers them from moderate to high levels of stimulation. People who score high on the Disinhibition scale may have a nervous system with a regulatory threshold level set to permit high levels of sensory input.

REFERENCES

Blackburn, R. Sensation seeking, impulsivity, and psychopathic personality. *Journal of Consulting & Clinical Psychology*, 1969, *33*, 571–574.

Buchsbaum, M. Neural events and the psychophysical law. *Science*, 1971, *172*, 502.

Buchsbaum, M., Goodwin, F., Murphy, D., & Borge, G. AER in affective disorders. *American Journal of Psychiatry*, 1971, *128*, 51–57.

Buchsbaum, M., & Pfefferbaum, A. Individual differences in stimulus intensity response. *Psychophysiology*, 1971, *8*, 612–622.

Dell, P., Bonvallet, M., & Hugelin, A. Mechanisms of reticular deactivation. In G. E. W. Wolstenholme & M. O'Connor (Eds.), *The nature of sleep*. London: Churchill, 1961. Pp. 86–107.

Eysenck, H. J. *The biological basis of personality*. Springfield, Illinois: Charles C Thomas, 1967.

Gray, J. A. *Pavlov's typology*. New York: The MacMillan Co., 1964.

Knispel, J. D., & Siegel, J. Tegmental stimulation: Aversive effects on behavior and modulation of visual evoked potentials. *Brain Research*, 1972, *37*, 317–321.

Knispel, J. D., & Siegel, J. Habituation of aversive reticular stimulation effects on evoked potentials. *Brain Research*, 1973, *56*, 340–344.

Koella, W. P., & Ferry, A. Cortico-subcortical homeostasis in the cat's brain. *Science*, 1963, *142*, 586–589.

Moruzzi, G., & Magoun, H. W. Brain stem reticular formation and activation of EEG. *Electroencephalography & Clinical Neurophysiology*, 1949, *1*, 445–473.

Neary, R. S., & Zuckerman, M. Sensation seeking, trait and state anxiety and the electrodermal orienting reflex. *Psychophysiology*, 1973, *10*, 211. (Abstract)

Nebylitsyn, V. D. *Fundamental properties of the human nervous system*. New York: Plenum Press, 1972.

Teplov, E. M. Problems in the study of general types of higher nervous activity in man and animals. In J. A. Gray (Ed.), *Pavlov's typology*. New York: MacMillan Co., 1964. Pp. 3–156.

Thorne, G. L. The sensation-seeking scale with deviant populations. *Journal of Consulting & Clinical Psychology*, 1971, *37*, 106–110.

Winer, B. J. *Statistical principles in experimental design*. New York: McGraw-Hill Book Co., 1962.

Zuckerman, M. Theoretical formulations: I. In J. P. Zubek (Ed.), *Sensory deprivation: Fifteen years of research*. New York: Appleton-Century-Crofts, 1969. Pp. 407–432.

Zuckerman, M. Dimensions of sensation seeking. *Journal of Consulting & Clinical Psychology*, 1971, *36*, 45–52.

Zuckerman, M. Sensation seeking and habituation of the electrodermal orienting response. *Psychophysiology*, 1972, *9*, 267–268. (Abstract)

Zuckerman, M., Bone, R. N., Neary, R., Mangelsdorff, D., & Brustman, B. What is the sensation seeker? Personality trait and experience correlates of the sensation seeking scales. *Journal of Consulting & Clinical Psychology*, 1972, *39*, 308–321.

Zuckerman, M., Kolin, E. A., Price, L., & Zoob, I. Development of a Sensation-Seeking Scale. *Journal of Consulting Psychology*, 1964, *28*, 477–482.

Zuckerman, M., & Link, K. Construct validity for the Sensation Seeking Scale. *Journal of Consulting & Clinical Psychology*, 1968, *32*, 420–426.

Zuckerman, M., & Lubin, B. *Manual for the Multiple Affect Adjective Check List (MAACL)*. San Diego, Calif.: Educational & Industrial Testing Service, 1965.

From S. B. G. Eysenck and H. J. Eysenck (1967). Perceptual and Motor Skills, *24,* 1047–1053, *by kind permission of the authors and Southern Universities Press*

SALIVARY RESPONSE TO LEMON JUICE AS A MEASURE OF INTROVERSION

SYBIL B. G. EYSENCK AND H. J. EYSENCK[1]

Institute of Psychiatry, University of London

Summary.—50 men and 50 women were administered the EPI and tested with respect to the increment in salivation produced by putting 4 drops of pure lemon juice on the tongue for 20 sec. It was found that in both groups introversion correlated approximately 0.7 with increase in salivation; there was no correlation with neuroticism. When a commercial product was substituted for pure lemon juice, all correlations became insignificant, possibly due to the weaker concentration of the product. The results are explained (and were predicted) in terms of an hypothesis relating introversion to cortical arousal.

The hypothesis has been put forward (Eysenck, 1963, 1964, 1967) that introverts are characterized by a state of higher cortical arousal; it appears that there is both direct evidence, e.g., from EEG studies (Savage, 1964; Marton & Urban, 1966) and indirect evidence (Eysenck, 1967) to support this notion. One deduction from such an hypothesis would lead one to expect that under conditions of equal stimulation effector output would be greater for introverts than extraverts. Several studies have in fact verified this deduction, among them an experiment by Corcoran (1964) in which he showed that salivary output of introverts in response to stimulation by four drops of lemon juice placed on the tongue was significantly greater than salivary output by extraverts. This interesting study is suggestive rather than conclusive because of the small number of Ss employed (two groups of 11 and 12 Ss, respectively, were used) and because of the uncertain status of the personality inventory used (the Heron two-part personality measure). Furthermore, the correlations found (0.62 and 0.70 for the two groups, using Kendall's *tau* and Spearman's *rho,* respectively) are unusually high for physiological measures when correlated with personality variables. In addition, Corcoran failed to find any differences between introverts and extraverts when using citric acid instead of lemon juice, although this stimulant was as effective as lemon juice in promoting salivation. In view of all these possible criticisms it seemed desirable to repeat Corcoran's study with adequate numbers of Ss and with a more widely recognized measure of personality.

FIRST EXPERIMENT

Subjects

Fifty male and 50 female volunteers, paid for their services, constituted our sample; these Ss had come to the laboratory for the day in order to carry out a

[1]We are indebted to the Research Fund of The Maudsley and Bethlem Hospitals for the support of this investigation. We are also grateful to Mrs. N. Humphery for assistance with the testing.

variety of experimental studies and knew nothing about the purpose of this experiment. Ages ranged from 20 to 40, with the mean slightly below 30; most were employed (in the case of the men) or housewives (in the case of the women). Few were students. All had been given the EPI (Eysenck & Eysenck, 1964) routinely on entering the laboratory, and the tester did not at any time know the scores achieved. No measure of intelligence was given, but from previous testing of similar samples it was surmised that their IQ would have been around 110 on the average.

Procedure

The experimental procedure was adapted from that used by Corcoran. Standard cotton-wool dental swabs were used throughout. One of these was picked up with a pair of tweezers and placed on *S*'s sublingual salivary gland. It was removed after a period of 20 sec., placed in a class container and put aside. Another swab was then positioned, 4 drops of lemon juice dropped on *S*'s tongue, and the pad removed after 20 sec. and placed in another glass container. Both containers were then weighed with, and later without, the swabs inside, the difference constituting the score. The swabs were very uniform in weight, with a mean of .2134 gm. ($SD = .0001$ gm.).

Results

Mean salivation of the 100 *S*s in the experiment was 0.3091 gm. on the first trial, and 0.7541 gm. on the second trial, giving a mean difference score of 0.4450 gm. Extraversion and neuroticism scores were correlated with first trial salivation (without lemon), second trial salivation (with lemon), the difference between trials, i.e., additional salivation due to lemon juice and the ratio of first and second trial. The product-moment correlations are given in Table 1. It will be seen that men and women give very similar results, so that the combined correlations may be taken as representative. None of the correlations between salivation and N are significant, while all the relevant correlations with E are significant at the .001 level. Figures relating to the first trial indicate slightly greater salivation of the introverts; this may be due to the presence of the swab,

TABLE 1

PRODUCT-MOMENT CORRELATIONS BETWEEN E AND N AND AMONG FOUR SALIVATION SCORES

	E			N		
	Women	Men	Combined	Women	Men	Combined
First Trial	−.12	−.44†	−.24*	−.10	−.11	−.08
Second Trial	−.68‡	−.76‡	−.71‡	−.21	−.04	−.09
Difference	−.74‡	−.73‡	−.73‡	−.18	.00	−.06
Ratio	.44†	.62‡	.52‡	−.08	−.01	−.08

*$p < .05$.   †$p < .01$.   ‡$p < .001$.

SALIVATION TO LEMON AND INTROVERSION

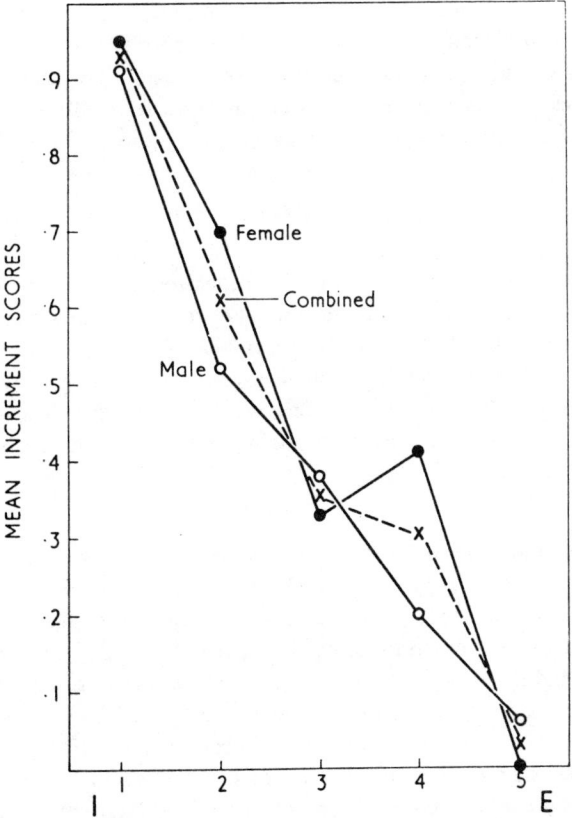

FIG. 1. Mean increase in salivation scores from Trial 1 to Trial 2 as a function of introversion-extraversion, for 50 males, 50 females, and the combined group

acting as an extra stimulus. The values for the second trial indicate that the presence of the lemon juice has stimulated introverts far more than extraverts. Correlations involving the difference between first and second trial are no higher than those involving the second trial alone; this suggests that the first trial might have been dispensed with. Ratios are less discriminative than are differences, or second-trial values by themselves; this is not surprising in view of the fact that first- and second-trial correlations are negative.

Inspection of the scatter plots failed to suggest any departure from linearity of regression. Fig. 1 shows the relation between extraversion and difference (mean increment) scores in diagrammatic form. The E scores for males and females separately were arranged in order and divided into 5 groups from low to high; these 5 groups were numbered from 1 to 5 and are shown on the abscissa. Their mean increment scores are shown on the ordinate. Male Group 1 was then combined with female Group 1, male Group 2 with female Group 2, and so forth up to male group and female Group 5; these constitute the combined groups in the figure. It will be seen that there is a very regular progression of incremental scores with greater introversion, and it will also be seen that sex differences are quite small; none were in fact statistically significant. Our results, therefore, are in good agreement with those reported by Corcoran (1964).

SECOND EXPERIMENT

Method

Corcoran (1964) reported high reliabilities for the test, although it is not clear from his paper whether these apply to first testing, second testing, or both. In any case, his Ss were small in number ($N = 11$). It seemed desirable to carry out another study to investigate the retest reliability of the procedure. Twenty-four Ss, similar in every way to those described in connection with the first experiment, were tested twice, with a period of exactly 24 hr. intervening.

Results

Product-moment correlations were calculated and gave the following results: for the first trial $r = 0.33$; for the second trial $r = 0.71$; for the mean difference scores, $r = 0.60$. These values are rather lower than those reported by Corcoran and are if anything rather lower than the correlations between salivation scores and E scores. It is possible that here, as often in the case of psychophysiological measures, repetition introduces new variables which make the value of retest reliability determinations suspect. On the first occasion Ss did not know that they were to be given lemon juice, so that its administration may have had some shock effect; on the second occasion they did, of course, know what was coming, and this knowledge might have some effect on their behaviour. One might postulate that repeated administration could have the effect of conditioning Ss to think of lemons and imagine the administration of lemon juice even on the first trial of the second administration; this might be the case particularly with introverted Ss who have been reported to form conditioned responses more easily (Eysenck, 1967).

For the sake of completeness another experiment concerned with reliability should be mentioned, although this was planned rather as a trial run for the study just described. Ss were largely members and students in the Department, and it seemed likely that their knowledge of the properties of lemon juice and in some cases the purpose of the experiment would make their responses more variable than might be the case with naive Ss. This proved to be the case; for 25 Ss the product-moment correlations were as follows: for the first trial $r = 0.48$; for the second trial $r = 0.50$; for the mean difference $r = 0.47$. All these values are significant at the $p < .02$ level, but, except for the first, they are lower than those of the other reliability study. It is, of course, not known whether the professional knowledge of many of these *S*s was indeed responsible for these low reliabilities, or whether some other source was influential; it seems clear that further work on repeated administration of the test, directed at disclosing some of the reasons for its low reliability, would be in order. At the same time, it must of course be realized that lack of high retest reliability in a test does not prevent reasonably high validity of that test on the occasion of its first administration. Validity cannot exceed reliability only when the repeated administration of the test does not involve new factors working against the recurrence of identical scores.

Third Experiment

Method

Corcoran (1964) failed to find any relationship with E scores when using citric acid instead of lemon juice, and it seemed desirable to discover whether other substances than fresh lemon juice would have similar effects, or whether the effect was rather specific. The experiment described at the beginning of the paper was therefore repeated twice more, on samples of 27 and 20 *S*s respectively, using a commercial preparation of lemon juice called "Jif," bottled in a plastic container resembling a lemon. This product consists entirely of pure lemon juice preserved with sulphur dioxide, 450 parts per million. The juice is of Mediterranean origin and appears subjectively weaker than the fresh juice used in Exps. 1 and 2, possibly because of dilution by the preservative.

Results

The two experiments with the "Jif" juice differed slightly one from the other. In the first, four drops were used and a 20-sec. period of measurement was retained; this experiment was an exact replica of the first (pure lemon) experiment. The product-moment correlation of the difference score with E was —0.02; none of the correlations of first or second trial with either E or N was significant. In the second experiment, 6 drops were used for a period of 30 sec., on the hypothesis that perhaps the "Jif" juice was weaker than fresh lemon juice and therefore had less effect. The correlation between difference score and E was again insignificant ($r = -.12$), as were all the other correlations with E and N. It does not seem that "Jif" juice produces the same effect as does fresh lemon juice, and in this respect it resembles citric acid. It is not at all clear why there should be such marked differences among substances superficially alike, at least as far as their taste and their salivation-instigating properties are concerned, and further work on the classification of such substances, and their relations with personality, is obviously required. Until this point is cleared up the value of the original hypothesis on which these studies were based must remain in some doubt.

Is the hypothesis tenable that perhaps the "Jif" juice was too weak to produce sufficient salivation to be effective? The mean increment in salivation (difference score) produced by the pure lemon juice was .4450 gm. for the 100 Ss of our first experiment; 4 drops of "Jif" on the tongue for 20 sec. produced .2372 gm. of saliva, and 6 drops of "Jif" on the tongue for 30 sec. produced .4354 gm. For the 20-sec. group the hypothesis of too weak a solution might thus be tenable; for the 30-sec. group the position is not altogether clear. *Total production* of saliva due to extra stimulation is equal to that of the pure lemon group, but *rate of production* of saliva is, of course, only ⅔ as great, as equal amounts are produced over a period 50% longer. If rate is the crucial variable, then weakness of the solution may be the correct explanation of our data. This explanation would not, however, apply to Corcoran's citric acid data, where salivation produced appears to have been just as strong over unit time as when pure lemon juice was used.

DISCUSSION

The data are too straightforward to require much discussion. Our results bear out Corcoran's findings and demonstrate that introverted Ss react more strongly with salivation to stimulation of the taste buds with pure lemon juice; they also tend to show a marked similarity of reaction in men and women, and a linear regression over the whole range of extraversion scores. The correlations are remarkably high, even higher than Corcoran's, possibly due to the fact that a better measure of extraversion was used in our studies. As our study was in many ways a replication of his (in fact a double replication, as we used two independent samples, one of men, the other of women), and as he replicated his original findings himself, there seems to be little doubt that the findings are not a chance effect but deserve to be taken seriously. As a personality measure this test has many obvious advantages; it is objective, quick, easy to perform, and has low visibility, in the sense that few Ss would guess the purpose of the procedure, which could be incorporated with medical checks or other procedures. Another advantage seems to be that it is quite independent of neuroticism and may thus be regarded as a relatively pure measure of extraversion-introversion.

It should perhaps be emphasized that the technique of administration of the test, although not difficult, has to be learned. Ss have to be taught to curl their tongues upward, so that the drops of lemon juice do not roll off; swallowing the juice during the experiment produces interesting effects (Eysenck & Eysenck, 1966) but ruins the measurement of personality. Care has to be taken to avoid mentioning the word "lemon" or leaving actual lemons visible in the room. A very accurate chemical weighing scale is required, and the routine of weighing practiced. Swabs have to be inserted accurately and quickly, and timing has to be accurate in spite of preoccupation with other activities, such as inserting the swab, etc. Utmost precision is required because of the very slight differences in weight with which one is dealing. Disturbing influences have to be kept to a minimum, as spatial inhibition (Eysenck, 1957) is very powerful in reducing salivary secretion (Eysenck & Yap, 1944). Care has to be taken that the swabs used are nearly identical in weight. It is only when all sources of error are carefully removed that experimental results can be replicated.

REFERENCES

CORCORAN, D. W. J. The relation between introversion and salivation. *American Journal of Psychology*, 1964, 77, 298-300.

EYSENCK, H. J. *The dynamics of anxiety and hysteria.* London: Routledge & Kegan Paul, 1957.

EYSENCK, H. J. The biological basis of personality. *Nature*, 1963, 199, 1031-1034.

EYSENCK, H. J. Biological factors in neurosis and crime. *Abhandlungen der Deutschen Akademie der Wissenschaften zu Berlin.* 1966, 2, 169-175.

EYSENCK, H. J. *The biological basis of personality.* Boston: Thomas, 1967.

EYSENCK, H. J., & EYSENCK, S. B. G. *Manual of the Eysenck Personality Inventory.* San Diego: Educational & Industrial Testing Service, 1964.

EYSENCK, H. J., & YAP, P. M. Parotid gland secretion in affective mental disorders. *Journal of Mental Science*, 1944, 90, 595-602.

EYSENCK, S. B. G., & EYSENCK, H. J. Physiological reactivity to sensory stimulation as a measure of personality. *Psychological Reports*, 1967, 20, 45-46.

MARTIN, M., & URBAN, I. An electroencephalographic investigation of individual differences in the processes of conditioning. In *Proceedings of 18th International Conference of Experimental Psychology*, 1966. Pp. 106-109.

SAVAGE, R. D. Electro-cerebral activity, extraversion and neuroticism. *British Journal of Psychiatry*, 1964, 110, 98-100.

Accepted April 24, 1967.

From M. J. F. Blake and D. W. J. Corcoran (1972). Aspects of Human Efficiency, 5, 261–272, *by kind permission of the authors and Hodder and Stoughton Limited*

Introversion-Extraversion and Circadian Rhythms

M. J. F. Blake, D. W. J. Corcoran
MRC Applied Psychology Unit, Cambridge

In a sudden fit of humour, Kleitman, in the 1939 version of 'Sleep and Wakefulness', commented that there are more marriages broken from incompatible temperatures than incompatible temperaments. He cannot have known at the time just how closely temperature and temperament might turn out to be linked. In the 1963 edition of the same book a longer and more sober treatment is made (p. 161) 'There are two distinct types of body temperature and efficiency curves with the peak reached early in the waking period in one and later in the other. In addition there are intermediate gradations between the extremes... There are advantages and disagvantages in being a morning or an evening person. Evening persons are likely to want to remain awake late at night when everyone goes to bed, and in turn they are inefficient during the early working hours of the day... The existence of distinct 'morning' and 'evening' types is also an everyday observation, among students particularly, some preferring to study late at night and sleep late in the morning, while others go to bed early and study early in the morning. As we were able to establish in some subjects, 'morning' people have their temperature peaks early in the day... and the opposite, of course, applies to 'evening' people'.

Most writers comment upon the very wide individual differences in the circadian rhythm, in terms of the biochemical, physiological and performance changes which are observed over the twenty-four hour period, as well as the ease with which the rhythms can be changed in some subjects compared to the difficulty experienced with others. It is, of course, one thing to appraise (or complain of) the wide variability from experiments, and quite another to relate such variation in data to some independent measure of personality. This paper summarises work which has succeeded in doing just this. The external measure which has been found to discriminate morning people from evening people is a scale of introversion-extraversion. The one used in the majority of the experiments quoted here was the one developed by Heron (1956), although the Eysenck scales have also been used and yield equally valid results. The work we shall describe is not great in bulk, but we think it is important both from a theoretical and a practical standpoint.

EXPERIMENTAL STUDIES

The first clue that introversion-extraversion might be related to performance at different times of day emerged in data published by Colquhoun (1960). The

Blake and Corcoran

experiments were conducted upon a vigilance task not unlike industrial inspection. There were altogether seventeen groups of subjects tested, with six subjects per group. Several different experimental conditions were compared, and it so happened that some groups were tested during the morning and a comparable number in the afternoon.

The scores achieved by the individuals in each group were correlated with their scores of introversion on the Heron scale and the pattern of relationships shown in Table 1 emerged. Although each individual correlation was non-significant, since it was based on so few scores, the overall pattern of positive correlations during the morning and negative correlations in the afternoon and the change in relationship from pre to post lunch periods were found to be reliable at an acceptable level of confidence. Despite the satisfactory level of significance the possibility that introverts perform better than extraverts in the morning and extraverts better than introverts in the afternoon seemed at the time an unlikely phenomenon which clearly needed confirmation.

Table 1. *Values of 'tau' for 17 groups of subjects. From Colquhoun (1960).*

Combinations of Experimental Conditions

Time of Test	A	B	C	D	E	F	G	H	I	J
10 a.m.	+0.50	+0.69	0	+0.45	+0.55	+0.16	+0.41	+0.41	–	–
12.30 p.m.	–0.44	–	–	–	–	–	–	–	–0.33	–
3 p.m.	–0.50	–0.83	–0.50	0	+0.36	0	–	–	–	–0.36

Colquhoun and Corcoran (1964) used a concellation task previously employed by Corcoran (1962). This task, which consisted simply of cancelling out all the letters 'e' in a passage of prose, has been shown to correlate very highly with introversion. In the 1962 experiment the cancellation task was conducted under two different conditions of incentive. In the 'low motivation' condition subjects were requested simply to complete as much of the material as possible in 15 minutes: in the high motivation condition the experimenter commented from time to time on their achievement. Under low motivation speed of performance correlated highly with introversion but under high motivation the direction of the relationship was reversed (Fig. 1). So, both the change from morning to afternoon and the introduction of an incentive served to change the direction of the relationship between introversion-extraversion and performance. It was, therefore, confidently expected that if the 'time of day effect' was real it would be observable on the task of cancellation. Other considerations (Corcoran 1962) lead us to the expectation that the measure of performance which would be sensitive would be speed of performance rather than accuracy.

Initially, in the Colquhoun and Corcoran study two groups of subjects were tested. They were seated around a circular table (in sets of six at a time, either at 08.30 (morning group) or at 13.30 (afternoon group). A single experimenter simply handed out the sheets of prose and requested that the subjects read through the sheets crossing out every letter 'e' they could find as rapidly as possible, during the following 15 minutes. *No differences were evident between the groups either in terms of the overall levels of performance or in the extent*

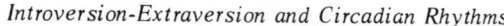
Introversion-Extraversion and Circadian Rhythms

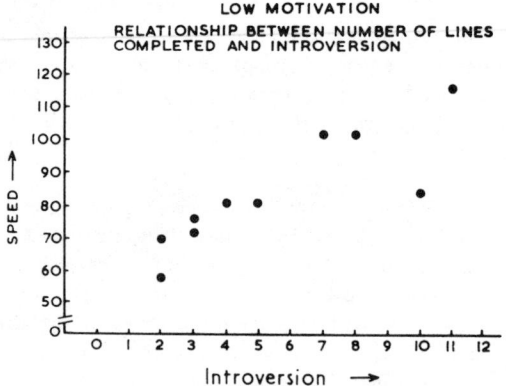

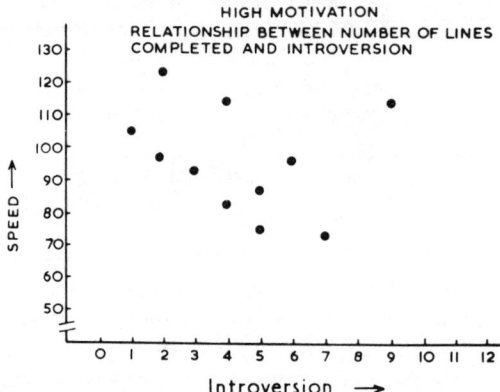

Figure 1. Relationships between introversion, motivational level, and performance.

to which the results correlated with introversion-extraversion score.

On examining the conditions under which these very disappointing results had been obtained, it became clear that the social situation itself might have influenced the results. Each subject had been able to see how well the others were doing, and since such 'knowledge of results' was well known to boost the performance of extraverts (Corcoran 1962, 1965) it could easily have been the case that during the morning extraverts worked considerably faster than they would have done if the subjects had been isolated.

Accordingly, two further groups of subjects were tested, but on this occasion each subject was seated in a room of his own, totally isolated from other subjects, and visited from time to time by one of the experimenters as he worked. This experiment yielded the expected results; in the morning group introverts completed more of the material than extraverts, whereas in the afternoon group there was no significant relationship between introversion and speed. It was

Blake and Corcoran

further observed that the performance of the extraverted members of the afternoon group was significantly higher than that of the morning extraverts, whereas the afternoon introverts performed at a lower level than the morning introverts (Fig. 2). *Clearly, to obtain a relationship between introversion and performance on this task it was necessary to test subjects in the morning and in
isolation.*

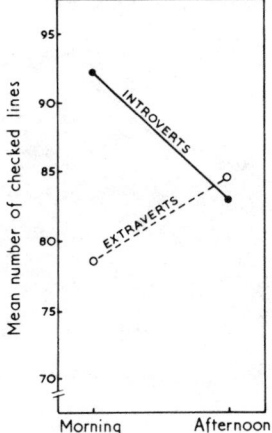

Figure 2. Mean output scores of introverts and extraverts on a letter cancellation task at different times of day in isolated testing conditions.
From Colquhoun and Corcoran (1964).

Pátkai (1969) selected two groups of subjects on the basis of a questionnaire
designed to discriminate those people who preferred to work in the morning
from those who were happier working in the evening. Various tasks were administered at different times of day and an analysis of adrenalin output was
also made. The inter-relationships between the tasks will not be discussed in
detail here, but it was found that reaction time performance related to preferred
time of day and to output of adrenalin at different times. The finding of primary
interest in the present context was that morning types were significantly more
introverted than afternoon types according to their scores on the Maudesley
Personality Inventory. This result, therefore, conforms well to the previous
findings of Colquhoun and Corcoran and is especially significant, since it
indicates that the previous findings were not limited to Naval Ratings tested
in Cambridge.

In an early study Blake (1967) measure the oral temperatures of extraverts and
introverts over the twenty-four hour period. The extravert group comprised
subjects with a score less than 4 on the Heron scale, and the introvert group
subjects with scores greater than 4. The differences in the two temperature
curves are striking (Fig. 3). Introverts appear to show a more rapid increase in
body temperature from 0400 hours for about ten hours until approximately 1400
hours. From 1400 to about 1900 there is no difference between the body tempera-

tures, but whereas the temperature of introverts tends to flatten between 1800 and 2000 hours that of extraverts continues to rise to reach a peak value at least an hour later than in introverts. Thereafter the two curves fall at identical rates, but the tenth of a degree difference evident at 2000 hours is maintained. until 0400 when the two curves converge. The major difference between the curves is therefore one of phase.

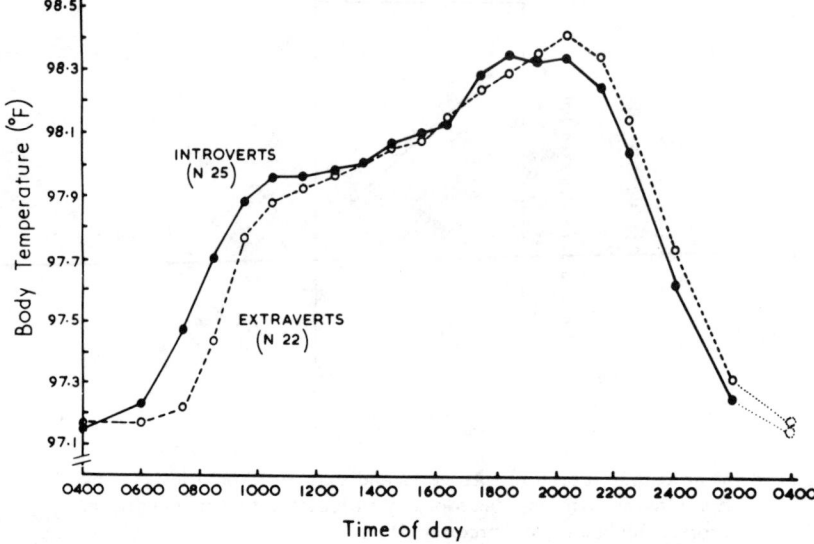

Figure 3. Circadian rhythm of body temperature in introverts and extraverts. From Blake (1967).

The experiments reported by Colquhoun and Corcoran had two major deficiences. One was that *different* groups of subjects were tested at the different times of day and the other was that no physiological index such as body temperature had been included in the experiment. Blake had reasoned that if the differences in circadian performance of introverts and extraverts were to be of practical value, they must be demonstrated upon the same group of subjects at the different times of day, and secondly, that if the explanation of the findings were to be expressed in terms of arousal levels (as was attempted in the Colquhoun and Corcoran paper) then an independent physiological measure should be incorporated.

Blake (1971) administered a wide variety of tasks at intervals throughout the working day, always taking temperatures before and after the task. The data shown in Fig. 4 are typical. Fig. 4(a) shows measures of the relative temperatures of the subjects used in the experiment. As in Fig. 3 introverts have the higher temperatures during the morning, little difference exists during the afternoon and extraverts have the higher evening temperatures. Performance at the cancellation task (Fig. 4(b)) follows much the same course as the temperature. Introverts begin the day with a greater output and end with a poorer level of performance. Although introverts appear in this figure to show less 'post-lunch' effect (see Hockey and Colquhoun's paper in this symposium) this is not a general finding. The extent of the post lunch dip is (to judge from other similar findings) unrelated to the personality difference.

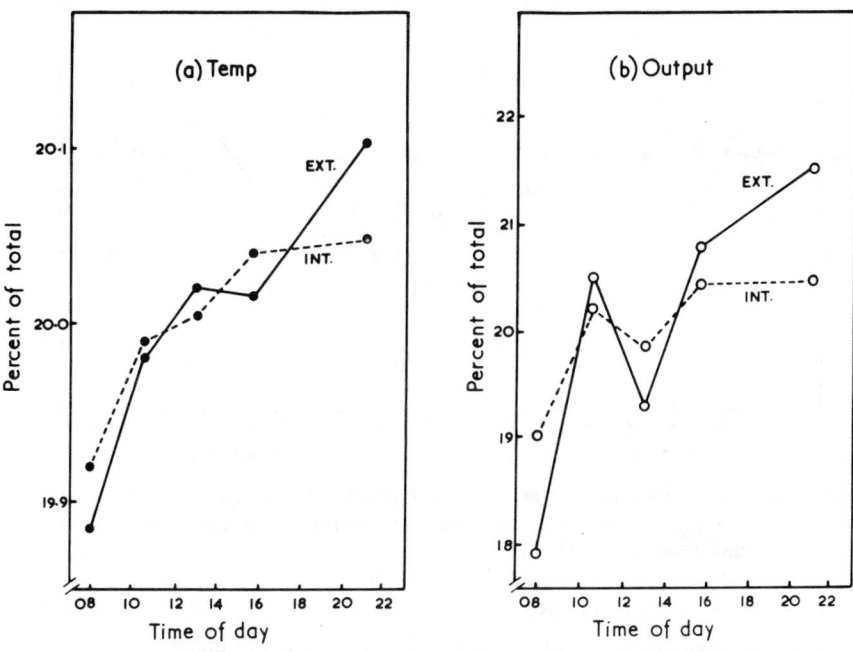

Figure 4. Within-day variations in measures of relative body temperature and cancellation output in introverts and extraverts. From Blake (1971).

Probably the most crucial of Blake's experiments, from a theoretical standpoint, involved the use of 'knowledge of results'. One of the earliest findings at the Applied Psychology Unit on the relation of introversion to performance was that extraverts improve their performance when they are given a continuous feedback of how well they are doing from the experimenter. This technique has been used largely on a serial reaction task, but had also been used in Corcoran's cancellation experiment, which we examined earlier. Blake fed knowledge of results to subjects doing the cancellation task at different times of day. The results are shown in Fig. 5. It can be seen in this Figure that knowledge of results benefits extraverts only in the morning (when their temperature is low relative to introverts). From about 1600 onwards the incentive is associated with a deterioration in the performance of extraverts. In fact the results suggest that extraverts are the more labile, in that they respond markedly to the incentive, but that his effect may be either beneficial or detrimental.

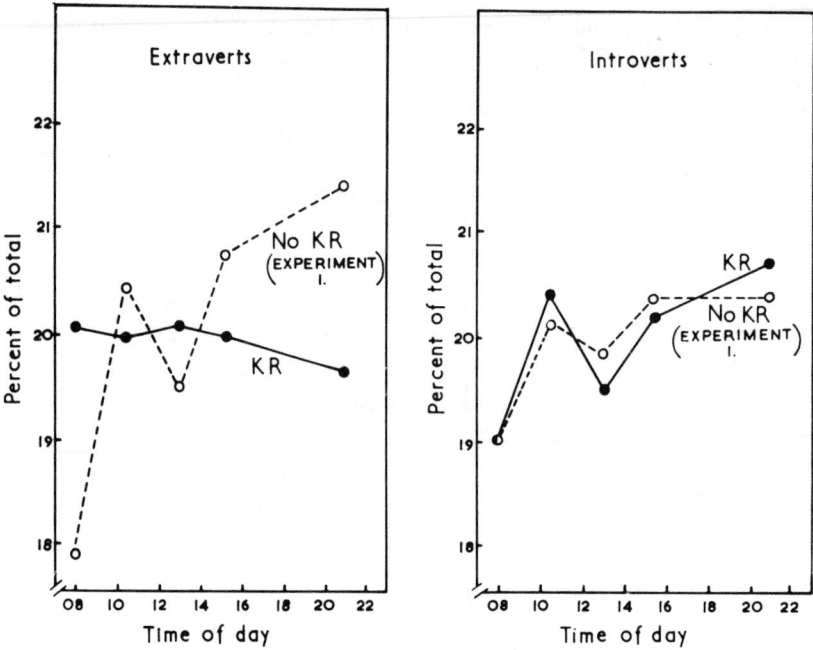

Figure 5. Effect of knowledge of results on measures of relative
cancellation output in introverts and extraverts at different times of
day. From Blake (1971).

THEORETICAL IMPLICATIONS

Perhaps the simplest theory which might be suggested to account for the time
of day differences in performance and body temperature between extraverts and
introverts, is a 'social' one. The extravert does on the whole conform to the
popular notion of a socialite. His answers to questionnaire items, if we can
believe them, certainly suggest that he enjoys parties and other social events.
During the normal working day there is certainly in the Navy ample opportunity
for social interaction, but during the evening one has the choice of being alone
or seeking further social stimulation. If one opts to socialise during the evening one necessarily expends more energy at this time and one tends to stay up
later than one would do if one stayed at home. Assuming that in the normal
course of events rhythms will exist, and that all that can be tampered with is
the *phase* of the rhythm, it follows that a person who tends to socialise in the
evenings will also tend to develop a later peak in his temperature rhythm than
one who does not. If he is an hour out·of phase with the non-socialite it will
take him about an hour more to reach his temperature peak during the day. Thus
the data illustrated in Fig. 3, which shows extraverts out of phase with introverts, can be easily explained by assuming (reasonably) that extraverts are
more sociable than introverts. In addition to explaining the temperature curves
the 'social' theory can also explain why introverts perform at a higher level

Blake and Corcoran

than extraverts in the morning and why the reverse holds in the evening. It cannot, however, account for the interaction between knowledge of results, time of day and extraversion. For example, if extraverts are simply livelier in the evening one might expect them to perform well when an additional incentive is added, but in fact they do not. In some manner evening liveliness is made *less* effective by increased incentive.

An alternative possibility is that the tendency for extraverts to enjoy a night life is not the *cause* of phase difference, but its *effect*. In other words the level of arousal of the extravert in the evening may make him more prone to go out, rather than engage in a more sedentary pursuit. If this latter interpretation is accepted, and it is also accepted that the time of day difference between introverts and extraverts is a primary biologically determined phenomenon, then the implication is that there exists, in introverts and extraverts, a difference in whatever mechanism it is that controls the *rate* of awakening during the early part of the day. But the exact nature of this difference is a matter of conjecture.

Colquhoun and Corcoran (1964) ventured an explanation of their findings, which in the face of Blake's results is quite untenable. It was suggested that introverts were characterised by higher levels of arousal than extraverts *throughout the day*. At early times during the day introverts were assumed to arrive at an optimal level of arousal, say at IM in Fig. 6, and extraverts at this time to be at a somewhat lower level, say at EM. Later in the day, a general increase in arousal occurs and extraverts reach an optimal level, say at EA, but introverts become hyper-aroused, occupying the position on the arousal continuum at IA. Thus, the performance levels reached by the types change over from morning to afternoon. This explanation clearly fails to account for the cross-over in the temperature graphs (Fig. 3). Obviously it becomes a little awkward to explain why extraverts have higher body temperatures than introverts during the later

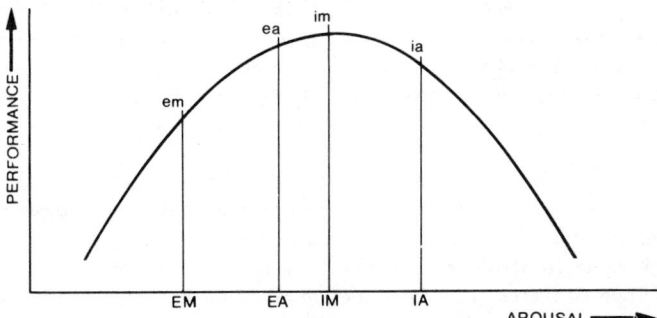

Figure 6. Postulated 'inverted-U' relationship between performance and arousal. I = introverts, E = extraverts, M = morning, A = afternoon. From Colquhoun and Corcoran (1964).

parts of the day, if it is assumed that introverts are more highly aroused at all times. It also fails to account for the findings of the knowledge of results experiment. If introverts are always higher in arousal than extraverts, then although the addition of an incentive in the morning would be expected to improve the performance of extraverts more than introverts, *this should also be the case at the later time of day*. Yet quite the reverse effect was observed at the later time.

The theory proposed by Eysenck (1967) does better. Eysenck suggested that introverts differ from extraverts in terms of their arousal *threshold*, that is introverts require less stimulus input to set the arousal system into an active state.

On arising the man is subject to all the various *zeitgebers*. There is light, noise, a rise in ambient temperature, social stimulation and so on. The *zeitgebers* are stimulus inputs and as such should act as arousing factors. If the introvert is assumed to possess a lower arousal threshold than the extravert, he would clearly be expected to respond to the *zeitgebers* at a more rapid rate, which is exactly what the temperature curves indicate.

However, although it is more successful in accounting for the phase differences in temperature between introverts and extraverts, Eysenck's theory comes to grief (like all other existing theories) over the knowledge of results experiment. If introverts are characterised by lower thresholds of arousal, then the addition of an incentive like knowledge of results *at any time* should always effect a change in their performance which is greater than that shown by extraverts. Also if *threshold* of arousal differentiates introverts and extraverts, extraverts should *never* respond more to knowledge of results, either beneficially or otherwise. However, in view of the success of Eysenck's theory in accounting for the phase difference, it is worth adding to his 'threshold of arousal' theory the extra postulate (invoked by Corcoran (1962, 1965) and Colquhoun and Corcoran (1964)) that *arousal level and performance are related according to an inverted U function*. The addition of the two theories makes the explanation of the data more complicated, but it does account for all the existing work which has shown time of day effects.

The 'threshold of arousal plus inverted U' theory might be stated somewhat as follows. Due to the arousing influences of the morning *zeitgebers*, introverts attain a level of arousal near optimum an hour or so before extraverts; this faster rise being due to the lower *threshold* of arousal characterising the introverts. Thus when measures of performance are taken in the morning introverts show the higher levels, but when an incentive is added at this time extraverts tend to improve, because their arousal level is sub-optimal. (This part of the theory accounts for the higher performance levels of introverts in the morning and the improvment in the performance of extraverts when knowledge of results is used in the morning.) As a result of their 'early rise', arousal level begins to fall in introverts about an hour before that of extraverts in the evening. At

Blake and Corcoran

this time let it be assumed that extraverts are in fact optimally or even hyper-aroused. If this is the case the addition of an incentive will increase their hyper-arousal even further and performance under incentive conditions will therefore fall relative to that of introverts. (This part of the theory accounts for the higher levels of performance in extraverts in the evening and the tendency for them to deteriorate relative to introverts when an incentive is introduced into the situation at this time.)

Although this theory may sound complicated enough to account for almost any finding, it cannot represent the whole picture, because it fails to account for various negative results. Many experiments support the notion that introverts differ from extraverts in terms of some arousal function (Corcoran 1962; Eysenck 1967), but *none* other than the studies reported here have suggested that extraverts have at any time of day higher levels of arousal than introverts. No doubt it could be argued that, since workers have frequently failed to report the times of day at which the subjects were tested, such considerations were ignored, and one must admit that during the normal working day (to judge from the temperature readings) introverts are either higher or equal in arousal level to extraverts. Thus on average one might expect the experimental results to support the conclusion that introverts have a higher level of arousal (whether this be due to the existence of lower thresholds or not would be largely irrelevant). So the argument might go, were it not for several studies reported in which time of day *has* been controlled and *has* been shown to have no effect whatsoever upon the findings.

The results of these studies support the notion that both in the morning *and* later in the afternoon introverts for some reason have the higher levels of arousal or lower thresholds of arousal.

The first of these studies was conducted as part of the reliability assessment of the salivation test (Corcoran 1964). Whether the test was conducted in the morning or the afternoon, introverts salivated more to lemon juice than introverts. Furthermore, neither the gross output of saliva nor the relationship with introversion was affected by testing in the early hours of the morning after 45 hours or so of sleeplessness.

Davis, Hockey and Taylor (1969) allowed subjects to switch on auditory inputs of various kinds whilst they were engaged on a task. Extraverts tended to use the audio inputs more frequently than introverts (supporting the notion that introverts were normally high enough in arousal not to need the extra stimulation). *This effect occurred independently of the time of testing.*

Finally Gale in his EEG work (1969) showed differences between introverts and extraverts again compatible with the notion that introverts had higher levels of arousal, and again the results were unaffected by the time of day at which the readings were taken (personal communication).

Thus it would appear that only in some studies is it found necessary to invoke the notion of a *change* in the relative positions of introverts and extraverts along the arousal continuum.

We are, therefore, at a disturbing though interesting phase in the understanding of the mechanism which differentiates introverts and extraverts. Almost all existing work on the topic suggests that some general difference exists in the arousal mechanism; most of it indicates that introverts are higher in arousal than extraverts whatever the time of day at which readings are taken, yet the work summarised here suggests that circadian rhythms are certainly involved.

REFERENCES

Blake, M. J. F. (1967) Relationship between circadian rhythm of body temperature and introversion-extraversion. *Nature, 215,* 896–897

Blake, M. J. F. (1971) Temperament and time of day. *In* Colquhoun, W. P. (ed.), *Biological rhythms and human performance.* London: Academic Press (in press).

Colquhoun, W. P. (1960) Temperament, inspection efficiency and time of day. *Ergonomics, 3,* 377–378.

Colquhoun, W. P. & Corcoran, D. W. J. (1964) The effects of time of day and social isolation on the relationship between temperament and performance. *Brit. J. Soc. Clin. Psychol., 3,* 226–231.

Corcoran, D. W. J. (1962) Individual Differences in Performance after Loss of Sleep. Unpublished Ph. D. Thesis, University of Cambridge, England.

Corcoran, D. W. J. (1964) The relationship between introversion and salivation. *Amer. J. Psychol., 77,* 298–300.

Corcoran, D. W. J. (1965) Personality and the inverted-U relation. *Brit. J. Psychol., 56,* 267–273.

Davis, D. R., Hockey, G. R. J. & Taylor A. (1969) Varied auditory stimulation, temperament differences and vigilance performance. *Brit. J. Psychol., 60,* 453–457.

Eysenck, H. J. (1967) The biological basis of personality. Boston: CC Thomas.

Gale, A., et al. (1969) *Brit, J. Psychol., 60,* 209–223.

Heron, A. (1956) A two-part personality measure for use as a research criterion. *Brit. J. Psychol., 47,* 243–251.

Pátkai, P. (1969) Interindividual differences in diurnal variations in alertness, performance and adrenaline excretion. *Rep. Psychol. Lab. Univer. Stockholm*, No. 273.

ACKNOWLEDGEMENTS

1. To Academic Press for permission to reproduce the diagrams shown as Figs 4 and 5.

2. To Taylor and Francis Ltd for permission to reproduce the data shown as Table 1.

3. To MacMillan Journals Ltd for permission to reproduce the diagram shown as Fig 3.

4. To Cambridge University Press for permission to reproduce the diagrams shown as Fig 2 and Fig 6.

DISCUSSION

Aschoff: Were the introverts and extraverts who show differences in morning temperatures awakened at the same time?

Corcoran: The subjects were aroused at 6.30 a.m., and, on the days when the temperatures were taken, they all rose at the same time. However, for all we know, on *other* days extraverts may have got back into bed after the Petty Officer had left the room!

Hartemann: What is the practical significance of your findings in the light of the fact that there is no *general* correlation between introversion and performance?

Corcoran: I agree that the practical significance of the relationship between personality and diurnal rhythm of performance is limited. A marginal improvement in overall level of output might be obtained by selecting introverts for morning work and extraverts for evening work, but probably only for long boring repetitive tasks. For other kinds of tasks it would not be possible to make this prediction.

Aschoff: A comment with regard to problems of personality: Among over 100 subjects, kept in isolation and showing 'free running' circadian rhythms, we found that the tendency for internal desynchronization was greater in subjects with a higher degree of neuroticism.

Corcoran: The relationship between neuroticism and internal rhythms you mention is most interesting. In the Cambridge laboratory we rarely find relationships between neuroticism and measures of performance of any kind. When they do occur they usually turn out to be non-repeatable.

From D. W. J. Corcoran (1965). British Journal of Psychology, *56, 267–273, by kind permission of the author and Cambridge University Press*

PERSONALITY AND THE INVERTED-U RELATION

By D. W. J. CORCORAN

Medical Research Council, Applied Psychology Research Unit, Cambridge

Difficulties with the postulated inverted-U relationship between performance and arousal are discussed, with emphasis upon individual differences in level of arousal. Predictions concerning the behaviour of highly aroused and less aroused subjects are made and tested in two experiments by relating changes in performance associated with increased and decreased levels of arousal to introversion score. Introverts behaved as highly aroused subjects were expected to and extraverts as less aroused subjects.

Many workers have found the assumption of an inverted-U relation between performance and level of arousal to be useful. Some (e.g. Hebb, 1955; Malmo, 1959; Duffy, 1949, 1957) have used the relation as an aid to theory, while others (e.g. Freeman, 1940; Courts, 1942; Schlosberg, 1954; Stennett, 1957) have found that the relation fits their data. The assumption is, however, loose and ill-defined since with a U function direct prediction of the value on one axis from knowledge of the other is not always possible. It is the purpose of the present paper to show how this difficulty may be overcome and to demonstrate that some of the predictions the assumption yields may be valid.

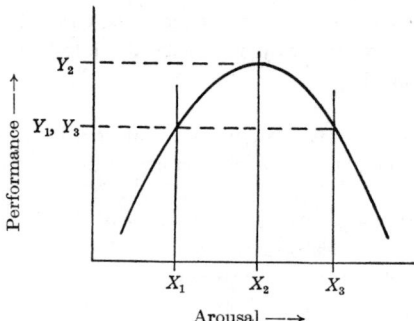

Fig. 1. Performance level Y_1, Y_3 would result from arousal levels X_1 or X_3. Given values Y_1, Y_3 it is possible to determine whether arousal level is at X_1 or X_3 by manipulating level of arousal and noting the directional change in performance.

An inverted-U relation implies that for any given value of performance except the optimal there will be two possible values of arousal. So that although level of performance is predictable, given level of arousal, level of arousal cannot be ascertained merely from knowledge of performance. However, there are instances in which the latter prediction is possible. Suppose level of performance was initially at Y_1 in Fig. 1, that with increased arousal performance rose to Y_2 and with a further increase dropped to Y_3 (where $Y_3 = Y_1$). Given only the value Y_1/Y_3, level of arousal could be either at X_1 or X_3. It is possible to decide which of the levels of arousal gave rise to performance level Y_1 either by increasing level of arousal or by decreasing it. If

D. W. J. Corcoran

arousal is lowered then Y_3 will increase, but Y_1 will decrease; similarly Y_1 will increase and Y_3 decrease if level of arousal is raised. Thus level of arousal can be predicted from level of performance, provided that the former is *varied* and the resulting performance level compared with that before level of arousal was changed.

Individual differences in arousal

The method suggested to determine level of arousal when level of performance only is given can be applied to discover which members of a group of subjects are operating at high levels of arousal and which at low levels. A group of subjects who are high in arousal may be considered to occupy a position along the abscissa of Fig. 2 somewhere to the right of the low arousal group. Although the following

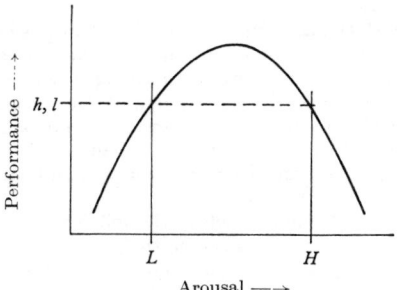

Fig. 2. Groups L and H both perform at h, l. By manipulating level of arousal it is possible to determine which group is at H and which at L.

arguments apply to any pair of positions along the abscissa we shall, for convenience, locate the high arousal group at H and the low at L, such that the level of performance of both groups is h, l. It is possible to discover which group has the high level of arousal either by decreasing the level of arousal of all subjects or by increasing it, since if level of arousal is decreased H's performance will improve by ascending the curve but L's performance will decline. Similarly, H's performance will decline and L's performance improve if the level of arousal of both is increased. The two groups may be differentiated by these methods no matter what positions they occupy along the arousal dimension, provided that H is to the right of L. Thus, for example, if H were at the optimal position and L somewhat lower, L would improve more than H if arousal were increased and decline more if arousal were decreased.

The following experiments were designed to test the validity of the foregoing argument. These experiments required (1) a method of changing arousal level, and (2) a technique for classifying subjects according to whether they would be likely to be operating at a high or low level of arousal. Deprivation of sleep was used to manipulate level of arousal (Corcoran, 1964*a*). The second requirement was met by relating the results to scores of introversion, since there is some evidence indicating that level of arousal may be related to degree of introversion (Shagass & Kerenyi, 1958; Claridge, 1961; Corcoran, 1962, 1964*b*; Colquhoun & Corcoran, 1964).

Personality and the inverted-U relation

EXPERIMENT I

Method

Task, subjects and procedure

The 'five-choice serial-reaction task' (Leonard, 1959) was used. The subject was seated in a sound proof cubicle, facing a display of five bulbs arranged in a pentagon on a board slightly inclined from the vertical. On the table before him was a board on which were inset five circular brass disks, each $1\frac{1}{2}$ in. in diameter. The disks were set in spatially equivalent positions to the five bulbs. The subject was instructed to tap the disk corresponding in position to the bulb which was alight at the time. By tapping the disk, the light was switched off and another bulb lit. The sequence in which the bulbs light repeats itself after 100 taps, and was thus effectively unpredictable. The apparatus was designed to yield three separate measures of performance: hits, the number of times the subject tapped the disk corresponded to the light; errors, the number of times an incorrect disk had been tapped; and gaps, the number of times an interval of $1\frac{1}{2}$ sec. had elapsed between responses.

An 'incentive' condition (HM) was used as a method of increasing level of arousal. Sleep deprivation was used as a de-arouser. The incentive was created by the following instructions: 'There is no time limit to this task; when you can finish depends how well you do. You have to make 3000 correct taps, and as soon as you have done this you can stop. You will be told when this figure has been attained. Errors do not count towards the total'. In the LM condition the subjects were simply requested to carry out the task for half an hour; they would usually make about 2000 hits during this time. All subjects worked for half an hour irrespective of number of hits.

Twelve naval ratings were tested under each of the following four conditions, according to a 2×2 latin-square design: (*i*) after normal sleep on the previous night, and under normal (low incentive) conditions (S/LM); (*ii*) after normal sleep, and after being given the instructions designed to result in a high level of incentive (S/HM); (*iii*) after losing sleep on the previous night and with low incentive (NS/LM); (*iv*) after loss of one night's sleep and with high incentive (NS/HM).

The Heron scale of introversion-extraversion (Heron, 1956) was administered to all subjects by laboratory staff unconnected with the present work. The scores on the Heron test showed that the subjects were on average slightly extraverted, having a mean score of 2·6 with an S.D. of 1·68.

Results and discussion

Spearman rho correlations were computed between introversion-extraversion and twenty-four measures of performance. The measures and the correlations are recorded in Table 1. In Table 2 are recorded the data relevant to the effects of increased incentive.

Table 1. *Correlations between introversion and measures of performance at the five-choice serial-reaction task, after loss of sleep (NS) and normal sleep (S), under conditions of low (LM) and high (HM) motivation*

Comparison no.	Condition	Gaps	Hits	Errors
1	S/LM	−0·29	0·68*	+0·11
2	S/HM	−0·16	0·45	−0·23
3	NS/LM	−0·72*	0·79*	−0·01
4	NS/HM	−0·51	0·18	+0·16
5	S/LM-S/HM	−0·26	0·43	+0·03
6	NS/LM-NS/HM	−0·63*	0·59*	+0·12
7	S/LM-NS/LM	+0·76*	0·38	−0·05
8	S/HM-NS/HM	+0·51	0·02	+0·05

$* P < 0.05$

D. W. J. Corcoran

The results of statistical significance in Table 1 may be summarized as follows. (*a*) Introverts made more hits than extraverts under S/LM and NS/LM conditions and scored fewer gaps under NS/LM conditions. (*b*) Extraverts deteriorated more from loss of sleep in terms of gaps under LM conditions, but improved more from the incentive, both in terms of gaps and hits. The two latter findings were significant only under the NS condition (see Table 2).

Table 2. *Performance at the five-choice serial-reaction task. Mean scores of the six most introverted subjects (I) and six most extraverted (E) after loss of sleep (NS) and normal sleep (S) under conditions of low (LM) and high (HM) motivation*

		Gaps					Hits			
		I			E			I			E	

	LM	HM		LM	HM		LM	HM		LM	HM
S	32·8	24·5	S	92·8	65·8	S	2932·8	2981·8	S	2205·8	2640·8
NS	107·0	33·8	NS	562·8	300·3	NS	2197·6	2393·8	NS	1124·2	2186·5

The results can be condensed into three main findings. (i) Introverts performed the task rather better than extraverts. If we accept the terminology and assumptions presented in the introduction, we may deduce from this finding that the task situation as a whole proved to be a relatively low in arousal value, since only under such conditions would a group operating at a high level of arousal be expected to perform better than one operating at a low level. (ii) The arousing procedure probably benefited extraverts more than introverts. This finding proved to be reliable only under NS conditions in the present experiment, but since other experiments have shown the effect after normal sleep (Corcoran, 1962), the generalization is probably warranted. (iii) Extraverts were probably the most affected by the de-arousing procedure. This result was found to be statistically significant only under LM conditions in terms of gaps.

The effect upon performance of changing level of arousal was shown to be about what one would expect on the basis of the inverted-U relationship. The less aroused subjects (if we can equate these with the extraverts) were more affected by lowering arousal, but improved relative to the highly aroused subject when level of arousal was increased. The results were far from conclusive, however, and the following further experiment was therefore carried out.

Experiment II

The task used in Expt. I was better performed by introverts. It was deduced from this finding that the nature of the task and the testing situation as a whole resulted in a suboptimal level of arousal, since under no other condition would a group high in arousal be expected to perform better than one which is low. Similarly, if a group is operating at a super-optimal level of arousal those subjects within the group who are low in arousal should perform the best, since they will be closer to the optimum. The aim of the following experiment was to investigate the effect of a de-arousing procedure upon groups who, it was hoped, were at post-optimal levels. On the basis of the Yerkes–Dodson principle, it would seem reasonable to choose a difficult task since these may be characterized by a low optimal level of arousal. A difficult task

Personality and the inverted-U relation

was therefore chosen, and the subjects were also put under stress, so that the low optimum level of arousal plus the arousing situation might be expected to result in a group who were operating at a high level of arousal. The effect to be expected from a reduction in arousal in such a situation is clear: the more aroused subjects should show more improvement than the less aroused.

METHOD

Task, subjects and procedure

A modified triple tester was used for this experiment. This apparatus consisted of a revolving brass drum with a celluloid cover. The cover was perforated with circular holes of $\frac{1}{4}$ in. diameter, arranged in such a way as to leave a passage free from holes. This passage wound spirally from left to right following a winding course. A pointer, controlled by means of a steering wheel, had to be kept within the passage as the drum revolved. When the pointer left the passage, it immediately made contact through the holes with the surface of the brass drum. This completed a circuit which included a counter and an error was scored. The error score thus indicated the approximate proportion of the time which the pointer was off track.

Subjects were tested under three separate conditions. (1) The drum was set to revolve at such a speed that the trial was completed in 40 sec.; the view of the oncoming track was restricted; each error was punished by a blast of about 100 db. white noise through earphones. (2) Conditions were identical to those described in 1, but three full sessions were allowed as practice before the first scored session. (3) Conditions were identical to those described in 1, but only the click of the error counter was heard through the earphones when an error occurred. These three conditions made up part of a larger investigation, which included other experimental conditions irrelevant to the present discussion.

A session consisted of ten trials; in each trial the pointer had to be kept in a position from the start of the passage on the left, through three and a half revolutions of the drum to end on the right. Three sessions were conducted on three consecutive mornings between 7·30 a.m. and noon.

Eighteen subjects were tested during a 60 hr deprivation of sleep: on the first morning (Day 1) they worked after sleeping normally on the previous night; on the second morning (Day 2) they had lost their normal sleep on the previous night; on Day 3 they worked after two nights' loss of sleep. Six subjects carried out the task under each of the three conditions (1), (2) and (3).

Results and discussion

The error scores were converted into normal deviates in order to make the scores more comparable under the three sets of conditions. Table 3 presents the introversion and extraversion scores of the subjects employed in the present experiment.

Table 3. *Introversion and extroversion scores: mean scores and ranges for subjects in Expt. II* ($n = 18$)

Group		n	Mean	Range
NS	*I*	9	6·2	4–9
	E	9	2·0	1–3

The converted tracking scores are presented in Table 4 in which the changes in performance over the 3 days can be seen. Extraverts show a consistent decline over the sleep deprivation, whilst introverts improve to an almost equal extent. These trends in performance differ significantly when assessed by the Mann–Whitney test ($U = 8$, $P = 0·002$).

These were not exactly the results expected, since the task was designed to be hyper-arousing to all subjects, so that all were expected to show an improvement in performance but the more aroused to the greater extent. The less aroused (if we can

D. W. J. Corcoran

equate these subjects with the extraverts) deteriorated rather than improved with loss of sleep. The results therefore suggest that the less aroused subjects were initially at a suboptimal level of arousal.

Table 4. *The converted scores of extraverts* $(n = 9)$ *and introverts* $(n = 9)$
on each day of sleep deprivation for the tracking task

	Day 1		Day 2		Day 3	
	Mean	Range	Mean	Range	Mean	Range
Introverts	-0.21	-1.96 to $+1.59$	$+0.40$	-0.86 to $+1.88$	$+0.70$	-0.42 to $+1.43$
Extraverts	$+0.19$	-1.14 to $+1.22$	-0.41	-1.44 to $+1.10$	-0.72	-1.71 to $+0.46$

The results may in fact indicate that a phenomenon rather like that shown in Fig. 2 was operating. In discussing the implication of the situation illustrated in Fig. 2 it was pointed out that the knowledge of level of performance alone was insufficient to determine level of arousal and that arousal level had to be changed in order to determine at which of the points (H or L) the subject had been operating. In the present experiment, initial level of performance was not very different and by manipulating level of arousal it was possible to ascertain which 'type' operated at H and which at L.

Conclusions

It was suggested in the introduction that information could be gained about the level of arousal at which a subject was operating by increasing or decreasing his level of arousal and noting the direction of the corresponding change in performance. The experiments were an attempt to demonstrate that this could be done. However, the results demonstrated the validity of the argument only to the extent that the groups used as external criteria were valid ones. In other words the argument has been shown to be valid provided that introverts are in general more highly aroused than extraverts. Although the results of many experiments showing differences between introverts and extraverts can be easily *interpreted* to be due to different levels of arousal, this hypothesis is far from proven.

Assuming, however, that the criterion groups were valid, the experiments showed (a) that the performance of the less aroused subject deteriorates when the general level of arousal is decreased, (b) that the performance of the more aroused subject is less affected than that of the less aroused subject when arousal generally is decreased and may even improve if the initial level of arousal is past the optimum.

References

Claridge, G. S. (1961). Arousal and inhibition as determiners of the performance of neurotics. *Brit. J. Psychol.* **52**, 53–4.

Colquhoun, W. P. & Corcoran, D. W. J. (1964). The influence of time of day and social isolation on the relationship of temperament to performance. *Brit. J. soc. clin. Psychol.* **3**, 226–31.

Corcoran, D. W. J. (1962). Individual differences in performance after loss of sleep. Unpublished Ph.D. Thesis, University of Cambridge.

Corocoran, D. W. J. (1964a). Changes in heart rate and performance as a result of loss of sleep. *Brit. J. Psychol.* **55**, 304–14.

Corcoran, D. W. J. (1964b). The relationship between introversion and salivation. *Amer. J. Psychol.* **77**, 298–300.

Courts, F. A. (1942). Relationships between muscular tension and performance. *Psychol. Bull.* **39**, 347–67.

Duffy, E. (1949). A systematic framework for the description of personality. *J. abnorm. soc. Psychol.* **44**, 175–90.

Duffy, E. (1957). The psychological significance of the concept of arousal or activation. *Psychol. Rev.* **64**, 265–75.

Freeman, G. L. (1940). The relation between performance level and bodily activity level. *J. exp. Psychol.* **26**, 602–8.

Hebb, D. O. (1955). Drives and the CNS (Conceptual Nervous System). *Psychol. Rev.* **62**, 243–54.

Heron, A. (1956). A two part personality measure for use as a research criterion. *Brit. J. Psychol.* **47**, 253–41.

Leonard, J. A. (1959). Five choice serial reaction apparatus. A.P.U. 326. Med. Res. Council Appl. Psychol. Res. Unit, Cambridge.

Malmo, R. B. (1959). Activation: A neuropsychological dimension. *Psychol. Rev.* **66**, 367–86.

Schlosberg, H. S. (1954. Three dimensions of emotion. *Psychol. Rev.* **61**, 81–5.

Shagass, C. & Kerenyi, A. B. (1958). Neurophysiological studies of personality. *J. nerv. ment. Dis.* **126**, 141–7.

Stennett, R. G. (1957). Performance level and level of arousal. *J. exp. Psychol.* **54**, 54–61.

(*Manuscript received* 11 *April* 1964)

PART III

PAIN, SENSORY DEPRIVATION, AND SENSATION SEEKING

Psychology has to deal with more complex matters than simple sensory stimulation, and most personality theorists have concentrated on such complex sources of stimulation, including social situations and other sources of higher-order input. However, this choice may be mistaken; science usually begins with the simple, and goes on to the complex only when it has succeeded in formulating laws which reduce the observed invariances to some quantitative form. So also in this book we shall proceed from the physiological to the simplest form of psychological reaction, going on to more complex forms of conduct only with the greatest hesitation. The question asked in this section relates simply to the effects on extraverts and introverts respectively of different kinds of sensory stimulation, ranging from a minimum (sensory deprivation) to a maximum (pain). The general hypothesis linking personality and sensory stimulation was stated originally by Eysenck (1963), and we are quoting below (Fig. 2) a diagram showing the postulated relation between level of stimulation (abscissa) and hedonic tone (ordinate). To put the hypothesis quite briefly, we assume that levels of stimulation which are too high or too low are both productive of negative hedonic tone (aversion), while levels of stimulation which are intermediate are productive of positive hedonic tone (pleasure). This view, which goes back to Wundt at least, is of course not new, and in its general form simply echoes common sense.

What produces a relationship with personality theory is the added hypothesis that introverts prefer a lower level of stimulation than ambiverts, extraverts a higher level. This hypothesis is mediated by the assumption of higher resting levels of arousal in introverts; if sensory stimulation is registered in the cortex to a degree which is a joined function of the objective level of intensity of the stimulation and of the arousal existing in the cortex at the time of arrival of the neural message, then identical intensities of input will be experienced as stronger by introverts than by ambiverts, and as weaker by extraverts than by ambiverts. In this way the optimum level of stimulation (OL) in Fig. 2 is displaced towards the left for introverts, and towards the right for extraverts. Similarly, at points A and B, respectively, the ambivert will experience indifference, while at A introverts will have positive, extraverts negative hedonic tone. At point B this relationship is inverted, with introverts experiencing negative and extraverts positive hedonic tone. If this were so then it would seem to follow that sensory stimulation of intensity A would be sought by introverts, and avoided by extraverts, while sensory stimulation of intensity B would be avoided by introverts, and sought by extraverts. These predictions are obvious deductions from the theory, and should not be difficult to support or disprove.

Another deduction from the theory would seem to be that introverts would tolerate sensory deprivation better, while extraverts would tolerate pain produced by

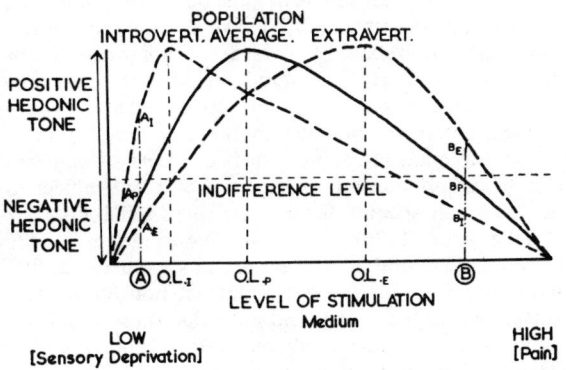

FIG. 2 Hedonic tone as a function of level of sensory stimulation

extreme sensory stimulation better. The concept of pain is too obvious to discuss (Beecher, 1959; Melzack, 1973); that of sensory deprivation has been well reviewed in Zubek (1969). Barnes (1975) has recently summarized the literature on the prediction that extraverts would be more tolerant of pain than introverts, and also the associated prediction that their pain thresholds would be higher. "In summary, the overall tests of significance conducted in this paper confirmed the association between extraversion on the one hand, and pain tolerance on the other." The literature on sensory deprivation has not been similarly summarized recently, and unfortunately it is subject to complexities from which that on pain tolerance is fortunately free.

Consider for instance a report by Tranel (1962), which is often quoted as disproving the hypothesis that introverts tolerate sensory deprivation better than extraverts. Measurement of toleration often simply means measuring the duration during which subjects are kept under the deprivation conditions, i.e. from the beginning of the experiment until the time when the subject asks to be released. However, there are other ways in which failure to tolerate the sensory deprivation conditions may manifest itself. In the Tranel experiment, for instance, subjects were instructed to remain in the isolation chamber, not to move about, not to go to sleep, and not to indulge in day dreaming. "Reactions of extraverts were characterized by remaining in the room for the specified period of time, but while in the room this group tended to violate instructions, to engage in some form of pleasant reverie, to go to sleep, and to move about while awake. . . . The study emphasized the importance of selecting criteria of tolerance for perceptual isolation." If we take the simple criterion of length of stay, then the prediction is apparently disconfirmed. If we look at the behaviour of the subjects during the period of the experiment, the prediction is clearly confirmed. The extraverted group, lacking external stimulation, supplied this stimulation themselves (by moving about, or by day dreaming), or went to sleep, thus neatly avoiding a state of low stimulation experience. Had the experimenter failed to observe the behaviour of his subjects (and many experimenters lack this careful attention to detail) the outcome would have been a quite unwarranted conclusion that the hypothesis was infirmed. All reports of sensory deprivation experiments should be read with this proviso in mind: duration of exposure is not the only, and may be an invalid, measure of tolerance of sensory deprivation.

Another source of possible confusion in these experiments is selection of subjects through volunteering. Most experiments (particularly in the U.S.A.) are conducted on volunteer students; the possibility exists that certain personality types are more likely to volunteer, or to volunteer for certain types of experiment, than others. McLaughlin and Harrison (1973) did indeed find that high N–high E subjects volunteered significantly more frequently for experiments said to involve electric shock. Volunteers altogether were more extraverted, but those

volunteering for other types of experiments were less extraverted than those volunteering for the shock experiment—itself a confirmation of the sensation-seeking tendencies of the extravert hypothesized. Francis and Diespecker (1973) failed to find any differences in extraversion for volunteers for a sensory deprivation experiment. There is not enough information on this point to be dogmatic, but the danger exists that volunteer subjects may be unrepresentative of the population sampled, and of course much more so of the general population.

The last paper reprinted in this section presents some unusual features which may justify comment. In the first place, it uses a particularly interesting technique of verification which deserves imitation, in that instead of using a questionnaire E score to correlate with a predicted empirical outcome on a particular laboratory test, it uses the correlation between two laboratory tests, both of which are theoretically measures of different aspects of extraversion, to demonstrate this relationship. Petrie, Collins and Solomon (1960) have used a test of kinaesthetic figural after-effects as their measure of extraversion, following the arguments presented originally by Eysenck (1955) for the association between these two variables. Petrie has modified the original method of measurement; her methodology and major findings have been described in her recent book (Petrie, 1967), and a brief description is also given in the article here reprinted.

Petrie's work isolates reducers, moderates, and augmenters, corresponding to extraverts, ambiverts, and introverts, on the basis of their reactions to the kinaesthetic figural after-effect experiment; reducers are disposed to seek out and react positively to complex and intense stimulus situations, while augmenters tend to seek out and favour quiet and simple stimulus situations. Petrie's original work was replicated by several independent observers (Poser, 1960; Ryan and Foster, 1967; Sales, 1971, 1972; Sweeney, 1966.) However, in recent years several authors failed to replicate her findings, and also found low test–retest reliability of her scores (e.g. Weintraub et al., 1973a, 1973b). This has led to a virtual abandonment of Petrie's method, on the basis of psychometric considerations reflecting the belief that unreliable tests cannot possess validity. However, this proposition involved "true" reliability, an ideal concept which cannot be measured directly but only inferred; test–retest reliability is one way of estimating "true" reliability, and low test–retest reliabilities may be susceptible to alternative explanations. Thus practice effects, which can bias scores on later administrations of a test subject to learning, may account for low test–retest reliability.

Baker et al. (1976) have shown that in the case of the kinaesthetic figural after-effect test this is indeed so; first scores are valid, later (retest) scores are not. Baker et al. analyse published studies and show that those which use only first test scores are almost 100% supportive; it is studies using retest scores which fail to support the hypothesis. Baker et al. further reanalyse the Weintraub et al. studies in which subjects were tested on seven different occasions. On each occasion the subject carried out four preinduction (pretest) judgments of the width of the T block, followed by a 60 sec. induction (rubbing) period, followed in turn by four postinduction (test) judgments of the block's width. The reanalysis shows that the effects of the first day's experiment are very lasting; subsequent pretest judgments are more like postinduction test judgments than preinduction test judgments made on the first day! Thus there are very long-term effects of the experimental procedure which make test–retest reliability calculations improper; indeed, Petrie had all along insisted on the existence of such long-term effects, and had incorporated this hypothesis into her experimental method, by asking subjects to keep their hands completely unoccupied for 45 min. before the start of the experiment. (This feature of kinaesthetic figural after-effect measurement may also be responsible for the many non-confirmative studies which followed the original Eysenck experiment.) We would seem justified in using the Petrie test in future work, provided only original test scores are taken into account (or a method is found which would enable us to eliminate the learning effects apparently incorporated into this test).

The theoretical explanation of the observed relationship between extraversion and "reducing" in the KAE type of experiment (and between "reducing" and other extraversion-related behaviours like criminality, smoking, sensory deprivation intolerance, pain tolerance, alcoholism, etc.) has changed from Eysenck's original hypothesis, which was based on Köhler's satiation-inhibition theory. Petrie (1967) uses instead a hypothesis which stresses an important attentional process, namely the way in which the intensity of ongoing stimulation is modulated in one's experience. Reducers *attenuate* the intensity of incoming stimulation; this enables them to tolerate high intensity stimulation but makes them uncomfortable when environmental stimulation is minimal (e.g. under sensory deprivation). Augmenters, on the other hand, *magnify* the intensity of incoming stimulation; thus they show intolerance of high level stimulation, but a marked capacity to cope with very low stimulus intensity. This accords perfectly with the other experiments in this chapter, and finds a ready explanation in the arousal type of theory presented in the previous chapter. KAE measures are direct estimates of the direction taken by an individual's sensory modulation, and consequently of considerable importance theoretically. The fact that stimulant and depressant drugs affect the KAE in predictable ways, as shown in the experiment by Gupta here reproduced, adds to the interest of the phenomenon.

REFERENCES

BAKER, A. H., MISHARA, B. L., KOSTIN, I. W., and PARKER, L. Kinesthetic aftereffect and personality: a case study of issues involved in construct validation. *Journal of Personality and Social Psychology*, 1976, in press.

BAKER, A. H., MISHARA, B. L., KOSTIN, I. W., and PARKER, L. When reliability fails, must a measure be discarded? *Journal of Research in Personality*, 1976, in press.

BARNES, G. E. Extraversion and pain. *British Journal of Social and Clinical Psychology*, 1975, *14*, 303–308.

BEECHER, H. K. *Measurement of subjective responses.* Oxford: Oxford University Press, 1959.

EYSENCK, H. J. Cortical inhibition, figural after-effect and theory of personality. *Journal of Abnormal and Social Psychology*, 1955, *51*, 94–106.

EYSENCK, H. J. (Ed.). *Experiments with drugs.* London: Pergamon, 1963.

FRANCIS, R. D. and DIESPECKER, D. D. Extraversion and volunteering for sensory isolation. *Perceptual and Motor Skills*, 1973, *36*, 244–246.

McLAUGHLIN, R. D. and HARRISON, N. W. Extraversion, neuroticism and volunteer subject. *Psychological Reports*, 1973, *32*, 1131–1134.

MELZACK, R. *The puzzle of pain.* Harmondsworth: Penguin, 1973.

PETRIE, A. *Individuality: pain and suffering.* Chicago: University of Chicago Press, 1967.

PETRIE, A., COLLINS, W., and SOLOMON, P. The tolerance for pain and for sensory deprivation. *American Journal of Psychology*, 1960, *73*, 80–90.

POSER, E. Figural after-effect as a personality correlate. Proceedings of the XVIth International Congress of Psychiatry. Amsterdam: North Holland Publishing Company, 1960, pp. 748–749.

RYAN, E. D. and FOSTER, R. Athletic participation and perceptual reduction and augmentation. *Journal of Personality and Social Psychology*, 1967, *6*, 472–476.

SALES, S. Need for stimulation as a factor in preferences for different stimuli. *Journal of Personality Assessment*, 1972, *36*, 55–61.

SALES, S. Need for stimulation as a factor in social behavior. *Journal of Personality and Social Psychology*, 1971, *19*, 124–134.

SWEENEY, D. R. Pain reactivity and kinesthetic after-effect. *Perceptual and Motor Skills*, 1966, *22*, 763–769.

TRANEL, N. Effects of perceptual isolation in introverts and extraverts. *Journal of Psychiatric Research*, 1962, *1*, 185–192.

WEINTRAUB, D. and HERZOG, T. The kinesthetic after-effect: ritual versus requisites. *American Journal of Psychology*, 1973a, *86*, 407–423.

WEINTRAUB, D., GREEN, G., and HERZOG, T. Kinesthetic aftereffects day by day: trends, task features, reliable individual differences. *American Journal of Psychology*, 1973b *86*, 827–844.

ZUBEK, J. P. *Sensory deprivation: fifteen years of research.* New York: Appleton-Century-Crofts, 1969.

From R. D. Francis (1969). Perceptual and Motor Skills, *28*, 534, *by kind permission of the author and Southern Universities Press*

INTROVERSION AND ISOLATION TOLERANCE

R. D. FRANCIS

University College, Wollongong N. S. W.

An argument relating introversion, sensory acuity and isolation tolerance has been presented by Eysenck (1967). The empirical data given here support that hypothesis; the evidence is from a variety of sources.

All Ss mentioned in this study completed the Cattell 16 P.F. test. Computation of the extraversion scores was as prescribed in the manual. A group of 18 Ss was tested for toleration of isolation by the immersion-in-water method. From this group 6 Ss with the highest toleration times were called high tolerators ($M = 2$ hr. 47 min., $SD = 18$ min.) and 6 Ss with the lowest toleration times were called low tolerators ($M = 51$ min., $SD = 15$ min.). Six college students (and a comparison group) were selected on their self ratings of being well able to withstand isolation in everyday situations, such as being kept in waiting rooms, being confined to bed, etc. Seven steelworkers (and a comparison group), 4 miners, and 5 reclusive priests were selected because their callings involved substantial isolation. The latter 2 groups are obvious choices; the former group was used in order to diversify the sample to include industrial-manufacturing settings.

TABLE 1
EXTRAVERSION SCORES OF TOLERATION GROUPS

Samples	High tolerators			Low tolerators			t^*	p
	N	M	SD	N	M	SD		
Exp. group	6	4.38	1.54	6	6.93	2.24	2.34	<.02
Self-defined	6	2.93	1.20	6	8.08	.92	8.30	<.001
Steelworkers	7	4.85	2.11	7	6.16	2.48	1.07	n.s.
Miners	4	2.45	1.35		Australian		4.55	<.01
Reclusive priests	5	2.27	2.40		norms		3.05	<.02

*One-tailed test.

In each case the groups who could bear isolation had lower extraversion scores. From the data, summarized in Table 1, the conclusion is drawn that introverts are best able to tolerate various forms of isolation. These data should also help resolve the ambiguity outlined by Tranel (1962).

REFERENCES

EYSENCK, H. J. *The biological basis of personality.* Springfield, Ill.: Thomas, 1967.
TRANEL, N. N. The effects of perceptual isolation on introverts and extraverts. *Dissert. Abstr.*, 1962, 23, 726-727.

Accepted March 20, 1969.

From G. F. Reed and J. C. Kenna (1964). Perceptual and Motor Skills, *18*, 182, *by kind permission of the authors and Southern Universities Press*

PERSONALITY AND TIME ESTIMATION IN SENSORY DEPRIVATION

G. F. REED AND J. C. KENNA

University of Manchester

Despite interest in "biological clocks" there is abundant evidence that our estimation of time may profitably be viewed as cue-learned behavior. Sturt (5) argued against William James' (3) view that the estimation of a period of time is determined by affective tone as well as the number of occurrences within the period. Sturt found that the duration of an interval was judged according to the number of "mental events" it contained, by which she meant all experiences, whether due to external or internal stimuli.

Under S.D. conditions, where external stimuli are reduced, the number of mental events experienced will be directly related to personality. By definition the introvert's psychic energy is normally directed toward himself, whereas the extravert is more attentive to external cues. It may be predicted, therefore, that under S.D. the extravert will suffer a relatively greater diminution of mental events. Thus, according to Sturt's theory, both introvert and extravert will tend to judge the duration of a given interval of S.D. as being shorter than it is by clock time but the extravert's error in estimation will be greater than the introvert's.

Ten normal Ss with scores on the Maudsley Personality Inventory Extraversion scale of 30 and above and 10 normal Ss with scores of 20 or less were asked to judge when 15 min. had elapsed (method of production) under normal and under S.D. conditions [described in (4)]. In every case both estimates were made on the same day; the order of conditions was reversed for half of each personality group. No significant difference was found between the group estimates under normal conditions ($M_{EXT} = 13.3$; $M_{INT} = 15.0$).

Under S.D. conditions errors in estimation were significantly greater; furthermore, all but one S made positive errors. In other words, clock time of 15 min. would be judged by 19 Ss to be shorter than this. This offers support for the experimental prediction and is in line with previous findings over short intervals (e.g., 1, 2). Although all errors were in the same direction, there was a pronounced difference between groups in size of error ($M_{EXT} \pm SD = 29.8$ min. ± 11.92; $M_{INT} \pm SD = 19.9 \pm 6.95$, $p = 0.025$, 1-tail Mann-Whitney U).

The larger errors made by the extraverts also accord with the experimental prediction, suggesting that the extravert, because of his higher dependence on external cues is more affected in his time estimates under S.D. than is the introvert.

REFERENCES

1. BANKS, R., & CAPPON, D. Effect of reduced sensory input on time perception. *Percept. mot. Skills,* 1962, 14, 74.
2. COHEN, S. I., SILVERMAN, A. J., BRESSLER, B., & SHMAVONIAN, B. Problems in isolation studies. In P. Solomon, *et al.* (Eds.), *Sensory deprivation.* Cambridge, Mass.: Harvard Univer. Press, 1961. Pp. 114-129.
3. JAMES, W. *Principles of psychology.* Vol. I. London: Macmillan, 1901.
4. REED, G. F., & KENNA, J. C. Sex differences in body imagery and orientation under sensory deprivation conditions of brief duration. *Percept. mot. Skills,* 1964, 18, 117-118.
5. STURT, M. *The psychology of time.* London: Kegan Paul, 1925.

Accepted January 30, 1964.

From D. Schalling (1971). Scandinavian Journal of Psychology, *12*, 271–281, *by kind permission of the authors and Almqvist and Wiksell*

TOLERANCE FOR EXPERIMENTALLY INDUCED PAIN AS RELATED TO PERSONALITY

DAISY SCHALLING

Karolinska Institute, Stockholm, and Psychological Laboratories,
University of Stockholm

SCHALLING, D. Tolerance for experimentally induced pain as related to personality. *Scand. J. Psychol.*, 1971, *12*, 271–281.—Relations between responses to noxious electrical stimulation (pain thresholds and tolerance levels) and personality variables were studied in a group of 26 students. Method of stimulation increase was found to be an important factor. When continuous stimulation increase was applied, the pain measures were significantly related only to scores in the Solidity scale of the Marke-Nyman Temperament inventory, low Solidity (extravert-impulsive) subjects showing high pain tolerance. When stimulation was increased in discrete steps (shocks), the pain measures were significantly related to scores in neuroticism–psychasthenia and extraversion scales, psychasthenic subjects being less and extravert subjects more tolerant of the stimulation. These results are consistently in the expected directions and are well in line with the implications of the personality concepts. Pain thresholds and tolerance levels were significantly correlated and showed similar patterns of correlation with the personality variables.

A few studies have been reported on relations between tolerance for experimentally induced pain and personality variables, but no consistent picture has emerged. One reason may be that different stimulation methods give different results (Davidson & McDougall, 1969 a). Electrical stimulation appears to be a suitable method for differential research (for a review, see Schalling, 1970 a).

In a previous study from this laboratory (Schalling & S. Levander, 1964), using electrical pain stimulation, it was found that a group of delinquents rated as predominantly anxiety-prone showed significantly lower pain tolerance than a group of predominantly psychopathic delinquents. However, this result was not confirmed in a later study (S. Levander, 1966). This discrepancy could of course be due to various factors. Although the subjects were taken from the same prison and classified on the basis of a similar rating procedure, the groups may still differ between the two studies, as the reliability of clinical ratings is not high. However, the group which was rated as more anxiety-prone in the latter study showed a significantly higher frequency of anticipatory spontaneous fluctuations in skin conductance than the more psychopathic group, which may be assumed to indicate higher anxiety (Schalling & S. Levander, 1967).

A difference between the two studies was that continuous stimulation increase was applied in the first study, whereas in the second, shocks of increasing current strength were given. Finally, an important factor may be the change of stimulator made in order to achieve a better control of the stimulation. The sensation created by the new stimulator appeared more dull and monotonous and less unpleasant. It was concluded that in further exploring the relations between pain responses and personality, a more effective noxious stimulation should be applied.

DAISY SCHALLING

The main purpose of the present study was to analyse responses of normal subjects to electrical stimulation, as related to personality. A new stimulator which appeared to satisfy the requirement of giving a more unpleasant sensation was used, and both continuous and shock stimulation were applied. The choice of personality variables was influenced by the hypothesis of Eysenck (1967), stating that extravert and psychopathic subjects are more tolerant to pain stimulation than introvert, due to a more rapid growth of cortical inhibiton and a consequent tendency towards attenuation of sensory input. Some support for this assumption was obtained by Lynn & Eysenck (1961), using continuous thermal stimulation. They found significant positive correlations between a pain endurance measure and Extraversion in the Maudsley Personality Inventory (MPI). Significant negative correlations were obtained between the pain measure and Neuroticism in MPI, although lower. Petrie, Collins & Solomon (1960) also reported a relation between endurance for thermal pain stimulation and Extraversion. In contrast, Levine, Tursky & Nichols (1966) did not find any significant correlations between MPI Extraversion and Neuroticism, and pain tolerance, using electrical stimulation. They ascribed the discrepancy between their results and those of Lynn & Eysenck (1961) to the fact that they increased the stimulation in discrete steps whereas Lynn & Eysenck applied continuous increase of stimulation. However, the lack of agreement could also be due to the fact that Levine et al. used electrical and Lynn & Eysenck thermal stimulation. Low correlations between measures obtained by these two types of stimulation were recently reported by Davidson & McDougall (1969a). It should be noted that these authors (Davidson & McDougall, 1969a, b) found a low but significant correlation between pain tolerance, and MPI Extraversion ($r = 0.26$) and the Manifest Anxiety scale ($r = -0.27$), when they applied electrical pain stimulation in shocks but not when thermal stimulation was used.

In the present study, the Marke-Nyman Temperament (MNT) inventory was used, in which two extraversion–introversion scales are comprised. For reasons outlined elsewhere (Schalling & Holmberg, 1970), it is assumed that one of these scales, Solidity, is related to the impulsiveness aspect of extraversion and to psychopathy. The main hypothesis was that the pain measures would be positively correlated with extraversion-impulsiveness. In addition, some neuroticism scales were included, on the assumption that they would be negatively correlated with the pain measures. For a discussion of these personality concepts, see Schalling (1970b).

METHOD

The data reported in the present paper were collected in connection with a study of habituation of skin resistance responses to auditory stimuli. Only the relevant parts of the experimental procedure will be described in detail.

Subjects

The subjects were 26 students, 8 men and 18 women, aged 20–35 years (Md = 22.6). Each subject participated in two sessions. The pain stimulation was carried out during the first session and the personality inventories were given during the second session.

Apparatus

An apparatus for electrical stimulation was constructed with the aim of making the quality of the stimulation more unpleasant than apparently had been the case with the stimulator used in an earlier study, in which alternating current of sine wave shape was used. It was assumed that for a given stimulus intensity, the degree of unpleasantness would be greater for a type of stimulation in which a train of spikes substituted the sine wave. In that way, large fibers with a short refractory period cannot fire more than once a spike, while small pain fibers with a long refractory period fire on each spike. It should be mentioned that in the first pain study from this laboratory (Schalling & S. Levander, 1964), trains of irregular spikes were created by chopping direct current mechanically, a procedure which gave rise to a markedly unpleasant kind of sensation.—Further, the rms (effective) value should be as low a fraction of the amplitude as possible in order to minimize the effects of extraneural tissue.

In the new stimulator, current pulses with interpulse intervals of 20 msec and pulse durations of 2 msec were produced with the aid of a thyristor. The peak value of the current pulses was used as an estimate of current strength.

There was a stable relationship between pulse amplitude and rms value. Through the use of a constant current circuit, the performance was unaffected by variations in the subject's skin resistance. The pulse form and amplitude were stable over a wide range of subject impedance. The time of stimulation was controlled with an electronic timer. In preliminary experiments, the sensation created by this stimulator appeared to be more unpleasant and to give a more pricking, aching and squeezing sensation than that created by the earlier stimulator (for details, see S. E. Levander & Schalling, 1970).

The current was fed into two 30 cm^2 stainless steel electrodes in two glass cups filled with 0.9% NaCl solution, which was kept at approximately 30°C. After inspection for possible cuts or abrasions, two fingers of the non-dominant hand were immersed into the two cups up to the second joint and were immobilized by tape. The use of fluid electrodes ensures a relatively low skin impedance (Tursky & Watson, 1964).

Procedure

The subjects were seated in a comfortable reclining chair in a quiet room. Instructions regarding the pain stimulation were given via tape recorder. It was emphasized that the stimulation might be unpleasant but was not dangerous. The subjects were asked to indicate first, when the stimulation became unpleasant (Pain Threshold) and second, when they could not tolerate any further stimulation (Tolerance Level). They were requested to try to tolerate as much as possible.

After seven minutes of hydration, 10 *current detection threshold measurements* were made with a method of ascending limits. The pain measurements were then started. Two types of stimulation increase were applied on each subject. In the *Continuous* (C) stimulation increase condition, the current strength was automatically increased at a constant rate of 0.4 mA/sec by means of a mechanical device. Measurements were made of the point at which the subject reported that the stimulation was unpleasant (*Pain Threshold*), and at which he reported that he could not tolerate any further increase (*Tolerance Level*). Three such sets of measurements were made with an interval of 3 min between measurements (PT$_1$, PT$_2$, PT$_3$ and TL$_1$, TL$_2$, TL$_3$). In the *Discrete steps* (DS) stimulation increase condition, shocks with a duration of 0.5 sec were administered with intervals of 15 sec. The current strength was increased with intervals of 15 sec. The current strength was increased in steps of 0.5 mA for the first nine shocks and 1 mA for the following. This was continued until the PT and TL were reached. The procedure was repeated three times. Condition C and Condition DS were given alternatively first and second to every other subject. Between the conditions, galvanic skin responses to a series of 21 tones were recorded. These data will be reported separately.

Personality Inventories

The Marke-Nyman Temperament inventory (MNT). The MNT is a Swedish personality inventory, constructed on the basis of a personality model by Sjöbring (see Nyman, 1956; Coppen, 1966). Three scales with 20 items each are included: *Validity* (psychasthenia, neuroticism vs. energy, dominance), *Stability* (extraversion vs. introversion, low emotional involve-

DAISY SCHALLING

ment, low sociability) and *Solidity* (extraversion vs. introversion, impulse control, restraint). Solidity is assumed to be related to the extraversion–impulsiveness factor and to psychopathy (Eysenck & Eysenck, 1963; Schalling & Holmberg, 1970). It should be noted that the MNT scales have a reversed scoring as compared to the Eysenck EPI scales, so that *low* scores in Validity correspond to *high* Neuroticism and *low* scores in Stability and Solidity to *high* Extraversion.

The Psychasthenia scale. A scale containing those of the Cattell 16 PF scales that differentiated between a group of psychasthenic patients and a control group (Idestrŏm & Schalling, 1970) was used in a modified 55-item version, based on an item analysis.

The Manifest Anxiety scale. A short form of the Taylor Manifest Anxiety Scale with 20 items was used (Bendig, 1956).

The Situational Unpleasantness Sensitivity inventory (SUS). A preliminary version of this instrument was used by Schalling & S. Levander (1964). The inventory contains 36 items consisting of short descriptions of various unpleasant situations. The subject is asked to rate on a seven point scale the degree of unpleasantness that he would experience in each situation. Items have been divided into four separate scales on the basis of item content. This subdivision has received support in a factor analysis (Schalling, Rissler & Edman, 1971). The scales were denoted *Anticipation scale* (e.g., "lining up for a vaccination"), *Pain scale* (e.g., "having a tooth pulled with freezing"), *Thrill scale* (e.g., "being caught in a storm while in a sailboat") and *Boredom scale* (e.g., "waiting for a train that is several hours late").

The SUS inventory takes into account not only the self-reported reaction of the subject, but also the type of situation for which these reactions are reported. In this respect, it is similar to the S–R Inventory of Anxiousness (Endler, Hunt & Rosenstein, 1962).

RESULTS AND DISCUSSION

Treatment of data

The mean of the last five current detection thresholds in the series of 10 obtained before the pain stimulation was used as the *current detection threshold* measure.

Pain measures were the means of the three *Pain Thresholds* (PT) and the three *Tolerance Levels* (TL) obtained in the two conditions (C and DS).

The conductance of extraneural tissues and the area of the electrodes will affect the current density in the nerves and thus influence the intensity of the stimulating current. In order to minimize the influence of interindividual differences in peripheral factors, PT and TL were expressed as multiples of the current detection threshold (Schalling & S. Levander, 1964). However, since it appears, that current detection thresholds of the type used are sensitive to threat of shock (Schalling, S. E. Levander, Dahlin & Jurborg, 1967), and since they may be assumed to be influenced by response criteria (Clark, Rutschman, Link & Brown, 1963), PT and TL are also reported in terms of absolute current strength (mA).

Since there were no significant differences with regard to sex or order of condition in the pain measures, these factors were not treated separately.

Characteristics of the pain measures

The intercorrelations between the three separate measurements of PT and TL were high and significant both for Condition C and DS (Table 1). Thus at least within one experimental session, the individual pain measures were stable.

In both conditions PT and TL tended to increase from the first to the third measurement. Analyses of variance for trend yielded significant effects only for PT ($F = 7.76$, df $= 2/50$,

TOLERANCE FOR EXPERIMENTALLY INDUCED PAIN

TABLE 1. *Test–retest correlation coefficients for successively obtained Pain Thresholds and Tolerance Levels (n = 26).*

	Pain thresholds			Tolerance levels		
Condition	$r_{1,2}$	$r_{1,3}$	$r_{2,3}$	$r_{1,2}$	$r_{1,3}$	$r_{2,3}$
Continous stimulation increase	.87	.80	.89	.98	.96	.97
Discrete steps stimulation increase	.76	.80	.98	.96	.94	.96

$p < 0.001$ for PT in Condition C; $F = 6.62$, $df = 2/50$, $p < 0.01$ for PT in Condition DS). Corresponding F values for TL were 1.07 and 0.27, both nonsignificant. The differences between successive PT measures were significant except for PT_2–PT_3 in Condition C. The differences between successive TL measures were not significant.

The correlations between mean PT and TL (mA) was 0.61 in Condition C and 0.79 in Condition DS, both significant ($p < 0.01$). In an earlier study (Schalling & S. Levander, 1964) with continuous stimulation increase, the correlation was 0.86. With a similar method, Clark & Bindra (1956) obtained a correlation of 0.63.

Continuous as compared to Discrete steps stimulation increase

The correlation between the mean PT measures obtained in Condition C and those obtained in Condition DS were 0.64 (mA) and 0.65 (multiples). The corresponding correlations for mean TL were 0.82 and 0.83. All correlations were significant ($p < 0.001$).

Means and standard errors of pain measures obtained in the C and DS conditions are shown in Table 2. The means of the measures in Condition DS were significantly higher than those in Condition C ($p < 0.001$). The variance was also significantly higher in Condition DS (for PT, $p < 0.001$, for TL, $p < 0.05$). The coefficients of variation were for PT and TL in Condition C 188 and 192, in Condition DS 162 and 186, respectively.

The relative importance of stimulus duration and intensity cannot be determined on the basis of the present data. The combined effect of these factors on ratings of unpleasantness

TABLE 2. *Means and standard errors for Pain Thresholds (PT) and Tolerance Levels (TL), expressed in milliampères and in multiples of the current detection threshold (n = 26).*

Pain measures	Continuous stimulation increase condition		Discrete steps stimulation increase condition		
	M	S.E.	M	S.E.	t
PT (mA)	2.55	0.26	4.34	0.53	4.37***
PT (multiples)	3.05	0.33	5.18	0.63	4.35***
TL (mA)	5.93	0.60	7.85	0.83	4.00***
TL (multiples)	7.11	0.75	9.34	1.00	3.99***

*** $p < 0.001$.

TABLE 3. *Intercorrelations among scores in personality inventories* ($n = 26$).

Variables	1	2	3	4	5	6	7	8	9
1 Validity (MNT)	—	−.24	−.33	−.66***	−.63***	−.59**	−.49**	−.44*	−.14
2 Stability (MNT)		—	.46*	.41*	.17	.34	.34	−.04	.35
3 Solidity (MNT)			—	.43*	−.01	.34	.47*	.40*	.19
4 Psychasthenia				—	.64***	.58**	.45*	.18	.01
5 Manifest Anxiety					—	.57**	.27	.15	.10
6 Anticipation (SUS)						—	.76***	.37	.37
7 Pain (SUS)							—	.38	.38
8 Thrill (SUS)								—	.38
9 Boredom (SUS)									—

* $p < 0.05$.   ** $p < 0.01$.   *** $p < 0.001$.

has been studied by Ekman, Frankenhaeuser, S. Levander & Mellis (1966) and by Ekman, Fröberg & Frankenhaeuser (1968). Perceived unpleasantness was a simple logarithmic function of stimulus duration (up to 3.00 sec tested). Unpleasantness was found to be a power function of stimulus intensity (up to 4 multiples of the sensation threshold). If a constant rate of current increase is used (as in the present study), a certain stimulus intensity will involve the same duration, which makes interindividual comparisons possible. However, the

TABLE 4. *Product-moment coefficients of correlation between Pain Thresholds (PT) and Tolerance Levels (TL), expressed in milliampères (mA) and in multiples of the current detection threshold, and scores in personality inventories* ($n = 26$).

V = Validity (MNT), St = Stability (MNT), So = Solidity (MNT), Pt = Psychasthenia, MA = Manifest Anxiety, A = Anticipation (SUS), P = Pain (SUS), T = Thrill (SUS), and B = Boredom (SUS). C = Continuous, DS = Discrete steps stimulation increase.

Condition	Pain measure	Inventory scales								
		V	St	So	Pt	MA	A	P	T	B
C	PT (mA)	.22	−.26	−.44*	−.15	.07	−.15	−.24	−.23	.00
	PT (multiples)	.27	−.29	−.47*	−.17	.05	.18	−.25	−.22	.03
	TL (mA)	.20	−.28	−.36	−.18	−.04	−.30	−.37	−.27	−.04
	TL (multiples)	.27	−.32	−.40*	−.23	−.07	−.34	−.38	−.27	−.00
DS	PT (mA)	.50**	−.46*	−.54**	−.49*	−.26	−.61**	−.58**	−.52**	−.38
	PT (multiples)	.54**	−.48*	−.58**	−.50**	−.26	−.64***	−.59**	−.52**	−.36
	TL (mA)	.47*	−.32	−.35	−.46*	−.32	−.53**	−.48*	−.37	−.27
	TL (multiples)	.51**	−.35	−.40*	−.48*	−.33	−.56**	−.49*	−.38	−.24

* $p < 0.05$.   ** $p < 0.01$.   *** $p < 0.001$.

influence of duration versus intensity will not be identical for different stimulus values in Condition C. Thus, if interest is focused on stimulus parameters, pain measures obtained with continuous and discrete steps stimulation increase are not comparable.

Intercorrelations among personality variables

The intercorrelations among the personality variables are shown in Table 3. The Validity, Psychasthenia, and Manifest Anxiety scales were significantly intercorrelated, forming a cluster of neuroticism–psychasthenia variables. As might be expected, the Situational Unpleasantness Sensitivity scales, especially the Anticipation scale, were related to this cluster and also to the extraversion–introversion variable Solidity.

Correlations between pain measures and personality variables

The correlations between the mean PT and TL and the personality variables are shown in Table 4. They were consistently in the expected directions. With the *Continuous* (C) stimulation increase, the only significant correlations obtained were negative correlations between Solidity and the two pain measures, more extravert-impulsive subjects showing higher tolerance for continuously increased electrical stimulation than did less extravert subjects (as mentioned, scoring in Solidity is reversed as compared to extraversion scales). Plotting did not reveal any systematic non-linear relationships between the pain measures and the other personality variables. With the *Discrete steps* (DS) stimulation increase, Validity, Psychasthenia, and Anticipation and Pain Unpleasantness Sensitivity showed consistent significant correlations with the pain measures in the expected direction. Thus, subjects with high scores in the neuroticism–psychasthenia variables were more sensitive than those with low scores to electrical stimulation when given in shocks. The correlations between PT in Condition DS and the two extraversion–introversion scales, Stability and Solidity, were also significant, significance levels being highest for Solidity. No significant correlations were obtained between the pain measures and the Manifest Anxiety scale, which is in agreement with findings by Nichols & Tursky (1967).

The relations between Solidity and the separate pain measures in the two conditions are illustrated in Fig. 1, in which the separate PT and TL measures are shown for subjects above and below the median value for Solidity.

When subjects above and below the median value in Solidity were compared by t-test with regard to the single pain measures, there were consistent significant differences for PT in both conditions ($p < 0.01$) and for TL in Condition DS ($p < 0.05$). A corresponding comparison between subjects above and below the median value in Validity yielded significant differences for PT and TL only in Condition DS ($p < 0.05$). Thus the pattern of correlation results was supported.

For Condition DS both Solidity and Validity were evidently of importance. When both variables were taken into account by multiple correlations, there was some increase over the single variable correlations, for PT (mA) 0.64 ($p < 0.01$) and for TL (mA) 0.51 ($p < 0.05$). Corresponding multiple correlations for the data from Condition C were very similar to the single Solidity correlations.

With regard to TL, the results obtained in Condition DS are in agreement with the findings by Davidson & McDougall (1969a). It appears that tolerance for electrical pain

DAISY SCHALLING

stimulation, given in shocks, tends to be related both to neuroticism and to extraversion variables. However, in the study by Davidson & McDougall (1969 a), personality variables were significantly correlated only with Tolerance Levels, not with Pain Thresholds, whereas in the present study, personality variables were related to both PT and TL, and most consistently to PT. Although there were certain methodological differences between the two studies (e.g., dry electrodes were used by Davidson & McDougall), it is not clear in what way these factors could be related to the discrepancy in results.

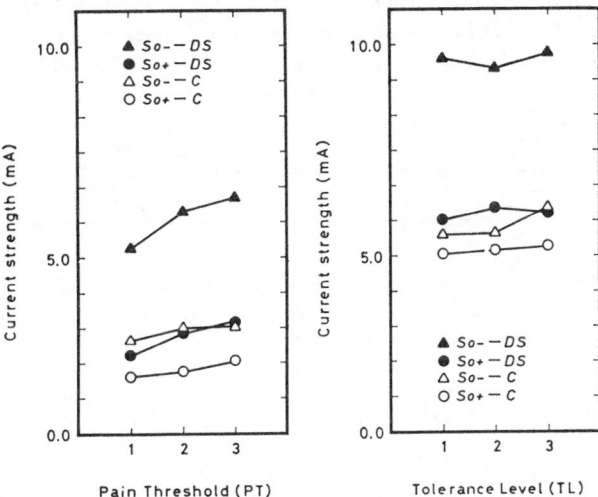

FIG. 1. Three consecutive measurements of Pain Threshold and Tolerance Level, obtained with Continuous (C) and Discrete (DS) stimulation increase in two groups comprising subjects with scores below and those with scores above the median value in Solidity. So- = low Solidity, extravert-impulsive; So+ = high Solidity, introvert.

Differences between conditions as related to personality

In Condition DS the coefficients of correlation between the pain measures and the personality variables were all significantly larger than the corresponding correlations in Condition C, except for Stability and Solidity and, as regards TL, for the Situational Unpleasantness Sensitivity scales. It should be noted that higher correlations could be expected in Condition DS, as the pain measures in this condition had larger variability. The correlations between the pain measures and the personality variables were consistently higher in Condition DS than in Condition C also when rank correlation methods were used, except with regard to Solidity, for which both sets of correlations were high.

In the total group, the mean PT and TL were significantly higher in the DS than in the C condition (Table 2). Thus, the general trend was that higher pain measures were obtained when stimulation was increased in discrete steps. This may be partly due to the longer duration of the stimulation and consequent cumulative effects in Condition C.

However, a closer analysis revealed that the differences between conditions with regard to TL were systematically related to the personality variables. When the group was divided into subgroups comprising subjects with scores below the median value and those with scores above the median value for each personality variable (Table 5), it was found that the TL measures in Condition DS were markedly and significantly higher than those in Condition C (*t*-test for correlated samples, $p < 0.001$) only for subjects with low scores in neuroticism-psychasthenia variables (high Validity, low Psychasthenia and low Manifest Anxiety) and for extravert subjects (low Stability, low Solidity). However, in the groups comprising introvert subjects and high neuroticism-psychasthenia subjects, there were no significant differences in TL between the conditions. Further, significant differences ($p < 0.001$) were obtained for subjects with low scores in the SUS Anticipation, Pain and Thrill scales, but not for those with high scores.

TABLE 5. *Means, standard deviations, and t-tests for Tolerance Levels (mA) obtained with Discrete steps stimulation increase (DS) and with Continuous stimulation increase (C) in sub-groups comprising subjects with scores below the median value (low, $n = 13$) and above the median value (high, $n = 13$) in neuroticism and extraversion variables.*

Groups	DS		C		
	M	S.D.	M	S.D.	t
High neuroticism groups					
Low Validity (MNT)	6.75	3.89	5.77	3.48	2.09
High Psychasthenia	6.19	4.01	5.46	3.63	1.68
High Manifest Anxiety	6.93	4.06	6.00	3.31	1.73
Low extraversion groups					
High Stability (MNT)	6.83	5.13	5.33	3.70	1.58
High Solidity (MNT)	6.18	4.66	4.85	3.37	1.63
Low neuroticism groups					
High Validity (MNT)	8.94	4.41	6.09	2.76	3.71**
Low Psychasthenia	9.51	3.88	6.40	2.48	4.25**
Low Manifest Anxiety	8.77	4.02	5.86	2.71	4.08**
High extraversion groups					
Low Stability (MNT)	8.87	2.42	6.33	2.07	5.45***
Low Solidity (MNT)	9.52	3.07	7.01	2.43	5.16***

** $p < 0.01$.   *** $p < 0.001$.

The DS–C differences in TL were significantly larger in groups of subjects with low scores in neuroticism-psychasthenia variables than in groups of subjects with high scores (*t*-test for independent samples, $p < 0.01$ for differences between high and low Psychasthenia groups, $p < 0.05$ for Validity and Manifest Anxiety groups). This was true also for the Anticipation scale groups ($p < 0.05$). There were no significant DS–C differences in TL between groups of subjects with high and low extraversion-scores.—The PT measures were significantly higher in the DS as compared to the C condition for all subgroups.

The findings described above indicate that higher pain tolerance in the DS than in the C condition is found only in non-psychasthenic stable individuals with low anxiety.

Pain measures as multiples of current detection thresholds

The correlations between the current detection thresholds and the PT and TL were low and nonsignificant in both conditions. The pattern of correlations with the personality variables was essentially the same when the pain measures were expressed in terms of absolute current strength (mA) as when they were expressed in multiples of the current detection threshold. Thus, at least in this group which was homogeneous from sociocultural, age and ethnic points of view, correction for differences in current detection thresholds did not greatly influence relations between pain measures and personality variables.

CONCLUSIONS

The results in the present study support the assumption of Levine et al. (1966), that the method of stimulation increase is of importance for the relations between experimentally induced pain and personality. With continuous stimulation increase, low Solidity (extravert-impulsive) subjects tolerated more stimulation than introverts, confirming the main hypothesis. Since Solidity appears to be related to psychopathy (Schalling & Holmberg, 1970), this finding is in line with an earlier study on delinquents (Schalling & S. Levander, 1964). The results are of interest in view of recent hypotheses of a more efficient attenuation o noxious sensory input in psychopaths (Hare, 1970). They are also in line with Eysenck's model (Eysenck, 1967), implying a more rapid growth of cortical inhibition in extraverts. It may be assumed that continuous stimulation increase favors such a growth. However, a problem which cannot be solved on the basis of the present data, is whether the Eysenck Extraversion scale, comprising both impulsiveness and sociability items, would be correlated with the pain measures in the same way as the Solidity scale, in which emphasis lies on impulsiveness and monotony-avoiding behaviour (Schalling & Holmberg, 1970).

When stimulation was increased in discrete steps, extravert subjects were less sensitive than introvert subjects, although pain tolerance in this case was also, in line with the hypothesis, related to neuroticism–psychasthenia variables, and to Anticipation and Pain Unpleasantness Sensitivity. This is of interest in view of the common assumption that anticipation of future pain is an important factor for pain tolerance (Sternbach, 1968). When noxious stimulation is given in shocks, the subject must decide during an interval before the stimulus if the next stimulus will be tolerable or not. Thus anticipation probably plays a greater role, and the situation may be more anxiety–provoking, than when continuous stimulation is used. This interpretation is consistent with the finding that the TL measures in Condition DS were significantly higher than those in Condition C only for subjects with low scores in neuroticism-psychasthenia scales and in the Anticipation Unpleasantness Sensitivity scale.

Interpretation of correlations in a small group of subjects as in the present study must be made with caution. Only consistent, replicated results which are in line with hypotheses and with theoretical assumptions can be accepted as valid.

As the generality of pain tolerance across different types of stimulation has recently been questioned (Davidson & McDougall, 1969a), it must be emphasized that the results in the present study may be restricted to electrical stimulation conditions. However, the efficacy of electrical pain stimulation in recent analgesic research (Wolff, Kantor & Laska, 1969) is a promising finding. In future research, relations between responses to electrical stimulation and other pain variables, including clinical pain responses, should be further explored.

The assistance of G. Edman, B.A., and A. Eriksson, B.A., in collecting the data is gratefully acknowledged. The electrical stimulator was constructed by G. Tollet and S. E. Levander.

Thanks are due to Professor B. Frankenhaeuser for advice and to Professor R. D. Hare for reading and commenting on a preliminary version of the manuscript. The experiment was carried out at the Department of Psychiatry, Karolinska sjukhuset.

REFERENCES

BENDIG, A. W. (1956). The development of a short form of the Manifest Anxiety Scale. *J. Consult. Psychol.*, *10*, 384.

CLARK, J. W. & BINDRA, D. (1965). Individual differences in pain thresholds. *Canad. J. Psychol.*, *10*, 69–76.

CLARK, W. C., RUTSCHMAN, L., LINK, R. & BROWN, C. J. (1963). Comparison of flicker-fusion thresholds obtained by the methods of forced-choice and limits on psychiatric patients. *Percept. & Mot. Skills*, *16*, 19–30.

COPPEN, A. (1966). The Marke-Nyman temperament scale: an English translation. *Brit. J. Med. Psychol.*, *39*, 55–59.

DAVIDSON, P. O. & McDOUGALL, C. E. A. (1969a) The generality of pain tolerance. *J. Pscyhosom. Res.*, *13*, 83–89.

DAVIDSON, P. O. & McDOUGALL, C. E. A. (1969b). Personality and pain tolerance measures. *Percept. & Mot. Skills*, *28*, 787–790.

EKMAN, G., FRANKENHAEUSER, M., LEVANDER, S. & MELLIS, I. (1966). The influence of intensity and duration of electrical stimulation and subjective variables. *Scand. J. Psychol.*, *7*, 58–64.

EKMAN, G., FRÖBERG, J. & FRANKENHAEUSER, M. (1968). Temporal integration of perceptual response to supraliminal electrical stimulation. *Scand. J. Psychol.*, *9*, 83–88.

ENDLER, N. S., HUNT, J. McV. & ROSENSTEIN, A. J. (1962). An S-R inventory of anxiousness. *Psychol. Monogr.*, *76*, No. 17.

EYSENCK, H. J. (1967). *The biological basis of personality.* Springfield, Ill.: Charles C. Thomas.

EYSENCK, S. B. G. & EYSENCK, H. J. (1963). On the dual nature of extraversion. *Brit. J. Soc. Clin. Psychol.*, *2*, 46–55.

HARE, R. D. (1970). *Psychopathy: Theory and research.* New York: Wiley.

IDESTRÖM, C.-M. & SCHALLING, D. (1970). Objective effects of dexamphetamine and amobarbital and their relations to psychasthenic personality traits. *Psychopharmacologica*, *17*, 399–413.

LEVANDER, S. (1966). Reactions to electrical pain stimulation. Unpublished thesis. The University of Stockholm.

LEVANDER, S. E. & SCHALLING, D. (1971). Notes on a method for noxious electrical stimulation, suitable for differential research. (In preparation.)

LEVINE, F. M., TURSKY, B. & NICHOLS, D. C. (1966). Tolerance for pain, extraversion and neuroticism: Failure to replicate results. *Percept. & Mot. Skills*, *23*, 847–850.

LYNN, R. & EYSENCK, H. J. (1961). Tolerance for pain, extraversion and neuroticism. *Percept. & Mot. Skills*, *12*, 161–162.

NICHOLS, D. C. & TURSKY, B. (1967). Body image, anxiety and tolerance for experimental pain. *Psychosom. Med.*, *29*, 103–110.

NYMAN, G. E. (1956). Variations in personality *Acta Psychiat., et Neurol. Scand.*, Suppl. no. 107.

PETRIE, A., COLLINS, W. & SOLOMON, P. (1960). The tolerance for pain and for sensory deprivation. *Am. J. Psychol.*, *73*, 80–90.

SCHALLING, D. (1970a). Personality and tolerance for experimentally induced pain. A review. *Rep. Psychol. Lab., Univ. Stockholm, 1970*, No. 305.

SCHALLING, D. (1970b). Contributions to the validation of some personality concepts. *Rep. Psychol. Lab., Univ. Stockholm*, Suppl. 1.

SCHALLING, D. & HOLMBERG, M. (1970). Extraversion in criminals and the "dual nature" of extraversion. Some comments based on results in inventories. *Rep. Psychol. Lab., Univ. Stockholm, 1970*, No. 306.

SCHALLING, D. & LEVANDER, S. (1964). Ratings of anxiety-proneness and responses to electrical pain stimulation. *Scand. J. Psychol.*, *5*, 1–9.

SCHALLING, D. & LEVANDER, S. (1967). Spontaneous fluctuations in skin conductance during anticipation of pain in two delinquent groups differing in anxiety proneness. *Rep. Psychol. Lab., Univ. Stockholm*, No. 238.

SCHALLING, D., LEVANDER, S. E., DAHLIN, Y. & JURBORG, B. (1967). Effects of experimentally induced threat on thresholds for electrocutaneous stimulation and conductance level. Unpublished manuscript.

SCHALLING, D., RISSLER, A. & EDMAN, G. (1971). Factor analysis and similarity analysis of items in the Situational Unpleasantness Sensitivity inventory. (In preparation.)

STERNBACH, R. A. (1968). *Pain. A psychophysiological analysis.* New York: Academic Press.

TURSKY, B. & WATSON, P. D. (1964). Controlled physical and subjective intensities of electric shock. *Psychophysiology*, *1*, 151–162.

WOLFF, B. B., KANTOR, T. G. & LASKA, E. (1969). Response of experimental pain to analgesic drugs. *Clin. Pharmacol. & Therapeut.*, *10*, 217–228.

From A. Gale (1969). Behaviour Research and Therapy, 7, 265–274, *by kind permission of the author and Pergamon Press*

"STIMULUS HUNGER": INDIVIDUAL DIFFERENCES IN OPERANT STRATEGY IN A BUTTON-PRESSING TASK

ANTHONY GALE

Department of Psychology, University of Exeter

(*Received* 4 *March* 1969)

Summary—In a free operant situation, where four different sound reinforcements could be obtained to reduce mild sensory deprivation, extraverts maintained a higher response rate than introverts and made more changes among stimulation sources but without obtaining a higher total duration of sound stimulation. There was no difference for stimulus preference between the personality groups; but both groups showed greatest preference for a 30 db white noise reinforcement as opposed to three variants of a 60 db 4,000 Hz tone. The results of earlier studies are interpreted in the light of these findings and the difficulties of providing direct experimental measures of "stimulus hunger" and sensory reinforcement are also considered. Eysenck's (1967) model of the neurophysiological substrates of extraversion-introversion is extended to account for "stimulus hunger".

EXTRAVERTS are "stimulus hungry" (Eysenck, 1967) and when given the opportunity to seek for stimulation, they will do so (Howarth, 1964; Weisen, 1965). This stimulus-seeking characteristic is implied by several items on the 'E' scale of the Eysenck Personality Inventory (1964) and by many of the extravert traits as specified by Eysenck and Eysenck (1963). Extraverts are more inclined than introverts to describe themselves as seeking more frequent and greater amounts of stimulation (Cooper and Payne, 1967). Extraverts and introverts may also be distinguished on a number of sensory measures, the differences being in part accountable for in terms of "stimulus hunger". Extraverts have higher sensory thresholds (Smith, 1968), higher pain thresholds (Haslam, 1966), greater tolerance for pain (Lynn and Eysenck, 1961) and greater intolerance for sensory deprivation (Petrie, Collins and Solomon, 1960). Stimulus hunger is attributable to a chronically lower level of cortical excitation in extraverts (Eysenck, 1967). Because of lower levels of cortical excitation, stimuli must be of greater physical intensity to reach perceived threshold. Thus to obtain equivalent subjective reports of stimulus intensity for the two personality groups, the physical intensity of the applied stimulus must be greater for extraverts. Eysenck (1963) presents a model relating level of sensory input and hedonic tone as a function of personality; this model caters for all the above findings in relation to sensory thresholds and degree of tolerance for pain and sensory deprivation.

The inferior performance of extraverts on vigilance tasks (Bakan, Belton and Toth, 1963) and the manner in which such performance may be improved, is also explicable in terms of low cortical excitation and stimulus hunger (Gale, in preparation, and see below). Indeed, Davies and Hockey (1966) find that high intensity white noise (which reduces stimulus hunger and raises cortical excitation) had a facilitatory effect on the visual vigilance performance of extraverts. An alternative explanation of the vigilance decrement may be made by reference to involuntary rest pauses (I.R.P.'s) induced by a higher level of cortical inhibition and the generation of reactive inhibition (Eysenck, 1967). Since vigilance tasks typically involve a complex interaction over time of both sensory and response processes, the most satisfactory explanation of individual differences in performance is likely to employ both the concepts of cortical excitation and cortical inhibition.

Direct evidence of chronically lower cortical excitation in extraverts is provided by E.E.G. studies. The occipital E.E.G. is higher in voltage than that of introverts, both when the eyes are closed and external visual stimulation is absent (Savage, 1964) and when the eyes are open in the presence of continuous monotonous stimulation (Gale, Coles and Blaydon, in press). This higher voltage E.E.G. in extraverts may also be interpreted as an indication of a chronically lower level of reticulo-cortical arousal, which is in itself one of the determinants of cortical excitation (Moruzzi and Magoun, 1949; Eysenck, 1967).

On Howarth's (1964) task, extraverts were more active in button pressing, both before and after satiation. Weisen's (1965) task was an operant conditioning procedure where reinforcement for button-pressing was either a 3-sec period of light and sound stimulation ("onset" condition) or a 3-sec period of relief from light and sound stimulation ("offset" condition). Extraverts pressed more frequently in the onset condition and introverts more frequently in the offset condition. Thus the number of presses in both the Howarth and Weisen studies is a direct measure of the amount of stimulation obtained. (In Howarth's study, any stimulation obtained is said to be by virtue of the act of button-pressing itself (Eysenck, 1967)).

However, it is possible that button-pressing and obtained stimulation are to a certain degree dissociable. In a free operant situation where S may impose his own "schedule" on the task, different Ss may obtain identical total amounts of sensory reinforcement and yet employ different response strategies. Thus Ss may press frequently for short bursts of stimulation even when an identical period of stimulation might be obtained by one continuous press. Such a procedure allows for a distinction between the response characteristics of the situation (button pressing) and the sensory characteristics (reinforcement). Thus predictions concerning individual differences may be made both on the basis of reactive inhibition (generated by continuous button-pressing) and on the basis of stimulus hunger (generated by sensory deprivation). According to Eysenck (1957) extraverts generate reactive inhibition to response tasks more rapidly than introverts. In the case of forced continuous tapping, extraverts, because of the rapid generation of reactive inhibition, show a significantly higher number of I.R.P.'s (Spielmann, 1963).

Thus it may be predicted for example, that extraverts will alter their button-pressing stategy over time; for as stimulus hunger increases with continued exposure to sensory deprivation, so also does reactive inhibition increase (to the very operant response which leads to a reduction of stimulus hunger). Indeed, in certain circumstances, the effects of reactive inhibition to the operant response may become so much stronger than the need for stimulation that performance of the operant response is considerably reduced (Jensen, 1966).

This experiment is designed to measure differences in button pressing strategy over time, between extraverts and introverts, in a free operant situation.

SUBJECTS

The Ss were 36 undergraduate students at the University of Exeter (average age 18 years 11 months). Two groups of Ss were selected on the basis of E.P.I. (1964) score: an extravert group (mean E score 16·6; standard deviation 1·7; range 14–21) and an introvert group (mean E score 7·1; standard deviation 2·4; range 2–10). The groups were matched for Neuroticism, no S having an N score greater than 11 (standard deviation for both groups was 2·5; combined range 6–11). Each personality group contained 9 males and 9 females.

APPARATUS AND PROCEDURE

S sat in a dimly lit corner of a darkroom, separated from E by a suspended blanket. Facing S was a black console, from which protruded the knobs of four morse keys. The four keys were connected both to four pens on a four-channel pen recorder (run continuously at 1·5 cm per sec) and to four signal lights. Thus, when S pressed a particular key, the corresponding pen on the recorder was displaced for the duration of the press and at the same time, the appropriate signal light warned the E to present one of four sound reinforcements to S. The reinforcements (provided by a Peters Audiometer) were as follows: (a) 30 db white noise (broad band); (b) 60 db 4,000 Hz (continuous); (c) 60 db 4,000 Hz (modulated at 2 cps) and (d) 60 db 4,000 Hz (modulated at 3 cps). Both the pre-test instructions and the sound reinforcements were delivered to S through earphones, binaurally.

S (having removed his watch) was instructed to sit quietly for a "considerable period of time" and not to talk to E. Stimulation would be available at all times if S pressed the keys; the same sound being associated with the same key throughout the experiment. Not more than one key was to pressed by S at any one time and stimulation would only be available for the duration of the press. S was asked to use his preferred hand only. In the absence of automated apparatus, there would be a delay of approximately 1·5 sec before stimulation occurred, therefore, rapid pressing would be to no avail. (As soon as S pressed and prior to the selection by E of the appropriate stimulation source, the output to S's earphones was temporarily disconnected). S could press as frequently as he wished on any of the four keys, or not press at all, there being no obligation to press. S was then asked to repeat these instructions. A testing period of 14 min then followed. Equal numbers of Ss in each experimental group were tested at one of two times (9 a.m. and 5 p.m.).

RESULTS

The two personality groups are not differentiated in terms of Total Listening Time (Table 1), although the group means are in the predicted direction (Fig. 1). However, the total number of presses is greater for extraverts ($p < 0.01$; Table 2; Fig. 2). Mean listening time per press (Total listening time per S divided by his total number of presses) is shorter for the extravert group ($t = 1.61$, $p < 0.05$, one-tail). Extraverts also make more Changes between stimuli ($p < 0.05$; Table 3; Fig. 3). However, the mean time spent on any one particular source, without changing to a new source, (but including repeated presses on the same source) is not different for the two groups. The only variable yielding an effect over time is Changes (Table 3; Fig. 3) which reduced over time for both groups. There are no significant interactions between Personality and Time. Since total possible listening time was fixed and S was allowed only one source of stimulation at any one time, the four sources of stimulation were not independent. It was therefore not possible to. test for stimulation preference by means of an analysis of variance, varying the stimulation sources within one design. Chi-square comparisons for stimulus preference between groups and between stimulation sources yield no difference in source preference between the two groups. However, both groups show a strong tendency to rank stimulation source (a) (white noise) first; $\chi^2 = 24.5$, $p < 0.001$.

ANTHONY GALE

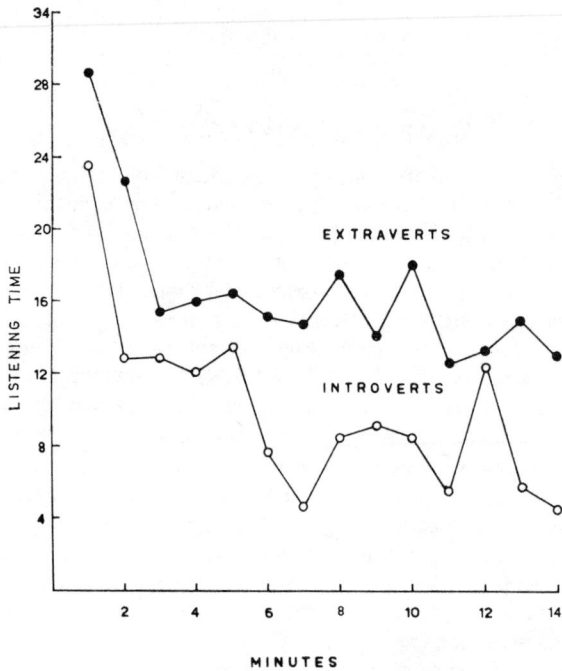

FIG. 1. Mean listening time. See Table 1.

DISCUSSION

The major difficulty in interpreting the results of this study lies in the definition of "stimulation". In terms of the stimulation *provided*, the extravert group do not obtain significantly more sound reinforcement than the introvert group. However, the extraverts adopt a *different strategy* in obtaining stimulation; they press more frequently, change

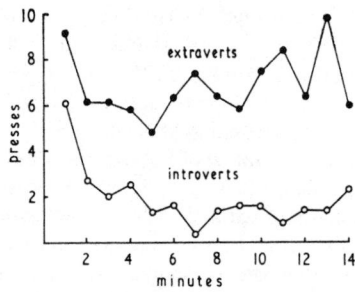

FIG. 2. Mean number of presses. See Table 2.

STIMULUS HUNGER

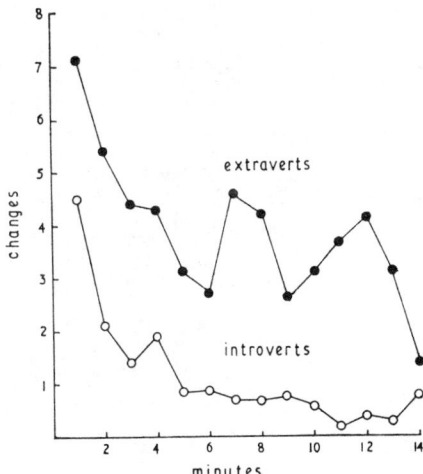

FIG. 3. Mean number of changes between stimulation sources. See Table 3.

between stimuli more frequently and their average listening time per press is shorter. This outcome is predictable in terms of Eysenck's (1957) construct of reactive inhibition. Stimulation is contingent upon *continuous* pressing; but *relief* from continuous pressing allows for dissipation of reactive inhibition. Moreover, since there is in this experimental procedure a minimum delay of 1·5 sec between presses, there is little opportunity for reactive inhibition to generate to repeated rapid pressing (which was predicted by Howarth (1964) but not demonstrated; but which is demonstrated in a *paced* pressing task by Spielman (1965)).

On the other hand the present results are also predictable in terms of stimulus hunger. It may be argued that alternation of "press"–"no-press"–"press" ("sound reinforcement on", "sound reinforcement off", "sound reinforcement on"), provides a richer source of sensory stimulation than continuous press (continuous sound reinforcement). The sensory reinforcement provided in this study is certainly of lower hedonic value than the coloured lights and music employed by Weisen (1965). (The preference for white noise, which subjectively, provides a continuously changing input, is intuitively reasonable.) The view that interrupted stimulation is more satisfactory as a reducer of stimulus hunger is further supported by electrophysiological evidence. The maximum electrical response to continuous stimulation at the receptors, occurs at onset; "Phasic receptors respond to a prolonged stimulus by initiating a burst of rapid nerve discharges. The rate of firing decreases rapidly with time and may reach zero". (Grossman, 1967).

We may conclude therefore that extraverts, by adopting their strategy of frequent pressing and changing between sources, do in fact obtain *more* stimulation from our experimental procedure. Direct support for this assertion may be provided by an experimental procedure where S is given the opportunity to obtain identical sound stimulation from either of two sources; one requiring continuous press (as in the present study), the other requiring only a brief press (as in the Weisen study). It is predicted that extraverts would show a preference for the latter since such a procedure would not only provide more varied stimulation but would also be less conducive to the generation of reactive inhibition.

ANTHONY GALE

TABLE 1. ANALYSIS OF VARIANCE FOR LISTENING TIME, VARYING PERSONALITY
(P) AND TIME (T)

Source	d.f.	S.S.	M.S.	F
Total	503	1,832,250·554		
Between subjects	35	79,715·054		
P	1	5,513·669	5,513·669	N.S.
S/P	34	74,201·385	2,182·393	
Within subjects	468	1,752,535·500		
T	13	9,013·192	693·322	N.S.
PT	13	1,200·970	92·382	N.S.
ST/P	442	1,742,321·338	3,941·903	

TABLE 2. ANALYSIS OF VARIANCE FOR PRESSES, VARYING PERSONALITY (P) AND
TIME (T)

Source	d.f.	S.S.	M.S.	F
Total	503	28,582·427		
Between subjects	35	16,022·069		
P	1	3,006·669	3,006·669	7·854*
S/P	34	13,015·400	382·805	
Within subjects	468	12,560·358		
T	13	539·288	41·48	N.S.
PT	13	320·858	24·681	N.S.
ST/P	442	11,700·212	26·471	

*$p < 0.01$.

The Howarth (1964) study appears to contradict this assertion since in fact extraverts press rapidly *and* at a high rate. But Howarth's task is of only 2 min duration and is insensitive, unlike the Spielmann (1965) study, to the measurement of pauses *during* pressing.

In the present study, extraverts are not differentially affected by Time. There are two reasons for the absence of this interaction. Firstly, sensory deprivation is only mild and of relatively short duration (14 min) and therefore presses and listening time do not *increase* during exposure as a result of excessive stimulus hunger. Secondly, the unpaced nature of the task is unlikely to allow for the generation of reactive inhibition and therefore pressing does not *reduce* over time, as a result of reactive inhibition. Thus *S*s may maintain a strategy which supports an equilibrium between the opposing influences of these two variables. The significant main effect for Time in the analysis of Changes (Table 3) is attributable to initial learning of the association between individual sound reinforcements and their manipulanda. Sheffé tests show that the major difference lies between the 1st and 3rd min.

TABLE 3. ANALYSIS OF VARIANCE FOR CHANGES, VARYING PERSONALITY (P)
AND TIME (T)

Source	d.f.	S.S.	M.S.	F
Total	503	10,134·968		
Between subjects	35	6,022·825	895·999	
P	1	895·999		5·942*
S/P	34	5,126·826	150·789	
Within subjects	468	4,112·143		
T	13	632·468	48·651	6·358†
PT	13	98·056	7·543	
ST/P	442	3,381·619	7·651	

*$p < 0.05$.
†$p < 0.005$.

The question arises as to whether it would be more parsimonious to limit predictions to one construct, for it may be argued that given both the reactive inhibition and stimulus hunger constructs a logical see-saw develops where *any* outcome may be accountable for. The stimulus hunger construct was devised largely to account for "stimulation seeking" behaviour by extraverts. It is difficult to set up conditions adequate to the task of quantifying stimulus hunger without employing an operant procedure. This of course involves a response measure, which in turn raises the necessity of predictions based on reactive inhibition. Studies on differential tolerance to sensory deprivation (where typically no relief of stimulus hunger is available) provide an alternative source of information; but such studies have failed to present consistent data (Zubek, 1964). It would seem inevitable therefore that predictions concerning stimulus hunger *must* presuppose the necessity for predictions concerning reactive inhibition. As Eysenck points out, it is difficult to predict the outcome of even very straightforward experimental procedures without calling upon a number of hypothetical constructs (Eysenck, 1965).

We have omitted to mention that Eysenck (1963, 1967) not only asserts that extraverts are "stimulus hungry", but that introverts are "stimulus aversive". Apart from the data derived from Weisen's (1965) "offset" condition, there is little direct evidence to support this view. In the present study, the introvert group were in fact active, although given the opportunity to refrain totally from obtaining sound stimulation. But the experimental design does not provide for a *range* of stimulation, from "moderate" (through "tolerable") to "intense". Moreover, it is also difficult to ascertain at what point on the arousal continuum the two groups were placed prior to obtaining stimulation. Thus the results cannot be fitted with great confidence onto Eysenck's (1963) hedonic tone model. Moreover, the four stimulation sources are difficult to rank in terms of richness; had this been the case, we would have predicted that when introverts *did* press, it would have been for milder or less complex stimulation. Thus the question of "stimulation aversion" in introverts remains open and is not answered by this study.

ANTHONY GALE

Eysenck (1967, p. 245) does not provide a sound theoretical basis for a relationship between low cortical excitation and stimulus seeking. In other words, why should extraverts work to *raise* cortical excitation; or alternatively, if extraverts are low-aroused, why do they not simply just fall asleep? We propose here a tentative model to explain this link between cortical excitation and stimulus hunger. This model is derived in part, from the arousal theory of Berlyne (1960) and extends Eysenck's (1967) neurophysiological model. Berlyne asserts that arousal should be considered as a drive, subject like other drives to homeostatic principles. Thus individuals have an optimum arousal level for functional efficiency and states of arousal either above or below this optimum are unsatisfactory. Berlyne uses "unsatisfactory" in an hedonic sense where the origins of the discomfort caused by deviations from optimum arousal level are homeostatic and presumably not physiologically dissimilar from other basic drives. We propose that the *adjustment* to obtain optimum level might be (a) homeostatic, (b) analogous to an acquired drive or (c) task or situation specific (see below). These alternatives are not of course mutually exclusive.

Several studies support the view that extraverts are chronically low-aroused (below optimum) and introverts chronically high-aroused (above optimum) (Colquhoun and Corcoran, 1964; Corcoran, 1965; Eysenck, 1967; Gale Coles and Blaydon (in press)). Moreoever, this chronic level has a physiological basis; it is determined by the level of reticulo-cortical bombardment (Eysenck, 1967). In order to relate this view to "stimulus hunger", we must postulate secondly, a system designed to raise arousal level in extraverts or reduce arousal level in introverts in order to maintain the optimum level and sustain functional efficiency. Thus introverts reduce arousal by *avoiding* stimulation and extraverts raise arousal by *seeking* stimulation. A physiological basis for this function resides in the cortico-reticular relationship; both inhibitory and excitatory effects of the cortex on the reticular system have been demonstrated. The cortex can raise or lower reticular arousal directly (Bremer and Terzuolo, 1953; French, Hernandez-Peon and Livingston, 1955; Sharples and Jasper, 1956; Hugelin and Bonvallet, 1957; Magoun, 1964) by either increasing sensory input or setting up "filters" against input at receptor level and thereby reducing sensory input via the collaterals to the A.R.A.S. (Hernandez-Peon, Sherrer and Jouvet, 1956; Sokolov, 1960). Moreover, there is an abundance of evidence for both positive and negative feedback loops between cortex and A.R.A.S. (Routtenberg, 1966). Thus, following Eysenck (1967) two types of arousal are postulated—reticular arousal (high or low) and cortical arousal (high or low). The former consists of an innate predominance or inhibitory function in extraverts and an innate predominance or excitatory function in introverts. The latter consists of acquired techniques, mediated by the cortex, to support functional efficiency and maintaining optimal arousal in the manner stated. An analogy may be drawn here with Thorpe's (1960) notion of "hard" and "soft" clocks; the former innate, the latter modifiable by experience. Or again, with Kleitman's (1939) notion of the ontogenetic development of "wakefulness of choice" as opposed to "wakefulness of necessity" (Morgan, 1965). Both personality types learn how to mitigate against the effects of an inherently maladaptive level of reticular arousal; extraverts by seeking stimulation and raising reticular arousal, introverts by avoiding stimulation and reducing reticular arousal. The extent of stimulus hunger (or aversion) at any particular time is determined by the sensory "richness" of the environment, and the level of functional efficiency required of the individual.

How does such a theory cope with the findings on vigilance? Perception of the "wanted" signal presupposes an efficient level of arousal. But the repetitious and monotonous nature of the regular "unwanted" signal is conducive to habituation, inhibition, and Pavlovian sleep. The mechanisms for such inhibition reside at reticular level (Oswald, 1960; Moruzzi, 1964; Lynn, 1966). Thus not only does the extravert start the vigilance task at a low level of arousal, but the task itself is de-arousing. But the extravert subject must avoid sleep (since sleep in a vigilance task is punished); he therefore searches for stimulation within the experimental environment in order to raise arousal. In group tasks, such stimulation is readily available and the extravert is able to sustain functional efficiency by observing his fellow subjects (Colquhoun and Corcoran, 1964); the presence of the experimenter also provides a source of extraneous stimulation (Broadbent, 1959). But when continuous stimulus seeking is necessary, as in the more typical vigilance task (which approximates more closely to sensory deprivation) a vicious circle develops and signals are missed. However, once arousal has been raised as a result of the search for stimulation, performance might recover. Explanations of the vigilance decrement have focussed largely upon the initial decrement and often neglect to explain the final spurt in performance reported in several studies (Broadbent, 1959, 1964). This final spurt might be accountable for in terms of conditions conducive to this sort of cyclic variation in arousal.

Although individual differences in vigilance performance are considered to be well established, there is in fact a paucity of evidence to support the earlier findings (McGrath, Harabedian and Buckner, 1968). The ideal testing ground for the theory presented above would be a vigilance task, where additional stimulation is available (Bakan, Belton and Toth, 1963) but where physiological monitoring provides a direct (or at least, operational) measure of basal arousal, within-task fluctuations of arousal (Eason, Beardshall and Jaffee, 1965; Daniel, 1967) and their relationship to both stimulus seeking and vigilance performance.

REFERENCES

BAKAN P., BELTON J. A. and TOTH J. C. (1963) Extraversion-introversion and decrement in an auditory vigilance task. In *Vigilance: A Symposium* (Edited by D. N. BUCKNER and J. J. McGRATH). McGraw-Hill, New York.
BERLYNE D. E. (1960) *Conflict, Arousal and Curiosity*, McGraw-Hill, New York.
BREMER F. and TERZUOLU C. (1954) Contribution à l'étude des mechanismes physiologiques du maintien de l'activité vigile du cerveau. Interaction de la formation réticulée et de l'écorce cérébrale dans le processus du réveil. *Archs int. Physiol.* 62, 157-178.
BROADBENT D. E. (1959) *Perception and Communication*, Pergamon Press, Oxford.
BROADBENT D. E. (1964) Vigilance. *Br. med. Bull.* 20, 17-21.
COOPER R. and PAYNE R. L. (1967) Extraversion and some aspects of work behaviour. *Person. Psychol.* 20, 45-57.
COLQUHOUN W. P. and CORCORAN D. W. J. (1964) The effects of time of day and social isolation on the relationship between temperament and performance. *Br. J. Soc. clin. Psychol.* 3, 226-231.
CORCORAN D. W. J. (1965) Personality and the inverted—U-relation. *Br. J. Psychol.* 56, 267-274.
DANIEL R. S. (1967) Alpha and theta E.E.G. in vigilance. *Percept. mot. Skills* 25, 697-703.
DAVIES D. R. and HOCKEY G. R. (1966) The effects of noise and doubling the signal frequency on individual differences in visual vigilance performance. *Br. J. Psychol.* 57, 381-389.
EASON R. G., BEARDSHALL A. and JAFFEE S. (1965) Performance and physiological indicants in a vigilance situation. *Percept. mot. Skills* 20, 3-13.
EYSENCK H. J. (1957) *The Dynamics of Anxiety and Hysteria*, Praeger, New York.
EYSENCK H. J. (1963) *Experiments with Drugs*, Pergamon Press, New York.
EYSENCK H. J. (1965) A three-factor theory of reminiscence. *Br. J. Psychol.* 56, 163-181.
EYSENCK H. J. (1967) *The Biological Basis of Personality*, Thomas, Springfield.
EYSENCK S. B. G. and EYSENCK H. J. (1963) The validity of questionnaires and rating assessments of extraversion and neuroticism and their factorial validity. *Br. J. Psychol.* 54, 51-62.
FRENCH J. D., HERNANDEZ-PEON R. and LIVINGSTON R. B. (1955) Projections from cortex to cephalic brainstem (reticular formation) in monkey. *J. Neurophysiol.* 18, 74.
GALE M. A. (in preparation) The relationship between vigilance performance, button pressing and physiological reactivity.
GALE M. A., COLES M. G. H. and BLAYDON J. (in press) Extraversion-introversion and the E.E.G.

ANTHONY GALE

GROSSMAN S. P. (1967) *A Textbook of Physiological Psychology*, John Wiley, New York.
HASLAM D. R. (1967) Individual differences in pain threshold and level of arousal. *Br. J. Psychol.* **58**, 139–142.
HERNANDEZ-PEON R., SCHERRER H. and JOUVET M. (1956) Modification of electrical activity in cochlear nucleus during "attention" in unanaesthetized cats. *Science, N.Y.* **123**, 331–332.
HOWARTH E. (1964) Differences between extraverts and introverts on a button-pressing task. *Psychol. Rep.* **14**, 949–950.
HUGELIN A. and BONVALLET M. (1957) Tonus cortical et contrôle de la facilitation motrice d'origine réticulaire. *J. Physiol.* **49**, 1171.
JENSEN A. R. (1966) The measurement of reactive inhibition in humans. *J. gen. Psychol.* **75**, 85–94.
KLEITMAN N. (1939) *Sleep and Wakefulness*, Univ. of Chicago Press, Chicago.
LYNN R. (1966) *Attention, Arousal and the Orientation Reaction*, Pergamon Press, Oxford.
LYNN R. and EYSENCK H. J. (1961) Tolerance for pain, extraversion and neuroticism. *Percept. mot. Skills* **12**, 161–162.
MAGOUN H. W. (1964) *The Waking Brain*, Thomas, Springfield.
McGRATH J. J., HARABEDIAN A. and BUCKNER D. N. (1968) Review and critique of the literature on vigilance performance. Technical Report 206-1 Los Angeles: Human Factors Research.
MORGAN C. T. (1965) *Physiological Psychology*, McGraw-Hill, New York.
MORUZZI G. (1964) Reticular influences on the E.E.G. *Electroenceph. clin. Neurol.* **16**, 2–17.
MORUZZI G. and MAGOUN H. W. (1949) Brain stem reticular formation and activation of the E.E.G. *Electroenceph. clin. Neurol.* **1**, 455–473.
OSWALD I. (1962) *Sleeping and Waking*, Elsevier, Amsterdam.
PETRIE A., COLLINS W. and SOLOMON P. (1960) The tolerance for pain and for sensory deprivation. *Am. J. Psychol.* **123**, 80–90.
ROUTTENBERG A. (1966) Neural Mechanisms of Sleep: changing view of reticular formation function. *Psychol. Rev.* **73**, 481–499.
SAVAGE R. D. (1964) Electro-cerebral activity, extraversion and neuroticism. *Br. J. Psychiat.* **110**, 98–100.
SHARPLESS S. and JASPER H. H. (1956) Habituation of the arousal reaction. *Brain* **79**, 655–680.
SMITH S. L. (1968) Extraversion and sensory threshold. *Psychophysiology* **5**, 293–300.
SOKOLOV E. N. (1960) Neuronal models and the orienting reflex. In *The Central Nervous System and Behaviour* (Edited by M. A. BRAZIER), J. Moon, New York.
SPIELMANN J. (1963) The relation between personality and the frequency and duration of involuntary rest pauses during massed practice. London. Unpublished. Ph. D. Thesis.
THORPE W. H. (1960) Sensitive periods in the learning of animals and men: a study of imprinting with special reference to the induction of cyclic behaviour, in *Current Problems in Animal Behaviour* (Edited by W. H. THORPE and O. L. ZANGWILL), Cambridge Univ. Press, Cambridge.
WEISEN A. (1965) Differential reinforcing effects of onset and offset of stimulation on the operant behaviour of normals, neurotics, and psychopaths. Univ. of Florida. Unpublished Ph. D. Thesis.
ZUBEK J. P. (1964) Prolonged sensory and perceptual deprivation. *Br. med. Bull.* **20**, 38–43.

From E. J. Ludvigh, III and D. Happ (1974). British Journal of Psychology, *65*, 359–365, *by kind permission of the authors and Cambridge University Press*

EXTRAVERSION AND PREFERRED LEVEL OF SENSORY STIMULATION

By ELEK J. LUDVIGH, III AND DEBORAH HAPP

Department of Psychology, Michigan State University, East Lansing, Michigan, U.S.A.

Based on the work of Eysenck (1967), the present study hypothesizes a positive correlation between extraversion scores and the amount of ambient illumination and sound necessary to provide optimum hedonic tone and to create a slightly unpleasant level of hedonic tone. The subjects were 120 male undergraduates at Michigan State University. The results support the existence of a positive correlation between extraversion and sensory-seeking behaviour hypothesized by Eysenck (1967), but suggest that the relationship between the variables is due to differences between introverts and extraverts as to what constitutes an *excessive* level of stimulation.

All of us have, at times, felt overwhelmed by sensory stimulation and a need to get away from it all. Those of us who are clinical or counselling psychologists have probably noticed our clients frequently express a need to get 'far from the madding crowd'. This need to reduce stimulation may be considered a neurotic need to escape or, at least in part, a manifestation of an attempt to maintain 'sensoristasis' (Schultz, 1965), a homeostatic balance with respect to sensory stimulation.

This study investigates the correlation between the extraversion–introversion dimension and the need for, or avoidance of, sensory stimulation.

In an early study concerned with introversion and sensory deprivation tolerance, Petrie *et al.* (1960) found that subjects who tolerated sensory deprivation well were significantly more introverted than subjects who tolerated sensory deprivation poorly. Studies by Tranel (1962) and Reed & Kenna (1964) contradicted the findings of Petrie *et al.* (1960). Tranel found that subjects classified as introverts by the Myers–Briggs Type Indicator tolerated sensory deprivation significantly less well than did extraverts. Reed & Kenna found that subjects classified as introverts by the Maudsley Personality Inventory perceived a given period of sensory deprivation as being longer than it seemed to subjects classified as extraverts.

Two studies of sensory deprivation tolerance and the extraversion–introversion dimension have been conducted by Rossi & Solomon. The first (1965) found that introverts, as classified by the Myers–Briggs Type Indicator, tolerated sensory deprivation slightly, but not significantly, less well than did extraverts, while the second (1966) found no difference in tolerance between the groups. In a subsequent study, Reed & Sedman (1964) found that all subjects reporting depersonalization during a brief sensory deprivation period scored significantly lower on the Maudsley Personality Inventory extraversion scale than did those who had not experienced depersonalization. Ludvigh (1970) found that there was no significant difference between introverts and extraverts, as measured by the Eysenck Personality Inventory, in manifest need for sensory stimulation in a sensory deprivation situation.

These experimental findings contradict the view (Eysenck, 1967) that introverts tolerate sensory deprivation better than extraverts.

ELEK J. LUDVIGH, III AND DEBORAH HAPP

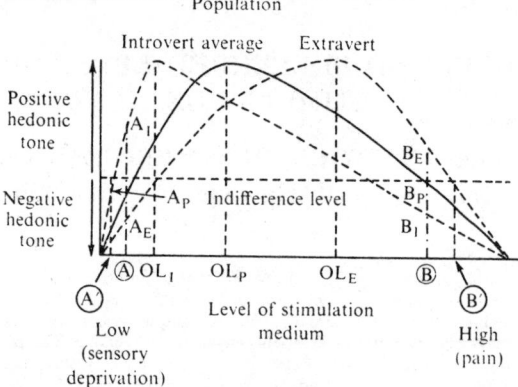

Fig. 1. Relation between level of sensory input and hedonic tone as a function of personality.

Eysenck (1967) offers two postulates explaining the general relationship he feels exists between personality and cortical inhibition–excitation phenomena:

(1) Human beings differ with respect to the speed with which excitation and inhibition are produced and the speed with which inhibition is dissipated. These differences are properties of the physical structures involved in making stimulus-response connexions.

(2) Individuals in whom excitatory potential is generated slowly and in whom excitatory potentials so generated are relatively weak are thereby predisposed to develop extraverted patterns of behaviour . . . Individuals in whom excitatory potentials so generated are strong are thereby predisposed to develop introverted patterns of behaviour . . . Similarly, individuals in whom reactive inhibition is developed quickly, in whom strong reactive inhibitions are generated, and in whom reactive inhibition is dissipated slowly, are thereby predisposed to develop extraverted patterns of behaviour; . . . conversely, individuals in whom reactive inhibition is developed slowly, in whom weak reactive inhibitions are generated, and in whom reactive inhibition is dissipated quickly are thereby predisposed to develop introverted patterns of behaviour.

Based on the foregoing, Eysenck hypothesizes that the sensory thresholds of introverts are lower than those of extraverts 'because of the higher efficiency of performance associated with cortical excitation' (Eysenck, 1967). Extrapolating from this hypothesis, 'the theory linking introversion with low sensory thresholds (and small j.n.d.'s) has been extended by Eysenck to pain tolerance and sensory deprivation tolerance in the following manner' (Eysenck, 1967).

The hypothesized relationship indicated in Fig. 1 is explained quite simply by the following four hypotheses derived as corollaries from the main cortical excitation–inhibition hypothesis. (1) Very low and very high levels of stimulation produce negative hedonic tone. (2) Positive hedonic tone develops only at intermediate levels of sensory stimulation. (3) Any amount of stimulation is experienced as effectively higher by introverts than by extraverts. (4) The optimum level of stimulation for introverts is lower than that for ambiverts which is also lower than that for extraverts.

Extraversion and preferred level of sensory stimulation

An examination of the research and theory related to Eysenck's general cortical excitation–inhibition hypothesis suggests a number of points relevant to the above four corollary hypotheses. First, studies by Lindsley (1961) and Cofer & Appley (1965) suggest that internal arousal processes can substitute for, or at least modify, the need for external stimulation, implying that studies related to sensoristasis should control for internal arousal.

Second, Fiske & Maddi (1961) and Jones and his associates (Jones *et al.*, 1961; Jones & McGill, 1967) suggest that the nature of the sensory stimulation is as important in determining its arousal value as its objective stimulus strength.

Third, the work of Zuckerman *et al.* (1968), Zuckerman *et al.* (1967) and Schubert (1964) point to the possibility that true sensory deprivation situations may have high arousal value and thus should be considered as potentially at the high rather than at the low end of the sensory stimulation continuum.

Hypothesis

The basic assumption underlying the author's extraversion–introversion sensoristasis hypothesis is that, other things being equal, Eysenck's hypothesis that extraversion is positively correlated with stimulus hunger is correct.

The hypotheses derived from this assumption are:

H_1. There is a positive correlation between extraversion scores and the amount of ambient illumination and sound which is necessary to provide optimum hedonic tone.

H_2. There is a positive correlation between extraversion scores and the amount of ambient illumination and sound which is necessary to create a slightly unpleasant level of hedonic tone.

METHOD

Subjects

One hundred and twenty male undergraduate students drawn from an introductory psychology class at Michigan State University served as subjects for the experiment. They were screened for auditory–visual abnormalities and stimulant or depressant drug use.

Experimental room

The experimental room was an 8×10 ft. windowless, well-insulated room equipped with a 6×25 in. one-way mirror installed in the door to enable the experimenter to observe unobtrusively the subject's activity. The room temperature was controlled at 72° F. and had 'normal' fluorescent lighting of 300 watts when lighting was not being controlled by the subject.

The furnishings consisted of a comfortable armchair and a 2 ft. × 18 in. table placed beside the right arm of the chair. A small bookcase with some miscellaneous equipment was located behind the chair, out of the subject's view. Apart from these furnishings and the apparatus to be described in the following section, the room was devoid of anything which could be of any interest to the subject.

Apparatus

The apparatus consisted for a 600-watt incandescent light source equipped with a 10-step, calibrated, continuously variable dimmer, placed on a 2×4 in. box on the table beside the subject's armchair. Each step represented an increment of 1 j.n.d. A remote control switch in series with the dimmer enabled the experimenter to turn the subject-controlled light source on and off at will from outside the experimental room.

Also on the table was a tape recorder with a 10-step, calibrated volume knob which, like the

ELEK J. LUDVIGH, III AND DEBORAH HAPP

light source, was calibrated in 1 j.n.d. increments and had a remote control on–off switch. An intercom placed on the bookshelf behind the subject enabled the experimenter to monitor any verbalizations by the subject.

Materials

Paper-and-pencil tests used were the Eysenck Personality Inventory (Eysenck & Eysenck, 1963) and the Contact Personality Factor (Cattell *et al.*, 1954). Both tests were used to measure the degree of extraversion. An additional measure was the Abnormal Arousal Questionnaire (AA Questionnaire) constructed by Ludvigh to check for possible abnormal internal arousal states and to serve as a screening device for subjects' possible perceptual handicaps and drug use.

Testing

On reporting for the experiment, the subject was successively given the Eysenck Personality Inventory and Contact Personality Factor. When these tests were completed, the period of optimum level of stimulation was begun.

Optimum level portion

The subject was seated alone in the dark, sound-insulated experimental room for an adaptation period of 1 min. At the end of this, the experimenter turned on the variable light source in the room for 30 sec. During this period the subject adjusted the light to the level most comfortable for him. At the end of the 30-sec. 'light on' period, the experimenter simultaneously turned out the lights and turned on the sound (background music) for 30 sec. As with the light, the subject adjusted the sound to his most comfortable, or optimum, level.

At the end of the 30 sec. 'sound on' period, the experimenter turned on the lights in the experimental room, entered it and recorded the settings made by the subject. The experimenter then left the room and the entire procedure described above was repeated.

Following the recording of the second set of preferred light and sound levels, the same basic procedure was repeated except that the light and sound were adjusted simultaneously to an optimum level.

Subsequent to recording the subject's optimum level of light and sound in conjunction, each of the above three trials was repeated with the modification that the subject adjusted the stimuli to a level slightly too high for comfort.

Abnormal Arousal Questionnaire and debriefing period

After completing the last part of the experiment, the subject was escorted from the experimental room and asked to fill out the AA Questionnaire. On completing this, he was given a debriefing sheet and was informed that he had completed the experiment.

RESULTS

Pearson product-moment correlations were computed for the variables of interest. Six subjects whose AA Questionnaire data revealed auditory–visual abnormalities or stimulant–depressant drug use were eliminated from the data analysis, resulting in an n of 114. Correlations which have direct bearing on the hypothesis are presented in Table 1.

H_1, which postulated a positive correlation between extraversion and amount of sensory stimulation preferred to produce optimum hedonic tone, did not receive statistical support.

H_2 postulated a positive correlation between extraversion and amount of stimulation necessary to produce slight discomfort. Of the six applicable correlations, all are in the predicted direction, two are significant at the 0·10 level, and two are significant at the 0·01 level. While the correlations are not of high magnitude, there is significant statistical support for this hypothesis.

Extraversion and preferred level of sensory stimulation

Table 1. *Correlations between extraversion scores and laboratory measures of preferred and slightly unpleasant levels of sensory stimulation – for all subjects ($n = 114$)*

Variable	Contact personality factor	Eysenck Personality Inventory
Optimum period		
Level of light	0·008	− 0·009
Level of sound	0·167	0·021
Level of light and sound in conjunction	0·127	− 0·045
Slightly unpleasant period		
Level of light	0·124	0·105
Level of sound	0·234***	0·163*
Level of light and sound in conjunction	0·229***	0·154*

* $P < 0·10$ ** $P < 0·05$ *** $P < 0·01$.

Table 2. *Correlations between extraversion scores and laboratory measures of preferred and slightly unpleasant levels of sensory stimulation for subjects with normal internal arousal states ($n = 62$)*

Variable	Contact personality factor	Eysenck Personality Inventory
Optimum period		
Level of light	0·008	0·052
Level of sound	0·210	− 0·078
Level of light and sound in conjunction	0·241**	0·068
Slightly unpleasant period		
Level of light	0·101	0·191
Level of sound	0·254**	0·200
Level of light and sound in conjunction	0·241**	0·233*

* $P < 0·10$ ** $P < 0·05$ *** $P < 0·01$.

Earlier, the view was presented that if subjects with abnormal internal arousal states were included in the sample, they might mask an existing correlation between extraversion–introversion and sensoristatic variables. Based on this belief, another correlation analysis was conducted after eliminating all subjects whose deviation from the norm on any one of the four variables of the AA Questionnaire related to arousal was greater than $1\frac{1}{2}\sigma$. To further ensure a subsample with a minimum of confounding variation, all subjects with scores of $1\frac{1}{2}\sigma$ above the mean on the lie scale of either the Contact Personality Factor or Eysenck Personality Inventory were also eliminated. This provided a sample of 62 subjects defined as 'normal'.

Inspection of Table 2 reveals findings quite similar to those for the entire sample. Again H_2 is supported while H_1 fails to receive statistically significant support. Worthy of note, however, is the fact that, while H_1 is not clearly supported by the data, it comes much closer to receiving support than it did for the sample as a whole. Specifically, for the six relevant correlations based on the Eysenck Personality Inventory and Contact Personality Factor scores, five are in the predicted direction, one is significant at the 0·05 level and one barely fails to reach the 0·10 significance level.

ELEK J. LUDVIGH, III AND DEBORAH HAPP

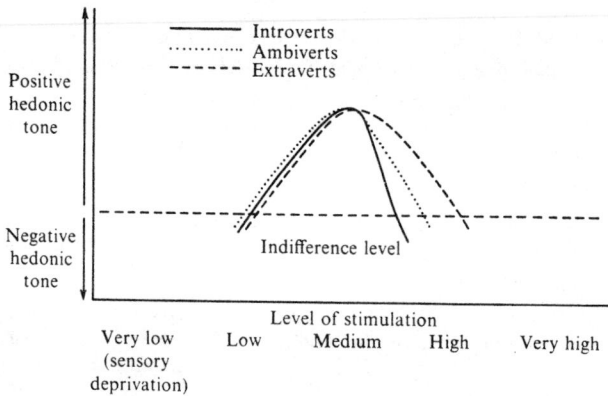

Fig. 2. Relation between level of sensory input, hedonic tone and the extraversion–introversion dimension based on obtained data.

DISCUSSION

Of considerable importance is the finding that the hypothesized relationship between the extraversion–introversion dimension, level of sensory stimulation and hedonic tone holds up considerably better for negative levels of hedonic tone than for optimum levels. That is, the data from the present study suggest that while extraverts and introverts may not be significantly different in preferred level of stimulation, they do differ on what constitutes an uncomfortably high level of stimulation. Since even the highest absolute levels of stimulation used in the present study did not exceed those encountered in daily life, the implications of the present findings are similar to that of Eysenck's original hypothesis. Thus differences which Eysenck explains in terms of optimum levels of stimulation can be explained equally well in terms of unpleasant levels of sensory input.

While the general shape of the curves observed in the present study was similar to those proposed by Eysenck, differences in level of sensory input between extraverts and introverts would be greater in the negative hedonic tone area than at optimum levels. Thus the present study suggests that the relationship can best be shown as in Fig. 2.

Implications of Fig. 2 are somewhat limited because of the small magnitude of the differences involved. It does, however, seem justifiable to say that level hedonic tone is approximately normally distributed over amount of sensory input. Additionally, it appears that there is a significant positive correlation between extraversion and amount of sensory stimulation necessary to produce feelings of slight discomfort.

A final note on Fig. 2 is that where there are no applicable data, no assumptions as to the nature of the relationship are made. The graph is thus incomplete and must remain so until carefully controlled studies are conducted, investigating extraversion–introversion sensoristasis differences at both extreme ends of the sensory stimulation continuum.

Extraversion and preferred level of sensory stimulation

REFERENCES

CATTELL, R. B., KING, J. E. & SCHUETTLER, A. K. (1954). *C.P.F. (form B)*. Champaign, Ill.: Institute for Personality and Ability Testing.

COFER, C. & APPLEY, M. (1965). *Motivation: Theory and Research*. New York: Wiley.

EYSENCK, H. J. (1967). *The Biological Basis of Personality*. Springfield: Thomas.

EYSENCK, H. J. & EYSENCK, S. B. G. (1963). *Eysenck Personality Inventory (Form A)*. San Diego, Calif.: Educational and Industrial Testing Service.

FISKE, D. W. & MADDI, S. R. (1961). A conceptual framework. In D. W. Fiske & S. R. Maddi (eds.), *Functions of Varied Experience*. Homewood, Ill.: Dorsey Press.

JONES, A. & McGILL, D. W. (1967). The homeostatic character of information drive in humans. *J. exp. Res. Person.* **2**, 25–31.

JONES, A., WILKENSON, H. J. & BRADEN, I. (1961). Information deprivation as a motivational variable. *J. exp. Psychol.* **62**, 126–137.

LINDSLEY, D. B. (1961). Common factors in sensory deprivation, sensory distortion and sensory overload. In P. Solomon *et al.* (eds.), *Sensory Deprivation*. Cambridge, Mass.: Harvard University Press.

LUDVIGH, E. (1970). Extraversion and need for sensory stimulation. (Unpublished master's thesis, Michigan State University.)

PETRIE, A., COLLINS, W. & SOLOMON, F. (1960). The tolerance for pain and for sensory deprivation. *Am. J. Psychol.* **73**, 80–90.

REED, G. & KENNA, J. (1964). Sex differences in body imagery and orientation under sensory deprivation of brief duration. *Percept. mot. Skills* **18**, 117–118.

REED, G. & SEDMAN, G. (1964). Personality and depersonalization under sensory deprivation conditions. *Percept. mot. Skills* **18**, 659–660.

ROSSI, A. M. & SOLOMON, P. (1965). Note on reactions of extraverts and introverts to sensory deprivation. *Percept. mot. Skills* **20**, 1183–1184.

ROSSI, A. M. & SOLOMON, P. (1966). Effects of sensory deprivation on introverts and extraverts: a failure to find reported differences. *J. psychiat. Res.* **4**, 115–125.

SCHUBERT, D. S. P. (1964). Arousal seeking as a motivation for volunteering: MMPI scores and central nervous system stimulant use as suggestive of a trait. *J. proj. Tech.* **28**, 337–340.

SCHULTZ, D. P. (1965). *Sensory Restriction: Effects on Behaviour*. New York: Academic Press.

TRANEL, N. (1962). Effects of perceptual isolation on introverts and extraverts. *J. psychiat. Res.* **1**, 185–192.

ZUCKERMAN, M., PERSKY, H., LINK, K. E. & BASU, G. K. (1968). Experimental and subject factors determining responses to sensory deprivation, social isolation and confinement. *J. abnorm. Psychol.* **73**, 183–194.

ZUCKERMAN, M., SCHULTZ, D. P. & HOPKINS, R. T. (1967). Sensation seeking and volunteering for sensory deprivation and hypnosis experiments. *J. consult. Psychol.* **31**, 358–363.

(*Manuscript received* 3 *January* 1973; *revised manuscript received* 15 *October* 1973)

From A. B. Hill (1975). British Journal of Psychology, *66*, 9–13, *by kind permission of the author and Cambridge University Press*

EXTRAVERSION AND VARIETY-SEEKING IN A MONOTONOUS TASK

By A. B. HILL

University of Keele

It is hypothesized on the basis of Eysenck's theory of extraversion that extraverts should build more variety into their performance at a monotonous task than introverts. The performance of a group of extraverts ($n = 16$) and a group of introverts ($n = 16$) on a simple repetitive task was compared. Comparisons were made on two measures of response variety: firstly, a simple measure of number of alternations among possible responses and, secondly, a measure of variety taken from information theory – the average entropy of the set of responses made. The hypothesis was confirmed on both measures. The results are interpreted as adding further support to Eysenck's work linking differences in extraversion to differences in arousal.

According to Eysenck (1957, 1967) inhibitory neural processes occur more quickly and strongly in the extravert, who is thus characterized by having a lower level of chronic arousal in the ascending reticular activating system than the introvert. If this is correct, it may be deduced that the extravert will require more external stimulation than the introvert to maintain an optimal level of cortical arousal.

A monotonous task offers only limited stimulation and it may be expected that the functional value of this stimulation for the maintainance of cortical arousal will decline more rapidly in the case of extraverts. If cortical arousal falls below its optimal level then, according to Hebb (1955), performance will be impaired. Eysenck (1963) has suggested that extraverts should show poorer performance on monotonous tasks, and evidence supporting this point can be seen in the vigilance studies of Bakan (1959) and Tarrière & Hartemann (1964).

Mackworth (1969), reviewing vigilance studies, has suggested that under certain conditions the introduction of irrelevant stimulation into a monotonous task may have beneficial effects on performance by aiding recovery of habituated responses. For this to occur the additional stimulation must be arousing but not distracting. In the conventional vigilance task there is little the subject can do to obtain greater stimulation from the task itself, although he may seek additional stimulation (and so increase his level of arousal) by going outside the task, e.g. by talking, singing, etc. If subjects were engaged in a monotonous task which permitted a certain amount of variation in the way responses were made, and so permitted subjects to derive greater stimulation from the task, it may be hypothesized, on the basis of the discussion above, that extraverts would exhibit a greater variety of response than introverts. In other words, it may be hypothesized that extraverts will build more variety into their responses on a monotonous task because doing so would tend to increase stimulation and so go some way to maintaining an optimal level of cortical arousal.

Eysenck & Levey (1965) showed that in a task where subjects were required to look at a pair of pictures (seeing one at a time) extraverts exhibited shorter inspection periods before alternation, a point which was taken as indicating that extraverts showed greater alternation. This study provided only weak support for Eysenck's

A. B. HILL

inhibition/arousal theory, because extraverts only showed significantly greater alternation behaviour at the beginning of the task whilst the theory predicts the difference in degree of alternation should have increased as the task was continued. Although the task used by Eysenck & Levey was not chosen as an especially monotonous one their comments on the behaviour of subjects suggests it may have been perceived as such. They report that some subjects tried to engage the experimenter in conversation, some played games by counting items in the pictures, etc. It seems reasonable to consider that such behaviour may have been an attempt to increase the amount of stimulation received by varying responses. Further evidence that extraverts tend to seek additional stimulation is provided by Farley & Farley (1967). They found a significant correlation between extraversion and sensation-seeking as measured by the Sensation-Seeking Scale of Zuckerman *et al.* (1964).

The work reported here represents a direct attempt to test the hypothesis that extraverts will exhibit greater response variety than introverts in their performance on a monotonous task.

METHOD

Subjects

Thirty-two male undergraduate students served as subjects. They were selected using Form A of the EPI (Eysenck & Eysenck, 1964) so that half were strongly extraverted (scores of 17 or above on the E scale) and half were strongly introverted (scores of 7 or below on the E scale). All subjects had scores in the middle range on the Neuroticism scale and a *t* test showed the difference between mean N scores for the two groups was not significant at the 5 per cent level of confidence.

The task

The task used was one in which the subject was required to pick up and place push pins in a partially but not fully prescribed manner. Subjects were tested individually in a quiet, drab room containing only a table and a chair each for the experimenter and subject. Seated at the table, the subject was confronted with a 10×8 in. sheet of paper pinned to a piece of chip-board. The paper was marked out into 50 cells (five columns and ten rows). Each cell contained three circles of approximately $\frac{1}{8}$ in. diameter arranged in the form of an equilateral triangle of side 1 in. On the table in front of the subject were three more pieces of board placed side by side, each containing 110 red push pins. The pins in each board were colour coded with small spots of paint in a manner invisible to the subject. The colour coding enabled the experimenter to identify at the end of the experiment which of the three pin beds each 'placed' pin had come from.

Procedure

To counterbalance time of day effects which Colquhoun & Corcoran (1964) have shown affect the performance of extraverted and introverted subjects differently, half the extraverts and half the introverts were tested in the morning, and the remainder of each group was tested in the afternoon.

The subject was instructed to pick up a pin from the left-hand bed and place it in one of the three circles forming the triangle in cell (1,1). Having done that he was instructed to pick up a pin from the middle bed and place it in one of the two remaining circles in the first cell and to follow that by placing a pin from the right-hand bed in the remaining circle. In this way all three circles in the cell (1,1) were filled. The subject was then asked to fill the other 49 cells. It was emphasized that the pins should always be picked up in the same sequence – left, middle, right – but that they might be placed in any way the subject chose provided he filled each cell before going on to the next. Subjects were instructed to work row by row and were asked to keep silent during the course of the experiment. They were also asked to use only their preferred hand in picking up and placing the pins.

Extraversion and variety-seeking in a monotonous task

During each experimental session the experimenter watched the subject's performance (without directly overlooking him) to ensure the instructions were adhered to. Each subject filled 300 cells in total. This required six 'placing' boards and the experimenter removed filled boards and replaced them with fresh ones with a delay of only a second or two.

The measurement of response variety

Because the pins from the three beds were colour-coded and because subjects were instructed to pick up the pins in the order left, middle, right, it was possible to determine after each experimental session how the subject had filled each cell. Using the letters A, B and C to stand for the three locations (circles) in each cell and the numbers 1, 2 and 3 to stand for the pins from left-hand, middle and right-hand beds respectively, it can be seen that there were six possible ways of filling each cell. These six response patterns are shown below:

A1	B2	C3
A1	C2	B3
B1	A2	C3
B1	C2	A3
C1	A2	B3
C1	B2	C3

Two measures of response variety were calculated for each subject. Firstly, the number of changes in response pattern over the first, second and final hundred trials. The disadvantage of this measure is obvious. Any given variety 'score' may be the result of alternation between the minimum number of response patterns (two) or the result of alternation between the maximum number of response patterns (six) or some number in between. Thus variety measured in terms of simple alternation takes no account of the range of response patterns used or the frequency with which each pattern is used. Following Ashby's (1956) identification of response variety with response entropy, a second measure of response variety was calculated in terms of entropy. This was achieved by applying the information theory measure of entropy (Attneave, 1959) to the results. This second measure was thus based upon the probability of occurrence of each of the six response patterns shown above. It is not contended that this eliminated the 'range and frequency of pattern usage' problem inherent in the simple alternation measure, but it may have lessened it.

RESULTS

Table 1 shows the mean number of changes in response pattern and the mean response entropy for extraverted and introverted subjects. As the distributions of both measures of variety showed signs of being positively skewed (six introverted subjects had zero variety scores over the entire 300 trials) non-parametric analyses were carried out.

Mann–Whitney U tests showed that in each block of trials, and also in the overall

Table 1. *Mean response variety for extraverts and introverts*

Trials	Mean no. of changes in response pattern		Mean response entropy in bits	
	E	I	E	I
1–100	15·7	9·4*	1·606	0·623*
101–200	17·1	8·9*	1·725	0·584*
201–300	20·3	11·2*	1·814	0·706*
All	53·1	29·5**	1·853	0·712**

* $P < 0.01$; ** $P < 0.001$ (Mann–Whitney U; one-tailed test).

A. B. HILL

results, extraverts exhibited significantly higher levels of response variety than introverts.

DISCUSSION

The overall results show that extraverts do tend to build more variety into their responses on a monotonous task than introverts. In the absence of any better alternative explanation, this may be considered as an attempt to increase the amount of stimulation received and so maintain, or at least go some way towards maintaining, an optimal level of cortical arousal. This finding therefore provides strong, though indirect, support for Eysenck's theory linking differences in extraversion–introversion to differences in cortical arousal.

Further support for Eysenck's view can be seen in the fact that the mean response variety of extraverts, however measured, showed a progressive increase over the course of the experiment. In the case of the introverts, mean response variety did not increase progressively through the experiment, although variety in the last block of trials was slightly greater than in the first block.

This finding in a progressive increase in response variety among extraverts (which was not present in the Eysenck & Levey study) is particularly interesting as it may point to the importance of methodology in this area. In the present experiment the task was specially chosen not only to be repetitive and monotonous but to offer the possibility for the subject to introduce subtle but measurable variations in response. It is difficult to see how objective measures of response variation other than alternation could have been assessed with the Eysenck & Levey task, yet it is precisely these subtle variations which may be important as sources of stimulation to the subject.

The results in Table 1 show good accord between the two measures of response variety used in the experiment. This suggests that the information theory measure of entropy may have some potential value as a means for measuring individual differences in extraversion and research on these lines is proceeding.

REFERENCES

ASHBY, W. R. (1956). *An Introduction to Cybernetics*. London: Chapman & Hall.
ATTNEAVE, F. (1959). *Applications of Information Theory to Psychology*. New York: Holt, Rinehart & Winston.
BAKAN, P. (1959). Extraversion–introversion and improvement in an auditory vigilance task. *Br. J. Psychol.* **50**, 325–332.
COLQUHOUN, W. P. & CORCORAN, D. W. J. (1964). The effects of time of day and social isolation on the relationship between temperament and performance. *Br. J. soc. clin. Psychol.* **3**, 226–231.
EYSENCK, H. J. (1957). *The Dynamics of Anxiety and Hysteria*. London: Routledge & Kegan Paul.
EYSENCK, H. J. (ed.) (1963). *Experiments with Drugs*. London: Macmillan.
EYSENCK, H. J. (1967). *The Biological Basis of Personality*. Springfield, Ill.: Thomas.
EYSENCK, H. J. & EYSENCK, S. B. G. (1964). *The Eysenck Personality Inventory*. London: University of London Press.
EYSENCK, H. J. & LEVEY, A. (1965). Alternation in choice behaviour and extraversion. *Life Sci.* **4**, 115–119.
FARLEY, F. & FARLEY, S. V. (1967). Extraversion and stimulus-seeking motivation. *J. consult. Psychol.* **31**, 215–216.

Extraversion and variety-seeking in a monotonous task

HEBB, D. O. (1955). Drives and the CNS (conceptual nervous system). *Psychol. Rev.* **62**, 243–254.

MACKWORTH, J. F. (1969). *Vigilance and Habituation*. Harmondsworth: Penguin Books.

TARRIÈRE, C. & HARTEMANN, F. (1964). Investigation into the effects of tobacco smoke on a visual vigilance task. *Ergonomics* **7**, 525–530.

ZUCKERMAN, M., KOLIN, E. A., PRICE, L. & ZOOB, I. (1964). Development of a sensation-seeking scale. *J. consult. Psychol.* **28**, 447–482.

(Manuscript received 4 July 1973; revised manuscript received 18 February 1974)

From B. S. Gupta (1974). Psychopharmacologia (Berl.), *36*, 275–280, *by kind permission of the author and Springer-Verlag*

Stimulant and Depressant Drugs
on Kinaesthetic Figural After-Effects

B. S. Gupta

Department of Psychology, Guru Nanak University, Amritsar, India

Received July 23, 1972; Final Version 17 January, 1973

Abstract. The effects of dexedrine, phenobarbitone and extraversion on kinaesthetic figural after-effects (KFAE) were examined. Forty five graduate and postgraduate students served as subjects. The subjects were randomly assigned to three drug treatments (stimulant, depressant and placebo) at each level of extraversion (high, average and low). A 3×3 factorial design was replicated five times. The study supports the following conclusions: 1. extraverted subjects have greater KFAE than introverted and average subjects; 2. phenobarbitone leads to greater KFAE and dexedrine reduces this effect; 3. introverted and average on E subjects do not show expected trends in KFAE under the influence of dexedrine; 4. variability (standard deviation) remains unaffected under the influence of centrally stimulant and depressant drugs.

Key words: Kinaesthetic Figural Afer-Effects — Dexedrine — Phenobarbitone.

According to Köhler and his associates (Köhler, 1940; Köhler and Wallach, 1944; Köhler and Dinnerstein, 1947) the figural after-effects (FAE) occur due to satiation, Eysenck's (1947, 1952, 1960a, 1967a, 1967b) theory of personality, based on the excitation/inhibition balance, proposes that satiation is built up more strongly and quickly and persists longer in extraverts than introverts. The theory suggests that after-effects, under equal conditions of stimulation, develop quicker, appear more strongly and persist longer in extraverts than introverts (Eysenck, 1955, 1956, 1960b, 1967b). Eysenck (1960b, 1963, 1967a, 1967b) also postulates that depressant drugs, by producing extraverted behaviour patterns, produce FAE more strongly and quickly; whereas stimulant drugs, by producing introverted behaviour patterns, produce FAE weakly and slowly. By connecting the two hypotheses, he (1960b, 1963, 1967b) has proposed that the susceptibility to the action of drugs is determined by the individual's temperamental characteristics. This concept probably was first emphasized by McDougall (1929), who says:

"... the marked extraverted personality is very much susceptible to the influence of alcohol... The introvert on the other hand is much more resistant to alcohol..."

B. S. Gupta

Eysenck (1967b) also states that the neuroticism (N) dimension of personality probably does not exert its effect in normal subjects under unstressed conditions. In a study of verbal conditioning by Gupta and Singh (1971) the results indicated that N exerted little influence.

The present study was designed to investigate the effects of dexedrine, a central stimulant, phenobarbitone, a central depressant, and the extraversion (E) dimension of personality on kinaesthetic figural aftereffects (KFAE). It was decided to select KFAE for this study because of the clear-cut results emerging from previous inquiries, as well as a means of avoiding the necessity to maintain fixation associated with visual tasks (Eysenck and Easterbrook, 1960a, 1960b). A dose of 10 mg for dexedrine and 100 mg for phenobarbitone was used. Calcium tablets were used as placebo. Similar doses used in a previous study (Gupta, 1970) were found to produce significant effects on performance. A Hindi translation of the MPI (Eysenck, 1959; Das, 1961) was used to obtain E scores.

Method

Subjects. The subjects (Ss) were graduate and post-graduate male students of different colleges and university teaching departments, between the ages of 21—25 years. They were drawn from a group of 1500 persons and were assigned to the following three personality groups, each consisting of 15 Ss (5 Ss were assigned randomly to each drug condition):

E+	39 +
E	26 to 28
E-	15 —

The selection of the extreme groups was done on the basis of Mean $\pm$ 1.5 SD of E scores (E Mean = 26.8; E SD = 7.9). The average group, i.e. E, ranged between Mean $\pm$ 0.1 SD. The Mean and SD of 1500 subjects were used for grouping the subjects.

Apparatus. The inspection (I) and test (T) figures were 2.5 and 1.5 in. in width respectively. These were made of aluminium but were otherwise the same as those used by Klein and Krech (1952), Eysenck (1955), Jaffe (1956), Eysenck and Easterbrook (1960b), and McEwen and Rodger (1960). An adjustable comparison scale in units of 0.05 in. (Satinder, 1964, 1966), was used for measuring KFAE.

Design. First a basal or pre-inspection point of subjective equality (PSE$_1$) was established which served as a control measure. After an inspection period of 60 sec another point of subjective equality (PSE$_2$) was established. The PSEs were based upon four judgments. Each judgment was followed by a one minute rest period. The method of average error, with a counterbalanced design of abba, was used. The procedure for measuring the KFAE was that adopted by Christman (1954) and Satinder (1966).

Procedure. The S was taken to the experimental room one hour after the oral administration of the drug. The latency period of the drugs was determined on the basis of the pilot observations regarding the time of peak effect of the drugs. The tablet, whether drug or placebo, was given by an assistant, and the experimenter had no knowledge of what each S had received until after the experiment had been concluded.

Stimulant and Depressant Drugs on Kinaesthetic Figural After-Effects

The S was seated on a stool between two tables, 34 in. in height, on which the figures were placed. The I and T figures were placed 3 in. apart on the right hand side, the T figure being nearer to S, and the comparison figure 22 in. away from T figure, on the left hand side of S. All the three figures were parallel to one another and at the same level from the ground. The PSE$_2$ was determined after S had inspected the I figure by making 60 movements in one minute at a rate of one movement per second. The movements were timed with the help of an electric metronome. The S was blindfolded throughout.

Results

The predicted effect of one minute stimulation by a larger block in place of standard is a displacement of the cerebral projection of the contours of the standard so as to make it seem relatively smaller. This is reflected in a smaller setting of the variable stimulus. The extent of KFAE was measured as PSE$_1$ minus PSE$_2$. The values thus obtained were subjected to analysis of variance (Edwards, 1968); the results of which are reported in Table 1.

Table 2 shows the means and SDs of various drug treatments within each of the extraversion groups.

Table 1. Results of analysis of variance

Source	df	Variance	F	P
Drug Treatments (T)	2	0.1670	55.6667	0.01
Extraversion (E)	2	0.0678	22.6000	0.01
T × E	4	0.0051	1.7000	n.s.
Within	36	0.0030		

Table 2. Means and SDs of drug treatments within each of the extraversion groups

E group	Placebo		Dexedrine		Phenobarbitone	
	Mean	SD	Mean	SD	Mean	SD
E+	0.27	0.04	0.14	0.06	0.42	0.07
E	0.15	0.03	0.11	0.05	0.28	0.05
E−	0.13	0.02	0.08	0.04	0.25	0.06

Discussion

The results of analysis of variance (Table 1) reveal that extraversion and the drugs, dexedrine and phenobarbitone, are significant variables for KFAE. The variance due to extraversion was analysed further by t-test. The results afford a good support for Eysenck's (1955, 1956, 1967a, 1967b) theory by revealing that Ss scoring high on E scale (possessing a high basic level of cortical inhibition and low basic level of cortical excitation) show significantly greater KFAE than their counterparts

B. S. Gupta

scoring low on this scale (possessing a low basic level of cortical inhibition and high basic level of cortical excitation). Moreover Ss high on E have also been found to have greater KFAE than Ss scoring average on E, whereas no such differences have been found to exist between Ss scoring low and average on E. Similar analysis of the variance due to drug treatments, indicates that phenobarbitone, a central depressant, leads to greater KFAE while dexedrine, a central stimulant, inhibits this tendency The results are, therefore, in conformity with Eysenck's (1960b, 1963, 1967a, 1967b) drug postulates. The results, though more pronounced and clear-cut, are also in agreement with those of Poser (1958), Eysenck and Easterbrook (1960b), and Costello (1962).

The non-significant F-ratio for the interaction of extraversion and drug treatments does not support the Eysenckian contention that individuals differ in their susceptibility to drug effects. The results in this section are not in accord with our previous findings on verbal conditioning (Gupta, 1970; Gupta and Singh, 1971). However, the t-test was applied to evaluate the significance of differences among the various means (Table 2) of drug and E groups. The results reveal that E^+ subjects differ significantly from E or E^- subjects, in the expected direction under the influence of phenobarbitone ($P < 0.05$) and placebo ($P < 0.01$) and not under the influence of dexedrine. And, moreover, the mean KFAE score, under decedrine, being a central stimulant, for each of the E groups, was expected to be significantly less than the corresponding mean value under placebo. This seems to be true for E^+ subjects ($P < 0.05$) in whom the basic cortical excitation level is already low. The similar trend, however, has also been observed for E and E^- groups though the results are non-significant statistically. The introverted subjects, who possess a high degree of cortical excitation, are assumed to be highly aroused people (Claridge, 1967; Davies and Tune, 1970; Gray, 1964, 1967, 1968, 1970; Nebylitsyn and Gray, 1972; Passingham, 1970). Such persons are already at the optimal level of performance (Eysenck, 1967c). Further increase in their excitation or arousability level, by the centrally stimulant drug, activates the inhibitory centres of the brain (Davies and Tune, 1970) and leads either to impairment in performance or the facilitating effect of the drug is masked. This seems to have happened with our E and E^- subjects who do not show expected trends in KFAE under the influence of dexedrine.

Differences between SDs of various drug treatments within each of the E groups were also tested by t-test (SDs in all the groups are given in Table 2) and found to be non-significant in all the cases except the placebo and phenobarbitone treatments of E^- group (differences significant at 0.05 level). Thus SDs remain unaffected by drugs, though in our previous study (Gupta, 1970) SDs tended to increase under the influence of drugs.

Stimulant and Depressant Drugs on Kinaesthetic Figural After-Effects

References

Christman, R. J.: Shifts in pitch as a function of prolonged stimulation with pure tones. Amer. J. Psychol. **67**, 484—491 (1954)

Claridge, G. S.: Personality and arousal. London: Pergamon Press 1967

Costello, C. G.: The effects of meprobamate on kinaesthetic figural after-effects. Brit. J. Psychol. **53**, 17—26 (1962)

Das, G.: Standardization of Maudsley Personality Inventory (MPI) on an Indian population. J. Psychol. Res. **5**, 7—9 (1961)

Davies, D. R., Tune, G. S.: Human vigilance performance. London: Stapples Press 1970

Edwards, A. L.: Experimental design in psychological research (3rd ed.). New York: Holt, Rinehart and Winston, Inc 1968

Eysenck, H. J.: Dimensions of personality. London: Routledge and Kegan Paul 1947

Eysenck, H. J.: The scientific study of personality. London: Routledge and Kegan Paul 1952

Eysenck, H. J.: Cortical inhibition, figural after-effect, and the theory of personality. J. abnorm. soc. Psychol. **51**, 94—106 (1955)

Eysenck, H. J.: Reminiscence, drive and personality theory. J. abnorm. soc. Psychol. **53**, 328—333 (1956)

Eysenck, H. J.: Manual of maudsley personality inventory. London: University of London Press 1959

Eysenck, H. J.: The structure of human personality (2nd ed.). London: Methuen 1960a

Eysenck, H. J. (Ed.): Experiments in personality (2 vols.). London: Routledge and Kegan Paul 1960b

Eysenck, H. J. (Ed.): Experiments with drugs. New York: Pergamon 1963

Eysenck, H. J.: The dynamics of anxiety and hysteria (3rd imp.). London: Routledge and Kegan Paul 1967a

Eysenck, H. J.: The biological basis of personality. Springfield, Ill.: Ch. C. Thomas 1967b

Eysenck, H. J.: Intelligence assessment: a theoretical and experimental approach. Brit. J. educ. Psychol. **37**, 81—98 (1967c)

Eysenck, H. J., Easterbrook, J. A.: Drugs and personality. IX. The effect of stimulant and depressant drugs upon visual figural after-effects. J. ment. Sci. **106**, 845—851 (1960a)

Eysenck, H. J., Esaterbrook, J. A.: Drugs and personality. X. The effects of stimulant and depressant drugs upon kinaesthetic figural after-effects. J. ment. Sci. **106**, 852—854 (1960b)

Gray, J. A.: Pavlov's typology. London: Pergamon Press 1964

Gray, J. A.: Strength of the nervous system, introversion-extraversion, conditionability and arousal. Behav. Res. Ther. **5**, 151—170 (1967)

Gray, J. A.: The physiological basis of personality. Advanc. Sci. **24**, 293—305 (1968)

Gray, J. A.: The psychophysiological basis of introversion-extraversion. Behav. Res. Ther. **8**, 249—266 (1970)

Gupta, B. S.: The effect of extraversion and stimulant and depressant drugs on verbal conditioning. Acta psychol. (Amst.) **34**, 505—510 (1970)

Gupta, B. S., Singh, S. D.: The effect of extraversion, neuroticism and a depressant drug on verbal conditioning. Indian J. exp. Psychol. **5**, 15—17 (1971)

B. S. Gupta

Jaffe, R.: The influence of visual stimulation on kinaesthetic figural after-effects. Amer. J. Psychol. **69**, 70—75 (1956)

Klein, G., Krech, D.: Cortical conductivity in the brain injured. J. Personality **21**, 118—148 (1952)

Köhler, W.: Dynamics in psychology. New York: Liveright 1940

Köhler, W., Dinnerstein, D.: Figural after-effects in kinaesthesis. In: Miscellanea psychologica, A. Michotte, Ed., pp. 196—200. Louvain: Publications 1947

Köhler, W., Wallach, H.: Figural after-effects: an investigation of visual processes. Proc. Amer. Phil. Soc. **88**, 265—357 (1944)

McDougall, W.: The chemical theory of temperament applied to introversion and extraversion. J. abnorm. soc. Psychol. **24**, 293—309 (1929)

McEwan, P., Rodger, R. S.: Some individual differences in figural after-effects. Brit. J. Psychol. **51**, 1—8 (1960)

Nebylitsyn, V. D., Gray, J. A.: (Eds.) The biological bases of individual behaviour. New York: Academic Press 1972

Passingham, R. E.: The neurological basis of introversion-extraversion: Gray's theory. Behav. Res. Ther. **8**, 353—366 (1970)

Poser, E.: Kinaesthetic figural after-effects as a measure of cortical excitation and inhibition. Amer. Psychol. **13**, 334—335 (1958)

Satinder, K. P.: Another device for the study of kinaesthetic figural after-effects. J. Psychol. Res. 8, 92—93 (1964)

Satinder, K. P.: Effects of intermodal stimulation on figural after-effects. Brit. J. Psychol. **57**, 1—5 (1966)

B. S. Gupta, Ph. D.
Department of Psychology
Guru Nanak University
Amritsar, India

From A. Petrie, W. Collins, and P. Solomon (1960). American Journal of Psychology, *73*, 80–90, *by kind permission of the authors and The University of Illinois Press*

THE TOLERANCE FOR PAIN AND FOR SENSORY DEPRIVATION

By Asenath Petrie, Walter Collins, and Philip Solomon,
Harvard Medical School

Varied reactions to pain have long been noted by investigators. There is a tendency to assume that these variations are due to differences in the control of the experience, but the work discussed in this paper suggests that the differences are inherent in the experience of pain itself.

Just as there are great differences in visual sensitivity between blindness and the acute normal vision of youth, so sensitivity for pain can vary in degree. A man with incurable cancer can be relieved from pain by pre-frontal lobotomy, but the cause of the pain is still there, though he has ceased to suffer from it. Apart from the relief from pain that lobotomy brings, there are individual differences in algesic sensitivity. Some people sense.pain acutely, others dimly, and still others scarcely feel it at all.

Sensory pain characteristically accompanies an excess of stimulation, whereas the stress of sensory deprivation (lack of stimulation) and monotony (lack of change in stimulation) are associated with a dearth of stimulation. Sensory deprivation is also borne differently by different persons; there are those for whom such deprivation creates great stress and also those for whom the stress is but minor.

The hypotheses of the present study are these. (1) Those aspects of personality that are changed by a pre-frontal lobotomy differentiate persons with high and low tolerance for pain. (2) Differences in tolerance for pain are paralleled by differences in perception. (3) Differences in tolerance for sensory deprivation are paralleled by differencs in perception that are the reverse of those associated with tolerance for pain.

Method and Procedure

Subjects. Altogether, 78 Ss were used in this study. They were divided as follows: 42 were patients undergoing different degrees and kinds of pain as a result of surgery or bronchoscopy; 19 were undergoing experimental pain; and 17 were undergoing sensory deprivation. The Ss undergoing experimental pain and deprivation were paid by the hour; the others were not paid.

* Received July 1, 1959, and accepted for prior publication December 29, 1959. This work was made possible by the active coöperation of the Boston Sanatorium and Beth Israel Hospital, Boston, with the collaboration of the Boston City Hospital. It was supported in part by the National Institute of Mental Health (M2641), the Lasker Foundation, and the Office of Naval Research.

TOLERANCE FOR PAIN AND SENSORY DEPRIVATION

Methods of assessing tolerance for pain and for deprivation. The patients in this study experiencing clinical pain were grouped according to their tolerance for pain (caused by comparable trauma) by three judges independently—a physician, a surgeon, and a nurse—who, in coming to their decisions, took into consideration (1) the patients' demands for analgesic drugs; (2) their sleeplessness as said to be caused by the pain; (3) the physical signs; and (4) the patients' statements of their experiences. The patients were interviewed by the physician on two occasions while they were in pain.

The *Ss* in the experimental group were subjected to pain caused by heat. Their thresholds for pain had been determined by Dr. Ulric Neisser,[1] with an adaptation of the Hardy-Wolff-Goodell dolorimeter, an instrument that concentrates radiant heat upon the skin.[2] The measurements are of temperature; the higher temperatures arise from longer exposure to the stiumulus. The temperature as which *S* first sensed pricking pain and the temperature at which he could no longer endure the pain were determined. For this second measurement, *S* was instructed to endure the pain as long as he possibly could. The difference between these two thresholds was used as a measure of *S*'s algesic tolerance—a new measure which we may call *tolerance for pain*. The group of experimental *Ss* was divided into thirds with low, medium and high tolerance for pain. The scores measuring tolerance for pain were about normally distributed in the population studied.

Tolerance for sensory deprivation and monotony was measured in 17 *Ss* who had volunteered to remain in a tank-type respirator under conditions inducing some sensory deprivation.[3] Our *Ss* took part in two investigations by Wexler, Mendelsohn, Leiderman, and Solomon.[4] The length of time that *S* was willing to remain in the respirator was used by us as the measure of his tolerance.

TOLERANCE FOR PAIN IN RELATION TO PERSONALITY

Broadly speaking, a person after pre-frontal lobotomy is more like a psychopath and less like a depressive. He is not a psychopath, but all his personality scores are changed in this direction. He might be said to be more 'extraverted.' Evidence for this statement comes from our studies of 100-odd patients with excisions of different extents in the pre-frontal regions of the brain.[5]

---

[1] Ulric Neisser, Temperature thresholds for cutaneous pain, *J. appl. Physiol.,* 14, 1959, 368-372.

[2] J. D. Hardy, H. G. Wolff, and Helen Goodell, *Pain Sensations and Reactions,* 1952, 67.

[3] The effects of sensory deprivation were first described by W. H. Bexton, Woodburn Heron, and T. H. Scott, Effects of decreased variation in the sensory environment, *Canad. J. Psychol.,* 8, 1954, 70-76. Subsequent experiments induced sensory deprivation by immersion in water; see J. C. Lilly, Mental effects of reduction of ordinary levels of physical stimuli on intact healthy persons, *Psychiat. Res. Reports,* 5, 1956, 1-28.

[4] J. H. Mendelson and J. M. Foley, A mental abnormality in poliomyelitis patients treated in a tank-type respirator, *Trans. Amer. neurol. Assoc.,* 81, 1956, 134-138; Donald Wexler, Jack Mendelson, P. H. Leiderman, and Philip Solomon, Sensory deprivation: a technique for studying psychiatric aspects-of stress, *A.M.A. Arch. neurol. Psychiat.,* 79, 1958, 225-233.

[5] Asenath Petrie, *Personality and the Frontal Lobes,* 1952, 96-99; also, Effects of

PETRIE, COLLINS, AND SOLOMON

In the present study of personality and its relations to tolerance for pain, we utilized the Maudsley Personality Inventory, the scores of which distinguish the psychopath from the depressive.[6] We used this inventory with three separate groups of patients at two Boston hospitals—the Boston Sanatorium and the Beth Israel Hospital. The patients had been subjected to (1) major chest surgery; (2) minor surgery, or (3) bronchoscopy. In addition, we used it (4) with volunteers subjected to experimental thermal pain and (5) on the first group of 10 vounteers who had been subjected

TABLE I

E-SCORES ON THE MAUDSLEY PERSONALITY INVENTORY FOR FIVE CLASSES
OF *S*s FURTHER DIVIDED INTO SUB-GROUPS ON THE BASIS OF TOLERANCE
FOR PAIN AND TOLERANCE FOR SENSORY DEPRIVATION

Class of Stress	*N*	Most tolerant sub-group	Least tolerant sub-group	Direction of difference
Pain from:				
Major chest surgery	16	24.9*	21.3	+
Minor surgery	9	25.9	18.5	+
Bronchoscopy	17	27.4	26.5	+
Experimental pain	13	28.67	23.57	+
Sensory deprivation	10	28.50	31.80	−

* Higher E-scores characterize the patient after lobotomy and the more psychopathic patient. The difference between sub-groups is significant at the 5%-level.

to sensory deprivation. The *S*s represented the extremes of tolerance and intolerance for pain; those moderately tolerant of pain were omitted from consideration.

In all five groups, our predictions were borne out. The scores are summarized in Table I. Results resembling those of a patient after lobotomy (the more 'psychopathic' scores) were found in the best tolerators, while those who suffered most had scores resembling a patient before lobotomy (the least 'psychopathic' scores). These relationships are reversed for the tolerance of sensory deprivation.

PERCEPTUAL SATIATION ASSOCIATED WITH TOLERANCE
FOR PAIN AND DEPRIVATION

With the experimental *S*s and with the slightly ill patients, we were able to explore some of the perceptual characteristics of the *S*s that are associated with the personality-type that tolerates pain. The important perceptual phenomenon in our study is the tendency, identified by Köhler and Wallach, for the intensity of a perception to be reduced in some persons

---

chlorpromazine and of brain lesions on personality, in H. D. Pennes (ed.), *Psychopharmacology*, 1958, 99-115.
[6] H. J. Eysenck, *The Dynamics of Anxiety and Hysteria*, 1957, 31.

after they have been stimulated for some time.[7] These investigators used the term *satiation* to describe this tendency and found individual differences in respect of it. It has been indicated that the susceptibility to satiation, as measured in one modality, like vision, is correlated with susceptibility to satiation in other modalities, like touch.[8]

The reduction in the subjective magnitude of a kinesthetic experience has, moreover, been shown to be related to the dimension of personality called *Introversion-Extraversion*. The more extraverted the personality, the greater the reduction.[9] The tendency toward reduced apparent size is also increased by certain types of brain injury.[10] Presumably the site of this phenomenon is central, not peripheral. The effect of brain-lesions is, however, apparently selective. Earlier work by Petrie shows that operations outside of the pre-frontal region which have no effect on sensitivity to pain, also have no effect on the tendency toward reduced size, nor any on some other measures related to extraversion.[11]

In this study we have measured satiability of kinesthetic size, adapting the apparatus first described by Köhler and Dinnerstein and subsequently used by other investigators.[12] S is first occupied for 45 min. answering questions, *and his hands are not used during this time*. We have introduced this resting period and consider it essential, as it permits the effect of whatever S handled prior to the testing session to wear off. Then S is blindfolded and feels with the thumb and forefinger of his right hand the width (38.1 mm.) of a test-object, a standard block of smooth, unpainted wood. Next, with the thumb and forefinger of his other hand, he feels a long tapered bar of similar unpainted wood and determines the place on the bar where it seems just as wide as the test-block. Movement back and forth along the bar is permitted, and the position of subjective equality for perceived width is thus fixed. The measurement is made four times in succession.

---

[7] Wolfgang Köhler and Hans Wallach, Figural after-effects, *Proc. Amer. phil. Soc.*, 88, 1944, 269-357. It should be made clear that certain of the after-effects reported by Köhler and Wallach are displacements that result in an enlargement of the apparent size of a figure. We are unable fully to confirm the results of Köhler and Wallach when Ss are grouped as Reducers and Non-reducers, in that the average effect on Reducers of stimulation with a large and a small block is to make them reduce while on the Non-reducers it is to make them enlarge. Details are being presented in a later paper. Ss of the two types should be separated in studying these two phenomena.

[8] Michael Wertheimer, Figural after-effect as a measure of metabolic efficiency, *J. Pers.*, 24, 1955, 56-73; Michael Wertheimer and Nancy Wertheimer, A metabolic interpretation of individual differences in figural after-effects, *Psychol. Rev.*, 61, 1954, 279-280.

[9] Eysenck, *op. cit.*, 156-159.

[10] G. S. Klein and David Krech, Cortical conductivity in the brain injured, *J. Pers.*, 21, 1952, 118-148.

[11] Petrie, Effects on personality of excisions in different regions of the brain with special reference to the relief of pain, *Proc. 14th int. Cong. Psychol.*, 1954, 167; Asenath Petrie, Walter Collins, and Philip Solomon, Pain sensitivity, sensory deprivation, and susceptibility to satiation, *Science*, 128, 1958, 1431-1433.

[12] Wolfgang Köhler and Dorothy Dinnerstein, Figural after-effects in kinesthesis, *Miscellanea Psychologica A. E. Michotte*, 1947, 196-220; Klein and Krech, *op. cit.*, 118-148; Eysenck, *op. cit.*, 155-156; Petrie, *Psychopharmacology*, 1958, 99-115.

PETRIE, COLLINS, AND SOLOMON

S is then given a wider test-block (63.5 mm.) which he rubs with his right-hand finger and thumb at a constant rate for 30 sec. The purpose of this rubbing of a wider block is to induce satiation if it is to occur. After the rubbing, he again equates the original test-block to the perceived equivalent width on the tapered bar, determining four equivalences.

Next the time of satiation-rubbing is increased, first to 60 sec., then to 90, then to 120, and four measurements of the subjective size of the test-object are made after each period of satiation. Thereafter, instead of rubbing to induce satiation, an empty interval is allowed to elapse, with measurements of the test-object after 15 min.

The second group of deprived *S*s were asked in addition to measure the larger block. They were given only one period of stimulation with the larger block and the whole process took 2 min.

We may call the persons who tend to reduce the size of the block subjectively after stimulation *Reducers,* contrasting them with the *Non-reducers* who accept the environment in its full intensity.

Our results support the hypothesis that the greatest tolerance for pain is shown by Reducers. We think that this tolerance for pain is partially due to the *S*s' tendency to reduce the effectiveness of stimulation. Thus a brief wave of intense pain could cause later pain to appear less severe. Indeed, our own experiments on satiability indicate that this diminution is a cumulative process which persists much longer than the stimulus that causes the reduction.

Experimental pain was induced in 19 *S*s by applying heat to the skin. Reducers were found to tolerate this pain best; Non-reducers poorly. The differences in satiability in the kinesthetic task between those who could and could not tolerate pain reached the 5% level of confidence after only 90 sec. of kinesthetic stimulation. An extreme Reducer diminished the apparent size of the wooden block by 30% after a further 90 sec. and this effect was still partially operative a quarter of an hour after all stimulation ceased (see Table II and Fig. 1). A pilot study of satiability in surgical patients who could sit up in a wheel chair also shows that tolerance for clinical pain is greatest in Reducers.

If we are right in explaining the tolerance of Reducers for pain as being partially due to a reduction in the intensity of stimulation, then this tendency to reduce should be a handicap in a situation where the environment starves the individual of sensory experience instead of bombarding him with it, as is the case for pain. Such sparsity of stimulation occurs in the experimental circumstances arranged to produce sensory deprivation or sensory monotony. Thus, being a Reducer should make for intolerance of sensory deprivation, because it would render the already limited stimulation even less effective.

Our findings on two different groups of 17 volunteers, all subjected to sensory deprivation, indicate that this relationship holds.[13] We find that it is Non-reducers who can better tolerate this starvation of stimulation as measured by the number of hours they are willing to remain in a tank-type respirator, while it is the Reducers who cannot for long accept this kind of stress. This difference is exactly the reverse of the behavior of these two types under the stress of pain. Results for the first group of 9 *S*s are given in Fig. 2 and Table II. In the second group of volunteers, the difference in satiability between the good and poor tolerators of deprivation

TABLE II

REDUCTION IN APPARENT SIZE OF BLOCK FOR FIVE GROUPS OF *S*s
DIFFERING IN TOLERANCE OF PAIN AND OF DEPRIVATION
(in millimeters)

	Pain						Deprivation			
Time of test	Least tolerant (N=7)		Moderately tolerant (N=6)		Most tolerant (N=6)		Least tolerant (N=4)		Most tolerant (N=5)	
	Mean	SE	Mean	SE	Mean	SE	Mean	SE	Mean	SE
After 30 sec. stimulation	0.81	1.07	0.42	1.68	2.46	1.47	1.26	0.95	−0.03	0.86
After 90 sec. stimulation	−0.42[a]	0.77	1.92	1.69	3.50[a]	1.64	1.74	0.75	−0.12	0.83
After 180 sec. stimulation	−0.09[ac]	0.56	2.97	1.81	4.95[a]	1.71	4.77[bc]	1.11	1.86[b]	0.70
After 300 sec. stimulation	0.96[ac]	0.87	3.36	1.82	5.28[a]	1.96	4.68[bc]	1.23	2.04[b]	0.63
After 15-min. rest	−0.42[ac]	0.46	0.72	1.24	4.02[a]	1.35	2.55[c]	0.69	1.83	1.19

Differences are significant between: [a] Least and most tolerant of pain; [b] Least and most tolerant of deprivation; [c] Least tolerant of pain and deprivation.

is significant beyond the 2% level of confidence. Indeed, if the two deprivation groups are combined, the difference in satiation after 120 sec. of stimulation is significant beyond the 1% level.

Contrasting attitudes concerning their pain were, moreover, expressed by those *S*s who were most and least tolerant of the stress of sensory deprivation. These two groups differed in their estimations of their tolerances for pain, in their estimations of their parents' attitudes towards the expression of suffering with pain, and in their evaluation of the pain they experienced in the respirator. Those who were unable to tolerate much deprivation believed themselves able to stand pain especially well and did not believe that the parental demand for self-control in their youth, control in the expression of suffering with pain, had been stringent. On the other hand, those persons who were able to stand sensory deprviation well did not think they could stand pain well and believed that the parental demand for self-control in the expression of suffering with pain had been unduly stringent.

Thus it appears that he who is least susceptible to deprivation is most susceptible to pain and that a pain or ache has a different value for a person according to his tendency to reduce the perceived intensity of sensation and his associated personality traits. To examine this generality further we decided to seek from the *S*s who had

[13] Philip Solomon, P. H. Leiderman, J. H. Mendelson, and Donald Wexler, Sensory deprivation, a review, *Amer. J. Psychiat.*, 114, 1957, 357-363.

PETRIE, COLLINS, AND SOLOMON

undergone deprivation subjective quantitative estimates of the pain they shared in common—the muscular pain associated with being confined in a respirator.

Each of 8 Ss was asked what proportion of his earnings from the experiment he would forego could he be relieved of the pain when required to repeat the rest of the experiment. Of the 4 Ss who stayed longest in the respirator one offered to take off 100% of his earnings for backache. Another offered 50%, a third 40%, and a fourth said that he had experienced mere discomfort rather than pain and that this had not been an important factor in his thinking.

In contrast to these offers, of the 4 Ss who stayed in the respirator the shortest period, one said he would never undertake the experience again for any amount of money, that the experience was infinitely worse than the most agonizing pain he could imagine. Two, who said they had left the respirator because of the pain,

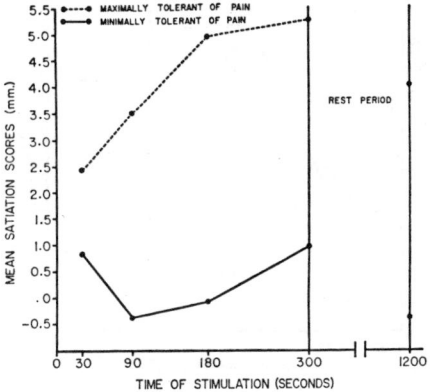

FIG. 1. DECREASE IN SIZE OF TACTUAL TEST-OBJECT FOR GROUPS WHO ARE MINIMALLY AND MAXIMALLY TOLERANT OF PAIN

would not forego any earnings to be relieved of it, and one agreed to forego 25% of his earnings.

It is clear that the absence of pain is more greatly valued by those Ss who tolerated sensory deprivation best; and they were the Ss who tend to be Non-reducers, who had their experience of pain undiluted. Implicit in these findings is the fact that the non-tolerators of deprivation are much more troubled by other aspects of the experience than by the pain, aspects that constitute the characteristic nature of the stress of sensory deprivation. Perhaps they, nevertheless, complain of pain because our culture regards pain as a proper signal of which to take notice and our language is rich in words for its description. These last two factors are absent, of course, in the stress of sensory deprivation.

Indeed, since pain is sensory, the Reducers might even need the pain of which they complain in the respirator, for it diminishes their sensory starvation and may protect them from hallucinatory substitutes. Two Ss in the group exposed to the most stringent conditions of deprivation had hallucinations, and they were the only Ss who did not report experiencing any pain in the respirator. This finding, therefore, supports the hypothesis that pain, in reducing sensory starvation, also reduces the need to produce hallucinatory experience.

CLINICAL MEDICINE AND SATIABILITY

Clinical medicine provides us with many instances of behavior under pain which could be well explained by a theory of satiability. For example, Dr. Travell of Cornell has reported to me that patients do not complain of pain if an injection of novacaine is made while an area is painful, that is to say, when, according to our theory, some satiation has taken place; yet plenty of complaints are made if such an injection is given in an area that is no longer painful. Dr. Gray, of the Harvard Medical School, has similarly reported that electrical treatment in a new area of the body results in the patient's thinking it is more painful than in the previous area

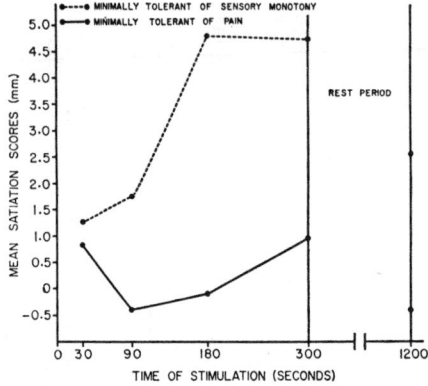

FIG. 2. DECREASE IN SIZE OF TACTUAL TEST-OBJECT FOR GROUPS WHO ARE MINIMALLY TOLERANT (1) OF SENSORY DEPRIVATION AND (2) OF PAIN

treated. In the new area, according to our theory, he has had no satiation for his pain, and therefore finds it greater. Every good nurse knows, moreover, that she can give injections, without causing pain, by counter-irritation—by firmly pinching the area before she inserts the needle.

TIME AND SATIABILITY

Besides satiability, there is another perceptual characteristic that changes after a pre-frontal lobotomy and in respect of which suggestive differences exist in contrasting Ss who are most and least tolerant of experimental pain. This is, moreover, again a difference that is reversed for those who who are most and least tolerant of deprivation. It is a difference in the perception of time. A minute is experientially lengthened after a pre-frontal lobotomy and, as a corollary, the time spent over a task tends to be underestimated. This altered perception of time is also characteristic of the good tolerator of pain and of the poor tolerator of deprivation.

The mean difference between the good and poor tolerators of pain in the reproduction of 60 sec. is 7.8 ($SE = 4.3$) sec. and between the good and poor tolerators of deprivation it is -6.6 ($SE = 7.1$) sec. If the scores of the poor tolerators of pain and the good tolerators of deprivation are combined and contrasted with the rest of the group, a difference of this size in this direction reaches the 5% level of confidence.

Everyone experiences periods full to the brim and periods curiously empty. The full periods appear to fly past when we are in them, but, when we look back at them, we feel they surely must have taken longer than they actually did. The empty periods, on the other hand, appear to be passing slowly while we are in them, but retrospectively, they seem shortened. It might, therefore, he predicted that the Reducer should experience time which is relatively empty for him, because of his tendency to reduce his perception of the environment and judge it as passing more slowly than does the Non-Reducer. This difference is, indeed, just what we have found.

Another characteristic of the good tolerator of pain and the poor tolerator of deprivation, one that parallels the change after pre-frontal lobotomy, is that such an S is more interested in, least worried about, and most happy about the present in contrast to the past and future. Details have been presented elsewhere as to how this change in the perception of the passage of time might contribute to tolerance for pain, as would also a loss of preoccupation with the past and future.[14] Such a patient would be dealing only with present pain and in a more contracted form.

Brief reference may be made to two studies in progress which amplify the findings reported here. First, children's characteristic behavior with pain and their intolerance of perceptual monotony and confinement have caused us to suppose that a tendency to reduce the perceived intensity of sensation might be a characteristic of childhood. Our pilot study suggests that such is the case. Secondly, the results of our preliminary study of 25 alcoholics, who were contrasted with 50 non-alcoholic patients, indicate that there is among the alcoholics a predominance of the personality type of the Non-reducer—of those who suffer much from the insults of the perceptual environment. This relation, taken in conjunction with the fact that alcohol was one of the first anesthetics to be used, suggests that alcohol might cause an increase in the tendency to 'reduce.' We have now found, in a pilot study with 28 members of a hospital staff, that, under the influence of alcohol, the Non-reducers tend to become Reducers.

Discussion and Conclusions

The results of the experiment support these hypotheses: (1) The aspects of personality changed by pre-frontal lobotomy differentiate those who can tolerate pain well from those who suffer greatly with pain. (2) Individual differences in tolerance for pain are paralleled by differences in

[14] Petrie, *Psychopharmacology*, 1958, 99-115; *Proc. 14th int. Cong. Psychol.*, 1954, 167.

perception, especially in the tendency subjectively to reduce the intensity of sensation and in the perception of time. (3) Individual differences in the tolerance for sensory deprivation are also paralleled by these differces in perception, but the direction of the difference is reversed.

Satiability may contribute to each of these tolerances. Indeed, the tendency to reduce the perceived intensity of sensation may be in part the mechanism of tolerance for pain, in that an intermittent bigger wave of pain causes subsequent pain to be perceived as less intense. The tendency to reduce could also be in part the mechanism of the intolerance of sensory deprivation in that it would cause the limited stimulation available to be perceived as even less intense. The sensations of a Reducer would be more diminished, as a result of his previous sensations, than would those of a Non-reducer. One may think of the Reducer as being, in his day-to-day life, subjected to some sensory deprivation: the greater his tendency to reduce, the greater his deprivation. The results of our experiment suggest that the intensity of his sensory experience (including pain) is mitigated because of his tendency to reduce—his tendency to diminish the apparent size of the object. This person is intolerant of further deprivation. At the other end of the spectrum are those whose incoming perceptions are least diminished by previous perception, who have their pain and other sensations 'neat' and undiluted, in whom pain is cumulative, and who more readily tolerate sensory deprivation. Thus different kinds of resistance appear to be needed for tolerating the stress of pain and the stress of sensory deprivation.

Experimental and actual sensory deprivation is never complete and is, indeed, at times a consequence of monotonous stimulation. Just as contrast and change are the conditions of attention, so monotony is in fact psychologically the equivalent of diminution in sensory input. We know that the process of habituation on the psychological level is accompanied by the nervous system's cutting off monotonous stimulation. For example, touch fibers adapt rapidly and respond only to change of pressure. Pain is, however, an exception in that it is not quickly blocked out[15] and under ordinary conditions complete habituation for it rarely occurs.[16] In sensory monotony or deprivation the non-adaptation to any pain that may be present results in a diminution of the sensory starvation: the pain provides 'sensory nourishment.' He who in sensory deprivation is starved of sensation may find that pain, as a sensation, constitutes an alleviation of his stress.

---

[15] E. D. Adrian, *Basis of Sensation,* 1928, 101.
[16] K. M. Dallenbach, Pain: History and present status, this JOURNAL, 52, 1939, 331-347; L. J. Stone and K. M. Dallenbach, Adaptation to the pain of radiant heat, this JOURNAL, 46, 1934, 229-242.

PETRIE, COLLINS, AND SOLOMON

This view gains support from our finding that those most tolerant of deprivation estimate the pain they experience under these conditions as more intense than the pain experienced by those least able to tolerate deprivation. It may well be that the more intense experience of pain is also contributory to the ability of Non-reducers to tolerate experimental deprivation. The fact that only those without pain experienced hallucinations is surely most relevant.

Findings that animals brought up in a restricted sensory and social environment behave as though some forms of pains are not noxious lend further support to this view. For such animals, the normal avoidance of pain is absent. A chimpanzee, whose tactual, kinesthetic, and manipulative experience had been restricted during the first 31 mo. of its rearing, on being subsequently pricked with a pin often responded by panting as chimpanzees do when they are being tickled and enjoying the stimulation.[17] A Scotch terrier who has been reared under conditions of extreme sensory deprivation will put his nose into the flame of a lighted match. This type of behavior does not occur for animals reared normally.[18] It is not impossible that such findings on the attractiveness of pain in sensory starvation may also turn out to have some relation to the origin of masochism in man. The main import of this paper is, however, the manner in which differences in perception are related to variation in the tolerance of pain and the tolerance of sensory deprivation.

---

[17] H. W. Nissen, K. L. Chow, and Josephine Semmes, Effects of restricted opportunity for tactual, kinesthetic, and manipulative experience on behavior of chimpanzee, this JOURNAL, 64, 1951, 485-507.
[18] Ronald Melsack and T. H. Scott, The effect of early experience on the response to pain, *J. comp. physiol. Psychol.*, 50, 1957, 155-161.

PART IV

PERSONALITY AND VIGILANCE

Vigilance, i.e. long-continued attention to periodically presented sets of stimuli into which occasional signals are interpolated to which special responses are required, is an experimental subject which has given rise to a large and varied literature (Buckner and McGrath, 1963; Davies and Tune, 1969; Stroh, 1971). It is of interest to students of personality because there is considerable evidence that the experimental conditions employed generate decreasing levels of arousal, as measured by psychophysiological methods (Carr, 1969; Becker-Carus, 1970; Davies and Krkovic, 1965; Gale, Haslum, and Lucas, 1972; O'Hanlon, 1965). Performance on the task typically deteriorates over time, and indices of arousal (EEG alpha, skin conductance, etc.) typically decline *pari passu*. There would appear to exist a direct link between physiological arousal and performance, and consequently it should be possible to use decline in performance as an index of arousal by means of which to test personality theories implicating arousal as a causal factor.

There are over a dozen studies which show that the predicted inferiority of extraverts on tasks of vigilance is apparent in connection with many different types of task; in addition to the papers reprinted below, we might mention the work of Bakan (1959), Bakan *et al.* (1963), Claridge (1960), Eysenck (1959), Hogan (1966), Harkins and Geen (1975), Tune (1966), Davies and Hockey (1966), and several of the authors mentioned above in connection with the electrophysiological measurement of vigilance decrement in arousal. Davies and Hockey (1966), in addition to personality, studied the effects of noise, signal frequency and time at work, using the "inverted-U hypothesis to integrate their results, with some measure of success". They concluded that "in spite of some difficulties of interpretation, an arousal theory of vigilance performance provides a reasonably parsimonious account of the present findings, although a conclusive test of its adequacy remains to be made". It is of course unrealistic to expect any test of a scientific

theory to be "conclusive"; theories are falsifiable, but cannot be proved to be correct. Nevertheless, the sentiment expressed is of course correct; the theory is still in an early state, and requires much more precise formulation before it can generate the requisite detailed predictions which would enable a more searching test to be made.

One aspect of such an improved theory which would have to take into account would be the difference between false alarm rate (FAR) and detection rate (Broadbent, 1971; Broadbent and Gregory, 1963). Small changes in the FAR can lead to large changes in detection rate, and these two measures are therefore not linearly related. As a consequence it is possible that in studies which use detection rate alone the major contributory factor to E–I differences is difference in FAR, which in turn produces differences in detection rate. Krupski, Raskin, and Bakan (1971), Carr (1969) and Tune (1966) did find that introverts make fewer false alarms, as well as detecting more signals. It is possible to use such data in the general paradigm of signal detection theory (Green and Swets, 1966), which makes use of two parameters to describe a subject's performance, d' and β. The former is a measure of the subject's ability to distinguish between signal and non-signal events, while the latter is a measure of the subject's criterion, i.e. the critical value of the likelihood ratio above which the subject reports a signal. Using these parameters enables us to make a distinction between a subject's ability to detect a signal, and his caution or bias in reporting the signal. The work of Tune (reprinted below) and of Harkins and Geen (1976) suggests that both factors are active in determining the inferior performance of extraverts on vigilance tests: they show less ability in signal detection, and they report more false positives. Tune suggests how these findings can be interpreted in terms of arousal theory. Altogether it may be said that vigilance experiments give some support to an arousal theory of E–I, although there are still some anomalies to be ironed out.

REFERENCES

BAKAN, P. Extraversion–introversion and improvement in an auditory vigilance task. *British Journal of Psychology*, 1959, *50*, 325–332.

BAKAN, P., BELTON, J., and TOTH, J. Extraversion–introversion and decrement in an auditory vigilance task. In: D. N. Buckner and J. J. McGrath (Eds.) *Vigilance: a symposium*. New York: McGraw Hill, 1963

BECKER-CARUS, C., Relationships between EEG, personality and vigilance. *Electroencephalography and Clinical Neurophysiology*, 1971, *30*, 519–526.

BROADBENT, D. E. *Decision and stress*. London: Academic Press, 1971.

BROADBENT, D. E. and GREGORY, M. Vigilance considered as a statistical decision. *British Journal of Psychology*, 1963, *54*, 309–323.

BUCKNER, D. N. and MCGRATH, J. J. (Eds.) *Vigilance: a symposium*. New York: McGraw Hill, 1963.

CARR, G. D. *Introversion–extraversion and vigilance performance*. Tufts University: Unpublished Ph.D. thesis, 1969.

CLARIDGE, G. S. The excitation–inhibition balance in neurotics. In: H. J. Eysenck (Ed.) *Experiments in personality, Vol. 2*. New York: Praeger, 1960.

DAVIES, D. R. and HOCKEY, G. R. J. The effects of noise and doubling the signal frequency on individual differences in visual vigilance performance. *British Journal of Psychology*, 1966, *57*, 381–389.

DAVIES, D. R. and KRKOVIC, A. Skin-conductance, alpha-activity, and vigilance. *American Journal of Psychology*, 1965, *78*, 304–306.

DAVIES, D. R. and TUNE, G. S. *Human vigilance performance*. New York: American Elsevier, 1969.

EYSENCK, H. J. Personality and problem solving. *Psychological Reports*, 1959, *5*, 592.

GALE, A., HASLUM, M. and LUCAS, B. Arousal value of the stimulus and EEG abundance in an auditory vigilance task. *British Journal of Psychology*, 1972, *63*, 515–522.

GREEN, D. and SWETS, J. Signal detection theory and psychophysics. New York: Wiley, 1966.

HARKINS, S. and GEEN, R. G. Discriminability and criterion differences between extraverts and introverts during vigilance. *Journal of Research in Personality*, 1976, *9*, 335–340.

HOGAN, M. J. Influence of motivation on reactive inhibition in extraversion–introversion. *Perceptual and Motor Skills*, 1966, *22*, 187–192.

KRUPSKI, A., RASKIN, D. and BAKAN, P. Physiological and personality correlates of commission errors in an auditory vigilance task. *Psychophysiology*, 1971, *8*, 304–311.

O'HANLON, J. F. Adrenaline and noradrenaline: reaction to performance in a visual vigilance task. *Science*, 1965, *150*, 507–509.

STROH, C. M. *Vigilance: the problem of sustained attention*. London: Pergamon, 1971.

TUNE, G. S. Errors of commission as a function of age and temperament in a type of vigilance task. *Quarterly Journal of Experimental Psychology*, 1966, *18*, 358–361.

From A. Krupski, D. C. Raskin, and P. Bakan (1971). Psychophysiology, *8*, 304–311, *by kind permission of the authors and the Society for Psychophysiological Research*

PHYSIOLOGICAL AND PERSONALITY CORRELATES OF COMMISSION ERRORS IN AN AUDITORY VIGILANCE TASK

Antoinette Krupski,

Michigan State University

David C. Raskin,

University of Utah

and Paul Bakan

Simon Fraser University

ABSTRACT

To determine correlates of the tendency to make errors of commission in a vigilance task, 31 Ss worked at a task of listening to recorded digits for 48 min and reported odd-even-odd digit sequences. Reports of "signals" where signals did not actually occur constituted commission errors. While S was engaged in the vigilance task skin conductance was continuously recorded. A measure of extraversion and neuroticism was available for each S. The tendency to make commission errors was associated with decrement in the detection of real signals over time, low GSR amplitude at detection points, and low initial orienting response. Commission errors were positively related to extraversion and unrelated to neuroticism. It was concluded that commission errors are made by Ss who are low in arousal level, subject to vigilance decrement, and likely to score higher on extraversion.

DESCRIPTORS: Arousal, Attention, Skin conductance, Extraversion, Galvanic skin response, Impulsivity, Orienting response, Signal detection, Vigilance. (A. Krupski)

A frequent observation in vigilance experiments is the occurrence of commission errors (CEs) or false positives. These errors occur when S reports a signal which has not in fact been presented to him. The main dependent variable in studies of vigilance is usually the detection of real signals, and the change in detection performance over time. However, the occurrence of commission errors in vigilance tasks has led to an interest in the etiology of these errors (Broadbent & Gregory, 1963a, 1963b; Jerison, 1967; McGrath, 1963). The literature on commission errors has recently been reviewed by Davies and Tune (1969).

The most systematic approach to the problem of CEs has been in the context

Address requests for reprints to: Professor Paul Bakan, Psychology Department, Simon Fraser University, Burnaby 2, B. C., Canada.

of the psychophysical theory of signal detection (Broadbent & Gregory, 1963a, 1963b, 1965). This approach treats CEs or false positives as a manifestation of a decision parameter called β (beta), a measure of caution or degree of reluctance to call any event a signal. This approach has recently come under severe criticism, however, because the traditional vigilance situation differs in important respects from the classical situation to which signal detection theory is applicable (Davies & Tune, 1969; Jerison, 1967). Jerison (1967) has argued that the application of the signal-detection model is psychologically unsound since values of β (beta) computed from vigilance data are not measures of caution, but are artifacts due to the pooling of observations made under different conditions of attentiveness during the vigil.

The presence of wide individual differences in the generation of commission errors has frequently been noted (Bakan, 1955; Wiener, 1963). This raises the problem of correlates of individual differences in the generation of commission errors. The present study was designed to explore some temperamental and physiological correlates of individual differences in the tendency to make commission errors in a vigilance task.

It was hypothesized that the kind of person who makes CEs or false positives is likely to be impulsive and at a chronically low level of physiological arousal. Since impulsivity is one of the components of extraversion (Eysenck & Eysenck, 1963b, 1969) it follows that extraversion should be positively correlated with CEs. The relationship between extraversion and low arousal has also been considered by Eysenck (1967).

There is evidence available relating both arousal and extraversion to performance in vigilance tasks. Measures of electrodermal activity have been shown to be related to detection measures. Generally, high levels of electrodermal activity (high arousal) are associated with little or no decrement in detection performance over time (Dardano, 1962; Ross, Dardano, & Hackman, 1959). High levels of extraversion are related to decrement in vigilance tasks, whereas low levels of extraversion (i.e., introversion) are associated with little change in performance over time (Bakan, Belton, & Toth, 1963; Claridge, 1967).

In the present study the relationship between commission errors and each of the following variables was explored: change in detection of true signals over time, galvanic skin response (GSR) amplitude, basal level of skin conductance, a GSR measure of the orienting response, and measures of extraversion and neuroticism.

METHOD

Subjects

Subjects were 31 male volunteers from an introductory psychology course. Their ages ranged from 18 to 21.

Apparatus

Zinc cup electrodes, $\frac{5}{8}$ inch in diameter, were used for recording. Cotton pads soaked in a 1 % zinc sulfate solution were placed within the cups and served as the electrolyte. GSR electrode placement was on the base of the left thumb and on the inside of the left forearm.

Skin resistance was continuously recorded on a Beckman Type RS Dynograph using a Beckman Type PGR coupler which utilizes a simple Wheatstone bridge circuit.

Vigilance Task

A copy of the vigilance tape developed by Bakan (1959) was employed. This tape is 64 min long and consists of digits which are spoken at the rate of one per second. The original tape was constructed by splicing to ensure uniformity. Each digit was recorded once, played on an endless tape, and recorded to produce multiple recordings of the same digit. Pieces from these multiple recordings were spliced together so that the sound of any digit was constant throughout the tape.

The original tape was duplicated on a Viking 433 recorder. It was recorded on one track while a tone was recorded on a second track at the onset of each signal. Although the tone was not audible to S, it served to trigger an audio switch which set off an event marker on the dynograph at the onset of each signal.

The tape began with a female voice saying, "The numbers will begin in 30 seconds," which was followed by 30 sec of silence and then the presentation of the first number. The tape was played back through a Dyna SCA-35 Stereo Control Amplifier to Sharpe stereo earphones which were worn by Ss.

Ss were instructed to detect odd-even-odd combinations of digits that were all different and successive, e.g., 943, 725. The tape was divided into four periods of 16 min and there were 10 signals, or odd-even-odd combinations presented during each period. Although the task appeared continuous to the S, there were actually four equivalent 16 min periods, differing only in the specific signals to be detected. The distribution of signals over time was the same in each period, the time between signals being 69, 152, 23, 181, 108, 102, 44, 13, 141, and 144 sec.

Ss were to press a button located in front of their right hand when they detected a signal. The button was connected to a second marker pen on the dynograph so that each detection response was recorded on the paper alongside the skin conductance recording. Consequently each S's record consisted of continuous recordings of skin conductance, detection responses, and critical detection points or signals. The paper speed was set at 1 mm/sec.

Procedure

Ss were tested individually in an experimental room which was adjacent to the recording room. A fan was used to mask noises from relays and other sources. When electrode placement was complete the S was asked to read instructions for the vigilance task. The last page of instructions consisted of a practice set where the S looked at a series of digits and was told to write down the appropriate odd-even-odd combinations. When S appeared to have completed the visual practice set, E asked if he had any questions. If S had no questions, the following instructions were read aloud:

The first part of this task is a practice period followed by a short rest. During the rest period you will be allowed to stretch and move around if you like. However, try to remain as still as possible while the practice and the actual test are going on. The electrodes, particularly those on the left side, are very sensitive to movement. So please try to keep movement, other than pressing the button, at a minimum. Get comfortable before the experiment begins. The actual test will follow the rest period. It will be identical in nature to the practice.

Earphones were placed on S and E left the experimental room and took her place in the recording room. The dynograph was turned on and if all appeared to be in working order the tape was begun. After the first 16 min period, the recording apparatus and tape were turned off and the earphones taken off S. He was told that the practice period was over and asked if he had any questions. If there were no questions, he was given about 5 min to stretch and relax before resuming the task. The S was not given specific knowledge of results, although he was told whether his performance was adequate or not. Ss who responded very often or did not respond at all during the practice were asked to verbally repeat the instructions. If the instructions were repeated correctly nothing more was said concerning S's performance. If, however, the S's report of the directions was inaccurate, E explained the procedure once again. This was found to be necessary in about 5 cases.

After the rest period, the earphones were replaced and tape recording was resumed as in the practice period, but for 48 min instead of 16. Continuous recordings of skin conductance were made during this time as well as during the practice.

At the end of 48 min, earphones and electrodes were removed and S was asked how many hours he had slept the previous night and if he was taking any drugs. All Ss had at least 6 hours of sleep the previous night and no one admitted to taking any drugs for at least 2 weeks prior to the experiment. At this time S was asked to complete the Eysenck Personality Inventory (Eysenck & Eysenck, 1963a).

Scoring

Number of correct detections for each test period constituted the vigilance score. Detection responses were scored if the S responded to a signal within 5 sec after it ended. A CE was scored each time S responded in the absence of a signal. Total number of CEs in 48 min was used as the CE score.

Both GSR amplitude and skin conductance base level were measured at each detection point. The GSR amplitude was calculated as the change in log conductance from onset to peak of the response (Raskin, 1969), and skin conductance base level was calculated in log conductance units. Each S's base level was then averaged for the entire 30 signals. Amplitude measures, defined as the size of non-zero responses (Prokasy & Ebel, 1967), required a somewhat different averaging technique. The amplitude of any response occurring between 1 to 6 sec after the last number of a detected signal was recorded. These amplitudes were then summed and divided by the total number of scored responses.

RESULTS

Three groups of 10 *S*s were formed on the basis of total number of CEs made during the 48-min vigilance task. These groups are referred to as the high, middle, and low CE groups. For this analysis one *S* was randomly eliminated to allow for groups of equal size.

Detection of True Signals

The course of signal detection over time for the three CE groups is shown in Fig. 1. The data was analyzed by a 2-factor mixed design (Bruning & Kintz, 1968) with three independent groups based on the number of CEs and three repeated measures of detections from the three 16 minute periods of the vigilance task. As can be seen from Fig. 1, the high CE group shows a marked and consistent decrement in detection of true signals over time; the middle CE group shows a less marked decrement, and the low CE group, in contrast, shows an increase in true signal detection over time. The interaction bearing on these differential trends over time (CE group $\times$ 16 min period) is significant at $p <$ .001 (F (4, 54) = 11.32).

The correlation between *total* number of true signal detections and number of CEs is .142; this is not statistically significant and is in line with the findings of others. The reason for the absence of any marked relationship between number of CEs and number of true signal detections is clear from Fig. 1. The low CE group starts out from a low level of signal detection in the first period and improves with time, whereas the higher CE groups start out with a higher level of

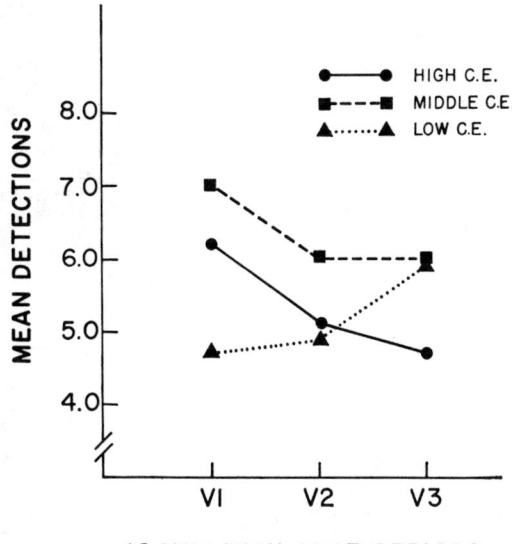

FIG. 1. The course of signal detection over time for groups differing in frequency of commission errors.

signal detection and then their detection performance deteriorates. Bakan et al. (1963) reported a similar finding in a comparison of introverts and extraverts. The extraverts showed the greater decrement over time, but their performance in the first part of the session was better than that of the introverts.

GSR Amplitude

An amplitude score was computed for each S. This was based on the average GSR amplitude for all points where a true signal appeared and was detected. GSRs at undetected signal points or spontaneous GSRs did not contribute to this score. The correlation between total number of CEs and mean GSR amplitude is $-.391$, significant at $p < .05$ (see Table 1). This means that the amplitude of GSR for high CE Ss is lower than for low CE Ss even when signal detection is controlled for by measuring GSR only for detected signals. The GSR amplitude did not change significantly throughout the task for any of the groups.

Orienting Response

An orienting response (OR) is defined as the initial GSR amplitude to the very first digit on the vigilance tape during the practice period. The correlation between number of CEs and the OR is $-.401$, significant at $p < .05$ (see Table 1). The OR is also significantly correlated with the other autonomic measures, the correlation with overall amplitude being .595 ($p < .01$), and the correlation with overall basal conductance being .397 ($p < .05$).

Basal Skin Conductance

A base level skin conductance measure was computed for each S, consisting of the mean log base conductance for all points at which a signal was presented. The correlation between total number of CEs and this measure of skin conductance is $-.304$; this is significant only at $p < .10$ (see Table 1). Basal skin conductance did not change significantly throughout the task for any of the groups.

Extraversion and Neuroticism

The correlation coefficient between total number of CEs and the extraversion score from the Eysenck Personality Inventory (EPI) is .326, just short of significance at the .05 level. Extraverted Ss are more likely to make CEs.

TABLE 1

Correlation coefficients between number of commission errors and some physiological and psychological measures

Measures	Correlations
Overall GSR Amplitude	$-.391$**
Orienting Response (GSR)	$-.401$**
Overall Basal Skin Conductance	$-.304$*
Extraversion	.326*
Neuroticism	$-.115$

* Significant at $p < .10$.
** Significant at $p < .05$.

Correlation coefficients were computed on impulsivity and sociability sub-scores of the EPI. The correlation between CEs and impulsivity score is .267 and the correlation between CEs and sociability is .194. Though neither of these correlations is statistically significant, they are both in the expected direction. The larger value of the impulsivity correlation suggests that this is the more important component of extraversion for the prediction of commission errors.

The correlation between CEs and the neuroticism measure of the EPI ($r = -.127$) was not significant.

DISCUSSION

The main purpose of this paper was to characterize the S who tends to make errors of commission (CEs) while engaged in a vigilance task. It has been shown that such Ss are more likely to show performance decrement in the detection of true signals. Also there is a consistent set of relationships between the tendency to make CEs and three measures of electrodermal activity: GSR amplitude, skin conductance base level, and a GSR measure of the orienting response. These measures can be conceived of as indicators of electrodermal arousal. Decrement in signal detection performance has in the past been shown to be related to measures of electrodermal activation (Dardano, 1962; Ross, Dardano, & Hackman, 1959). Low levels of electrodermal arousal are associated with marked vigilance decrements. This study indicates that CEs are related to *both* decremental performance and electrodermal activation or arousal.

The personality variable extraversion-introversion is related to decrement in vigilance performance (Bakan et al., 1963) and there is a considerable body of theory and research relating extraversion-introversion to behavioral arousal (Bakan, 1959; Blake, 1967; Claridge, 1967; Corcoran, 1965; Davies & Hockey, 1966; Eysenck, 1967; Gray, 1967; Haslam, 1967). This literature provides evidence for the relationship of extraversion to low behavioral arousal. The present study shows that CEs are related to vigilance decrement and low electrodermal arousal.

Furthermore, the almost significant correlation between CEs and extraversion suggests that this personality variable, and especially its impulsivity component, is also related to the making of CEs. Extraversion is considered by Eysenck (1963b, 1969) as a second order factor composed of the first-order factors of sociability and impulsiveness. Further support of this notion comes from a study by Kagan, Rosman, Day, Albert, and Phillips (1964). They found that impulsive children are more distractible and less attentive than non-impulsive children. Impulsive children also show patterns of heart rate response consistent with poor attentive behavior (Kagan & Rosman, 1964).

The S who is likely to make errors of commission may thus be characterized as lower in electrodermal arousal and subject to vigilance decrement over time. The significance of this cluster of variables for behavior in situations other than the vigilance task appears to be an area worthy of further research.

REFERENCES

Bakan, P. Discrimination decrement as a function of time in a prolonged vigil. *Journal of Experimental Psychology*, 1955, *50*, 387–390.

Bakan, P. Extraversion-introversion and improvement in an auditory vigilance task. *British Journal of Psychology*, 1959, *50*, 325–332.

Bakan, P., Belton, J., & Toth, J. Extraversion-introversion and decrement in an auditory vigilance task. In D. N. Buckner & J. J. McGrath (Eds.), *Vigilance: A symposium.* New York: McGraw Hill, 1963. Pp. 22–33.

Blake, M. J. F. Relationship between circadian rhythm of body temperature and introversion-extraversion. *Nature*, 1967, *215*, 896–897.

Broadbent, D. E., & Gregory, M. Division of attention and the decision theory of signal detection. *Proceedings of the Royal Society, Series B*, 1963, *158*, 222–231. (a)

Broadbent, D. E., & Gregory, M. Vigilance considered as a statistical decision. *British Journal of Psychology*, 1963, *54*, 309–323. (b)

Broadbent, D. E., & Gregory, M. Effects of noise and of signal rate upon vigilance analysed by means of decision theory. *Human Factors*, 1965, *7*, 155–162.

Bruning, J. L., & Kintz, B. L. *Computational handbook of statistics.* Glenview, Illinois: Scott Foresman & Co., 1968.

Claridge, G. S. *Personality and arousal.* Oxford: Pergamon Press, 1967.

Corcoran, D. W. J. Personality and the inverted U-relation. *British Journal of Psychology*, 1965, *56*, 267–274.

Dardano, J. F. Relationships of intermittent noise, intersignal interval, and skin conductance to vigilance behavior. *Journal of Applied Psychology*, 1962, *46*, 106–114.

Davies, D. R., & Hockey, G. R. J. The effects of noise and doubling the signal frequency on individual differences in visual vigilance performance. *British Journal of Psychology*, 1966, *57*, 381–389.

Davies, D. R., & Tune, G. S. *Human vigilance performance.* New York: American Elsevier, 1969.

Eysenck, H. J. *The biological basis of personality.* Springfield: Charles C Thomas, 1967.

Eysenck, H. J., & Eysenck, S. B. G. *Eysenck Personality Inventory.* San Diego: Educational and Industrial Testing Service, 1963. (a)

Eysenck, H. J., & Eysenck, S. B. G. *Personality structure and measurement.* London: Routledge and Kegan Paul, 1969.

Eysenck, S. B. G., & Eysenck, H. J. On the dual nature of extraversion. *British Journal of Social & Clinical Psychology*, 1963, *2*, 46–55. (b)

Gray, J. A. Strength of the nervous system, introversion-extraversion, conditionability and arousal. *Behavior Research & Therapy*, 1967, *5*, 151–169.

Haslam, D. R. Individual differences in pain threshold and level of arousal. *British Journal of Psychology*, 1967, *58*, 139–142.

Jerison, H. J. Signal detection theory in the analysis of human vigilance. *Human Factors*, 1967, *9*, 285–288.

Kagan, J., & Rosman, B. L. Cardiac and respiratory correlates of attention and an analytic attitude. *Journal of Experimental Child Psychology*, 1964, *11*, 50–63.

Kagan, J., Rosman, B., Day, D., Albert, J., & Phillips, W. Information processing in the child: Significance of analytic and reflective attitudes. *Psychological Monographs*, 1964, *78*, 1–37.

McGrath, J. J. Some problems of definition and criteria in the study of vigilance performance. In D. N. Buckner & J. J. McGrath (Eds.), *Vigilance: A symposium.* New York: McGraw Hill, 1963. Pp. 227–246.

Prokasy, W. F., & Ebel, H. C. Three components of the classically conditioned GSR in human subjects. *Journal of Experimental Psychology*, 1967, *73*, 247–256.

Raskin, D. C. Semantic conditioning and generalization of autonomic responses. *Journal of Experimental Psychology*, 1969, *79*, 69–76.

Ross, S., Dardano, J., & Hackman, R. Conductance levels during vigilance task performance. *Journal of Applied Psychology*, 1959, *43*, 65–69.

Wiener, E. L. Knowledge of results and signal rate in monitoring: A transfer of training approach. *Journal of Applied Psychology*, 1963, *47*, 214–222.

From D. R. Davies, G. R. J. Hockey, and A. Taylor (1969). British Journal of Psychology, 60, 453–457, by kind permission of the authors and Cambridge University Press

VARIED AUDITORY STIMULATION, TEMPERAMENT DIFFERENCES AND VIGILANCE PERFORMANCE

By D. R. DAVIES, G. R. J. HOCKEY* and ANN TAYLOR

Department of Psychology, University of Leicester

Three experiments are described which investigate the effects of varied auditory stimulation (VAS) on the visual vigilance performance of relatively introverted and relatively extraverted subjects and the preferences of these two groups for such stimulation. In Expt. I, 80 db VAS was found to be associated with a significantly lower commission error rate than was 50 db steady noise, but only in the case of the more extraverted subjects. VAS had no effect upon the detection rate, possibly because the task was too insensitive. In Expt. II a preference for VAS was found to a significantly greater extent among more extraverted subjects, while in Expt. III a preference for silence was found to a significantly greater extent among more introverted subjects.

In a previous study, Davies & Hockey (1966) found that the facilitating effect of high intensity white noise on visual vigilance performance was significantly greater for extraverts than for introverts; the Maudsley Personality Inventory or MPI (Eysenck, 1959) was used as a criterion of extraversion. This finding was interpreted in terms of differential levels of arousal, extraverts being thought of as chronically less highly aroused than introverts (Broadbent, 1963; Corcoran, 1965). There is evidence which suggests that, with increasing arousal, performance improves up to an optimal point and thereafter declines (Duffy, 1957, 1962; Malmo, 1959). Since noise is generally considered to raise the level of arousal (Broadbent, 1963; Davies, 1968), it was argued that the performance of subjects who enter the task situation at a low level of arousal should improve in noise to a greater extent than that of subjects who commence work at comparatively high arousal levels. It is reasonable to suppose that varied auditory stimulation (VAS) would exert similar effects on performance to those of intense white noise, since an increase in stimulus variety as well as in stimulus intensity can be thought of as arousing (Berlyne, 1960; Hebb, 1955). The first experiment to be described was designed to examine this possibility. Expt. I of the present study investigated the effects of VAS upon indices of vigilance performance, and sought to provide some evidence of the contribution of temperament differences to such effects. Expts. II and III were intended to examine the function of VAS for different temperament groups, and in particular to determine whether extraverts and introverts would differ systematically in their utilization of VAS when it was optionally available.

EXPERIMENT I

Method

Subjects. Twenty-eight university students (14 men, 14 women) served as subjects and were paid for their services. Subjects were tested individually; alternate subjects were assigned to each of the two experimental treatments, with the constraint that the two groups should contain

---

* Now at M.R.C. Applied Psychology Research Unit, Cambridge.

D. R. DAVIES, G. R. J. HOCKEY AND ANN TAYLOR

equal numbers of men and women. There was no systematic difference in the time of day at which groups were tested.

Apparatus. The type of task used has been described in greater detail elsewhere (Davies & Hockey, 1966). It consisted of a series of digits from 1 to 9 inclusive, which appeared, one at a time, on a 30-in. closed-circuit television screen in quasi-random order. Each digit remained on the screen for $\frac{2}{3}$ sec. Subjects were instructed to look for signals, defined as three successive odd digits that were all different, for example, 597, 135.

Procedure. The task lasted for 40 min., during which time 24 signals were presented, six in each 10-min. sub-period. The temporal distribution of signals in each sub-period was the same. Testing took place in a sound-deadened room, with an experimenter's room adjacent. Subjects sat in a padded chair, whose height and position were adjustable. The head-rest of the chair was 4 ft. from the television screen. At the beginning of the experiment they were given a typed list of instructions, were shown a sample of the task with no signals and were questioned about whether they understood what constituted a signal, being asked to give examples. They were also asked to remove their watches and were told that the task would not last longer than one hour. Subjects reported the detection of signals by pressing a button fixed to an arm of the chair. This button was connected to a loud bell in the experimenter's room; the bell was also clearly audible to the subject. The task was continuously followed on a television monitor by two experimenters, who had transcriptions of the task on which the incidence of signals was marked. Both correct detections and commission errors—that is, pressing the button in the absence of a signal—were recorded manually in the experimenter's room.

In the control condition subjects performed the task in relative quiet, most—although not all—external noise being masked by an electric wall fan. The ambient noise level in this condition, as measured by a noise level meter, was 50 db. In the VAS condition a tape-recording of varied sounds was played continuously to subjects via the amplifier of the television set. The noise level in this condition was approximately 80 db. It is very unlikely that the difference in the intensity of stimulation would confound the effects of variety of stimulation since intensities below 90 db rarely, if ever, significantly affect performance. The tape-recording consisted of 80×30-sec. segments of music and speech taken from records and from radio and television broadcasts. There were approximately equal amounts of music and speech. Each segment of sound was separated from the next by 3 sec. of silence. At the conclusion of the experiment subjects completed the MPI and Part II of the Heron Inventory which gives an 'unsociability' score (Heron, 1956). The MPI E scale was taken as a criterion of extraversion, Heron Inventory scores being used chiefly to corroborate MPI scores. Those subjects in each group whose MPI E scale scores were above the median were designated 'extraverts' and those who fell below the median were designated 'introverts'.

Results

Non-parametric analyses were applied to the experimental data since they were not normally distributed. The mean number of correct detections made by the VAS group was 22·70, representing 95 per cent of the possible total, and by the control group 21·48, representing 89 per cent. The difference between the scores of the two groups is not significant (Mann–Whitney U test, two-tailed; $P > 0.10$). The mean number of commission errors made by the VAS group was 2·20 and by the control group 4·77. This difference is significant (Mann–Whitney U test, two-tailed; $P < 0.02$).

χ^2 analyses of decrement were made, following a procedure adopted by Bakan *et al.* (1963); decrement was indicated by a subject detecting fewer signals in periods 3 and 4 than in periods 1 and 2. However, no significant difference was found between the control group and the VAS group on this measure ($\chi^2 = 0.18$; $P > 0.50$). Thus the two groups do not differ in the amount of decrement shown. As far as commission errors are concerned, the number made by both groups showed a steady and significant decline with time on task (Wilcoxon T test; $P < 0.01$ in each case).

Stimulation, temperament differences and vigilance performance

In terms of the criterion for extraversion mentioned above, there were seven extraverts (mean E scale score 35·50, S.D. 5·12; mean N scale score 19·00, S.D. 10·84) and seven introverts (mean E scale score 16·14, S.D. 3·57; mean N scale score 27·28, S.D. 10·96) in each of the two groups. Extraverts made significantly fewer commission errors in the VAS condition than in the control condition (Mann–Whitney U test, two-tailed; $P < 0.04$). Introverts, however, showed no such effect. No other comparisons between conditions were significant and no direct comparisons between introverts and extraverts, either in terms of mean performance levels or in terms of the amount of decrement shown, reached an acceptable level of significance.

EXPERIMENTS II AND III

Extraverts apparently prefer situations which are more 'stimulating' than those preferred by introverts (Weisen, cited by Eysenck, 1966). Zuckermann and his colleagues (cited by Cooper & Payne, 1967), employing a 'stimulus-seeking' questionnaire, have found that extraverts describe themselves as seeking stimulation more frequently and in greater amounts than do introverts. On the basis of this evidence and the 'stimulus hunger hypothesis' (Eysenck, 1967), it would be expected that given the opportunity extraverts would select segments of VAS more frequently, while introverts would prefer periods of silence.

One might expect temperament differences in the readiness with which subjects utilize the opportunity to modify the task situation, however, irrespective of the nature of the stimulation. To control for this possibility two 'choice' situations were devised, constituting Expts. II and III. In Expt. II subjects performed the task in quiet conditions but were able to request and obtain periods of VAS; in Expt. III they performed the task in VAS but were able to request and obtain periods of quiet.

EXPERIMENT II
Method

Subjects. In this experiment 28 university students (16 men, 12 women) acted as subjects and were paid for their services.

Apparatus and procedure. These were the same as in Expt. I, except that instead of the tape-recording being played either continuously or not at all, 30-sec. segments of the tape-recording were supplied on demand. Subjects were instructed that their main task was the detection of signals but that, if they wished, by pressing a button they could hear a 30-sec. segment of a tape-recording. The tape-recording was then described to them. It was stressed that the tape-recording was not part of the task, but was simply there for their use if they wanted it, and that pressing the button would give them 30 sec. of music or speech. At the conclusion of the experiment subjects were asked to complete the MPI and Part II of the Heron Inventory. Thirteen extraverts (mean E scale score 32·23, S.D. 6·18; mean N scale score 21·31, S.D. 9·37) and 15 introverts (mean E scale score 15·20, S.D. 8·13; mean N scale score 26·24, S.D. 7·54) were selected on the same basis as in Expt. I.

Results

Significantly more extraverts than introverts selected at least one segment of VAS ($\chi^2 = 4.08$; $P < 0.05$). The mean number of segments requested by introverts was 2·66 and by extraverts 5·14. However, no significant differences in the detection or commission error rates emerged, either overall or with time at work, although both

D. R. Davies, G. R. J. Hockey and Ann Taylor

temperament groups showed significant declines in the number of commission errors from the first half of the task to the second (Wilcoxon T test, two-tailed; $P < 0.05$ for introverts and $P < 0.02$ for extraverts).

Experiment III
Method

Subjects. In this experiment 22 university students (11 men, 11 women) acted as subjects and were paid for their services.

Apparatus and procedure. These were the same as in Expt. II except that subjects were instructed that while they performed the task a tape-recording of varied sounds would be played to them and that if they wished they could obtain 30 sec. periods of silence by pressing a button.

Subjects were classified as introverts and extraverts on the same basis as in Expts. I and II, except that two subjects whose MPI scores fell at the median were classified as introverts because of their high unsociability scores on Part II of the Heron Inventory. There were thus 10 extraverts (mean E scale score 34·60, S.D. 8·45; mean N scale score 24·00, S.D. 7·11) and 12 introverts (mean E scale score 14·16, S.D. 4·55; mean N scale score 18·32, S.D. 6·12).

Results

Significantly more introverts requested that the tape-recording be turned off on at least one occasion; seven out of 12 introverts and one out of 10 extraverts made such a request (Fisher exact probability test; $P = 0.048$). The mean numbers of such requests made by introverts was 5·67 and by extraverts 0·90. As in Expt. II, no significant differences in the detection or commission error rates were apparent, although once again both temperament groups showed significant declines in commission error rates from the first half of the task to the second (Wilcoxon T test, two-tailed; $P < 0.05$ for introverts and $P < 0.02$ for extraverts).

Discussion

In the present experiments, the only performance measure affected by VAS was the commission error rate. One reason for this, as already indicated, is that the task was perhaps too easy, detection rates being uniformly high, and there was thus little room for VAS to exert a beneficial effect on the number of correct detections. This may also account for the absence of a vigilance decrement in the control condition of Expt. I. However, there is in any case no evidence from previous studies (McGrath, 1960; Poock & Wiener, 1966) that VAS ever abolishes the vigilance decrement. In this respect VAS differs from high-intensity white noise, which has been shown to prevent decrement in the detection rate, at least in extraverted subjects (Davies & Hockey, 1966). The respective effects of VAS and white noise upon individual differences in vigilance performance may therefore merit further investigation.

The results of Expts. II and III provide some support for the 'stimulus hunger' hypothesis (Eysenck, 1967) and the findings of Weisen (cited by Eysenck, 1966) and Zuckerman (cited by Cooper & Payne, 1967). Significantly more extraverts than introverts select VAS when given the opportunity to do so and significantly more introverts than extraverts select silence when presented with a background of VAS. The implications of the 'stimulus hunger' hypothesis for arousal theory and task performance remain to be further investigated.

Stimulation, temperament differences and vigilance performance

REFERENCES

BAKAN, P., BELTON, J. A. & TOTH, J. C. (1963). Extraversion–introversion and decrement in an auditory vigilance task. In D. N. Buckner & J. J. McGrath (eds.), *Vigilance: a Symposium*, pp. 22–23. New York: McGraw-Hill.

BERLYNE, D. E. (1960). *Conflict, Arousal and Curiosity*. New York: McGraw-Hill.

BROADBENT, D. E. (1963). Possibilities and difficulties in the concept of arousal. In D. N. Buckner & J. J. McGrath (eds.), *Vigilance: a Symposium*, pp. 184–198. New York: McGraw-Hill.

COOPER, R. & PAYNE, R. L. (1967). Extraversion and some aspects of work behaviour. *Personnel Psychol.* **20**, 45–57.

CORCORAN, D. W. J. (1965). Personality and the inverted-U relation. *Br. J. Psychol.* **56**, 267–274.

DAVIES, D. R. (1968). Physiological and psychological effects of exposure to high intensity noise. *Appl. Acoustics* **1**, 215–233.

DAVIES, D. R. & HOCKEY, G. R. J. (1966). The effects of noise and doubling the signal frequency on individual differences in visual vigilance performance. *Br. J. Psychol.* **57**, 381–389.

DUFFY, E. (1957). The psychological significance of the concept of arousal or 'activation'. *Psychol. Rev.* **64**, 265–275.

DUFFY, E. (1962). *Activation and Behavior*. New York: Wiley.

EYSENCK, H. J. (1959). *The Manual of the Maudsley Personality Inventory*. London: University of London Press.

EYSENCK, H. J. (1966). Personality and experimental psychology. *Bull. Br. psychol. Soc.* **19**, no. 62, 1–28.

EYSENCK, H. J. (1967). *The Biological Basis of Personality*. Springfield, Ill.: Thomas.

HEBB, D. O. (1955). Drives and the C.N.S. (conceptual nervous system). *Psychol. Rev.* **62**, 243–254.

HERON, A. (1956). A two-part personality measure for use as a research criterion. *Br. J. Psychol.* **47**, 243–251.

McGRATH, J. J. (1960). The effect of irrelevant environmental stimulation on vigilance performance. *Project on Human Factors in Anti-submarine Warfare.* (Tech. Rep. no. 6. Personnel and Training Branch, Psychol. Sciences Division, Office of Naval Research.)

MALMO, R. B. (1959). Activation: a neuropsychological dimension. *Psychol. Rev.* **66**, 367–386.

POOCK, G. & WIENER, E. L. (1966). Music and other auditory backgrounds during visual monitoring. *J. industr. Eng.* **17**, 318–323.

(Manuscript received 10 December 1968; revised manuscript received 4 May 1969)

From R. I. Thackray, K. N. Jones, and R. M. Touchstone (1974). British Journal of Psychology, *65,* 351–358, *by kind permission of the authors and Cambridge University Press*

PERSONALITY AND PHYSIOLOGICAL CORRELATES OF PERFORMANCE DECREMENT ON A MONOTONOUS TASK REQUIRING SUSTAINED ATTENTION

By RICHARD I. THACKRAY, KAREN N. JONES AND
ROBERT M. TOUCHSTONE

*Aviation Psychology Laboratory, FAA Civil Aeromedical Institute,
Oklahoma City, Oklahoma, U.S.A.*

A serial-reaction task was used to study personality, as well as physiological, correlates of individual differences in performance decrement under low task-load conditions. Sixty subjects performed the task continuously for 40 min. Extraverted subjects showed increasing lapses of attention, while introverted subjects failed to show any evidence of a decline in attention. Of the two extraversion components (impulsivity and sociability), impulsivity was the component responsible for the obtained decrement. Heart-rate variability showed significant relationships with personality and with performance decrement, while mean heart rate did not.

In a previous study by Thackray *et al.* (1973), it was found that individuals who rated themselves as highly distractable in their daily lives were unable to sustain attention when required to perform a monotonous serial-reaction task demanding continuous attention. In contrast, low distractability subjects were able to perform the task in a superior manner with no evidence of a decline in attention. The obtained decrement took the form of increasingly variable response times with frequent gaps or pauses which various investigators have hypothesized to be a reflexion of declining task attention (Broadbent, 1971; Faulkner, 1962). The high and low distractability groups did not show differing patterns of decrement in either mean response time or frequency of errors.

Although it is fairly well established that extraversion also is related to performance decrement on monotonous, repetitive tasks (Bakan, 1959; Claridge, 1967; Corcoran, 1965; Davies & Hockey, 1966), a satisfactory explanation of why extraverts do more poorly than introverts on these tasks has not been developed. Using a factor-analytic approach, Eysenck & Eysenck (1963) have determined that extraversion is not a unitary dimension but rather consists of two main components, sociability and impulsivity. Since there is evidence that impulsivity is related to distractability (Kagan & Rosman, 1964), the findings of a relationship between distractability and performance decrement in the previous study by Thackray *et al.* (1973) might suggest impulsivity rather than sociability to be the component of extraversion most directly related to vigilance decrement. The findings of a vigilance study by Krupski *et al.* (1971) also suggest this possibility. Impulsivity and sociability subscores of the Eysenck Personality Inventory (Eysenck & Eysenck, 1968) were obtained and both found to be positively correlated with commission errors. While neither correlation was statistically significant, the higher value was obtained for impulsivity.

On the basis of this previous research, it was hypothesized that extraversion would be positively related to performance decrement on a serial-reaction task and that the obtained decrement would be primarily manifested in increased response varia-

R. I. Thackray, K. N. Jones and R. M. Touchstone

bility. It was further hypothesized that, of the two extraversion components (impulsivity and sociability), impulsivity would show the greater relationship with the obtained decrement.

A second aspect of the present study was to evaluate the use of heart-rate variability as a monitor of declining attention during monotonous performance. Evidence from a variety of studies suggests that this measure may be a sensitive physiological index of attention. Relative to resting conditions, heart-rate variability has been shown to decrease markedly when attention is initially directed to task stimuli (Kagan & Rosman, 1964; Thackray, 1969; Welford, 1968) or when changes in the direction of increased task load occur (Kalsbeek, 1968). To the extent that attention declines during performance on a monotonous task, this decline should be reflected in increased heart-rate variability.

While the previous study by Thackray *et al.* (1973) failed to establish a relationship between heart-rate variability and performance decrement, it was felt that the measurement intervals were too few to adequately assess whether or not a relationship existed. In the present study, heart-rate data were continuously recorded and computer-processed to provide a more adequate determination of possible relationships. It was hypothesized that heart-rate variability would show a progressive increase during the task session and that this increase would be positively correlated with performance decrement (increased response variability) on the serial-reaction task. Since Thackray *et al.* (1973) failed to obtain any evidence of a change in mean heart rate during performance on this task, no relationship between mean heart rate and performance decrement was expected.

Method

Subjects

Sixty paid college men served as subjects. None had any prior experience with the task used.

Apparatus

The same serial-reaction task employed in the previous study (Thackray *et al.*, 1973) was used in this study. This type of task appears ideal for studying the decrement function, since it provides repetitive and monotonous stimulation, demands continuous discrimination, involves only minor physical fatigue, yields essentially continuous measures of response time, provides immediate feedback to the subject, and gives a measure of errors as well as correct responses.

The subject's panel contained four lever-actuated microswitches arranged in a row 3 cm apart with a 1·9 cm diameter visual display centrally located over the keys. The visual display presented the numbers 1–4 corresponding to keys 1–4 as numbered from left to right. A tape reader was used to present the numerical stimuli to the subject. Stimuli consisted of a quasi-random series of numbers with the restrictions that no number occur twice in succession and that each number occur an equal number of times in the series. The series was 300 stimuli in length and repeated itself automatically.

Each time a given number appeared, the subject attempted to press the corresponding key. If a correct response was made, the tape reader advanced, a new number was presented, and the cycle continued. If an incorrect response was made, the visual stimulus did not change until the correct key was pressed. Elapsed time between responses was measured by means of a Welford Mark V SETAR (Welford Bioelectronics Enterprises) and the data punched on paper tape. Response times were identified as to whether they corresponded to correct or incorrect responses.

Heart rate was obtained from chest electrodes with the leads connected to a Beckman Type R Dynograph. Pulses from a cardiotachometer coupler were used as inputs to the SETAR for recording successive heart beats.

Personality and physiological correlates of performance decrement

Table 1. *Product-moment correlations between extraversion, neuroticism, impulsivity and sociability*

	1 Extraversion	2 Neuroticism	3 Impulsivity	4 Sociability
1		−0·33**	0·52**	0·75**
2			0·00	−0·40**
3				0·03

** $P < 0.01$.

Procedure

Upon arriving for the experiment, the subject was administered Form A of the Eysenck Personality Inventory (EPI). To minimize association between the inventory and the experiment, the subject was not told that the personality scale was relevant to the present experiment, and one experimenter administered the inventory while a different experimenter conducted the rest of the experiment.

Following completion of the inventory, the subject was taken to the experimental room, instrumented for physiological recording, and the task instructions were presented. Besides explaining the basic procedure, the instructions emphasized that the task should be performed as rapidly as possible but not at the expense of accuracy.

After the task instructions, the subject was given a 1-min. practice trial and then told that he was to work continuously for approximately 50 min. To prevent the subject's knowing that the task was almost over, the experiment was stopped after 40 rather than 50 min.

Measurement of the performance and physiological data

The performance data were computer-processed and the following data obtained for each subject for each successive 4-min. period of the session: (*a*) mean response time, (*b*) standard deviation of the response times (response variability), (*c*) number of incorrect responses.

For heart rate, a computer program was developed to yield two measures for each successive 4-min. period during the performance session. These measures were the mean rate and the standard deviation. Because of occasional muscle potential artifacts and premature contractions, the computer program was designed to reject any apparent heart-beat interval which, when converted to a beat per minute (bpm) basis, exceeded 160 bpm or fell below 30 bpm. In addition, any two successive heart beats which increased by more than 25 bpm or decreased by more than 46 bpm were also rejected. These limits were empirically determined from preliminary hand-scored analyses and were felt to represent values for this set of experimental conditions which would maximize rejection of artifacts and minimize rejection of 'valid' heart-rate data.

RESULTS

Personality variables

Mean scores on the EPI were 12·3, 9·4, 4·0 and 5·4 for the extraversion, neuroticism, impulsivity and sociability scales, respectively. Table 1 shows the intercorrelations of these measures. As expected, extraversion showed a significant positive correlation with both impulsivity and sociability. The significant negative correlation between extraversion and neuroticism, however, was not expected.

Although negative correlations between extraversion and neuroticism are frequently found, these are generally non-significant (Eysenck & Eysenck, 1968). Because a significant relationship was obtained between these two variables in the sample employed, neuroticism was separately examined even though it was not originally intended to do so. (Neuroticism has been frequently examined in vigilance-type studies and has typically shown no relationship to performance decrement

R. I. THACKRAY, K. N. JONES AND R. M. TOUCHSTONE

Table 2. *Mean response time, response variability (standard deviation) and frequency of errors for each 4-min. period of the task session*

(Data are for the total group of 60 subjects.)

	4-min. periods									
Variable	1	2	3	4	5	6	7	8	9	10
Mean response time (sec.)	0·78	0·80	0·80	0·80	0·80	0·80	0·80	0·80	0·82	0·82
Response variability (sec.)	0·16	0·19	0·21	0·21	0·23	0·24	0·25	0·27	0·28	0·29
Frequency of errors	4·8	6·8	7·2	7·2	8·4	8·4	9·6	9·6	10·0	9·6

(Davies & Tune, 1969).) For each of the four scales, the 15 subjects with the highest and lowest scores were identified. The high and low cut-off scores for each distribution were as follows: extraversion (15 and 10), neuroticism (12 and 6), impulsivity (5 and 3), and sociability (7 and 4).

Since the neuroticism, extraversion, impulsivity and sociability subgroups were each drawn from the same sample of 60 subjects, the total group data for each performance measure were analysed in order to provide reference data for the comparison of differential response patterns of the various subgroups. The data for mean response time, response variability and frequency of errors for the 60 subjects are given in Table 2. Analyses of variance conducted on each set of data yielded significant F values for the effect of 4-min. periods for mean response time ($F = 4·16; P < 0·01$), response variability ($F = 21·19; P < 0·01$) and frequency of errors ($F = 12·79; P < 0·01$). The only variable which did not reveal a progressive increase with time was mean response time, and the significant F value was apparently the result of slight increases at the beginning and end of the session.

Analyses of variance were then conducted on the performance data of each subgroup. Since the between-periods effects were significant in the analyses of variance conducted on the data for all 60 subjects, it is not surprising that the differences between periods were significant ($P < 0·05$) for all variables in each subgroup with the exception of mean response time for extraversion. This F value approached, but did not reach, significance at the 5 per cent level ($P < 0·10$). None of the group differences was significant, but significant interactions were obtained between groups and periods for mean response time on the extraversion factor ($F = 3·03; P < 0·01$) and for response variability on both the extraversion ($F = 2·77; P < 0·01$) and impulsivity ($F = 2·03; P < 0·05$) factors. Fig. 1, which displays mean response time for the high and low extraversion groups, shows generally increasing response times for the high group, but a mixed pattern for the low group. However, although the interaction was significant and differences between the high and low groups appear pronounced at some of the time periods, tests of simple effects of groups revealed none of the differences between the groups at any of the periods to be significant ($P > 0·05$). Fig. 2 shows the response variability patterns for the high and low extraversion and impulsivity groups. There is a continuous rise in variability among the high extraversion and impulsivity subjects during the experimental session with a relatively stable level of response variability among the low subjects. Tests of simple effects of periods revealed the differences between periods to be significant

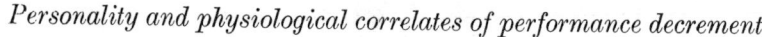

Personality and physiological correlates of performance decrement

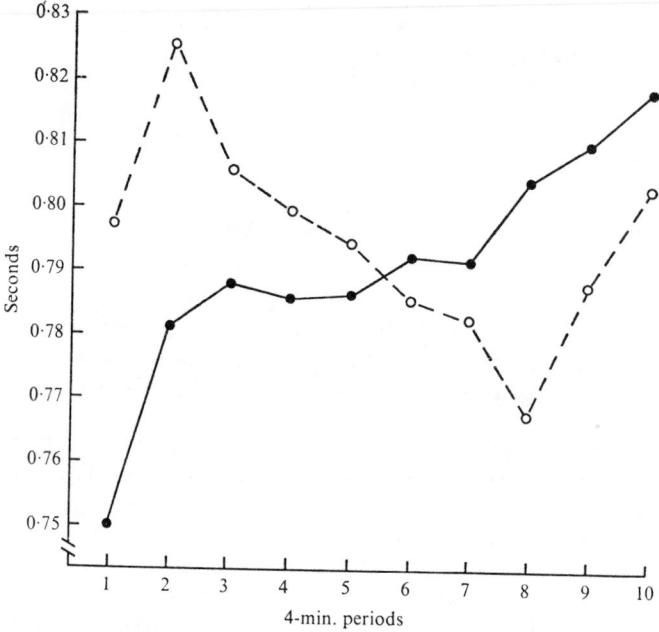

Fig. 1. Mean response times for the high (●) and low (○) extraversion groups across periods.

for the high extraversion ($F = 11·03$; $P < 0·001$) and high impulsivity ($F = 9·59$; $P < 0·001$) groups. There were no differences between periods for either the low extraversion ($F = 1·42$; $P > 0·05$) or low impulsivity ($F = 1·74$; $P > 0·05$ groups).

Heart-rate measures

As expected, heart-rate variability for the entire sample of 60 subjects showed a progressive, significant increase ($F = 20·64$; $P < 0·001$) during the session. Mean heart-rate showed a slight, but significant, decrease ($F = 2·54$; $P < 0·01$). These data are given in Table 3. Since the previous study by Thackray *et al.* (1973) failed to find any change in mean heart rate, further tests were conducted on mean heart rate. Scheffé tests (Edwards, 1960) revealed no difference between periods 1 and 8 ($F = 1·53$; $P > 0·05$) or between periods 1 and 10 ($F = 8·57$; $P > 0·05$). The only significant difference was obtained when the periods with the highest (period 2) and lowest (period 10) heart rates were compared ($F = 16·84$; $P = 0·05$).

Mean heart rate and heart-rate variability were separately correlated with performance variability for each of the 4-min. periods. None of the correlations of mean heart rate with performance variability was significant ($P > 0·05$). Heart-rate variability was not significantly correlated with performance during the first three periods, but showed significant ($P < 0·05$), increasing correlations during the remaining seven periods. The correlations for periods 4–10 were 0·26, 0·35, 0·34, 0·37, 0·36, 0·43 and 0·42, respectively.

Since both extraversion and heart-rate variability were found to be related to per-

R. I. Thackray, K. N. Jones and R. M. Touchstone

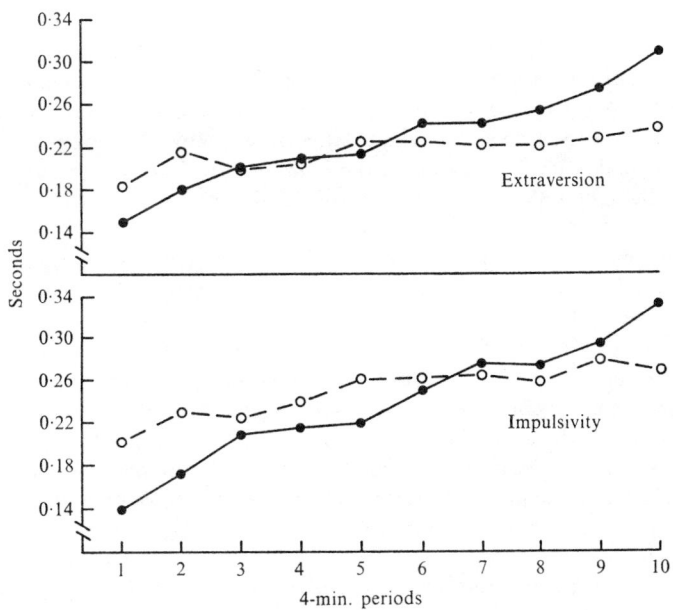

Fig. 2. Response variability for the high (●) and low (○) extraversion and impulsivity groups across periods.

Table 3. *Mean heart rate and heart-rate variability (standard deviation) for each of the 4-min. periods*

(Data shown are for all 60 subjects.)

Variable	4-min. periods									
	1	2	3	4	5	6	7	8	9	10
Mean heart rate (bpm)	73	74	73	73	73	73	73	73	72	72
Heart-rate variability (bpm)	4·4	4·6	4·6	4·8	5·2	5·5	5·5	5·7	5·9	5·9

formance variability, it would seem reasonable that extraversion might show some degree of relationship with heart-rate variability. In order to evaluate this, the difference between period 1 and period 10 was obtained for each subject's heart-rate variability scores and these values separately correlated with each of the personality variables. The resulting correlations were $0·30$ $(P < 0·05)$, $0·12$ $(P > 0·05)$, $0·30$ $(P < 0·05)$ and $0·06$ $(P > 0·05)$ for extraversion, impulsivity, sociability, and neuroticism respectively.

Discussion

Extraverts are known to exhibit more frequent pauses or blocks during performance on serial-reaction (Corcoran, 1965) and simple tapping (Spielmann, 1963) tasks than do introverts, and the present results support these previous findings. Of greater interest, however, was the predicted finding that impulsivity rather than sociability was the extraversion factor primarily responsible for the obtained decrement.

Personality and physiological correlates of performance decrement

Although both impulsivity and sociability were significantly correlated with extraversion, only the high and low impulsivity groups showed response variability patterns which were similar to those of the high and low extraverts. This cannot be attributed simply to a sampling bias in which a greater proportion of impulsivity than sociability subjects were drawn from the extraversion groups. The proportions were approximately equal, with 57 per cent of the high and low impulsivity subjects and 63 per cent of the high and low sociability subjects common to the two extraversion groups.

Neither errors nor mean response time showed any appreciable relationship with any of the personality variables. The lack of relationship between frequency of errors and any of the personality variables agrees with the lack of relationship between this measure and susceptibility to distraction obtained in the previous study (Thackray *et al.*, 1973). It would appear that an increase in error frequency during serial-reaction performance is either a poor index of declining attention or it reflects attentional processes unrelated to those manifested by increased response variability.

While the negative correlation between extraversion and neuroticism was not anticipated, this small, though significant, correlation does not alter interpretation of the results obtained. First, no relationships were found between neuroticism and any of the performance measures. And, second, although impulsivity showed no correlation with neuroticism, the decrement pattern obtained for impulsivity was essentially the same as that obtained for extraversion. Thus the negative correlation is interpreted to reflect a common factor not related to performance decrement on this type of task.

The finding of a generally increasing correlation between heart-rate variability and performance variability would appear to support previous findings of Ettema & Zielhuis (1971) that heart-rate variability increases with a reduction in the mental or attentional requirements of a task. Apparently this increase in heart-rate variability during monotonous task performance is more pronounced among extraverts than among introverts. Why heart-rate variability was found to be related to the sociability, but not to the impulsivity, dimension of extraversion is somewhat puzzling. On the basis of the performance data, one might have expected impulsivity to show the higher relationship. Further research is clearly needed to clarify the possibly quite different behavioural and physiological correlates of these two dimensions of extraversion.

The authors wish to gratefully acknowledge the assistance of Marilyn Dollar and Joe Bailey in scoring and analysing the data of this study.

REFERENCES

BAKAN, P. (1959). Extraversion–introversion and improvement in an auditory vigilance task. *Br. J. Psychol.* **50**, 325–332.

BROADBENT, D. E. (1971). *Decision and Stress*. London: Academic Press.

CLARIDGE, G. S. (1967). *Personality and Arousal*. London: Pergamon Press.

CORCORAN, D. W. J. (1965). Personality and the inverted-U relation. *Br. J. Psychol.* **56**, 267–273.

DAVIES, D. R. & HOCKEY, G. R. J. (1966). The effects of noise and doubling the signal frequency on individual differences in visual vigilance performance. *Br. J. Psychol.* **57**, 381–389.

DAVIES, D. R. & TUNE, G. S. (1969). *Human Vigilance Performance*. New York: American Elsevier.

R. I. Thackray, K. N. Jones and R. M. Touchstone

Edwards, A. L. (1960). *Experimental Design in Psychological Research.* New York: Holt.

Ettema, J. H. & Zielhuis, R. L. (1971). Physiological parameters of mental load. *Ergonomics* **14**, 137–144.

Eysenck, H. J. & Eysenck, S. B. G. (1968). *Eysenck Personality Inventory.* San Diego: Education and Industrial Testing Service.

Eysenck, S. B. G. & Eysenck, H. J. (1963). On the dual nature of extraversion. *Br. J. soc. clin. Psychol.* **2**, 46–55.

Faulkner, T. W. (1962). Variability of performance in a vigilance task. *J. appl. Psychol.* **46**, 325–328.

Kagan, J. & Rosman, B. L. (1964). Cardiac and respiratory correlates of attention and an analytic attitude. *J. exp. child Psychol.* **1**, 50–63.

Kalsbeek, J. W. H. (1968). Measurement of mental work load and of acceptable load: possible applications in industry. *Int. J. prod. Res.* **7**, 33–45.

Krupski, A., Raskin, D. C. & Bakan, P. (1971). Physiological and personality correlates of commission errors in an auditory vigilance task. *Psychophysiol.* **8**, 304–311.

Spielmann, J. (1963). The relation between personality and the frequency and duration of involuntary rest pauses during massed practice. (Unpublished Ph.D. thesis, University of London.)

Thackray, R. I. (1969). Patterns of physiological activity accompanying performance on a perceptual-motor task. FAA Office of Aviation Medicine Report no. AM-69-8.

Thackray, R. I., Jones, K. N. & Touchstone, R. M. (1973). Self-estimates of distractability as related to performance decrement on a task requiring sustained attention. *Ergonomics* **16**, 141–152.

Welford, N. T. (1968). Heart-rate variability during continuous performance. (Paper read to the American Association for the Advancement of Science, Dallas.)

(*Manuscript received* 21 *September* 1973; *revised manuscript received* 19 *December* 1973)

From M. E. Keister and R. J. McLaughlin (1972). Journal of Experimental Research in Personality, *6*, 5–11, *by kind permission of the authors and Academic Press*

Vigilance Performance Related to Extraversion—Introversion and Caffeine[1]

MICHAEL E. KEISTER[2] AND ROBERT J. MCLAUGHLIN

Southern Illinois University at Edwardsville

Sixty subjects who scored on the extremes of the introversion–extraversion dimension of the Eysenck Personality Inventory were tested on a vigilance task under either a drug (caffeine), placebo, or no drug condition. It was predicted and found that extraverts in the no drug condition showed a significant decrement in performance between the first and last third of the task. The introverts as predicted showed no decrement. As hypothesized, the drug produced differential effects on the two personality groups relative to their performance without the drug; the extraverts and introverts who were given caffeine showed no increment or decrement between the first and last third of the task.

Eysenck (1957, 1960, 1967) has developed a theory which postulates that there are two fundamental dimensions of personality: extraversion–introversion and neuroticism. From a large body of research evidence Eysenck has inferred the existence of the physiological substrata which underlie these behaviorally measured dimensions. A physiological predisposition to strong autonomic nervous system activation in the presence of anxiety-eliciting stimuli is hypothesized to be a major factor in the determination of level of neuroticism. Level of cortical arousal which is a function of rate of accrual and dissipation of inhibition is assumed to constitute the physiological basis differentiating extraverts and introverts. Individuals who have high cortical-activation levels are predisposed to introversion while those with relatively low activation levels tend toward extraversion. A high degree of extraversion is characteristic of individuals in whom inhibitory processes occur quickly, strongly, and persistently while excitatory processes occur slowly, weakly, and nonpersistently; a high degree of introversion is characteristic of individuals in whom the reverse is true. Eysenck (1967) has proposed that the differences between extraverts and introverts are a direct function of the level of activity in the ascending reticular-activating system.

A major portion of the empirical support for Eysenck's theory derives from physiological measures (e.g., EEG, cortical-evoked potentials) based on theoretical deductions which have been behaviorally inferred, measured, and tested. Unequivocal substantiation, alteration, or contradiction of the postulates from physiological data awaits further technological developments. Another means of identifying the relationship between cortical characteristics and behavior involves the attempted manipulations of cortical arousal level though the administration of drugs and measurement of concomitant behavioral data. Assessment of drug effects may be confounded by S variables, contextual variables, and the heterogeneity within classifications of drugs as stimulants or depressants (Trouton & Eysenck, 1960); yet when appropriate methodology is applied, drugs have proven to be a highly valuable adjunct to theory testing. Eysenck

[1] This research was supported by Research Grant 020408 from the Office of Research and Projects, Southern Illinois University, Edwardsville.

[2] Now at Saint Louis University, Saint Louis, MO

(1960) has proposed the following specific postulate from which numerous deductions have evolved:

> Depressant drugs increase cortical inhibition, decrease cortical excitation and thereby produce extraverted behavior patterns. Stimulant drugs decrease cortical inhibition, increase cortical excitation and thereby produce introverted behavior patterns (p. 106).

This postulate has resulted in a large number of testable hypotheses. The effects of stimulant and depressant drugs have been tested with conditioning paradigms (Franks & Laverty, 1955; Franks & Trouton; Willett, 1960) visual after-effects (Holland & Gomez, 1963; Paramesh, 1963) visual masking (Holland, 1963; Eysenck & Aiba, 1957) pursuit rotor performance (Eysenck, Casey, & Trouton, 1957) verbal learning (Eysenck 1957, 1960) and CFF thresholds (Aiba, 1963; Landis & Zubin, 1951). Results of these studies have shown general agreement with the prediction that stimulant drugs lead to greater arousal and hence to more introverted behavior, while depressant drugs lead to greater inhibition and hence to more extraverted behavior.

Another task which is particularly suitable for investigating the effects of drugs on performance is the vigilance task. Vigilance has been variously described as performance on monitoring tasks, attention over extended periods of time or as a state of readiness to detect and respond to certain specified small changes, occurring at random time intervals in the external environment. In terms of Eysenck's theory introverts are expected to be superior to extraverts in vigilance tasks because the persistently heightened arousal level of introverts facilitates vigilant attention and prevents performance decrements which result from inhibition increments and consequent lowered arousal. Bakan (1959) developed a vigilance task consisting of a tape recording of digits presented at the rate of one per second. The task for the subject was to detect any successive odd-even-odd sequence. Bakan found the performance of introverts to be significantly

superior to extraverts. Claridge (1960), using this same task, found that a dysthymic group (neurotic introverts) of subjects showed no performance decrement over time, whereas a hysteric group (neurotic extraverts) showed a large performance decrement. Bakan, Belton, and Toth (1963), also using this task, found that a significantly greater proportion of the extraverts and normals showed a performance decrement over time than the corresponding proportion of introverts. With regard to the effects of drugs on vigilance, Bakan (1961) found that subjects performing under the effects of meprobamate, a depressant, showed a tendency toward greater decrement than a no drug control. Treadwell (1960) has similarly found that depressants accelerate a performance decline.

The present study is designed to determine the difference between introverts and extraverts on the Bakan vigilance task (1959). This is essentially replicating the findings of previous studies which have supported the general hypothesis that heightened cortical arousal, characteristics of introverts, will minimize vigilance decrement. The effects of a stimulant, caffeine, are also being assessed in its effects on introversion–extraversion. The predicted effect of the caffeine is that the performance of extraverts in the drug condition will maintain the continued efficiency characteristic of the introverts. The introverts who are characterized by a heightened cortical arousal will show little if any facilitation from the administration of the caffeine. Degree of neuroticism will be controlled for rather than investigated as a relevant variable in this study as previous research has found this dimension unrelated to vigilance performance (Bakan, 1959).

METHOD

Subjects. The Eysenck Personality Inventory (Eysenck & Eysenck, 1964) was administered to 350 students enrolled in undergraduate psychology courses at Southern Illinois University, Edwardsville. Thirty *S*s who scored eight and below and 30 *S*s who scored 17 and above on the extraversion scale of the EPI and who agreed to participate were tested on the vigilance task. *S*s scoring six or above on the lie scale were excluded. Approximately half of each personality group were tested in the morning and half in the afternoon.

Materials. The vigilance task consisted of a 48-min tape recording of digits which were spoken at a rate of one per second. A series of 2880 digits were randomly generated by a computer which was programmed to produce no odd-even-odd sequence of digits. Thirty-two signals, comprised of odd-even-odd sequences (e.g., 927, 365), were interpolated into the series before it was recorded by a male voice. Ten signals occurred during the first 16 min of the tape, and 11 signals occurred during each of the second two 16-min periods. This vigilance task is essentially a replication of the task used by Bakan (1959).

Procedure. Each of the two 30-*S* personality groups was randomly subdivided into three groups of 10 *S*s. The *S*s were assigned on the basis of a predetermined random number sequence based on order of appearance at the laboratory to either a No Drug, Placebo, or Drug (caffeine) condition. *S*s in the drug condition ingested four 50-mg capsules of caffeine (powdered Bristol Meyers No Doz Stay-Alert Tablets) just before the pretest which was approximately 12–17 min before initiation of the actual task. The manufacturer suggests that two 100-mg tablets should achieve effectiveness in 15 min. The *S*s assigned to the placebo condition were given four 50-mg capsules of milk powder under the impression that they were being given caffeine.

All *S*s were required to sign a consent form to take caffeine including those *S*s assigned to the No Drug condition. Only four *S*s were unable or unwilling to sign the consent form. All *S*s were given identical instructions and pretest practice. The first practice task required *S* to identify and underline odd-even-odd sequences in a printed series of 300 digits. Each *S* was required to work on the task until he had detected at least four of the five signals. The second task consisted of a tape recording of 240 digits presented in a manner which was identical to the actual task. The practice tape was presented to each *S* and contained four signals. The *S*s were instructed to write down on a sheet of paper each of the odd-even-odd sequences detected. Upon completion of the practice task the *S*s commenced the actual task. The *S*s were tested individually and wore earphones during the task.

RESULTS

Means for the extraversion–introversion (E–I) and neuroticism (N) scores were calculated for each of the six drug-personality conditions. The mean scores were 18.7, 18.6, and 18.1 for the E No Drug, Placebo, and Drug conditions, respectively. For the I No Drug, Placebo, and Drug conditions the means were 5.5, 6.2, and 5.0, respectively. Table 1 shows the mean signals detected for each of the three 16-min

TABLE 1

MEANS AND STANDARD DEVIATIONS OF SIGNALS DETECTED PER PERIOD, TOTAL SIGNALS AND DECREMENT FROM FIRST TO THIRD PERIOD FOR E–I AND DRUG CONDITIONS

Period	Extraverts			Introverts		
	No drug	Placebo	Drug	No drug	Placebo	Drug
First						
Mean	5.9	5.4	6.5	5.3	6.5	5.6
SD	1.52	1.71	1.35	1.91	.97	2.32
Second						
Mean	6.6	5.9	6.6	6.5	5.8	6.9
SD	2.72	2.42	2.01	1.78	1.62	2.28
Third						
Mean	4.9	4.5	7.0	6.2	6.6	6.2
SD	2.42	2.51	1.56	2.10	2.59	2.74
Total						
Mean	17.4	15.8	20.1	18.0	18.9	18.7
SD	7.61	2.00	5.74	4.81	4.94	1.97
Decrement						
Mean	1.0	.9	−.5	−.9	−.1	−.6
SD	2.79	2.02	1.18	2.64	2.28	1.84

195

KEISTER AND MCLAUGHLIN

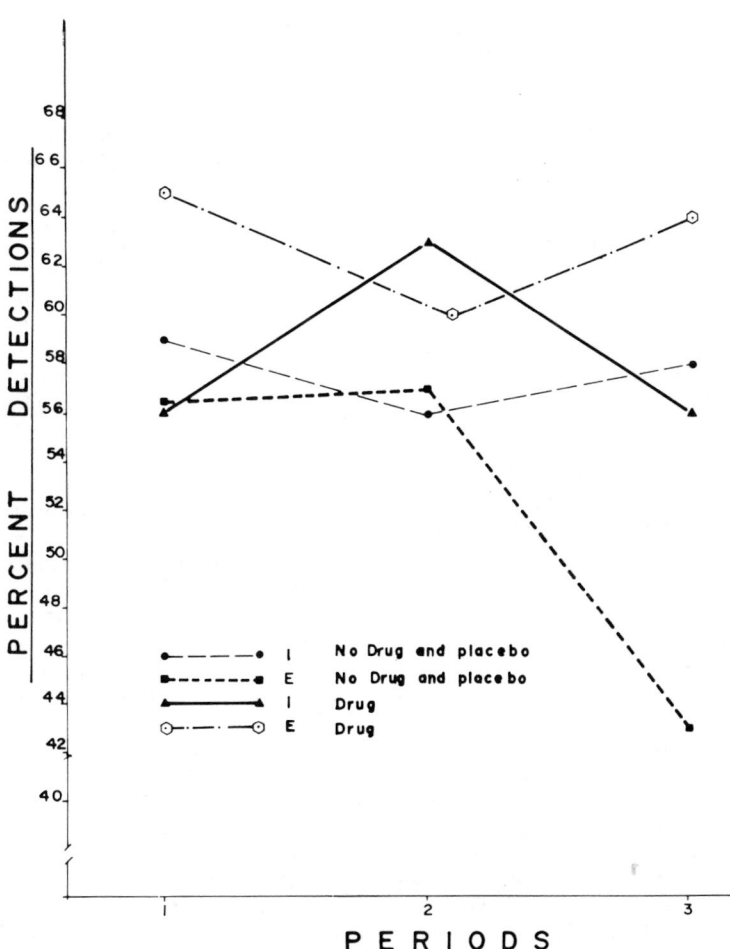

Fig. 1. Percentage of detection of signals in each of the three 16-min periods of the task for the Drug and the combined No Drug and Placebo conditions for E and I.

periods of the task, total scores and decrement scores for each of the six drug-personality conditions.

A three-way analysis of variance (personality type × drug condition × periods) was done on the number of signals detected. No significant main effects or interactions were obtained. A similar analysis was done excluding the E and I Drug conditions. Thus, a comparison was made for the E and I No Drug and Placebo conditions for the number of signals detected in each period of the task. This analysis

yielded no significant main effects but a significant interaction between E and I and signals detected per period ($F(2,72) = 3.70$, $p < .05$). Figure 1 shows the percentage of detection of signals per period. In the combined No Drug and Placebo conditions the significant interaction resulted from the discrepant scores in the third period. The Es detected only 42% of these signals while the Is detected 58%.

An analysis was made of the decrement scores for all six drug-personality conditions. The decrement score was obtained by subtracting the number of signals detected in the third period from the number detected in the first period. The mean decrement score for each condition is presented in Table 1. Negative decrement scores indicate an increase in the frequency of correct detections in the third period relative to the first. The Es in the No Drug and Placebo conditions manifested average decrements of 1.0 and 0.9 signals detected, respectively; whereas Is in the No Drug and Placebo conditions showed average increments of 0.9 and 0.1 signals, respectively. In contrast to this pattern, Es in the Drug conditions showed a mean increment of 0.5 as compared to a mean increment of 0.6 signals for Is in the Drug conditions. A two-way analysis of variance (personality $\times$ drug condition) yielded no significant main effects or interaction. There was a trend toward significance for the main effect of E-I with the Es showing a greater decrement score ($F(1,54) = 3.12$, $p = .08$). A comparison was made of the decrement scores for the E-I No Drug and Placebo conditions. This comparison showed a significantly greater decrement for the Es than for the Is ($t(38) = 1.91$, $p < .05$). The decrement score between the number of signals detected in the second period and the third period was analyzed for the E No Drug and Placebo conditions. A significant decrement was found for these conditions ($t(38) = 2.01$, $p < .05$). The E Drug and I No Drug, Placebo, and Drug conditions showed no significant increment or decrement between the second and third periods.

Mean N scores differed significantly between the E No Drug (7.8) and E Placebo (12.8) conditions ($t(18) = 3.65$, $p < .01$) and between the E Placebo (12.8) and I No Drug (8.8) conditions ($t(18) = 2.70$, $p < .05$). N scores were not significantly different for any other pairs of conditions, nor were they significantly different between the overall E and I groups whose mean N scores were 9.9 and 10.2, respectively. To determine the relationship between N and performance on this task, product-moment correlations were calculated between N and first period ($-.03$),

second period (.00), third period scores (.04), and the decrement score between the first and third periods ($-.07$). The results of this analysis indicate that the N score differences which did exist did not produce an influence on the vigilance scores which could confound the E-I and Drug condition effects.

DISCUSSION

The results support the prediction that there would be no differences between the introverts and extraverts on the first part of the task but that the introverts would be superior toward the end of the task. The decrement scores for the combined No Drug and Placebo conditions supported the prediction that the extraverts would show a significant decrement relative to the introverts.

Two arousal-based theories seem to be relevant as possible explanations of these data. The first emphasizes that increased arousal level resulting from caffeine effects might function to heighten the reinforcing effect on attentive behavior which results from the detection of individual signals which signifies task success. Extensive work on this theoretical model has been done by Holland (1963). Bakan (1959) has cited evidence for the reinforcing effect of signal detection during a vigilance task and has proposed a related explanation for the superior performance of introverts on vigilance tasks. During the task in which the occurrence of relatively infrequent signals serves as reinforcement for task attention, extraverts extinguish more rapidly than introverts. As the appropriate attentive response is weakened, inappropriate responses resulting from attention to irrelevant stimuli and drowsiness further reduce the relative strength of task-appropriate attention. Eysenck (1967) has summarized evidence that extraverts do condition less efficiently and show extinction more quickly than introverts.

The second explanation of these findings is that the continuous redundant task of listening to a long series of digits induces cortical inhibition which causes involuntary rest pauses and consequent missed signals.

Since extraverts are believed to be more susceptible to the accrual of cortical inhibition and less efficient at dissipating it than are introverts; they make more involuntary rest pauses. These two explanations are integrally related by their essential reliance on proposed differences between introverts and extraverts in the process of cortical excitation and of the accumulation and dissipation of inhibition. With regard to the present study, it is theorized that the effect of caffeine was to increase the cortical arousal of the extraverts and make them equal in performance to the introverts who characteristically function at a high arousal level.

There is a consideration relative to the findings of the present study which is warranted. Since the subjects were selected on the basis of extreme scores on the E-I dimension, the differences obtained on the vigilance task were not as great as might have been expected. This minimizes the likelihood that there is a strong, linear relationship between the entire E-I dimension and vigilance performance. There are two possible explanations for this. First, it is possible that the self-report inventory is not a highly reliable index of differences in cortical arousal. Second, it is possible that even if extreme differences in cortical arousal could be accurately measured, it would only bear a weak relationship to performance on a vigilance task, especially a task with a duration as short as 1 hr. Since there is evidence supporting the likelihood that cortical arousal is the physiological basis of differences in the E-I dimension (Eysenck, 1967), the second reason should appear more tenable at the present time.

REFERENCES

AIBA, S. The suppression of the primary visual stimulus. In H. J. Eysenck (Ed.), *Experiments with drugs.* New York: Pergamon Press, 1963.

BAKAN, P. Extraversion–introversion and improvement in an auditory vigilance task. *British Journal of Psychology,* 1959, **50**, 325–332.

BAKAN, P. Effect of meprobamate on auditory vigilance. *Perceptual and Motor Skills,* 1961, **12**, 26.

BAKAN, P., BELTON, J. A., & TOTH, J. C. Extraversion-introversion and decrement in an auditory vigilance task. In D. N. Buckner and J. J. McGrath (Eds.), *Vigilance: A symposium.* New York: McGraw-Hill, 1963.

CLARIDGE, G. S. The excitation-inhibition balance in neurotics. In H. J. Eysenck (Ed.), *Experiments in personality.* New York: Praeger, 1960.

EYSENCK, H. J. *The dynamics of anxiety and hysteria.* New York: Praeger, 1957.

EYSENCK, H. J. (Ed.), *Experiments in personality.* New York: Praeger, 1960.

EYSENCK, H. J. *Experiments with drugs.* New York: Pergamon, 1963.

EYSENCK, H. J. *The biological basis of personality.* Springfield, IL.: Thomas, 1967.

EYSENCK, H. J., & AIBA, S. Drugs and personality. V. The effects of stimulant and depressant drugs on the suppression of the primary visual stimulus. *Journal of Mental Science,* 1957, **103**, 661–665.

EYSENCK, H. J., CASEY, S., & TROUTON, D. S. Drugs and personality. II. The effects of stimulant and depressant drugs on continuous work. *Journal of Mental Science,* 1957, **103**, 645–649.

EYSENCK, H. J., & EYSENCK, S. B. G. *Eysenck personality inventory.* San Diego: Educational and Industrial Testing Service, 1964.

FRANKS, C. M., & TROUTON, D. Effects of amo- and eyelid conditioning. *Journal of Mental Science,* 1955, **101**, 654–663.

FRANKS, C. M., & TROUTON, D. Effects of amobarbital sodium and dexamphetamine sulphate on the conditioning of the eyelid response. *Journal of Comparative and Physiological Psychology,* 1958, **51**, 220–222.

HOLLAND, H. C. "Visual masking" and the effects of stimulant and depressant drugs. In H. J. Eysenck (Ed.), *Experiments with drugs.* New York: Pergamon, 1963.

HOLLAND, H. C., & GOMEZ, B. H. The effects of stimulant and depressant drugs upon visual figural after-effects. In H. J. Eysenck (Ed.), *Experiments with drugs.* New York: Pergamon, 1963.

HOLLAND, J. G. Human vigilance. In D. N. Buckner and J. J. McGrath (Eds.), *Vigilance: A symposium.* New York: McGraw-Hill, 1963.

LANDIS, C., & ZUBIN, J. Effect of thonzylamine hydrochloride and phenobarbital sodium on certain psychological functions. *Journal of Psychology,* 1951, **31**, 181–200.

PARAMESH, C. R. Introversion-extraversion and figural after-effects. *Indian Journal of Psychology,* 1963, **38**, 93–97.

EXTRAVERSION AND VIGILANCE

TREADWELL, E. The effects of depressant drugs on vigilance and psychomotor performance. *In* H. J. Eysenck, (Ed.), *Experiments in personality.* New York: Praeger, 1960.

TROUTON, D. S., & EYSENCK, H. J. The effects of drugs on behavior. *In* H. J. Eysenck (Ed.), *Handbook of abnormal psychology.* New York: Basic Books, 1960.

WILLETT, R. A. The effects of depressant drugs on learning and conditioning. *In* H. J. Eysenck (Ed.), *Experiments in personality.* New York: Praeger, 1960.

From J. Brebner and C. Cooper (1974). Journal of Research in Personality, *8*, 263–276, *by kind permission of the authors and Academic Press*

The Effect of a Low Rate of Regular Signals upon the Reaction Times of Introverts and Extraverts[1]

JOHN BREBNER AND CHRIS COOPER

University of Adelaide, Australia

In an RT (reaction time) task involving responding to infrequent, regular signals, extraverts produced higher proportions of missed signals and lengthened RT's than introverts did. This result was only obtained after some time on task and is evidence that inhibitory states are formed more rapidly in extraverted subjects under low stimulation conditions. In a more extended version of the task, mean RT was found to be longer in extraverted than introverted subjects in the second half of the experiment though there was no significant difference between the groups in the first half. These findings are complementary to data from previous studies showing that extraverts generate stronger inhibitory potential in continuous responding tasks, or that their characteristic arousal level may be lower than that of introverted subjects. The need to distinguish between the different explanatory constructs is discussed and a simple model amalgamating the major theoretical positions is outlined.

Attempts to explain behavior which we now characterize as introverted or extraverted have varied from the original humoral doctrine of Hippocrates, to Jung's (1923) analysis and Pavlov's (1927) explanation in terms of the balance of excitation which retained the original Hippocratic terminology. Pavlov's (1935) more complex interpretation, which attributed individual differences to three properties of the nervous system (strength, balance and mobility), was largely ignored in the English speaking world, until the 1960's. Eysenck's influential theory (Eysenck, 1955, 1957), while adopting Jungian terminology and formalized in terms of Hullian reactive inhibition, was based upon the earlier, simpler Pavlovian model rather than the later 1935 version.

Currently, two broad trends are evident in the research into introversion–extraversion. The first is the attempt to relate these individual differences to the arousal level or "arousability" of the person, for example,

[1] Requests for reprints should be sent to John Brebner, Department of Psychology, University of Adelaide, Adelaide, Southern Australia 5001.

the performance of extraverted subjects in a paired-associated recall task (Howarth & Eysenck, 1968) is interpreted in terms of the effect of arousal upon a process of consolidation. The second trend is a return to Pavlovian or neo-Pavlovian explanations of introverted or extraverted behavior patterns, Mangan and Farmer (1967) finding, for example, a significant correlation between extraversion and strength sensitivity of the nervous system as measured by Nebylitsyn (in Gray, 1965).

There is by now an impressive array of models, any one of which is capable of dealing with a large portion of the differences observed in these two groups. Cortical satiation, reactive inhibition, internal inhibition, strength sensitivity, equilibrium, sampling periods, arousal states: all of these and others occur as explanations of introversion–extraversion effects.

In this state of affairs the practice is widespread of adopting whichever explanation fits an obtained result regardless of differences between the source models. Differences between the original models are sometimes washed out by redefining their respective concepts in less specific terms, for example, Hull's W includes "mental work" (Eysenck, 1967, p. 78); "reactive inhibition" is another term that has been retained but is used as a less precise concept than originally. Difficulties arise in this sort of situation where shifting between theoretical models affects the conception of the mechanism underlying the changes in state of the individual; a problem exists, for example, as to when to refer to one mechanism rather than another. Confusion results, too, over what result is expected in a given experiment, or concerning the significance of what has been found. This is demonstrated clearly in the matter of tolerance for sensory deprivation. Eysenck predicts that introverts should have relatively greater tolerance for sensory deprivation (Eysenck & Eysenck, 1969, p. 51). The prediction is derived from the view that, for a given level of stimulation, introverts will produce a higher state of excitatory potential than extraverts. This result, however, has not always been observed. Tranel (1962) failed to show that introverts differed from extraverts in their tolerance of sensory deprivation. Rossi and Solomon (1965), in one study, found introverts experienced more discomfort than extraverts during isolation. Subsequently, however, these same workers (Rossi & Solomon, 1966) observed no differences between their subject groups in premature termination, verbal reports, self-ratings or records of movements during 3-hr isolation. Contrary again to these latter findings, Petrie, Collins, and Solomon (1960) did find extraverts less tolerant of sensory deprivation. What is important here is that explanations in terms of characteristic arousal levels, or reactive inhibition or Pavlovian mechanisms, can give different predictions. One can argue that sensory deprivation conditions will not provide the stimulating environment sought by the "stimulus hungry" extraverts to raise their characteristic low arousal level to some preferred level. This will be reflected in their poor tolerance of deprivation conditions. On a reactive inhibition view, however, the low *response* rates typically required of subjects in deprivation situations avoid the build up of any strong response-related negative drive-state (R-inhibition) in extraverts whose tolerance it could be argued would, therefore, be more akin to that of the introverts in this setting. A Pavlovian interpretation, if we equate our extraverted subjects with his "sanguine," dogs would be that, without a high degree of stimulation, irradiation of inhibition will occur in extraverts causing drowsiness and even sleep (see (Pavlov, 1928, Lecture 32)). If this occurred, the tolerance of deprivation could well be higher in extraverts since a comatose state is not sui generis an aversive state.

Similarly, the responsiveness of the individual provides further evidence of the need to clarify the theoretical foundations upon which differences in the performance of introverts and extraverts are based. Howarth (1964) observed that, if anything, extraverts tended to emit slightly more responses than introverts in a free response situation. If R-inhibition built up more quickly among these subjects, one would hypothesize that they should show more "involuntary rest pauses," with a consequent reduction of response rate relative to introverted subjects. Yensen (1967) found no trend for extraversion to correlate with response frequency in a task similar to Howarth's. With a change in explanatory construct to one in which extraverts are hypothesized to have a lower level of arousal than introverts or than they themselves prefer, however, it can be predicted that extraverts would seek more stimulation in order to maintain a balance between excitation and inhibition, and Gale (1969) and Phillipp and Wilde (1970) both confirm that extraverts maintain *higher* rates of response in a free response situation.

The purpose of exposing the incoherence of the literature in this review is to point out the danger of failing to distinguish between the processes postulated in the original reactive inhibition and the more recent models. Rather than merely illustrating this problem, however, a more constructive approach, and one which at the present time seems likely to prove necessary sooner rather than later, would set out to show how far the explanatory constructs of the various models can be amalgamated. Such an amalgamation can be achieved if, instead of assuming central excitation to derive only from stimulation and inhibition as a consequence of either the absence of stimulation or of high response rates, it is accepted that the central mechanisms are capable of being in one of two different states, excitation or inhibition, and that either can be induced by the demands for stimulus analysis (S-excitation or S-inhibition) or response organization (R-excitation or R-inhibition) acting upon the person. It is perhaps worth noting that, while stimuli or responses have individual excitatory or inhibitory effects, these are modified by the context in which they occur and which is created by the occurrence of other stimuli and the requirement for other responses.

Since perceiving any stimulus is a response, just as any response creates a set of stimuli, we should perhaps be clear from the outset that "stimulus-related" effects include the feedback from responses, so that "response-related" effects is a class of actions which does not include integrations of sensory information into percepts or concepts; these are retained in the "stimulus" category.

In some tasks it is difficult to know whether the effects on performance derive from S-effects or R-effects. For example, changes in performance which occur in vigilance tasks can be ascribed either to the development of S-inhibition related to the absence of signals, to a lack of R-excitation due to the lack of opportunity to respond, or to the generation of inhibition mediated by the observing response. Eysenck (1967, p. 84 *et seq.*) expresses the view that maintaining a state of readiness to detect and respond to small changes in the environment is an observing response, and that missed responses indicate "involuntary rest pauses" due to the build-up of reactive inhibition. Thus, for vigilance situations, although the observing response may be covertly rather than overtly made, an R-inhibition explanation can hold good. However, the possibility of S-inhibition existing separately from the effects of low arousal and R-inhibition has not been considered widely; consequently, the relative contribution of S- and R-inhibition has not been systematically investigated, although Eysenck seems to acknowledge an important difference between these inhibitory effects: "When . . . it is argued that a deficiency in performance is due to reactive inhibition, it is always open to the critic to hypothesize that this deficiency in performance is due rather to a lessening of excitation, and conversely" (Eysenck, 1967, p. 81).

The first experiment below is a reaction time task so structured as to minimize R-inhibition in order to find if the performance (in terms of prolonged RT's and missed signals) of extraverts was more detrimentally affected than that of introverts by inhibition resulting from the conditions of stimulation (S-inhibition) rather than the number of responses made. The way chosen to achieve this was to use a low response rate in association with a low but regular signal rate. A low response rate implies little R-inhibition will be generated, and that dissipation of inhibition will take place between responses. Thus R-inhibition should not contribute to any difference between the performance of introverts and extraverts. A low signal rate, on the other hand, acts to reduce the level of arousal, raising inhibitory potential. Differences in the performance of introverts and extraverts found in this situation would be expected to reflect the hypothesized differences in S-inhibition levels rather than differences in R-inhibition. It has been claimed above that this change which we refer to as S-inhibition is not necessarily the same as the characteristic differences in arousal level accepted by Eysenck. Extraverts may be "chronically underaroused" relative to introverts, but if so, differences in their performance should be evident right from the beginning of our experiment. S-inhibition, on the other hand, would be expected to build up as a function of the duration of the stimulus conditions, implying a gradual separation in the performance of the two groups.

Finally, if the need to maintain a state of readiness to detect and respond for prolonged periods is removed, but a low signal and a low response rate is retained, a method is provided for testing between an R-inhibition model and arousal or S-inhibition explanations. This may be achieved by presenting a signal for response at regular time intervals. In this case the individual need be prepared to detect and respond only during a relatively small proportion of the total time, attending only around the time a signal is due to arrive. In effect, he may control his "voluntary rest pauses" to occur between signals. To the degree that the observing response can be "switched off," R-inhibition would not be generated and would dissipate during the "off" periods. There is a problem in selecting the intertrial interval between signals for response, because there is little useful information on how long a time is needed for the R-inhibition generated by one response to dissipate completely. The signal rates used reflect the writers' conviction that under the conditions of the experiment this dissipation would be complete in less than 18 sec. This conviction was based on pilot work from which it seemed that performance would be improved rather than impaired by a higher response rate.

Eysenck (1967) equates early studies of monotony with those of vigilance when citing early evidence that extraverts are more affected by monotonous situations (Munsterberg, 1913; Thompson, 1929). While this may be reasonable for the examples cited, it is also theoretically important to distinguish situations demanding continued attention from those simply providing a low level of stimulation. The effect of extraversion in vigilance performance may be explained in R-inhibition terms, but if the present experiment shows a difference in performance between introverts and extraverts, this will confirm a separate case of S-inhibitory activity.

1. Extraverts would in particular, then, be expected to miss more signals than introverts as time on task increased.
2. Extraverts would be expected to produce relatively slower RT's as time on task increased.

These predictions were tested in Experiment 1 of the present study.

EXPERIMENT I

Apparatus

The RT apparatus consisted of one Racal timer with 10^{-4} sec accuracy, and a Morse key operated by the subject in response to the onset of a small neon lamp which was controlled by two interval timers serialized to give ISI of 18 sec and signal duration of 1 sec.

Subjects

Sixteen members of the introductory class in Psychology at the University of Adelaide took part in the experiment. Subjects were classified as extraverted or introverted from their scores on the M.P.I. Extraverts' scores ranged from 35–46, the modal age of these subjects being 19 yr. Introverts' scores ranged from 2–11, again with a modal age of 19 yr.

Procedure

Subjects were first introduced to the experimental booth and the nature of their task, "to respond as quickly as possible to this signal light which will come on every so often," was explained, while silver/silver chloride "stick-on" electrodes (Specialized Laboratory Equipment) were being fixed in a bioccipital configuration. (See Addendum for further comments.)

During the experiment the subject sat in a reclining position on a dental chair, and operated the response key with the index finger of the dominant hand. The dental chair was located inside a fine wire mesh booth within which the subject was screened from the apparatus and the experimenter who recorded RT. The subject performed the task for a period of 10 min before any RT was taken. The object of this setting in period was to avoid "warm-up" effects so that, for example, subjects had realized that signals occurred regularly, by the time RT was recorded. But the settling in period also served the additional functions both of avoiding any temporary lift in arousal which might be occasioned by beginning the experimental task, and of allowing any influence of the signal rate to have some effect upon performance before recording began so that any differences between the subject groups could be detected from the outset of recording.

Each subject provided 100 RT's. If a subject failed to respond within 4 sec of a signal occurring, he was deemed to have missed that signal. No instances were observed of any subject attempting to respond to a signal after the experimenter had judged the subject to have missed it. On completing the experiment, subjects were questioned about the experiment.

RESULTS

Missed signals. The present experiment could be accurately described as presenting subjects with a transit RT task (Slater-Hammel, 1958; Brebner, 1971) with a low signal rate. The essential feature of such tasks is that subjects can estimate the time of occurrence of a known signal, and with accurate judgement may achieve zero RT. With an intersignal interval as long as 18 sec, the level of speed in responding approximates more closely to a simple RT. Since signals are predictable, detection rates should be higher than if signals occurred at random time intervals.

In fact, half the subjects missed no signals. Those who did miss signals tended to be extraverts, and more signals were missed in the later stages of the experiment. Unfortunately, with such a high proportion of "tied" scores as was obtained, one cannot easily compare the performance of introverts and extraverts with any validity. However, it is the case that, with due correction for "ties," a Spearman rank correlation coefficient of $+.53$ is obtained between M.P.I. score and total number of signals missed. This value of r_s is significant at the 0.05 level, though one should be wary of interpreting correlational values when only extreme scorers are used. Even so, the trend is clearly in the predicted direction and one can consider the hypothesis that extraverts will tend to miss more signals than introverts to derive some support from these results.

As far as missing signals is concerned, it is interesting that of the introverts, only one, subject 8, reported experiencing a state resembling sleep. This subject volunteered that he had several times "had the sensation of having just wakened up." Among the extraverts on the other hand, subject 12 reported having fallen asleep, and subjects 10, 11, 13 and 15 that they had dozed, though they had not slept during portions of the experiment. Extending Pavlov's observation, that the "sanguine" dog required a reasonably high level of stimulation or else fell asleep, to human subjects seems quite possible. Tune (1969) did not find any difference in the sleep–wakefulness pattern of introverts and extraverts below the age of 40 yr, but even in uncontrolled nonlaboratory situations, older extraverts were found to sleep longer than their introverted counterparts.

Reaction times. On the hypothesis that extraverts generate more S-inhibition with a low signal rate than introverts do, one would expect the extraverted subjects to produce more long RT's as the experiment progresses. This general view was tested using ANOVA applied to the mean RT's in first and second halves of the experiment for both groups. The interaction between personality and halves of the experiment, however, proved not to be significant ($F(1,14) = 0.02$, $p > .05$). Table 1A gives the mean RT for each subject in both halves of the experiment. Inspection of Table 1A shows, not only that there is no systematic difference in the average level of speed with which the two groups respond to signals, but also that no such change in mean RT occurs within either group in the two halves of the experiment. However, these results do not clearly reflect what was happening to the distributions of RT's in the two groups of subjects during the experiment.

Table 2 shows the skewness of the RT distributions of subjects for both halves of the experiment. From Table 2 it appears that, in the first half

BREBNER AND COOPER

TABLE 1A
MEAN RT (MSEC) AND STANDARD DEVIATIONS IN THE
FIRST AND SECOND HALVES OF EXPERIMENT 1

	Introverts					Extraverts			
	First half		Second half			First half		Second half	
	$\bar{X}$		$\bar{X}$			$\bar{X}$		$\bar{X}$	
1.	295	57.2	281	39.0	9.	287	54.6	337	127.1
2.	262	37.7	278	52.3	10.	543	295.1	517	235.4
3.	283	89.8	298	100.1	11.	376	68.9	352	56.6
4.	375	67.6	247	63.2	12.	631	423.8	550	370.4
5.	367	53.0	407	127.3	13.	398	153.4	460	206.5
6.	327	70.5	342	68.5	14.	295	50.9	284	46.4
7.	340	102.7	342	54.0	15.	265	54.1	295	175.9
8.	362	182.3	379	140.3	16.	305	117.5	294	84.4
Group mean and σ	326	92.8	322	87.9		388	199.1	386	192.0

TABLE 1B
MEAN RT (MSEC) IN THE FIRST AND SECOND HALVES OF EXPERIMENT 2

1.	302	36.3	295	41.1	9.	426	67.2	440	63.3
2.	360	112.8	346	52.5	10.	369	88.2	357	54.3
3.	348	68.5	358	151.4	11.	501	154.0	529	107.6
4.	426	125.1	416	91.7	12.	358	97.8	441	145.7
5.	310	32.4	321	48.6	13.	265	44.8	284	49.5
6.	349	50.8	314	29.1	14.	461	107.3	507	97.0
7.	293	59.8	292	56.8	15.	352	225.3	426	199.3
8.	290	24.3	287	33.4	16.	325	62.3	329	69.8
Group mean and σ	335	72.6	329	73.6		382	119.2	414	84.7

of the experiment at least, there is no difference between groups in the skewness of distributions. A computer-run randomization test, which assigned the obtained scores randomly to the two groups 1000 times, made it possible to find an empirical probability distribution for differences between means for the given data. This test was applied to these data in preference to ANOVA since the underlying distribution of skewness measures is unknown and cannot be assumed to be normal. The randomization test showed that the two groups do not provide differently skewed distributions in the first half of the experiment ($p = 0.70$). The difference between the groups does, however, increase in the expected direction with time on task, and a clear trend toward greater positive skewing is shown for RT's obtained in the second half of the experiment from the extra-

I-E AND RT TO REGULAR SIGNALS

TABLE 2

Skew Values of RT Distributions in First and
Second Halves of Experiment 1

	Introverts			Extraverts	
	First half	Second half		First half	Second half
1.	1.20	0.45	9.	0.65	2.34
2.	0.78	0.79	10.	2.80	2.32
3.	1.60	2.25	11.	2.25	0.36
4.	1.83	1.00	12.	2.35	3.78
5.	1.28	1.65	13.	2.34	3.30
6.	0.35	−2.00	14.	0.25	1.33
7.	4.89	1.15	15.	0.19	6.44
8.	2.29	2.18	16.	1.43	2.98
Group mean	1.78	0.93		1.53	2.86

verted subjects. A randomization test on the skew values for the two groups in the second half of the experiment evidences a significant difference ($p = 0.02$).

This increase in positive skew in the second half of the experiment for the extraverted subjects only shows that these subjects were unable to maintain a consistently high level of performance throughout the task. This finding also suggests that the duration of the task may have been too short for the difference between the two groups to manifest itself in measures of central tendency. If this is so, then this result argues against any initial difference in the arousal levels of the two groups.

To some extent, treating cases where the subject failed to respond as "missed signals" rather than assigning them some arbitrary "reaction time," contributes to the present result. Nevertheless, it seems preferable to adopt this course rather than lumping the two different effects together as if they were the same phenomenon. However, since the hypothesized differences in the performance of extraverts and introverts are verified both for missed signals and also for changes in RT distribution, this indicates a higher degree of sensitivity on the part of the extraverts to the conditions of the experiment. Moreover, even allowing a "settling-in" period, the RT distributions of the two groups did not differ in the first half of the experiment, but a significant difference appeared in the latter half. This is evidence that it is the effect of the conditions of stimulation, and not any initial incomparability in arousal levels between the two groups, which leads to the observed difference in performance.

Summing up, the data on missed signals and the difference in RT distributions of the groups in the second half of the experiment are in line with the hypotheses under test, but no significant difference was observed in mean RT. The likeliest explanation for this result would seem to be that the task was only long enough for a "flow" of RT values from shorter to longer readings to commence, but was not sufficiently prolonged for measures of central tendency to be affected. On this basis a second experiment which required subjects to spend a longer time at the task was performed.

EXPERIMENT II

The second experiment can be briefly described as a computer controlled version of the one above with two major changes. First, subjects provided 180 RT readings at the same ISI of 18 sec as was used previously. The first 30 RT's were regarded as the "settling-in" period so that the experimental session comprised two halves each of 75 RT's. This increase in the number of readings obtained, and therefore of the time on task, was introduced in an attempt to strengthen the effects observed in the previous experiment. Second, EEG records were derived from a monopolar occipital configuration, the "active" electrode being located at 0_1 (in the International 10–20 electrode system), and the "indifferent" one on the left ear lobe, from an equal number of introverts and extraverts selected by chance (see Addendum).

Apparatus

Signal presentation and RT recording was controlled by a PDP 8L Computer. subjects operating a Morse key in response to the onset of a light emitting diode with a signal duration of 1 sec and a regular ISI of 18 sec.

Subjects

Sixteen members of the introductory class in Psychology at the University of Adelaide took part in the experiment. Subjects were classed as introverted or extraverted from their scores on the E.P.I. The change in test from the previous experiment was dictated by practical considerations of which test results were available, but it was hoped that some slight increase in validity might result from using the more recent inventory. Extraverts' scores ranged from 18–22, the modal age of these subjects being 19 yr. Introverts' scores ranged from 2–6, and again the modal age of the group was 19 yr.

Procedure

The procedure was the same as for the previous experiment except that it was explained that the task was computer controlled, lasted "about an hour," and that any noises outside the test room (mainly emanating from high-speed tape punches or related equipment) were irrelevant to the experiment and should be ignored.

RESULTS

Missed signals. As in the first experiment most of the misses were made by a few subjects, and these are among the extraverts. Bearing in mind that the same strictures noted in the previous experiment also apply here, a Spearman rank correlation coefficient of $+.69$ is obtained between E.P.I. score and number of signals missed, which is significant at the 0.01 level.

Reaction times. Table 1B shows the mean RT values obtained in the first and second halves of this second experiment. From Table 1B it is evident that with this lengthened task there is a systematic slowing in the performance of the extraverted subjects in the second half of the experiment. No such tendency exists in the group of introverts. ANOVA confirms this interpretation, the interaction between personality and halves of the experiment is significant ($F(1,14) = 8.76$, $p < .01$).

This result supports the interpretation of the first experiment. Increasing the duration of the task has strengthened the effect, and the central tendencies of the RT distributions now reveal the reduced performance of extraverted subjects in the latter stages of the experiment. Once again the absence of any difference between the groups in the early stages militates against any initial difference in arousal level between introverts and extraverts. Rather, the low signal rate leads to a lowering of the responsiveness of the extraverted group of subjects in the second half of the experiment which does not happen among the introverted subjects.

DISCUSSION

The results of these experiments argue against R-inhibition or characteristic arousal levels as the only explanations of the differences in performance of the two groups, and it seems useful to distinguish S-inhibition from these other possibilities. From the present data, such a change seems to be a matter of necessity rather than preference, since differences between groups only occur after a reasonable length of time on task. This has not always been the case with vigilance studies. In some cases, e.g., Bakan (1959) the two groups show differences at the beginning of the experiment. This small point raises the wider question of how far studies of introversion–extraversion are investigating the same thing. Differences due to R-inhibition should increase with time on task. Differences due to different *characteristic* arousal levels are expected right at the start of an experiment. Differences which arise more gradually in the absence of a high response rate, however, argue that the stimulus conditions of the task produced a stronger inhibitory effect on one group. This latter possibility, akin to Pavlovian irradiation of inhibition, seems to be the factor underlying the present results. Many of the findings in this area of personality difference can be accommodated within this model of the introvert as an individual more sensitive to stimulation who can be described as having a "weak" nervous system, i.e., a person who generates higher S-excitatory potential than the extravert given the same level of stimulation, and who is therefore less prone to S-inhibitory states than the extravert is. At the same time the extravert produces relatively greater R-excitatory potential for any given S-state, so that he is, as it were, "geared to respond" whereas the introvert is "geared to inspect." Where response demands are low and with low levels of stimulation or repetitive stimulation, the development of S-inhibition is favored, and extraverts would be expected to be more affected by these conditions than the introverts. This simple model can also generate predictions of similar performance between introverted and extraverted subjects, as well as predicting differences in their performance. In tasks where S- and R-excitatory potential is low, the extraverts' performance would be lowered by a relatively greater amount. In the opposite case where R-excitatory potential is high but S-excitatory potential is low the extraverts' performance would be relatively better until S-inhibition increased as a function of responding and acted to decrease the overall excitatory potential in the extraverted subjects.

This is speculative but it does offer one way of tying together the explanatory constructs of the major theories of introversion–extraversion. Whether these speculations derive support from future studies or not, the present study rules out R-inhibition and chronic arousal levels as the only explanations of the differences observed between introverted and extraverted subjects. Moreover, referring again to Pavlov's discussions of "sanguine" types of dogs, the result of the present experimentation with human subjects parallels the description in his Lecture 17 (Pavlov, 1928) where he notes that those dogs of the "sanguine" type which were the most vivacious, responsive and lively outside the experimental conditions were the ones which became drowsy earliest under the conditions of the experimental treatments which restricted responding.

The model offered above is not identical to any of the major theories. Rather it is an amalgamation of them which is capable of being collapsed to any one of the major positions. But its real virtue lies in linking the main explanations together into a simple, unitary model of introversion–extraversion.

ADDENDUM

It is necessary to record that all the subjects in the first experiment and half the subjects in the second (equally distributed through the introvert–extravert groups) were subjected to the extra stresses demanded by recording electroencephalographic activity, amounting to the prior application of two electrodes and a minor restraint on mobility. It was hoped that the record might provide objective information concerning fluctuations in the subjects' state of arousal; it being usually assumed that the presence of synchronized rhythms in the alpha band of frequencies registers "relaxation." However, on the one hand the functional significance of the reflection at the scalp of the alpha generator is complex and not understood (there may, for example, be more than one such generator (Walter *et al.* (1966)). There have been assertions that alpha rhythms imply a state of central inhibition (e.g. Magoun, 1963; Morrell, 1966) and the notion is basic in biologically based personality concepts (see Eysenck, 1967). However, the correlation of synchronized EEG activity with arousal or vigilance is complex (Becker-Carus, 1971; Berkhout, 1965) and with introversion–extraversion scores the correlation is not found in some studies (Werre & Barendregt, 1963; Dongier & Dongier, 1958; Fenton & Scotton, 1967) and in others runs contrary to prediction (Broadhurst & Glass, 1969). Another factor was fortuitously uncovered whose influence is not assessed; of the subjects "selected" for EEG recording in the second experiment, all those who were introverts had undergone some form of meditational training.

On the other hand, the value of the form of gross EEG analysis commonly used is open to question (Gale, Coles and Blaydon (1969) emphasize the dangers thereof in this context). The present experience with a sample of the EEG records was that an "alpha index" score (amount of time in a record where waves in the alpha frequency range were above some criterial amplitude) would have produced a misleading result in the sense that there appeared to be an increase of synchronization but progressively more of it fell below criterion. The appropriate form of data-processing, frequency spectral analysis, was not available. In view of these considerations, the analysis was not continued.

REFERENCES

BAKAN, P. Extraversion–introversion and improvement in an auditory vigilance task. *British Journal of Psychology*, 1959, **50**, 325–332.

BECKER-CARUS, C. Relationships between EEG personality and vigilance. *Electro-encephalography and Clinical Neurophysiology*, 1971, **30**, 519–520.

BERKHOUT. J. Comparative frequency distributions of large and small amplitude rhythms of the human electroencephalogram. *Electroencephalography and Clinical Neurophysiology*, 1965, **19**, 598–600.

BREBNER, J. The refractoriness of regular reponses. *Australian Journal of Psychology*, 1971, **23**, 3–7.

BROADHURST, A., & GLASS, A. Relationship of personality measures to the alpha rhythm of the encephalogram. *British Journal of Psychiatry*, 1969. **115**, 199–204.

DONGIER, M., & DONGIER, S. Quelques aspects de l'electreencephalogramme de nerveses. *Évolution Psychiatrique*, 1958, **1**, 1–18.

EYSENCK, H. J. A dynamic theory of anxiety and hysteria. *Journal of Mental Science*, 1955, **101**, 28–51.

EYSENCK, H. J. *The dynamics of anxiety and hysteria.* New York: Praeger, 1957.

EYSENCK, H. J. *Biological basis of personality.* Springfield, IL: Thomas, 1967.

EYSENCK, H. J., & EYSENCK, S. B. G. *Personality structure and measurement.* San Diego, CA: Knapp, 1969.

FENTON, G. W., & SCOTTON, L. Personality and the alpha rhythm. *British Journal of Psychiatry*, 1967, **113**, 1288–1289.

BREBNER AND COOPER

GALE, A. 'Stimulus hinges': individual differences in operant strategy in a button pressing task. *Behaviour Research and Therapy*, 1969, **7**, 265–274.

GALE, A., COLES, M., & BLAYDON, J. Extraversion–introversion and the EEG. *British Journal of Psychology*, 1969, **60**, 209–223.

GRAY, J. A. (Ed.). *Pavlov's typology*. New York: Pergamon, 1965.

HOWARTH, E. Differences between extraverts and introverts on a button-pressing task. *Psychological Reports*, 1964, **14**, 949–956.

HOWARTH, E., & EYSENCK, H. J. Extraversion, arousal and paired-associate recall. *Journal of Experimental Research in Personality*, 1968, **3**, 114–116.

JUNG, C. G. *Psychological types*. New York: Harcourt Brace & World, 1923.

MAGOUN, H. *The waking brain*. Springfield, IL: Thomas, 1963.

MANGAN, G. L., & FARMER, R. G. Studies of the relationship between neo-Pavlovian properties of higher nervous activity and western personality dimensions: the relationship of nervous strength and sensitivity to extraversion. *Journal of Experimental Research in Personality*, 1967, **2**, 101–106.

MORRELL, L. K. Some characteristics of stimulus-provoked alpha activity. *Electroencephalography and Clinical Neurophysiology*, 1966, **21**, 552–561.

MUNSTERBERG, N. *Psychology and industrial efficiency*. Boston: Houghton Mifflin, 1913.

NEBYLITSIN, V. D. *In* J. A. Gray (Ed.), *Pavlov's typology*. New York: Pergamon, 1965.

PAVLOV, I. P. *Conditioned reflexes*. London: Oxford, 1927.

PAVLOV, I. P. *Lectures on conditioned reflexes*. New York: International, 1928.

PAVLOV, I. P. *Conditioned reflexes and psychiatry*. New York: International, 1935.

PETRIE, A., COLLINS, W., & SOLOMON, P. The tolerance for pain and for sensory deprivation. *American Journal of Psychology*, 1960, **123**, 80–90.

PHILLIPP, R. L., & WILDE, G. J. Stimulation seeking behavior and extraversion. *Acta Psychologica*, 1970, **32**, 269–280.

ROSSI, A. M., & SOLOMON, P. Note on reactions of extraverts and introverts to sensory deprivation. *Perceptual and Motor Skills*, 1965, **28**, 1183–1184.

ROSSI, A. M., & SOLOMON, P. Effects of sensory deprivation on introverts and extraverts: a failure to find reported differences. *Journal of Psychiatric Research*, 1966, **4**, 115–125.

SLATER-HAMMEL, A. T. Psychological refractory period in simple paired responses. *Research Quarterly American Association for Health, Physical Education and Recreation*, 1958, **29**, 469–481.

THOMPSON, L. A. Measuring susceptibility to monotony. *Personnel Journal*, 1929, **8**, 172–197.

TRANEL, M. N. The effects of perceptual isolation on introverts and extraverts. *Dissertation Abstracts*, 1962, **23**, 726–727.

TUNE, G. S. The influence of age and temperament on the adult human sleep–wakefulness pattern. *British Journal of Psychology*, 1969, **60**, 431–441.

WALTER, D. O., RHODES, J. M., BROWN, D., & ADEY, W. R. Comprehensive spectral analysis of human EEG generator in posterior cerebral regions. *Electroencephalography and Clinical Neurophysiology*, 1966, **20**, 224–237.

WERRE, P. F., & BARENDREGT, J. T. Correlations between some electroencephalographic and psychological variables. *Confinia Psychiatrica*, 1963, **8**, 181–190.

YENSEN, R. Replication study of responsiveness on a simple five-button pressing task. *Perceptual and Motor Skills*, 1967, **25**, 965–966.

From G. S. Tune (1966). Quarterly Journal of Experimental Psychology, *18*, 358–361, *by kind permission of the author and the Longman Group Limited*

ERRORS OF COMMISSION AS A FUNCTION OF AGE AND TEMPERAMENT IN A TYPE OF VIGILANCE TASK

BY

G. S. TUNE

From the Medical Research Council, Unit for Research on Occupational Aspects of Ageing, Department of Psychology, University of Liverpool

Forty subjects monitored a 40 min. series of 10-sec. intervals containing digits (spoken at the rate of 1 per sec.), each followed by 10-sec. silence. The task was to report whether or not three consecutive and different odd digits occurred. Responses were forced. The results showed that there was no correlation between either age or temperament and the number of correct detections made. Older subjects, however, made more errors of commission, and were less able to distinguish wanted from unwanted events. The younger and introverted subjects appeared to be more cautious. The data is discussed in terms of the arousal theory of vigilance performance.

INTRODUCTION

Griew and Lynn (1960) have argued that older and extraverted subjects should be worse at vigilance tasks than younger and introverted subjects because they generate reactive inhibition faster and dissipate it more slowly. While it is well established that introverts do make more correct detections than extraverts (Bakan, 1959; Bakan, Belton and Toth, 1963), the evidence for an age difference in correct detections is not unanimous. Davies and Griew (1965) in a survey of the topic indicated that old people achieved similar detection scores to younger people. Surwillo and Quilter (1964), however, did show an age difference in performance in the Mackworth Clock test, but this emerged only after 45 min. on the task.

It has also been reported (Tune, 1966) that while older and younger subjects made comparable correct detection scores in a forced-choice response vigilance task, the former made many more errors of commission (reported many unwanted events as if they were in fact "wanted"). In an extreme case the effect of this response bias would be that subjects achieved a maximum correct detection score but also a maximum number of commissive errors. Obviously the more errors of this type a subject is prepared to make then the greater is the insurance against an error of omission. Such a response strategy would have the effect of masking, either partially or wholly, any individual differences which might be expected in the correct detection score. The question remains, however, as to whether or not there are temperament differences in the number of errors of commission subjects make. If the vigilance performance of older and extraverted subjects is comparable, as Griew and Lynn (1960) predicted, it is likely that these groups would make relatively large numbers of commissive errors. It is further likely that both age and temperament differences would not be apparent in the correct detection scores.

The present experiment was designed to examine these points in a vigilance task where forced-choice responses were required, and where errors of commission were not discouraged, where the performance of young, old, introverted and extraverted subjects could be compared.

PROCEDURE

Subjects listened to a tape recording of groups of 10 digits (the numbers 1 to 9 inclusive were used in a quasi-random order) each group being followed by 10 sec. silence. The task was to identify three consecutive, different and odd digits (e.g. 517, 93 5, etc.) occurring somewhere in the group (the exact location of the three "wanted" digits was randomized such that neither the first nor the last number in any group of 10 was the beginning or end of an odd-odd-odd triad). No more than one "wanted" triad occurred in any one block of 10 digits. Subjects were instructed to listen to all 10 numbers and then to place a tick in one of two columns on a prepared answer sheet. The two columns were headed "No" (a wanted combination of numbers did not occur) and "Yes" (a wanted combination did occur). In the latter case subjects were also encouraged to write the triad in a third column: it was emphasized, however, that this was unimportant (transcription errors were·not counted against a subject). Scores were assessed entirely in terms of the number of ticks placed in the "Yes" column. The subjects listened to 120 groups of 10 digits over a period of 40 min.: 27 of these contained a "wanted" triad. A brief practice session consisting of two groups of 10 digits (one with and the other without a "wanted" triad) was given in order to ensure that subjects understood the procedure. The experimenter remained with the subject for the first ½ min. of the task and then left.

Subjects. Forty subjects were used. These were classified as old (those over 50 years) or young (those of 49 years and under). They were further classified into introverts or extraverts by means of their score on Part 2 of the Heron (1956) inventory. A division was taken at the median score to ensure equal groups. There were thus four groups of 10 subjects (see Table I). In addition each group contained five men and five women.

RESULTS

Two response measures were taken from the raw data produced by each subject: these were (*a*) the number of "Yes" responses which were correct detections and (*b*) the number of "Yes" responses which were errors of commission. The distribution of "Yes" responses by type, age and temperament is shown in Table I. It is apparent that in the four groups the probability of making a correct detection was about the same. The error of commission scores, however, show a different picture. Spearman rank correlations were calculated therefore between the two response measures and the two independent variables and are given in Table II. These indicate that the older subjects made more

TABLE I

THE DISTRIBUTION OF "YES" RESPONSES BY AGE, TEMPERAMENT AND TYPE

	N	Mean age	Mean Heron 2 score	Correct detections	Errors of commission
Old Introverts ..	10	65·9	7·8	248	96
Old Extraverts ..	10	65·3	3·9	234	325
Young Introverts ..	10	35·5	9·3	246	16
Young Extraverts..	10	38·1	4·4	252	32
Totals	40	—	—	980	469

TABLE II

SPEARMAN RANK CORRELATIONS BETWEEN THE RESPONSE MEASURES AND THE INDEPENDENT VARIABLES

	ρ	$p <$ (two-tailed)
Age × Correct Detections ..	−0·046	NS
Age × Errors of Commission ..	+0·521	0·001
Age × d'	−0·498	0·01
Age × β	−0·417	0·01
Heron (2) × Correct Detections ..	+0·021	NS
Heron (2) × Errors of Commission ..	−0·352	0·05
Heron (2) × d'	+0·281	0·10
Heron (2) × β	+0·395	0·01

errors of commission whereas there was no relationship between age and correct detection score, although there was a slight tendency for the older people to make fewer (as shown by the negative sign of the correlation). Temperament was not significantly associated with correct detections although there was a tendency for high Heron 2 scorers (introverts) to make more. A low Heron 2 score on the other hand was significantly associated with a high error of commission score.

The probability of making a correct detection and the probability of making an error of commission were calculated for each subject and from these scores d′ and β were ascertained by reference to tables (Freeman, 1964). If the former is taken as a measure of signal discriminability and the latter as a measure of caution (Broadbent and Gregory, 1963), it is apparent from the correlations between these scores and the independent variables (Table II) that the older people and the extraverts were less able to discriminate signals from non-signals whereas the younger people and introverts were more cautious.

DISCUSSION AND CONCLUSIONS

It seems clear that although, in this experiment, there were no individual differences in correct detections, the older and extraverted subjects did exhibit similar performance. Increasing age and extraversion were both associated with large error of commission scores, an inability to distinguish wanted from unwanted events and a tendency to be incautious.

These results are apparently in agreement with some findings, that there is no age difference in detection scores (Davies and Griew, 1965), and apparently in conflict with others, that there are temperament differences in correct detection scores (Bakan, 1959). If errors of commission are considered, however, the picture is changed. It was emphasized in the introduction that such errors would tend to obscure individual differences in detection scores. This, it seems, is what happened here although the older and extraverted subjects tended to detect fewer wanted events than the younger and introverted.

The problem of why some groups made more errors of commission than others is not easy to answer. Although these data lend support to Griew and Lynn's reactive inhibition hypothesis, other accounts of vigilance performance must be considered.

Broadbent (1963) has argued that introverts are chronically aroused, hence extraverts may be regarded as underaroused. While there is little physiological evidence to support this view, it has been found useful in explaining temperament differences in vigilance performance (Broadbent, 1963). It is tempting to assume further, that older people are likewise underaroused (Tune, 1966). From this point of view it would be reasonable to infer that underaroused subjects would attempt to raise their arousal level to a suitable level by increasing their response information (alternating between the two types of response, "Yes" and "No," more readily). This would result in the underaroused groups making more commissive errors, as was found here. On the other hand, Welford (1965) has argued cogently that older subjects are in fact overaroused. What the effect of such a state would be on such subjects' error of commission score is not entirely clear. It is possible that overarousal might imply overactivity which could be exhibited in a tendency to alternate between response categories. If this was accepted, it would mean that over and underarousal were behaviourally indistinguishable since both would produce high numbers of commissive errors. For this reason it is perhaps more economical to regard older subjects as underaroused.

A second approach is to avoid speculation about arousal states, since the evidence regarding older people in this respect is not unequivocal, and to posit that older and extraverted subjects are inherently less cautious. This view implies that such groups could insure against low detection scores by reporting many events as wanted even when they were not. The fact that β, in this experiment, was negatively correlated with age, and positively with a high Heron 2 score (introversion) lends some support to the argument, although it conflicts with Craik (1965) who found that older subjects were more cautious than younger. These two approaches are not necessarily unrelated, for it is likely that arousal level and cautiousness are not independent of each other (Welford, 1962).

From the results of this experiment and what has been said some speculations may be made. The arousal approach seems to imply that errors of commission can be regarded as an index of need for information. This ties in well with the "sensoristasis" hypothesis (Schultz, 1965) and implies that subjects will seek information in order to perform adequately. Errors of commission should, therefore, increase with time spent on a progressively de-arousing task. Commissive errors should also distinguish between differential levels of arousal. The present data show that age correlated with errors of commission at a higher level of significance than did temperament. This is only slight

AGE, TEMPERAMENT AND ERRORS OF COMMISSION

evidence that age is more de-arousing than extraversion and more refined evaluations of this point need to be made.

I should like to thank Mr. R. Aldridge-Morris for carrying out some of the experimental work described here.

REFERENCES

BAKAN, P. (1959). Extraversion—Introversion and improvement in an auditory vigilance task. *Brit. J. Psychol.*, **50**, 325–32.

BAKAN, P., BELTON, J. A., and TOTH, J. C. (1963). Extraversion—Introversion and decrement in an auditory vigilance task. In BUCKNER, D. N., and MCGRATH, J. J. (Ed.), *Vigilance: A Symposium.* New York: McGraw Hill. Pp. 22–8.

BROADBENT, D. E. (1963). In BUCKNER, D. N., and MCGRATH, J. J. (Ed.), *Vigilance: A Symposium.* New York: McGraw-Hill. Pp. 192.

BROADBENT, D. E., and GREGORY, M. (1963). Vigilance considered as a statistical decision. *Brit. J. Psychol.*, **54**, 309–23.

CRAIK, F. I. M. (1965). *Age Differences in Confidence and Decision Processes.* Unpublished Ph.D. Thesis, University of Liverpool.

DAVIES, D. R., and GRIEW, S. (1965). Age and vigilance. In WELFORD, A. T., and BIRREN, J. E. (Ed.), *Behavior, Aging and The Nervous System.* Springfield: Thomas. Pp. 54–9.

FREEMAN, P. R. (1964). Table of d′ and β. *Med. Res. Coun., A.P.R.U.*

GRIEW, S., and LYNN, R. (1960). Construct "Reactive Inhibition" in the interpretation of age changes in performance. *Nature*, **186**, 182.

HERON, A. (1956). A two part personality inventory for use as a research criterion. *Brit. J. Psychol.*, **47**, 243–51.

SCHULTZ, D. P. (1965). *Sensory Restriction Effects on Behavior.* New York: Academic Press.

SURWILLO, W. W., and QUILTER, R. E. (1964). Vigilance, age and response time. *Amer. J. Psychol.*, **77**, 614–20.

TUNE, G. S. (1966). Age differences in errors of commission. (Unpublished paper.)

WELFORD, A. T. (1962). Arousal, channel-capacity and decision. *Nature*, **194**, 365–6.

WELFORD, A. T. (1965). Performance, biological mechanisms and age: a theoretical sketch. In WELFORD, A. T., and BIRREN, J. E. (Ed.), *Aging, Behavior and the Nervous System.* Springfield: Thomas. Pp. 3–20.

Manuscript received 10th June, 1966.

PART V

PERSONALITY AND PERCEPTUAL REACTIONS

Among the many possible interactions between general psychology and personality research, there has always been a particularly close one between perception and personality theory (Granger, 1953; Frith, 1973). Some of the tests resulting from this interaction have become more widely used than their reliability and validity might seem to warrant (e.g. the Rorschach test), but generally interest in perception has led to many intriguing approaches to the problem of personality measurement. The range of phenomena investigated is enormous, ranging from semi-physiological effects like the Pulfrich phenomenon (extraverts show stronger effects than introverts—unpublished data) to spiral after-effects (stable extraverts show less effect than unstable introverts—Janssen, 1973), and from magnitude-estimating behaviour (Cavonius et al., 1974) to the experiencing of time (introverts overestimate the duration of time—Buchwald and Blatt, 1974).

In this section we have concentrated on some of the more elementary phenomena of perception, particularly sensory sensitivity as indicated by threshold experiments. Earlier work had indicated that extraverts, as one would have expected from arousal theory, have higher thresholds for sensory stimuli (e.g. Dunstone et al., 1964; Smith, 1968); and reports on differences in visual and auditory sensitivity are included in our selection here. However, greater interest centres on another approach to the problem because this takes into account the additional hypothesis of transmarginal inhibition, or inverse-U shaped relation between arousal and performance. This work was pioneered in our laboratory by Frith (1967), and is here represented by several studies carried out by Shigehisa. (In addition to the two studies here reprinted, readers may like to consult Shigehisa, 1974; Shigehisa and Symons, 1973; and Shigehisa, Shigehisa, and Symons, 1973.) In these studies the author has used the hypothesis that raising arousal level by stimulation in one sensory channel will lead to a lowering of thresholds in other sensory channels, and has added the hypothesis that the effects will depend on the intensity of the induced stimulation in interaction with the personality of the subject. More particularly, if we measure the effects of auditory stimulation on visual thresholds, then the effect in lowering visual thresholds will be larger the stronger the auditory stimulation (Pavlov's Law of Strength). However, as intensities are increased beyond a certain limit, the Law of Transmarginal Inhibition will come into play, and further increments in intensity will have the opposite effect, i.e. will *raise* visual thresholds. This curvilinear effect interacts with personality, in the sense that the point at which sensory stimulation ceases to be effective in lowering thresholds will be lower for introverts than for ambiverts, and lower for ambiverts than for extraverts. In a whole series of studies Shigehisa has shown that this is actually so, whether we use visual stimulation to enhance auditory thresholds, or whether we use auditory stimulation to enhance visual thresholds. The precision of the effects is particularly impressive when it is realized that in previous work on intersensory threshold effects results were very variable, and often not replicable. Shigehisa is almost certainly right in thinking that this failure of previous work was due to the neglect of personality as a moderator variable. His work thus illustrates the point often made that personality is one of the variables which should be controlled, or at least measured, in all psychological experiments (Eysenck, 1967); if it is not, then the variance attributable to personality goes into the error variance, and makes it that much more difficult to discover main effects (and impossible, of course, to discover interaction effects).

The remaining extracts deal with preference judgments for colours and forms, testing hypotheses arising from the arousal model, namely that extraverts would prefer the more stimulating (strong) colours and (complex) forms. There has been much work done on the relationship between arousal and preference judgments for forms (Wiedl, 1975), and the results have tended to support such an interpretation; the study here reprinted extends this general approach to the personality field. Direct evidence is available to demonstrate the relation between arousal and colour preferences

(Wilson, 1966; Kourse and Welch, 1971), and arousal and complexity preferences (Gale *et al.*, 1975), to give support to the generality of these phenomena.

REFERENCES

BUCHWALD, C. and BLATT, S. J. Personality and the experience of time. *Journal of Consulting and Clinical Psychology*, 1974, *42*, 639–644.

CAVONIUS, C. R., HILZ, R., and CHAPMAN, R. M. A possible basis for individual differences in magnitude-estimation behaviour. *British Journal of Psychology*, 1974, *65*, 85–91.

DUNSTONE, J. J., DZENDOLET, E., and HELICKEROTH, O. Effect of some personality variables on electrical vestibular stimulation. *Perceptual and Motor Skills*, 1964, *18*, 689–695.

EYSENCK, H. J. The Biological Basis of Personality. Springfield: C. C. Thomas, 1967.

FRITH, C. D. The interaction of noise and personality with critical flicker fusion performance. *British Journal of Psychology*, 1967, *58*, 127–131.

FRITH, C. D. Abnormalities of perception. In: H. J. Eysenck (Ed.) *Handbook of abnormal psychology*. London: Pitman, 1973.

GALE, A., SPRATT, G., CHRISTIE, P., and SMALLBONE, A. Stimulus complexity, EEG abundance gradients and detection efficiency in a visual recognition task. *British Journal of Psychology*, 1975, *66*, 289–298.

GRANGER, G. V. Personality and visual perception: a review. *Journal of Mental Science*, 1953, *99*, 8–43.

JANSSEN, R. H. C. Spiral after-effect, extraversion and the EEG. Research Report, Psychiatrische Klinick, Rijsuniversiteit, Leiden, 1973.

KOURSE, J. C. and WELCH, R. B. Emotional attributes of color: a comparison of violet and green. *Perceptual and Motor Skills*, 1971, *32*, 403–406.

SHIGEHISA, T. Effect of auditory stimulation on visual tracking as functions of stimulus intensity, task complexity and personality. *Japanese Psychological Research*, 1974, *16*, 186–196.

SHIGEHISA, T., SHIGEHISA, P. M. J., and SYMONS, J. R. Effect of interval between auditory and preceding visual stimuli on auditory sensitivity. *British Journal of Psychology*, 1973, *64*, 367–373.

SHIGEHISA, T. and SYMONS, J. R. Reliability of auditory responses under increasing intensity of visual stimulation in relation to personality. *British Journal of Psychology*, 1973, *64*, 375–381.

SMITH, S. L. Extraversion and sensory threshold. *Psychophysiology*, 1968, *5*, 293–299.

WIEDL, K. H. Die Bedentung der Variablen Betrachtungszeit und Präferenzakzentuierung sowie individueller Differenzen für die Erforschung von Komplexitätspreferenz im visuellen Bereich. *Zeitschrift für experimentelle und angewandte Psychologie*, 1975, *22*, 316–346.

WILSON, G. Arousal properties of red versus green. *Perceptual and Motor Skills*, 1960, *23*, 947–949.

From R. M. Stelmack and K. B. Campbell (1974). Perceptual and Motor Skills, *38*, 875–879, *by kind permission of the authors and Southern Universities Press*

EXTRAVERSION AND AUDITORY SENSITIVITY TO HIGH AND LOW FREQUENCY

ROBERT M. STELMACK AND KENNETH B. CAMPBELL[1]

University of Ottawa

Summary.—The sensitivity of 10 extraverts, 10 ambiverts, and 10 introverts to auditory stimuli was determined by a signal detection procedure. Under the low-frequency condition, introverts were significantly more sensitive than extraverts. Under the high-frequency condition, extraverts showed a significant increase in sensitivity, the introverts tended to show a relative decrease in sensitivity. Results endorse Eysenck's proposed relation of extraversion and the reticular formation arousal system.

Eysenck (1967) has predicted that introverts, characterized by higher levels of cortical arousal or excitatory potential, ought to manifest greater sensory sensitivity than extraverts. This prediction has received support from Smith (1968) who found that introverts have lower absolute thresholds than extraverts for low-frequency auditory stimulation. Siddle, *et al.* (1969) presented evidence of a moderate relationship between introversion and lower absolute threshold to a visual stimulus, although neuroticism appeared to be a confounding variable.

An acknowledged limitation of these reports concerns the prospect that the threshold differences may reflect individual differences in response style, with introverts showing an anticipatory set. Hake and Rodwan (1966) have argued that such a bias would persist even in "corrected" guessing patterns. This weakness may be met by applying methods of analysis derived from the theory of signal detection (Green & Swets, 1966), which purport to provide measures of sensitivity relatively independent of the criterion or response factors which may influence psychophysical judgments.

Since the prediction of greater sensitivity for introverts constitutes a significant source of evidence linking the extraversion dimension to individual differences in cortical arousal, extension and refinement of previous findings were warranted. The present study tested the hypothesis that introverts have greater absolute auditory sensitivity than extraverts. A signal-detection analysis was employed. The sensitivity to both high- and low-frequency acoustic signals was determined.

METHOD

Subjects

From an initial sample of 48 volunteers, 30 female undergraduates, in the age range 18 to 22 yr., were selected on the basis of scores obtained on the

---

[1]This report is based on portions of a thesis submitted by the second author to the University of Ottawa in partial fulfillment of the requirements for the Master of Arts degree.

Eysenck Personality Inventory, Form A. The mean and standard deviation on the extraversion scale for the introverts were 4.80 and 1.87; for the ambiverts 11.70 and 0.95 and for the extraverts 17.20 and 1.23. The mean and standard deviation on the neuroticism scale were 13.80 and 2.48 for the introverts, 12.20 and 3.79 for the ambiverts, and 11.70 and 4.50 for the extraverts.

Apparatus

Testing took place in a moderately illuminated, anechoic Industrial Acoustics laboratory. *S* and *E* were separated by an insulated wall with a 2- $\times$ 3-ft. plate window mounted approximately in the center of the wall, through which *S* was observed. A Maico MA-24 research and clinical audiometer, consisting of twin audiometer channels and an accessory control section, was used to present the auditory stimuli. The monitoring headset and the test headset used standard MX 41/AR cushions. Each channel was calibrated to the corresponding earphone of the test headset. Intensity could be varied over the entire hearing threshold level range, from —5 to 110 db., ISO. A Lafayette Four Bank Timer monitored the onset and offset of the stimuli and a 6- $\times$ 4-in. signal box with a white ready light and red light which signaled an observation interval to *S*.

Procedure

S was taken into the soundproof testing laboratory and seated facing the warning lights, at about a 45° angle away from the viewing window. The headset was placed in position, care being taken to ensure that hair did not fall between the cushions and the ears. *E* left the test laboratory and entered the control room where the instructions were read into a microphone and fed into the test headset.

The general procedure followed the fixed-interval observation rating experiment described by Egan, *et al.* (1959). The *a priori* probability of occurrence of a signal during an observation interval was 0.50 and this information was provided to *S*. The instructions required *S* to decide whether or not a signal occurred during an observation interval and to indicate the degree of confidence in this decision according to the criterion positive, fairly sure or guess. The instructions stated that 1 sec. after the white light, the red light would appear, indicating an observation interval. The duration of the white light was 1.5 sec. with the last 0.5 sec. fixing the observation interval which was marked by the onset of the red light. The signal, when presented, also had a duration of 0.5 sec. with its onset and offset synchronous with the onset and offset of the red light. The interobservation interval was 5.0 sec. during which time *S* responded with her decision.

Following a series of 30 practice trials employing a 2000-Hz signal, a block of either 100 low-frequency (500 Hz) or 100 high-frequency (6000 Hz) signals were presented to the left ear, with 100 blank (noise) trials in a random

EXTRAVERSION AND AUDITORY SENSITIVITY TO FREQUENCY

order. Each frequency condition was presented 20 times at each of five levels of intensity (-3, -1, 1, 3, 5 db, ISO) in a random order. The order of presentation of the high- and low-frequency conditions was counterbalanced within groups.

Computation of the receiver operating characteristic (ROC) curve parameter, d*, was executed with EPCROC, a computer program developed by Ogilvie and Creelman (1968) which provides a maximum-likelihood estimation of ROC parameters for the rating method.

RESULTS

A measure of sensitivity (d*) to absolute levels of intensity, independent of the criteria adopted by S, was determined for the high- and low-frequency conditions for each S. The larger the value of d*, the greater the sensitivity.

A two-way analysis of variance with repeated measures indicated a significant Extraversion $\times$ Frequency interaction ($F = 4.85$, $df = 2/27$, $p < 0.05$). Analysis of the simple main effects for the low-frequency condition indicated significant differences between the extraversion groups ($F = 5.78$, $df = 2/50$, $p < 0.01$), with introverts showing greater mean sensitivity (4.27) than the extraverts (1.77) or the ambiverts (2.36). At the high-frequency condition, no significant differences were observed between the extraversion groups ($F = 1.52$). As shown in Fig. 1, the extraverts manifested a significantly greater sensitivity ($F = 3.97$, $df = 1/27$, $p < 0.07$) under the high-frequency condition

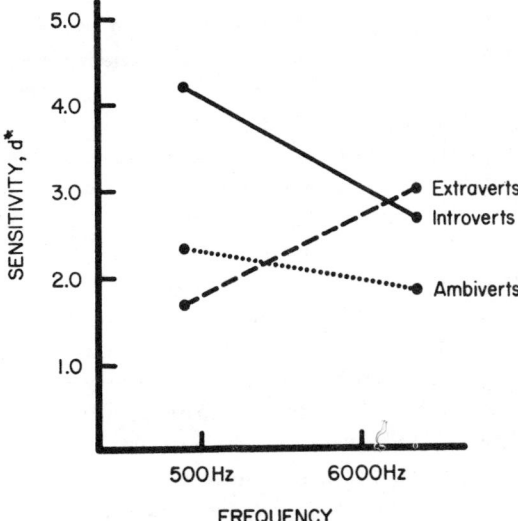

FIG. 1. Sensitivity to high and low frequencies for extraversion groups

(3.07) than under the low-frequency condition (1.77). The introverts obtained significantly greater sensitivity ($F = 5.45$, $df = 1/27$, $p < 0.05$) under the low-frequency condition (4.27) than under the high-frequency condition (2.75).

DISCUSSION

Eysenck (1967) has suggested that the hypothesized greater levels of cortical arousal or "excitation" which characterize introverts may be due to their lower threshold of reticular arousal. On the premise that reticular stimulation generally enhances the efficiency of sensory systems, introverts are expected to display greater sensitivity than extraverts to both the low- and high-frequency acoustic signals. Smith (1968) found that introverts had lower absolute thresholds to low-frequency (500-Hz) tones; the present results further indicate that, independent of the response criteria of the observer, the introverts show greater absolute sensitivity to low-frequency acoustic signals than extraverts.

An interesting result, however, is the significantly increased sensitivity of the extraverts under the high-frequency condition, where, in fact, the extraverts tended to be more sensitive than the introverts. Under the high-frequency condition, the introverts showed less sensitivity than under the low-frequency condition. These results are relevant to Eysenck's (1963) discussion of extraversion and the relationship between hedonic tone and strength of sensory stimulation. Eysenck develops the argument that the greater level of cortical arousal or "excitation" of the introvert leads not only to the prediction of greater sensitivity to low-intensity stimulation but also leads to the expectation that introverts would manifest lower intensity levels of optimal or preferred stimulation. The extraverts, on the other hand, are seen to prefer stronger more intense levels of stimulation.

With the present results, the increase in sensitivity to high-frequency tones for the extraverts and the decrease for the introverts suggests that introverts may have lower frequency levels of preferred stimulation as well as lower intensity levels. Evidence of the congruence of intensity and frequency in relation to hedonic tone has been presented by Guilford (1954) who observed that those individuals who preferred low levels of intensity also preferred low-frequency sound. It would seem that those individuals are introverts.

With regard to the excitation-inhibition hypothesis, the present results, implicating a selective mechanism, can be interpreted in terms of individual differences in a cortico-reticular loop which modulates cortical excitation and inhibition. The decrease in sensitivity from low to high frequency for the introverts may reflect a pre-excitatory inhibition (automatic gain control); the increase in sensitivity from low to high frequency for the extraverts would seem to involve an excitatory mechanism specific to high frequency.

Although a more precise statement of the dynamics of this process is beyond the scope of this report, some insight into the type of mechanisms involved may be inferred from evidence sketched by Eysenck (1967, p. 238). First, it is noted

EXTRAVERSION AND AUDITORY SENSITIVITY TO FREQUENCY

that frequency-specific adaptation remained in decorticate cats with intact medial geniculate bodies sending collaterals into the diffuse thalamic nucleus (Sharpless & Jasper, 1956). Second, it was suggested that under conditions of high activation the brain stem reticular and the unspecific thalamic systems may overshadow the differentiating functions of the thalamic nuclei (Samuels, 1959). In this context, it is necessary to assume that even a low-intensity high-frequency signal strongly activates, relative to low frequency, the reticular and unspecific systems, either directly or by specific afferent pathways via cortical projections. For the extravert, this increase in reticular activation facilitates sensitivity. For the introvert, characterized by a greater degree of excitatory potential, this increase in activation of the brain stem reticular and unspecific thalamic systems masks the differentiating function of the medial geniculate body and expresses itself as a decrease in sensitivity to high-frequency signals. This interpretation is, of course, speculative. Nevertheless, the present results endorse Eysenck's (1967) proposal relating extraversion and individual differences in the reticular formation arousal system.

REFERENCES

EGAN, J. P., SCHULMAN, A. I., & GREENBERG, G. Z. Operating characteristics determined by binary decisions and by ratings. *Journal of the Acoustical Society of America,* 1959, 31, 768-773.

EYSENCK, H. J. (Ed.) *Experiments with drugs.* London: Pergamon, 1963.

EYSENCK, H. J. *The biological basis of behavior.* Springfield, Ill.: Thomas, 1967.

GREEN, D. M., & SWETS, J. A. *Signal detection theory and psychophysics.* New York: Wiley, 1966.

GUILFORD, J. P. Systems in the relationship of affective value to frequency and intensity of auditory stimuli. *American Journal of Psychology,* 1954, 67, 691-698.

HAKE, H. W., & RODWAN, A. S. Perception and recognition. In J. B. Sidowski (Ed.), *Experimental methods and instrumentation in psychology.* New York: McGraw-Hill, 1966. Pp. 332-381.

OGILVIE, J. C., & CREELMAN, D. C. Maximum-likelihood estimation of receiver operating characteristic curve parameters. *Journal of Mathematical Psychology,* 1968, 5, 377-391.

SAMUELS, I. Reticular mechanisms and behavior. *Psychological Bulletin,* 1959, 56, 1-25.

SHARPLESS, S., & JASPER, H. H. Habituation of the arousal reaction. *Brain,* 1956, 79, 655-680.

SIDDLE, D. A. T., MOORISH, R. B., WHITE, K. D., & MANGAN, G. L. Relation of visual sensitivity to extraversion. *Journal of Experimental Research in Personality,* 1969, 3, 264-267.

SMITH, S. L. Extraversion and sensory threshold. *Psychophysiology,* 1968, 5, 296-297.

Accepted January 28, 1974.

From D. A. T. Siddle, R. B. Morrish, K. D. White, and G. L. Mangan (1969). Journal of Experimental Research in Personality, *3, 264–267, by kind permission of the authors and Academic Press*

Relation of Visual Sensitivity to Extraversion

DAVID A. T. SIDDLE, ROBERT B. MORRISH, KENNETH D. WHITE,
AND GORDON L. MANGAN

The University of Queensland

Visual sensitivity, operationally defined as the inverse of lower absolute threshold, and measured by a method similar to that described by Sokolov (1963) was related to extraversion as measured by the Eysenck Personality Inventory (Eysenck and Eysenck, 1964). Results indicated that there is a moderate relationship between sensitivity and introversion, although neuroticism appears to be a confounding variable.

Over the past 12 years, a considerable amount of research has been reported on the strength-sensitivity property of the excitatory process (Nebylitsyn, 1966a; Teplov and Nebylitsyn, 1966). Sensitivity has been theoretically linked with weakness; i.e., lack of strength or endurance of the nervous system, in that it is presumed to reflect the rapid destructibility of the hypothetical excitatory substances in the cells (Teplov, 1956). Strength, on the other hand, is identified with the limit of functional capacity of the cells, such limit being set at the threshold of transmarginal inhibition (TTI). In the visual modality, sensitivity is measured by the induced lower absolute threshold (LAT), and strength by a variety of classical Pavlovian indices such as extinction with reinforcement of the photochemical conditional reflex (PCR). An inverse relationship between strength and sensitivity has been clearly established (Nebylitsyn, 1966b).

Recently, a number of investigators (Eysenck, 1957, 1962, 1966; Gray, 1964, 1967; Mangan and Farmer, 1967) have attempted to relate Russian typological properties to Western personality dimensions. Eysenck (1966) contended that "the Pavlovian notion of 'strong' and 'weak' nervous systems, which has formed the basis for most of Teplov's experimental work, bears a striking similarity to the notions of extraverted personality types .... The

'weak' personality type appears to resemble the introvert, the 'strong' personality type the extravert" (p. 33). A recent paper (Eysenck and Eysenck, 1967a) suggested that the link might be the association of sensitivity with a high level of cortical arousal.

The linkage of extraversion-introversion with strength-sensitivity has received limited empirical support from Smith (1967) and Haslam (1966), who found that introverts had lower sensory (auditory and pain) thresholds than extraverts. At the other end of the dimension of response intensity, Eysenck and Eysenck (1967b) in a study of salivary responses to an acid stimulus, offered evidence which Gray (1967) interpreted as suggesting that introverts are weaker and thus reach TTI more quickly than extraverts.

The purpose of the present study is to relate sensitivity in the visual modality to extraversion. Sensitivity is measured by LAT, and extraversion by scores on Eysenck and Eysenck's (1964) Personality Inventory (EPI).

METHOD

Subjects

Subjects were 15 male undergraduate students (age range 18–25 years) whose extraversion (E) scores were obtained from individual administrations of Form A of the EPI. The mean E score was 11.86, S.D. = 6.16. High neuroticism (N) Ss were excluded. Since the mean N score of the population from which Ss were selected was 7.8, S.D. = 4.4, Ss with N scores higher than 11 were discarded.

'Contribution to a program of studies of the relationship between neo–Pavlovian properties of higher nervous activity and western personality dimensions.

VISUAL SENSITIVITY AND EXTRAVERSION

Apparatus

All experimental work was carried out in a sound-dampened room measuring $10 \times 5 \times 7$ feet (inside measurements) constructed inside a standard laboratory room.

The apparatus used for the determination of threshold sensitivity was constructed to provide a continuous measure of threshold, according to the design reported by Sokolov (1963), and based on the principle involved in the von Bekesy direct recording audiometer (von Bekesy, 1960).

A circular neutral density filter wedge (diameter 3.5 inches) mounted on a spindle, was revolved in front of a 6-volt light source at a speed of 1.3 rpm by a small a-c motor. After passing through the wedge, the light illuminated a 1.5-mm aperture inside the experimental room. A second 1.5-mm aperature, behind which was placed a red filter, served as a constant-intensity fixation point, situated slightly above the test spot. With S seated 4.5 feet away, the angular distance between the apertures was 2° 17′ (Rozhdestvenskaya, 1955), and when S fixated the red spot, the light from the test spot struck the fovea. The lower test beam was screened, thus ensuring that only light which had passed through the wedge illuminated the test aperture.

The wedge was scaled in terms of transmission

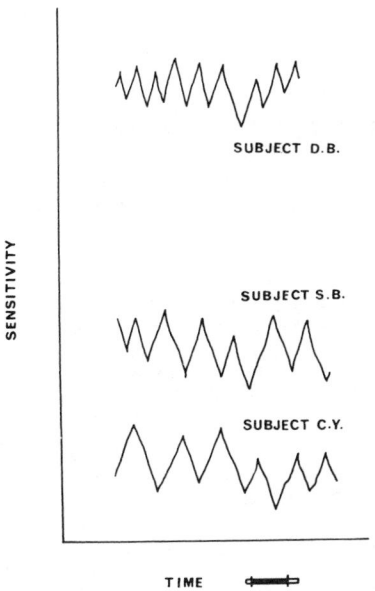

FIG. 1. Two sample records for sensitivity determination.

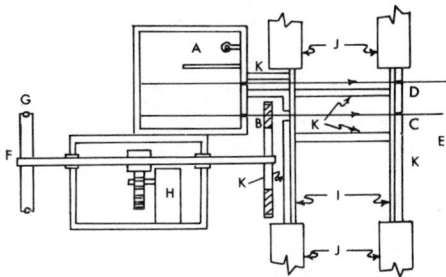

FIG. 2. Apparatus used in visual sensitivity determination (section through wedge axis). A, light box; B, neutral density filter wedge; C, 1.5-mm aperture (test spot at S's eye level); E, experimental room; D, fixation point (1.5 mm); F, rear wheel; G, cord to kymograph; H, a-c motor and gear system; I, transparent panels in walls; J, room walls; K, opaque screening.

rates which ranged from 80% at the lightest section to 0.00256% at the darkest section. A cord connected the wedge to a pen, and as the direction of the wedge was changed by the action of a microswitch and solenoid on a system of gears, this pen travelled up and down on moving paper carried by a Brodie-Starling kymograph. Since the pen reflected which section of the wedge was in front of the test aperture, a transmission rate could be assigned to any point on the recording paper. Sample records are shown in Fig. 1, and the apparatus in Fig. 2.

The subject was seated comfortably and provided with a switch for reversing the direction of the wedge. Adjustable chin and forehead rests eliminated head movements, and ensured that S's eyes were at the same level as the test spot. No apparatus noise could be heard by S during experimentation.

Procedure

The procedure was similar to that described by Sokolov (1963) in that the stimulus was constantly varied from subliminal to supraliminal intensity and vice versa. Subjects were dark-adapted for 45 minutes. At the beginning of each 1-minute trial, the stimulus lights were turned on, and S instructed to sit forward and locate the fixation point. The apparatus was then started. Each trial began with the test spot being supraliminal, and the wedge turning in such a direction that S's first button press occurred when the stimulus disappeared.

Intertrial interval was 2 minutes. Trials continued until the threshold stabilized for three consecutive trials; i.e., until intertrial differences in sensitivity disappeared.

RESULTS AND DISCUSSION

A threshold value, which was the midpoint of the area of uncertainty, was obtained by averaging the mean upper and lower transmission points for each S. Since these values were in terms of transmission rates, the higher the obtained value, the higher was the threshold and the lower the sensitivity.

Rank order correlation between sensitivity and extraversion gave a value of −0.52 ($p < .05$). This result thus expands the evidence (Haslam, 1966; Smith, 1967), cited by Gray (1967) in support of Eysenck's (1966) hypothesis that extraversion is negatively related to the sensitivity of the excitatory process.

Additional support is also available from three studies conducted in this laboratory in which the sensitivity-extraversion link was investigated, although this was in fact only a side-issue to the main experimental enquiry. In the first of these studies ($N = 10$), in which sampling procedures followed precisely those of the present study, rank order correlation between sensitivity and extraversion was −0.57 ($p < .01$). In the second ($N = 16$), and third ($N = 13$) studies, no Ss were excluded on the grounds of high N scores; in the third study, all Ss were female. In these two studies, rank order correlations between sensitivity and extraversion were −0.16 (NS) and −0.33 (NS) respectively. Thus, although only two of the four groups yielded significant correlations, all four were in the predicted direction.

It is possible that a high level of neuroticism obscures the relationship reported. In the two samples from which high N Ss were excluded, there is a significant correlation between sensitivity and extraversion; when high N Ss were included, however, the correlations, though still negative, are nonsignificant. Neuroticism thus appears to be a confounding variable in the relationship between sensitivity and extraversion, though further data will be necessary before any more definite conclusion can be reached.

REFERENCES

BEKESY, G. VON. *Experiments in hearing.* Translated by E. G. Wever (Ed.), New York: McGraw-Hill, 1960.

EYSENCK, H. J. *The dynamics of anxiety and hysteria.* London: Routledge and Kegan Paul, Ltd., 1957.

EYSENCK, H. J. Conditioning and personality. *British Journal of Psychology,* 1962, **53,** 299–305.

EYSENCK, H. J. Conditioning, introversion-extraversion, and the strength of the nervous system. In V. D. Nebylitsyn (Organizer), Symposium 9, *Physiological bases of individual psychological differences.* 18th Int. Congr. Psychol., Moscow: 1966. Pp. 33–44.

EYSENCK, H. J., AND EYSENCK, S. B. G. *Manual of the Eysenck Personality Inventory.* London: University of London Press, 1964.

EYSENCK, S. B. G., AND EYSENCK, H. J. Physiological reactivity to sensory stimulation as a measure of personality. *Psychological Reports,* 1967 (a), **20,** 45–46.

EYSENCK, S. B. G., AND EYSENCK, H. J. Salivary response to lemon juice as a measure of introversion. *Perceptual Motor Skills,* 1967 (b), **24,** 1047–1053.

GRAY, J. A. Strength of the nervous system as a dimension of personality in man. In J. A. Gray (Ed.), *Pavlov's typology.* Oxford: Pergamon, 1964. Pp. 157–287.

GRAY, J. A. Strength of the nervous system, introversion-extraversion, conditionability, and arousal. *Behavior Research and Therapy,* 1967, **5,** 151–169.

HASLAM, D. R. Individual differences in pain threshold and the concept of arousal. Unpublished Ph.D. Thesis, 1966, Bristol University. Cited by J. A. Gray, Strength of the nervous system, introversion-extraversion, conditionability, and arousal. *Behavior Research and Therapy,* 1967, **5,** 151–169.

MANGAN, G. L., AND FARMER, R. G. Studies of the relationship between neo-Pavlovian properties of higher nervous activity and Western personality dimensions: I. The relationship of nervous strength and sensitivity to extroversion. *J. of Experimental Research in Personality,* 1967, **2,** 101–106.

NEBYLITSYN, V. D. Some questions relating to the theory of the properties of the nervous system.

In V. D. Nebylitsyn (Organizer), Symposium 9, *Physiological bases of individual psychological differences.* 18th Int. Congr. Psychol., Moscow: 1966 (a). Pp. 23–32.

NEBYLITSYN, V. D. *Osnovniye svoistva nervnoi systemi cheloveka.* (Basic properties of the human nervous system). Moscow: Akademiya Pedagogicheskikh Nauk. RSFSR, 1966 (b). Unpublished English translation by M. Kravchenko, University of Queensland, 1968.

ROZHDESTVENSKAYA, V. I. An attempt to determine the strength of the process of excitation through features of its irradiation and concentration in the visual analyser. *Voprosi Psikhologii,* 1955, No. 3, pp. 90–98. In J. A. Gray (Ed.), *Pavlov's typology.* Oxford: Pergamon, 1964. Pp. 379–390.

SMITH, S. L. The effect of personality and drugs on auditory threshold when risk taking factors are controlled. Cited by J. A. Gray, Strength of the nervous system, introversion-extraversion, conditionability, and arousal. *Behavior Research and Therapy,* 1967, **5**, 151–169.

SOKOLOV, E. N. *Perception and the conditioned reflex.* Translated by S. W. Waydenfeld. Oxford: Pergamon, 1963.

TEPLOV, B. M. Problems in the study of general types of higher nervous activity in man and animals. In B. M. Teplov (Ed.), *Tipologicheskiye osobennosti vysshei nervnoi deyatelnosti cheloveka,* Vol. 1, 1956. English translation by J. A. Gray. In J. A. Gray (Ed.), *Pavlov's typology.* Oxford: Pergamon, 1964. Pp. 3–153.

TEPLOV, B. M., AND NEBYLITSYN, V. D. Results of experimental studies on properties of the nervous system in man. In A. Leontiev, A. Lurija, and A. Smirnov (Eds.), *Psychological research in the USSR.* English translation by D. Rottenberg. Moscow: Progress Publishers, 1966. Pp. 181–198.

From T. Shigehisa and J. R. Symons (1973). British Journal of Psychology, *64*, 205–213, *by kind permission of the authors and Cambridge University Press*

EFFECT OF INTENSITY OF
VISUAL STIMULATION ON AUDITORY SENSITIVITY
IN RELATION TO PERSONALITY

By T. SHIGEHISA and J. R. SYMONS

Department of Psychology, University of Aberdeen

Auditory thresholds were determined by a modified method of limits under 10 intensities of light (patterned or homogeneous). An analysis of variance of the data showed significant results for intensity conditions, personality type and the interaction of these parameters. Auditory sensitivity increased under weak, and decreased under strong, intensities of light in introverts. It increased under all intensities in extraverts, with greater increase at greater intensities, and increased under weak and medium intensities in ambiverts. The EPI E, but not N, scale scores and sensitivity increases correlated positively, at medium and strong intensities of light.

There has been constant interest in whether or not intersensory effects occur, as indicated by the reviews (Hartmann, 1935; Stern, 1935; Ryan, 1940; Gilbert, 1941; Harris, 1950; London, 1954; Symons, 1954; Bartley, 1958; Torii, 1962; Maruyama, 1964; Kravkov, 1966; Loveless *et al.*, 1970; Shigehisa, 1972). Since Urbantschitsch's experiment in 1883, evidence has accumulated indicating that the perception of visual, auditory, tactile, pressure, pain, olfactory and gustatory stimuli can be facilitated by simultaneous heteromodal stimulation, but there have also been reports to the contrary. Many of the results reported on this subject have been quite divergent and often contradictory, hence no generally tenable conclusions have emerged. One reason for the contradictory results may be that the exact function of the parameters involved in determining these effects are surprisingly unknown. A survey of the literature dealing with intersensory effects suggests that the intensity of the heteromodal stimulus and the subject variables may be involved in differentiating these divergent effects. However, recent works, which attempted to reconcile these inconsistencies, did not sufficiently explore the possibility that the intensity of the heteromodal stimulus could, perhaps depending on the personality variables, exert a direct effect on responses in the primary modality. Most sources have concluded instead that the effect can be either facilitatory or inhibitory, and have suggested that the direction of the effect may be influenced by either the intensity of the heteromodal stimulus or personality variables (see Shigehisa, 1972). Increase in intensity of the heteromodal stimulus may lead to effects that are the reverse of those induced by weaker intensities. Such a hypothesis has been labelled the 'law of inversion' in the Russian work. However, none of the studies on this subject thoroughly explored the possibility of this inversion experimentally while controlling the personality variables. It is possible that personality type is systematically related to the relationship between the intensity of the heteromodal stimulus and sensitivity in the primary modality.

The present study is an attempt to differentiate the conditions under which a heteromodal stimulus facilitates or inhibits sensitivity to the primary stimuli. In the preliminary experiments (Shigehisa, 1971), an increase in auditory sensitivity

T. Shigehisa and J. R. Symons

was typically found under weak heteromodal stimuli, and a decrease under strong stimuli. The subjects who showed a decrease in sensitivity under weak heteromodal stimuli were found to be more introverted than those who showed an increase. One possibility is that the process of intersensory influence as a function of heteromodal stimulus intensity varies with personality type. Unfortunately, the relationship between the intensity of the heteromodal stimulus, or the personality type, and sensitivity in the primary modality has never been reliably quantified so that the point of transition between intersensory facilitation and inhibition could be determined. However, such a possibility is consistent with the theoretical issues in the field, and certain pieces of evidence support this possibility.

The reticular activities of the brain stem have been shown to produce facilitation or inhibition of inputs in several sensory systems (Lindsley, 1960). Evidence indicates that the personality type may play an important role in these facilitatory and inhibitory mechanisms. Experiments by Corcoran (1965) suggest that there are differential sensory performances by two personality types, in that the performance of extraverts decreases, while that of introverts tends to increase, under the same sensory conditions. It seems that introverts have lower sensory thresholds, and show less inhibition to continued stimulation, while extraverts have higher thresholds and show greater inhibition to continued stimulation (Eysenck, 1967). It follows that a given intensity of heteromodal stimulation may be perceived as higher by introverts than by extraverts. The theory of Pavlovian transmarginal inhibition predicts that introverts will show a greater decrease in performance, or a decrease at lower intensities of stimulation, than extraverts. It is expected, therefore, that introverts will show a greater decrease in sensitivity to the primary stimulus, or a decrease at weaker intensities of a heteromodal stimulus, than extraverts.

It is a reasonable assumption that weaker visual stimuli increase auditory sensitivity, and that this effect can be reversed at greater intensities. It can be predicted further that this effect varies with the personality type. It follows, then, that the point of transition between facilitatory and inhibitory effects of visual stimulation may be systematically related to the personality type. At stronger intensities, a facilitatory effect is more likely to occur in extraverted subjects, and an inhibitory effect in introverted subjects. This leads to the assumption that a facilitatory effect is more likely to occur at weaker intensities in introverted subjects. It follows then that a facilitatory effect is more likely to occur at intensities which are intermediate between weak and strong, if subjects are neither introverted nor extraverted. It is hypothesized that absolute auditory sensitivity varies with the change in intensity of the simultaneous visual stimulus, and with the difference in the personality type. Sensitivity may be differentially affected by this intensity as a function of the personality type. It is these hypotheses that determine the design of the present experiments.

METHOD

Subjects

Thirty randomly selected students, 21 males and nine females, whose ages ranged from 18 to 33 yr., were used. They had hearing sensitivity within normal limits for the auditory stimuli used in this study, and reported negative histories of visual pathologies. First, the Eysenck Personality Inventory (EPI) (Eysenck & Eysenck, 1964) was administered. (Eight subjects,

Effect of visual stimulation on auditory sensitivity

whose E scale scores would have placed them in already completed groups, or whose L scale scores were above 4, were rejected.) Those ten subjects with E scale scores ranging from 4 to 8 were designated introverts or I (mean E scale score 6·70, S.D. 1·49; mean N scale score 12·30, S.D. 6·20), and those ten ranging from 14 to 20 were designated extraverts or E (mean E scale score 16·10, S.D. 1·79; mean N scale score 10·60, S.D. 5·62). The remaining ten subjects (range: 9–13) were designated ambiverts or A (mean E scale score 11·40, S.D. 1·08; mean N scale score 6·30, S.D. 4·25). All subjects served equally in the three experiments. (There was no correlation between auditory sensitivity change and the EPI N scale score, under any intensity of visual stimulation, hence the N scale score was disregarded in this study.)

Apparatus

A Békésy audiometer (Grason-Stadler, Model E800) was used for stimulus presentation and recording. The output of the system was calibrated by monitoring an appropriate voltage across the terminal of the earphone, and the tone frequency and attenuation rate were adjusted accordingly. A sound-proof chamber (Industrial Acoustics, 100 × 100 × 180 cm) was used for threshold determinations. Inside the chamber all furnishings and equipment, including stereo headphones (Sharp, HA–10), armchair and adjustable chinrest, were covered with plastic or rubber pads, and ambient noise level was less than 14 db SPL, at 250–8000 cps. The temperature was controlled between 20 and 22 °C and humidity between 35 and 45 per cent.

The light was uniformly projected from a 500 W. projector, through a green filter (Ilford, No. 604), on to a milk plastic screen measuring 60 × 38 cm (patterned visual stimulation), or on to the eyecups (homogeneous visual stimulation), from outside the chamber. The distance between projector lens and the screen was 120 cm, and between the screen and the subject's eyes 60 cm, i.e. 180 cm between the lens and eyecups. The brightness increments in the green light at the screen and eyecups were obtained using fixed filters, diaphragm and variac transformer. The light stimulus constituted ten intensity levels, as measured by a Gamma photometer (visually corrected photomultiplier), at the following candela per square metre: 0, 0·006, 0·06, 2·32, 14·45, 44·69, 98·99, 175·32, 299·08, 474·39. (These will be called, in this order, intensity levels 1–10.) These levels were chosen for ease of administration and for the comfort of the subjects within as wide an intensity range as feasible. The two eyecups used for producing homogeneous visual stimulation (Ganzfeld) were similar to those described by Hochberg et al. (1951). They were made from halved table-tennis balls of good diffusing power, trimmed and shaped to fit over the eyes with snug contact around the edges. Surgical tape assured strong support and a complete seal without irritating the skin.

Procedure

There was no systematic difference in the time of day at which groups were tested. The time and amount of sleep, meals and previous exercise were controlled as much as possible within the range of normal living, among the subjects. They were instructed to refrain from stimulants or depressants on the test day, such as coffee, tea, chocolate, alcohol, tranquillizers and sedatives. They were also asked to refrain from smoking for at least 2 hr. prior to testing. The subject, who had practised the whole procedure on the previous day, was seated comfortably in the darkened chamber facing the screen. He was instructed to place his head in the chinrest, to keep his eyes open and not to move his head throughout the testing. The grip button was held in his right hand, and he received the tones from the left ear.

A descending method of limits was used. The pure tones were pulsed at the rate of 2·5 interruptions per sec. with a constant frequency setting at 1000 Hz. The subject's task was to press the button three times successively when he first heard the tones (within the 3 sec. following a signal), to press it once when he did not hear, and to press twice when he was not certain. In each trial, immediately following the signal (4·5 V. buzzer, 250 msec.), the tones were presented for 3 sec. with simultaneous illumination of the screen or eyecups, except in the control condition (no light). Immediately after the subject's response to the tones, the tones and the light were terminated, hence the subject made each response under the light, and spent each inter-trial interval (30 sec.) in darkness. In each trial, the tones and light were terminated at the end of 3 sec. if the subject did not respond. The loudness of the tones was held constant in db in each trial, and was reduced over trials in 2 db steps, starting from 10 db above threshold. After 7 min. practice the initial starting-point was so adjusted, in each stimulus intensity condition, that

T. Shigehisa and J. R. Symons

Table 1. *Analysis of variance of auditory sensation levels*

Source	D.F.	Control s.s.	F	PVS s.s.	F	HVS s.s.	F
Between subjects	29	49·89	—	255·84	—	172·57	—
PT	2	2·21	0·63	126·96	13·31***	61·34	7·44**
Error (b)	27	47·68	—	128·88	—	111·23	—
Within subjects	60	38·07	—	181·93	—	152·71	—
IC	2	2·05	1·69	17·13	3·97*	9·09	3·32*
IC × PT	4	3·30	1·36	48·27	5·59***	71·21	13·28***
Error (w)	54	32·72	—	116·53	—	72·41	—
Total	89	87·96	—	437·77	—	325·28	—

* $P < 0.05$.   ** $P < 0.01$.   *** $P < 0.001$.

threshold determination included five consecutive hearing response trials, one or more not-certain trials, and three consecutive not-hearing trials. Hence each subject normally had nine or more trials for threshold determination at each intensity of light. The decibel level of the not-certain response, or mean of these responses if more than one occurred, or mean of the lowest hearing response and highest not-hearing response, was taken as threshold, in each determination. The main threshold determination began 8 min. after practice during which the subject experienced the visual stimulus.

Threshold was determined under the ten light intensities. The sequence of intensity conditions was from weaker to stronger, but the starting-point was counterbalanced among the ten intensities over the ten subjects in each personality group. In Expt. I, control, the same procedure was used as in the following experiments, except that each auditory threshold was measured in darkness. In Expt. II, patterned visual stimulation (PVS), the subject was asked to fixate the centre of the screen throughout the experiment. In Expt. III, homogeneous visual stimulation (HVS), the subject wore the eyecups comfortably, so as to avoid any contact with the eye-lashes. Subjects were tested in the order of Expts. I–III.

RESULTS

For each subject there were ten threshold measures, one at zero (control) light intensity and nine brightness increases. The thresholds were adjusted to give the raw data in terms of sensation level by taking the zero light condition threshold as the zero sensation level for that subject, i.e. his normal threshold of audibility, and subtracting from this the thresholds for the other nine light conditions. The means of the first three (0·006, 0·06, 2·32 cd m^{-2}), second three (14·45, 44·69, 98·99 cd m^{-2}) and third three (175·32, 299·08, 474·39 cd m^{-2}) light increments were then obtained. These will be referred to as 'weak', 'medium' and 'strong', respectively.

As shown in Table 1, an analysis of variance performed on the data of the visual stimulation experiments shows significant results for intensity conditions (IC), personality type (PT) and their interaction (IC × PT).

The significance of the intensity conditions variable indicates that auditory sensitivity varies with change in the visual stimulus intensity accompanying presentations of the auditory stimulus. Similarly, the significance of the personality variable indicates that auditory sensitivity under visual stimulation varies with the personality type. It is the interaction of light intensity levels with the personality type which is the primary concern of this study. The significant results for this interaction, in both visual stimulation experiments, indicate that auditory sensitivity is differ-

Effect of visual stimulation on auditory sensitivity

Table 2. Changes in auditory sensitivity (mean sensation level) at each light intensity

(Negative sensation level indicates a decrease in sensitivity.)

Light intensity level	Control Sensation level	t	PVS Sensation level	t	HVS Sensation level	t
	Group I					
2	−0·1	0·33	0·8	1·18	1·9	3·14*
3	0·4	0·89	1·3	1·95	2·1	4·38**
4	0·4	0·93	1·4	1·79	1·6	2·52*
5	0·6	1·26	−0·2	0·36	1·0	2·74*
6	−0·2	0·51	−0·6	0·87	0·1	0·17
7	0	0	−1·0	1·20	1·0	1·27
8	−0·9	2·09	−1·7	2·83*	−0·3	0·43
9	−0·5	0·89	−2·1	3·13*	−1·2	1·65
10	−0·3	0·71	−2·2	2·72*	−1·8	1·85
	Group A					
2	0·5	2·23	1·9	2·97*	1·1	1·82
3	0·3	0·64	2·1	4·38**	2·0	3·47**
4	0·1	0·23	1·5	2·05	1·5	4·05**
5	0	0	2·1	3·04*	1·8	2·86*
6	−0·2	0·45	0·9	0·95	2·1	3·04*
7	−0·6	1·11	1·1	1·86	1·6	2·22
8	−0·4	1·31	0·9	1·58	0·8	0·96
9	0·3	0·54	0·1	0·15	0·4	0·80
10	0·1	0·23	0·1	0·26	0·4	0·80
	Group E					
2	0·3	0·90	1·4	2·41*	1·5	3·48**
3	0	0	2·0	4·47**	1·9	3·62**
4	0·3	1·00	1·8	3·83**	0·9	1·58
5	0·4	1·81	2·1	3·96**	2·0	5·48***
6	0·1	0·56	2·7	5·40***	2·3	6·87***
7	0·5	1·47	3·3	7·86***	2·8	7·78***
8	0·2	0·61	3·0	7·69***	3·3	7·25***
9	0·2	1·00	3·1	5·25***	3·8	15·26***
10	0·4	1·82	2·9	5·09***	3·9	11·14***

t test gives significance of difference between any given level of intensity and baseline.
* $P < 0.05$.   ** $P < 0.01$.   *** $P < 0.001$.

entially affected by the intensity of the visual stimulus as a function of the personality type. An analysis of the data of the control experiment provides a check on the possibility of a practice or other temporal effect on the thresholds. The non-significance of the sequence effect in the control data corresponding to the intensity levels in the visual stimulation experiments, together with the non-significance of the personality type, and of the interaction of sequence and personality type, shows that there is no evidence of a practice or other temporal effect. The results of the control experiment make it possible to consider the data of the two experiments solely in terms of the light intensity levels and the personality type.

Evaluation of the hypothesized facilitatory effect at weak light intensities and the inhibitory effect at strong intensities for introverted subjects, graded facilitatory effects at all (or most) intensities for extraverted subjects, and the greater facilita-

T. SHIGEHISA AND J. R. SYMONS

tory effect at medium intensities for subjects who are neither introverted nor extraverted, was accomplished by means of t tests (two-tailed tests were used throughout this study). As can be seen from Table 2, auditory sensitivity increases at weak, and decreases at strong, intensities in I, it increases at weak or medium intensities in A, and it increases at all intensities, with greater increase at greater intensities, in E. (In E, the increase is greater at strong intensities than at weak or medium ($t = 5 \cdot 56, P < 0 \cdot 001; t = 4 \cdot 44, P < 0 \cdot 01$), and it is less at weak than at medium ($t = 4 \cdot 08, P < 0 \cdot 01$).)

Excepting the data for A under PVS, all these results are consistent with the hypothesized effects. The t tests performed on the data of the control experiment show that none of the sensation levels at any position of the threshold determination sequence for any group of subjects is significantly different from the corresponding zero sensation level. These results indicate that the data of each group of subjects in the two visual stimulation experiments can be considered solely in terms of the light intensity conditions.

There is a significant positive correlation between mean auditory sensation level and the EPI E scale score. Under PVS, individual coefficients are $r = +0 \cdot 563$ ($P < 0 \cdot 01$) at medium intensity, and $r = +0 \cdot 736$ ($P < 0 \cdot 01$) at strong intensity. Under HVS, $r = +0 \cdot 426$ ($P < 0 \cdot 05$) at medium intensity, and $r = +0 \cdot 725$ ($P < 0 \cdot 01$) at strong intensity (two-tailed tests). No significant correlation was found at any threshold determination position in the control experiment sequence. These results indicate that the greater the EPI E scale score, the greater the increase in auditory sensitivity, when the visual stimulus is medium or strong. No such correlation was found between auditory sensation level and the N scale score at medium or strong PVS ($r = +0 \cdot 129$ or $-0 \cdot 093$), or at medium or strong HVS ($r = +0 \cdot 179$ or $+0 \cdot 097$).

DISCUSSION

Intensity of visual stimulus and auditory sensitivity. The present results indicate that the physical intensity of a simultaneously applied visual stimulus affects sensitivity to a 1000-cycle pure tone, thus supporting the proposed hypothesis. Auditory sensitivity was affected by the intensity of the visual stimulus in such a way that the range of weak intensities provides for facilitation of sensitivity regardless of the personality type. The magnitude of facilitation increased as the intensity of the visual stimulus was increased from weak to medium, and then to strong in one type of subject, viz. E; and the facilitatory effect disappeared as the intensity was increased from weak to medium in another type of subject, viz. I. In I, an inhibitory effect occurred as the intensity of the visual stimulus was increased from medium to strong. These results agree with the general statement of the 'law of inversion' and provide further information on this inversion in relation to personality. The present results indicate a fruitful approach towards a more precise definition of the conditions which differentiate various types of intersensory effects from each other, by considering the function of the magnitude of the intensity change of the heteromodal stimulus in relation to personality.

The present results provide support for the view that: (1) weak visual stimuli increase auditory sensitivity, and this effect can be reversed at greater intensities

Effect of visual stimulation on auditory sensitivity

(in I); (2) weak visual stimuli increase auditory sensitivity, and this effect can be enhanced at greater intensities (in E); (3) weak visual stimuli increase auditory sensitivity, and this effect disappears at greater intensities (in A). These relationships between the intensity of the simultaneous visual stimulus and auditory sensitivity are related systematically to the personality type. It may be concluded that, in relation to auditory sensitivity, the intensity of the visual stimulus is a parameter involved in determining: (1) the point of transition between greater and less facilitatory effects, (2) the point of transition between facilitatory and inhibitory effects, and (3) the occurrence of these effects.

Personality type and the effect of visual stimulation. The present results support the hypothesis that auditory sensitivity varies with difference in the personality type, when measured under various intensities of a visual stimulus. The change in auditory sensitivity was affected by the personality type in such a way that sensitivity increases in E regardless of the intensity of the visual stimulus, and it increases at weaker and decreases at stronger intensities in I. The higher E scale score clearly provides for facilitation of auditory sensitivity regardless of the intensity of the visual stimulus. The lower E score, on the other hand, provides for inhibition of auditory sensitivity in regard to the intensity of the visual stimulus. When the visual stimulus was medium or strong, it was clearly shown that the greater the EPI E scale score (regardless of N scale score) the greater the increase in auditory sensitivity. These results on the sensory performance suggest some implications for the 'stimulus aversion–hunger' hypothesis (Eysenck, 1967). Although there is a clear distinction, in terms of scores on the personality inventory, among the three types of subject responsible for producing the facilitatory and inhibitory effects, it is difficult to state whether this distinction was fully responsible for producing the present results. For example, variations blurring this distinction may have occurred, particularly over the duration of the experimental session (which lasted for about 75 min.) and variables such as drowsiness or fatigue may have had some influence. However, the personality type, as here interpreted, is obviously involved in producing opposite types of response which persist for the duration of the experimental session, i.e. auditory sensitivity is facilitated in one type and is inhibited in another, when the intensity of the visual stimulus is increased up to a certain level.

In the present experiment, the same strong visual stimulus increased auditory sensitivity in E, exerted no influence in A and decreased sensitivity in I. These relationships between the personality type and auditory sensitivity were systematically related to the intensity of the visual stimulus. It may be concluded that the personality type is a parameter involved in determining: (1) the occurrence of the effects of visual stimulation, and (2) the point of transition between facilitatory and inhibitory effects, on auditory sensitivity.

The differential effect of intensity of the visual stimulus as a function of the personality type. The present results show that the intensity of a simultaneous visual stimulus affects absolute auditory sensitivity differently, in different personality types. Auditory sensitivity was affected by these two parameters in such a way that sensitivity was increased by the weaker, and decreased by the stronger, intensities in I. Sensitivity increased, however, at all intensities in E, with greater increase at greater intensities. These results indicate a differential effect from one intensity level of

15-2

T. Shigehisa and J. R. Symons

visual stimulation to another as we move from one personality type to another. They suggest that the point of transition between facilitatory and inhibitory effects, on auditory sensitivity, is at a weaker intensity of the visual stimulus in I than in E or A. In general, the results of the present study suggest that the changes in auditory sensitivity can be predicted by manipulating the level of intensity of the visual stimulus along the millilamberts scale and the type of personality along the EPI E scale.

The present results indicate the functional relationship between the intensity of simultaneous heteromodal stimulation and sensitivity in the primary modality, with personality type as a parameter. From these results, it is expected that the intensity of the heteromodal stimulus accounts for the transition between the effects of heteromodal stimulation on sensitivity in the primary modality, if only one personality type is involved. Similarly, it is expected that the personality type accounts for the transition between these effects, if only one intensity is used. Since I show an increase in auditory sensitivity at weak, and a decrease at strong, intensities, with E continuing to show increased sensitivity at increased intensities, the present findings may therefore offer a reasonable interpretation of those studies in the literature where personality type was not defined. For example, the curvilinear facilitatory effects reported by Levine (1958) using two subjects, and by Miller (1969) using five subjects can be readily accounted for in terms of the present hypotheses if we assumed their subjects were neither introverted nor extraverted. Similarly, the inversion effects reported by the Russian workers (e.g. Lazarev, 1905; Kekcheev, 1938) were possibly obtained with relatively introverted subjects. In this way, some of the negative reports in the literature could be understood in terms of these possibilities, as interpreted above.

The present results seem to suggest some practical implications. If indeed absolute auditory sensitivity is a reasonable response measure reflecting the efficiency of sensory activities, then it appears that one type of subject (i.e. extraverts) can operate most efficiently under bombardment from a fairly high level of irrelevant stimulation, while another type of subject (i.e. introverts) operates least efficiently under such sensory bombardment.

Conclusions

In conclusion, the results of the present study can be summarized as follows. (1) Absolute auditory sensitivity varies with change in the intensity of a simultaneous visual stimulus. (2) Auditory sensitivity varies with difference in the personality type, in terms of introversion–extraversion, when measured under a simultaneous visual stimulus at ten intensities. (3) Auditory sensitivity is differentially affected by the intensity of the simultaneous visual stimulus, as a function of the personality type. (4) Auditory sensitivity increases at weaker, remains unchanged at intermediate, and decreases at stronger, intensities of a visual stimulus, in introverted subjects. (5) Auditory sensitivity increases at weaker, intermediate, and stronger intensities of a visual stimulus in extraverted subjects, with greater increase at greater intensities. (6) Auditory sensitivity increases at weaker and intermediate, and remains unchanged at stronger, intensities of a visual stimulus in subjects who are neither

Effect of visual stimulation on auditory sensitivity

introverted nor extraverted. (7) The greater the EPI E scale score the greater the increase in auditory sensitivity, at intermediate and stronger intensities of a visual stimulus.

The many valuable suggestions and discussions with Professor Elizabeth D. Fraser, technical help of Mr J. Torrie, Chief Technician, and patient assistance of Mrs Phyllis M. J. Shigehisa are gratefully acknowledged.

REFERENCES

BARTLEY, S. H. (1958). *Principles of Perception*. New York: Harper.

CORCORAN, D. W. J. (1965). Personality and the inverted-U relation. *Br. J. Psychol.* **56**, 267–273.

EYSENCK, H. J. (1967). *The Biological Basis of Personality*. Springfield, Ill.: Thomas.

EYSENCK, H. J. & EYSENCK, S. B. G. (1964). *Manual of the Eysenck Personality Inventory*. London: University of London Press.

GILBERT, G. M. (1941). Intersensory facilitation and inhibition. *J. gen. Psychol.* **24**, 381–407.

HARRIS, J. D. (1950). *Some Relations between Vision and Audition*. Springfield, Ill.: Thomas.

HARTMANN, G. W. (1935). *Gestalt Psychology*. New York: Ronald Press.

HOCHBERG, J. E., TRIEBEL, W. & SEAMAN, G. (1951). Colour adaptation under conditions of homogeneous visual stimulation (Ganzfeld). *J. exp. Psychol.* **41**, 153–159.

KEKCHEEV, K. KH. (1938). On the influence of inadequate stimuli on the sensitivity of achromatic vision. V. The influence of muscular activity. *Biull. eksper. Biol. i Medits.* **5**, 432–436. Cited by London (1954).

KRAVKOV, S. V. (1966). Interaction of the sense organs. In A. Leontyev *et al.* (eds.), *Psychological Research in the USSR, I.* Moscow: Progress Publishers.

LAZAREV, P. P. (1905). On the mutual influence of visual and auditory excitations. *Physiologiste russe* **4**, 1–5. Cited by S. V. Kravkov (1966).

LEVINE, B. (1958). Sensory interaction: the joint effects of visual and auditory stimulation on critical flicker fusion frequency. (Unpublished doctoral dissertation, Columbia University.)

LINDSLEY, D. B. (1960). Attention, consciousness, sleep and wakefulness. In J. Field *et al.* (eds.), *Handbook of Physiology: Neurophysiology*, vol. III. Washington, D.C.: American Physiological Society.

LONDON, I. D. (1954). Research on sensory interaction in the Soviet Union. *Psychol. Bull.* **51**, 531–568.

LOVELESS, N. E., BREBNER, J. & HAMILTON, P. (1970). Bisensory presentation of information. *Psychol. Bull.* **73**, 161–199.

MARUYAMA, K. (1964). Intersensory effects in vision and audition. *Jap. J. Psychol.* **35**, 204–216. (In Japanese.)

MILLER, H. L. (1969). Effect of auditory stimulation on critical flicker fusion frequency. *J. exp. Psychol.* **81**, 365–369.

RYAN, T. A. (1940). Interrelations of the sensory systems in perception. *Psychol. Bull.* **37**, 659–698.

SHIGEHISA, T. (1971). Effect of intensity of simultaneous heteromodal stimuli on absolute auditory sensitivity. (Unpublished manuscript.)

SHIGEHISA, T. (1972). An investigation of intersensory effects. (Unpublished doctoral dissertation, University of Aberdeen.)

STERN, W. (1935). *Allgemeine Psychologie auf personalistischen Grundlage*. The Hague: Nijhoff.

SYMONS, J. R. (1954). An investigation of intersensory relationships. (Unpublished doctoral dissertation, University of Reading.)

TORII, N. (1962). Sensory interaction between vision and audition. *Bull. Jap. Res. Centre* **1**, 26–37. (In Japanese.)

URBANTSCHITSCH, V. (1883). Über den Einfluss von Trigeminus-Reizen auf die Sinnesempfindungen insbesondere auf den Gesichtssinn. *Arch. ges. Physiol.* **30**, 129–175.

(*Manuscript received* 9 *March* 1972)

From P. M. J. Shigehisa, T. Shigehisa, and J. R. Symons (1973). Japanese Psychological Research, *15*, 164–172, *by kind permission of the authors and the Japanese Psychological Association*

EFFECTS OF INTENSITY OF AUDITORY STIMULATION ON PHOTOPIC VISUAL SENSITIVITY IN RELATION TO PERSONALITY[1]

PHYLLIS M. J. SHIGEHISA[2], TSUYOSHI SHIGEHISA[2] AND JOHN R. SYMONS

Department of Psychology, University of Aberdeen

Visual thresholds were determined in 3 types of *S* by a modified method of limits under 5 intensities of a 1 KHz pure tone. An analysis of variance of the data showed significant results for personality group and its interaction with intensity conditions. Under medium and strong intensities of tone, visual sensitivity " decreased " in introverts, and " increased " in extraverts with a greater increase at strong than medium intensities. In ambiverts it increased under strong intensity only. Non-significance of the intensity effect suggested visual dominance over auditory stimulation. Significant correlations between EPI E (but not N) scale scores and sensitivity change indicated the more extraverted the *S* is, the greater the increase in visual sensitivity. The results supported the proposed hypotheses.

Sensory interaction can be said to occur when a stimulus in one modality is effective in altering sensitivity in another modality, either increasing it or decreasing it. Although intersensory effects have been acknowledged for over a century, a number of experiments showed that the effect of auditory stimulation on visual sensitivity could be either facilitatory or inhibitory, and confusing reports on the effects of stimulation in almost any modality on any other have accumulated in the literature (see reviews by Hartmann, 1935; Stern, 1935; Ryan, 1940; Gilbert, 1941; Harris, 1950; London, 1954; Symons, 1954; Bartley, 1958; Torii, 1962; Maruyama, 1964; Kravkov, 1966; Maruyama, 1969; Morinaga & Noguchi, 1969; Loveless, Brebner, & Hamilton, 1970; Shigehisa, 1972). It is only within the last decade or two that reliable investigation of the

variables involved in sensory interaction has been attempted. Although not in agreement as to its specific effects, a number of workers seem to have concluded that the " intensity " of the heteromodal stimuli is one of the main parameters involved in determining the occurrence of intersensory effects. (see Shigehisa, P.M.J., 1972; Shigehisa & Symons, 1973a). Symons (1963) obtained facilitatory effects for all heteromodal stimuli used except auditory, and, while acknowledging the contradictory evidence provided by previous studies, suggested three parameters which may differentiate facilitation from inhibition. Two of these parameters may be linked with intensity and personality variables. The suggestion that personality differences are involved in sensory interaction was not a new one although little experimental evidence has been produced for it (see, e.g. Börnstein, 1936; Gray, 1964).

Experiments by Corcoran (1965) suggest that sensory performances by two personality groups are different, in that the performance of extraverts decreases while that of introverts increases, under the same sensory conditions. It seems that in ex-

[1] The many valuable suggestions and discussions with Professor Elizabeth D. Fraser, and technical help of Messrs. A. E. Bursill, P. Kinnear, J. Torrie, J. Devanney and L. Gray are gratefully acknowledged.

[2] Now at the Department of Psychology, Taisho University.

traverts thresholds are higher to begin with and inhibition to continued stimulation is great, while in introverts thresholds are lower and inhibition to continued stimulation is less (Eysenck, 1967). It follows then that a certain intensity of heteromodal stimulation may be perceived as lower by extraverts than by introverts. It can be predicted further that extraverts will show a greater increase in performance, or an increase at greater intensities of stimulation, than introverts. It is expected, therefore, that extraverts will show a greater increase in sensitivity to the primary stimulus, or an increase at greater intensities of heteromodal stimulation, than introverts.

Using introversion-extraversion as one of the personality measures, Shigehisa (1972), and also Bursill & Shigehisa (1972), analyzed the effects of personality groups on absolute sensitivity under heteromodal stimulation of various intensities. Shigehisa & Symons (1973a) further examined the effects of two types of visual stimuli on auditory sensitivity while controlling the variables of personality difference and the intensity of the visual stimulus, over ten levels of light in cd m^{-2}. Both under patterned and homogeneous (Ganzfeld) visual stimulation, significant effects were obtained for intensity of the visual stimulus, personality group, and their interaction. The results demonstrated that introverts show facilitatory effects only at weak intensities, auditory sensitivity decreasing at strong intensities, and extraverts show increasing facilitation with increasing intensities of the visual stimulus. The auditory responses under increasing intensities of the visual stimulus over ten levels were found to be most reliable in introverts, and least in ambiverts, i.e., introverts had the highest test-retest reliability, ambiverts least (Shigehisa & Symons, 1973b). Unfortunately, apart from these studies, the relationship between the intensity of the heteromodal stimulus and sensitivity in the primary modality has never been reliably quantified, in relation to the personality group, so that the point of transition between intersensory facilitation and inhibition could be determined. However, such a possibility is not inconsistent with findings by Maruyama (1959a; 1959b) that a point of transition between facilitatory and inhibitory effects (of auditory stimulation on visual sensitivity) along the frequency of auditory stimulus, varies with individual subjects.

The present experiment was designed to examine whether the effects of these variables, intensity of heteromodal stimulus and personality, would hold when the primary modality was visual, and an auditory stimulus was used for heteromodal stimulation. In this way, common features of intersensory phenomena can be examined across modalities. It is predicted, therefore, that visual sensitivity varies with difference in intensity of simultaneous auditory stimulation or personality group. Furthermore, it is very likely that the effect of each parameter varies as a function of the other. Thus, it can be assumed that introverted subjects show an increase in visual sensitivity if the simultaneous auditory stimulus is relatively weak, and a decrease when it becomes stronger. And, it may be that extraverted subjects show a progressive increase in visual sensitivity at stronger intensities of the auditory stimulus. One possibility is that the intensity effect of auditory stimulation on visual sensitivity is less pronounced than that of visual on auditory, within a certain range of intensity, simply because of visual dominance over the auditory modality due to the greatest innervation density of the visual modality. This possibility is consistent with observations by Rock & Harris (1967), of visual dominance over somatic sensory and proprioceptive sensation.

The purpose of the present study is to examine these hypotheses.

METHOD

Subjects. Fifteen students at the University of Aberdeen, 10 males and 5 females, whose ages ranged from 18 to 33 years (median 19 : most subjects 18–20), were used according to the method employed by Shigehisa & Symons (1973a). They had visual sensitivity within normal limits for the stimuli used in this study, and reported no previous hearing defects. First, the Eysenck Personality Inventory or EPI[3] (Eysenck & Eysenck, 1964) was administered twice using Forms A and B. (Although the extraversion scale scores on the 2nd test using Form B were adopted, six subjects whose scores on both the extraversion (E) and neuroticism (N) scales varied by more than 5 points between the two tests, whose L scale scores were above 4, or whose E scale scores would have placed them in already completed groups, were rejected.) Those five subjects with E scale scores ranging from 3 to 7 were designated introverts (mean E scale score 5.00, *S.D.* 1.87 ; mean N scale score 15.20, *S.D.* 1.64), and those five ranging from 15 to 20 were designated extraverts (mean E scale score 17.00, *S.D.* 1.87 ; mean N scale score 11.20, *S.D.* 2.18). The remaining five *S*s (range : 9 to 13) were designated ambiverts (mean E scale score 11.20, *S.D.* 1.48 ; mean N scale score 4.60, *S.D.* 3.85). (There was no correlation between visual sensitivity change and the EPI N scale score, under any intensity of auditory stimulation, hence the N scale

---

[3] The EPI is a development of the Maudsley Personality Inventory or MPI (Eysenck, 1959). It is more useful than the MPI from many practical points of view, viz., it consists of two parallel forms (Form A and B), making possible retesting without interference from memory factors; its items have been carefully reworded so as to make them understandable even by subjects of low intelligence or education; the correlation between E and N on the MPI is marginally significant, but it disappears in the EPI; the EPI contains a lie or L scale to eliminate " desirability response set ", while the MPI contains no such scale; the test-retest reliability of the EPI is higher than that of the MPI; and so on.

score was disregarded in this study.)

Apparatus. The apparatus used for visual threshold determination and auditory stimulation was described in detail elsewhere (Symons, 1963 ; Shigehisa & Symons, 1973a). Basically, at one end of a sound-proofed room were a chair and a desk with a padded chin-rest, response key and black screens which restricted the field of view to the test area. At the other end of the room was the apparatus for visual threshold determination. This consisted of a black screen 150 cm long and 100 cm high, along the middle of which ran two parallel horizontal ridges between which two movable plates could slide apart to reveal a white square behind, first seen as a narrow vertical white line to which the *S* was required to respond. Separation of the plates was achieved by the rotation of a disc which comprised a 360° scale, one complete rotation of which separated the plates by 1 mm, so that readings of the widths of the white line could be obtained to 1/360th of a millimeter. The white line when revealed was 8.5 cm high, and the bottom of it was 120 cm above floor level. The distance between the white line and the *S*'s eyes was 300 cm.

A sound generator (Dawe 443B) with earphones was used for auditory stimulation. The generator was adjusted to produce a continuous pure tone of 1 KHz, with variable loudness and duration. The loudness of the tone at the earphone was calibrated in each experimental session using a Dawe sound-level meter (1415A). The illumination at the test area, measured by an EEL Lightmaster photometer, was $10.764 \, lm \, m^{-2}$, and the luminance measured by a Gamma photometer telescope with a 20′ subtend was $0.171 \, cd \, m^{-2}$.

Procedure. The *S*s were instructed to make themselves comfortable at the desk and to wait quietly in the experimental room. During this period, the *S*s were adapted to the dim light ($10.764 \, lm \, m^{-2}$) for 10 min. The *S*'s task was to press the key once as soon as the white line was seen against the black background, while keeping his head on the chin-rest. The *S* was told that tones would sometimes, but not always, be present in the earphone.

P. M. J. SHIGEHISA, T. SHIGEHISA AND J. R. SYMONS

He received the tones from the right ear only, and then was given practice at responding to the line, without the tone, until responses stabilized. The main threshold determination began 6 min after preliminary tone stimulation.

For visual threshold determination a modified ascending method of limits was used. Five tone intensity levels as measured by a Dawe sound-level meter were used at the following decibels: 0, 10, 35, 60 and 85. (These will be called, in this order, intensity levels 1 to 5.) These levels were selected as the best range possible, taking into account ease of administration and the comfort of the S. The sequence of intensity conditions was from weaker to stronger, but the starting-point was counterbalanced among the five intensities over the five Ss in each personality group. In each trial, immediately following the signal, the tone came on (except in the 0 dB condition) and the disc began rotating (at the rate of 5–6° per sec) for separation of the plates. Immediately after the S's response to the white line, rotation was stopped and the tones were terminated. The reading on the scale was then noted and the pointer returned to zero (starting-point). When 30 sec from the signal had elapsed, the whole procedure was repeated. According to individual differences in responding, the observation period varied from 5 to 16 sec among Ss. The S made each response under the tone stimulation, and spent each inter-trial interval in silence. Five trials were held at each intensity condition and then a rest of 1 min was given. A number of blank trials were given during the practice session, but on no occasion did a response occur; therefore blank trials were not used during the experimental session.

RESULTS

Each S made five responses at each intensity condition and the mean threshold for each condition was first calculated. There were five threshold measures for each S, one at zero (control) tone intensity and four loudness increases. The thresholds were then adjusted to give the raw data in terms of sensation level by taking the control condition threshold (0 dB) as the zero sensation level for that S, i.e., his normal threshold of visibility, and subtracting from this the thresholds for each of the four stimulus conditions.

As shown in Table 1, an analysis of variance performed on these data shows significant results for personality group and interaction of personality group with intensity conditions. However, the F for intensity effects did not reach significance, suggesting that visual sensitivity is not affected by the intensity of a simultaneous auditory stimulus within the range: 10—85 dB. The significance of the personality variable indicates that the change in visual sensitivity brought about by auditory stimulation varies with personality difference. Similarly, the significant results for interaction of tone intensity levels with the personality group indicate that visual sensitivity is differentially affected by the personality group as a function of the intensity of a simultaneous auditory stimulus.

As can be seen from Table 2, which shows the significance of the difference between any given level of intensity and the baseline, visual sensitivity in introverts decreases at medium and strong intensities; in ambiverts it decreases at the strongest intensity only; and in extraverts it increases at medium and strong intensities, with greater increase at strong than at medium. In extraverts the increase was greater at intensity level 5 than at 4 ($t=$ 3.48, $p<.05$), and also at 5 than at 2 ($t=$ 2.78, $p<.05$). In introverts, the decrease was greater at intensity level 5 than at 3 ($t=2.33$, $p<.05$), and also at 4 than at 2 ($t=2.16$, $p<.05$). In ambiverts, the increase was greater at intensity level 5 than at 3 ($t=2.53$, $p<.05$).

Table 3 indicates that visual sensation level in each personality group differed from that in each other group at each intensity condition. Firstly, it is important

Effects of Auditory Stimulation on Photopic Visual Sensitivity

TABLE 1

A summary of the results of an analysis of variance of visual sensation levels

Source	df	SS	MS	F
Between-Ss	14	1167.66		
PT	2	746.51	373.26	10.63**
error (b)	12	421.15	35.10	
Within-Ss	45	454.72		
IC	3	44.02	14.67	1.85
IC×PT	6	125.11	20.85	2.63*
error (w)	36	285.59	7.93	
Total	59	1622.38		

PT=personality type. IC=intensity condition.
* $p < .05$ ** $p < .01$

TABLE 2

Changes in visual sensitivity (mean sensation level in arbitrary units) at each tone intensity in three types of subject. A negative sensation level indicates a decrease in sensitivity. Summary of the results of one-tailed t tests

Group	Tone intensity level	Sensation level	t
I	2	−2.25	1.96
	3	−2.90	0.90
	4	−5.60	2.55*
	5	−5.80	2.59*
A	2	1.70	0.81
	3	0.05	0.05
	4	0.10	0.04
	5	3.15	3.78**
E	2	3.45	1.45
	3	5.75	3.87**
	4	5.90	2.60*
	5	11.65	3.99**

I=introverts A=ambiverts E=extraverts
* $p < .05$ ** $p < .01$

to note an increase in auditory sensitivity is greater in extraverts than in ambiverts at the strongest intensity; and secondly, the sensation level is greater in extraverts than in introverts at the weakest intensity. On the contrary, the visual sensation level

TABLE 3

Difference in visual sensitivity change between personality groups at each intensity condition of auditory stimulation
(Summary of the results of one-tailed t tests)

Difference between personality groups	Tone intensity level			
	2	3	4	5
I : A	1.65	0.87	1.74	3.75**
I : E	2.15*	3.22**	3.62**	4.74**
A : E	0.55	1.97*	1.75	2.80*

I=introverts A=ambiverts E=extraverts
* $p < .05$ ** $p < .01$

TABLE 4

Correlation of visual sensation level with the EPI E, or N, scale score

Tone intensity level	r	
	with E scale score	with N scale score
2	+0.469	−0.161
3	+0.569*	+0.024
4	+0.682**	−0.129
5	+0.744**	−0.275

* $p < .05$ ** $p < .01$ (Two-tailed tests)

is not significantly different between introverts and ambiverts when the tone intensity is within the medium range, and also between ambiverts and introverts, or extraverts, even if the tone intensity is the weakest.

A Pearson product-moment coefficient of correlation was calculated for each intensity condition of auditory stimulation. Table 4 summarizes correlation coefficients of mean visual sensation levels with the EPI E, and also N, scale scores. There is a significant positive correlation between visual sensation level and the EPI E scale score, at medium and strong tone intensities, as predicted. These results indicate that the greater the EPI E scale score, the greater the increase in visual sensitivity, when the auditory stimulus is medium or strong. No such correlation was found

P. M. J. SHIGEHISA, T. SHIGEHISA AND J. R. SYMONS

between visual sensation level and the N scale score at any intensity of auditory stimulation.

DISCUSSION

The present results indicate that the type of subject, based on scores on a personality inventory, does serve to differentiate the effects of auditory stimulation on visual sensitivity, thus supporting the proposed hypotheses. However, it is possible that introverts, ambiverts and extraverts as defined here would show different results if the range of intensities of auditory stimulation was extended. Although the intensity level of the tone did seem to differentiate the sensitivity changes within individual personality groups, the tone intensity did not differentiate visual sensitivity changes if the personality groups were disregarded. Thus, the interaction of tone intensity condition and personality group found in this study supports the general statement that visual sensitivity is differentially affected by personality group as a function of the intensity of the simultaneous auditory stimulus. It was clearly shown that a strong auditory stimulus produces a greater decrease in visual sensitivity than a medium stimulus in introverts, and it produces a greater increase than a weak or medium stimulus, in extraverts. The data for ambiverts indicated that at all intensities of tone, except the strongest, visual sensitivity is not affected by the simultaneous tone stimulation. Thus, we may conclude that the interaction effect of intensity of heteromodal stimulus with personality variables, found in previous studies (Shigehisa & Symons, 1973a; 1973b), holds when the primary modality is visual, and an auditory stimulus is used for heteromodal stimulation. The present results indicate that there are common features of intersensory phenomena between visual and auditory modalities, in terms of this interaction effect.

As predicted, visual sensitivity, under increasing intensity of simultaneous auditory stimulation, varied with difference in personality group, of one specific dimension. Furthermore, the effect of this personality variable varies as a function of the intensity of simultaneous auditory stimulation. In this context, it was shown clearly that introverted subjects show less increase (than do extraverted subjects) in visual sensitivity if the simultaneous auditory stimulus is relatively weak, and a decrease when it becomes stronger. It was also shown that extraverted subjects show a progressive increase in visual sensitivity at stronger intensities of an auditory stimulus. Furthermore, when the auditory stimulus was medium or strong, it was clearly shown that the greater the extravertedness (regardless of neuroticism) the greater the increase in visual sensitivity. These results on the sensory performance agree with the general statement of the "stimulus aversion-hunger hypothesis" (Eysenck, 1967).

The intensity effect of auditory stimulation on visual sensitivity was indeed less pronounced within the range of intensity used in the present experiment, than that of visual stimulation on auditory sensitivity found in a previous study (Shigehisa & Symons, 1973a), suggesting visual dominance over the auditory modality. This intersensory dominance phenomenon favors interpretation in terms of greater density of innervation in visual, than auditory or any other, modality leading to greater sensory activity (i.e., the visual modality is more sensitive) and this in turn reflects dominance of visual sensory activity over those in any other modalities. This visual dominance phenomenon resembles those intersensory phenomena reported by Washburn (1895), Klemm (1909), Grings & Kimmel (1959), Kimmel, Hill & Fowler (1962), Wilson & Wilson (1962), and Rock & Harris (1967), and would be best interpreted, in this way, by considering the visual modality as the center of perceptual integration.

The visual dominance effect, as revealed by the lack of significance of the intensity effect of the auditory stimulation, may be a result of the range of intensities employed in the present study. Within the range of intensities used, the effect of personality group, as well as dominance of the visual modality, may overshadow that of intensity of auditory stimulation. The significant interaction of intensity with personality effect found in the present study suggests that this indeed may have occurred.

Another important factor may be the interval between visual and preceding auditory stimuli used in this study. Shigehisa, Shigehisa & Symons (1973) examined the effects of interval between auditory and preceding visual stimuli on absolute auditory sensitivity. These authors found significant effects of interval, personality group and the interaction of these parameters, under the weak light. Interval effects were also significant under medium and strong light. In addition, a weak light increased, and a strong light decreased, auditory sensitivity when threshold determinations began 30 sec, but not more than about 8 min, after the light stimulation, in introverts. Kuroki (1937) and Child & Wendt (1938) originally examined these interval effects, but without regard to the intensity or personality variables. In the present study, this interval condition was equivalent to those in the previous studies (Shigehisa & Symons, 1973a; 1973b), hence it is reasonable to assume that the effect of this interval condition is involved in the effect of auditory stimulation if visual threshold determination begins at those intervals (see, Shigehisa, Shigehisa & Symons, 1973) in introverted subjects, in the light of the observed intersensory similarity between these modalities.

In relation to the personality effects, it should be pointed out that the noted N scale trend in which introverts were most neurotic, ambiverts least, and extraverts intermediate, may have been a causal factor in the effects obtained. However, although a similar trend was noted by Shigehisa & Symons (1973a), these authors found no correlation between auditory sensitivity change and EPI N scale score under any intensity of visual stimulation used. This lack of relation between the sensitivity change and the N scale score was confirmed in the present study. An interaction of E and N factors would not be expected since Eysenck's dimensions are purportedly orthogonal (Eysenck & Eysenck, 1964), but further experiments examining the role of the N factor in sensory interaction, might repay investigation.

The present results would indicate that the variable of personality difference is an important one to consider in the examination of intersensory effects, and its interaction with the intensity of the heteromodal stimulus may account for a number of the diverse results reported in the literature. Previous negative auditory results (Serrat & Karwoski, 1936; Burnham, 1941; Matthews & Luczak, 1944; Chapanis, Rouse & Schachter, 1949; Symons, 1963) may have obtained because the personality and intensity variables were confounded. However, it seems unlikely that this should have occurred in one experiment only of the many carried out in the Symons' study, since significant facilitatory effects were found in all other heteromodal stimulations apart from auditory. Nevertheless, in experiments where only a few subjects are used and personality type and intensity of the stimuli involved are not specified, the results should be interpreted with caution, especially in view of the highly significant interactions of these variables obtained in the present experiments as well as those by Shigehisa & Symons (1973a).

CONCLUSIONS

From the demonstrated effects of a

1 KHz pure tone at five intensity levels on absolute photopic visual sensitivity in three types of subject, it is concluded that: (1) Visual sensitivity, when measured under different intensities of a simultaneous auditory stimulus, varies with personality group. (2) Visual sensitivity is differentially affected by personality group as a function of the intensity of a simultaneous auditory stimulus. (3) Introverts show decreases in visual sensitivity at moderate and strong intensities of an auditory stimulus; ambiverts show an increase at strong intensity; and extraverts show increases at moderate and strong intensities, with greater increase at strong than moderate. (4) The greater the EPI E, but not N, scale score, the greater the increase in visual sensitivity at all but the weakest intensities of auditory stimulation. (5) There is a certain similarity between visual and auditory modalities in terms of effects of simultaneous stimulation in one modality on sensitivity in the other modality. (6) Visual dominance over the auditory modality is suggested. (7) These results support the proposed hypotheses.

References

BARTLEY, S. H. 1958 *Principles of Perception.* New York: Harper.

BÖRNSTEIN, W. 1936 On the functional relations of the sense organs to one another, and to the organism as a whole. *Journal of General Psychology*, **15**, 117–131.

BURNHAM, R. W. 1941 Intersensory effects and their relation to memory theory. *American Journal of Psychology*, **54**, 473–489.

BURSILL, A. E. & SHIGEHISA, T. 1972 Heteromodal stimulation, personality and the inverted-U function. *Bulletin of British Psychological Society*, **25**, 70.

CHAPANIS, A., ROUSE, R. O. & SCHACHTER, S. 1949 The effect of inter-sensory stimulation on dark adaptation and night vision. *Journal of Experimental Psychology*, **39**, 425–437.

CHILD, I. & WENDT, G. R. 1938 The temporal course of the influence of visual stimulation upon the auditory threshold. *Journal of Experimental Psychology*, **23**, 108–127.

CORCORAN, D. W. J. 1965 Personality and the inverted-U relation. *British Journal of Psychology*, **56**, 267–273.

EYSENCK, H. J. 1959 *The Manual of the Maudsley Personality Inventory.* London: University of London Press.

EYSENCK, H. J. 1967 *The Biological Basis of Personality.* Springfield, Ill.: Thomas.

EYSENCK, H. J. & EYSENCK, S. B. G. 1964 *Manual of the Eysenck Personality Inventory.* London: University of London Press.

GILBERT, G. M. 1941 Intersensory facilitation and inhibition. *Journal of General Psychology*, **24**, 381–407.

GRAY, J. A. 1964 *Pavlov's Typology.* Oxford: Pergamon Press.

GRINGS, W. W. & KIMMEL, H. D. 1959 Compound stimulus transfer for different sense modalities. *Psychological Report*, **5**, 253–260.

HARRIS, J. D. 1950 *Some relations between vision and audition.* Springfield, Ill.: Thomas.

HARTMAN, G. W. 1935 *Gestalt Psychology.* New York: Ronald Press.

KIMMEL, H. D., HILL, F. A. & FOWLER, R. L. 1962 Inter-sensory generalization in compound classical conditioning. *Psychological Report*, **11**, 631–636.

KLEMM, O. 1909 Lokalization von Sinneseindrücken bei disparaten Nebenreizen. *Psychologische Studien*, **5**, 73–162.

KRAVKOV, S. V. 1966 Interaction of the sense organs. In A. Leontyev, A. Luriya, & A. Smirnov (Eds.) *Psychological Research in the USSR. I.* Moscow: Progress Publishers. 218–266.

KUROKI, S. 1937 The influence of light stimulus upon hearing. *The Japanese Journal of Psychology*, **12**, 253–269. (In Japanese with English Summary).

LONDON, I. D. 1954 Research on sensory interaction in the Soviet Union. *Psychological Bulletin*, **51**, 531–568.

LOVELESS, N. E., BREBNER, J. & HAMILTON, P. 1970 Bisensory presentation of information. *Psychological Bulletin*, **73**, 161–199.

MARUYAMA, K. 1959a The effect of intersensory tone stimulation on absolute light threshold. *Tohoku Psychologica Folia*, **17**, 51–81.

MARUYAMA, K. 1959b Kōkakuiki ni oyobosu ikeikankakushigeki toshiteno onkyō no kōka. *Ohwaki Yoshikazu Kyōju Zaishoku 35 Nen Kinen Shinrigaku Ronbunshū.* Ohwaki Kyōju Zaishoku 35 Nen Kinen Shukugakai, 355–372.

Effects of Auditory Stimulation on Photopic Visual Sensitivity

(In Japanese)

MARUYAMA, K. 1964 Shikaku to chōkaku toni arawareru ikeikanseisōgosayō. *The Japanese Journal of Psychology*, **35**, 204–216. (In Japanese)

MARUYAMA, K. 1969 Kankakukansōgosayō. In Yagi Ben kanshū/Osaka Ryōji hen, Kōza Shinrigaku 3, Kankaku. Tokyo: University of Tokyo Press. (In Japanese)

MATTHEWS, B. H. C. & LUCZAK, A. K. 1944 *Some factors influencing dark adaptation.* (Report No. FPRC/577), London: Flying Personnel Research Committee.

MORINAGA, S. & NOGUCHI, K. 1969 Kanseikan no sōgokanren. In Wada Yōhei, Oyama Tadasu & Imai Shogo henshū, Kankaku Chikaku Shinrigaku Handbook. Tokyo: Seishinshobō. (In Japanese)

ROCK, I. & HARRIS, C. S. 1967 Vision and touch. *Scientific American*, **216**, 96–104.

RYAN, T. A. 1940 Interrelations of the sensory systems in perception. *Psychological Bulletin*, **37**, 659–698.

SERRAT, W. B. & KARWOSKI, T. 1936 An investigation of the effect of auditory stimulation on visual sensitivity. *Journal of Experimental Psychology*, **19**, 604–611.

SHIGEHISA, PHYLLIS M. J. 1972 The effect of various intensities of auditory stimuli on visual sensitivity in relation to extraversion. Unpublished master's dissertation, University of Aberdeen.

SHIGEHISA, T. 1972 An investigation of intersensory effects. Unpublished doctoral dissertation, University of Aberdeen.

SHIGEHISA, T. & SYMONS, J. R. 1973a Effect of intensity of visual stimulation on auditory sensitivity in relation to personality. *British Journal of Psychology*, **64**, 205–213.

SHIGEHISA, T. & SYMONS, J. R. 1973b Reliability of auditory responses under increasing intensity of visual stimulation in relation to personality. *British Journal of Psychology*, **64**, 375–381.

SHIGEHISA, T., SHIGEHISA, PHYLLIS M. J. & SYMONS, J. R. 1973 Effect of interval between auditory and preceding visual stimuli on auditory sensitivity. *British Journal of Psychology*, **64**, 367–373.

STERN, W. 1935 *Allgemeine Psychologie auf personalistichen Grundlage.* The Hague: Nijhoff.

SYMONS, J. R. 1954 An investigation of intersensory relationships. Unpublished doctoral dissertation, Universty of Reading.

SYMONS, J. R. 1963 The effect of various heteromodal stimuli on visual sensitivity. *Quarterly Journal of Experimental Psychology*, **15**, 243–251.

TORII, N. 1962 Shikaku to chōkaku no kanseikankōgosayō. Nippon Research Center Kenkyūkiyō, **2**, 26–37. (In Japanese)

WASHBURN, M. F. 1895 Ueber den Einfluss von Gesichtsassociation auf die Raumwahrnehmung der Haut. *Philosophische Studien (Wundt)*, **11**, 190–225.

WILSON, M. & WILSON, W. A. Jr. 1962 Intersensory facilitation of learning sets in normal and brain operated monkeys. *Journal of Comparative and Physiological Psychology*, **55**, 931–934.

(Received Oct. 13, 1973)

246

From R. M. Stelmack and N. Mandelzys (1975) Psychophysiology *12*, 536–540, *by kind permission of the authors and the Society for Psychophysiological Research*

Extraversion and Pupillary Response to Affective and Taboo Words

ROBERT M. STELMACK AND NATHAN MANDELZYS

University of Ottawa

ABSTRACT

The association of pupillary constriction with negative valence stimulation was explored within the context of Eysenck's theory of extraversion. Three groups of 11 introverts, ambiverts, and extraverts observed the auditory presentation of 12 affective, 12 taboo, and 24 matched neutral words. Introverts yielded the largest average pupil size under all conditions and the largest magnitude of change in pupil size from prestimulus level. The results support Eysenck's general statement relating extraversion and cortical arousal in its postulate of a higher level of arousal in introverts. The general hypothesis that the pupil constricts to unpleasant stimulation was not affirmed.

DESCRIPTORS: Extraversion, Pupillary response, Arousal.

Recent reviews (Hess, 1972; Goldwater, 1972; Janisse, 1973) have been instrumental in revealing the anatomy of the unresolved controversy attending the hypothesized association of negative valence stimulation and pupillary constriction. In addition to the methodological revisions which these reviews inspire, a number of issues emerged which are of considerable interest to the development of pupillometrics in particular, and to the explication of the physiological correlates of affective experience in general. One of the issues clouding the aversion-constriction hypothesis concerns the nature and extent of individual differences in pupillary reactivity. Although a number of authors have remarked on the wide range of individual differences in pupillary response to affective stimuli, attempts to relate this differential responsivity to personality differences have not been successful (cf. Janisse, 1973). The extraversion dimension of the *Eysenck Personality Inventory* (EPI), which has been successful in identifying individual differences in other physiological measures, may be usefully applied to this problem (Eysenck, 1967).

It has been proposed by Eysenck (1967) that introverts, as defined by the EPI, are characterized by higher chronic levels of arousal or arousability than extraverts. Although far from conclusive, evidence indicating that introverts display greater

sensory sensitivity (Smith, 1968; Siddle, Moorish, White, & Mangan, 1969; Stelmack & Campbell, 1974) and greater electrodermal reactivity (Mangan & O'Gorman, 1969; Coles, Gale, & Kline, 1971) generally support the proposal. Similar differences in arousal would be expected to be manifested in the pupillary response of introverts and extraverts to affective and taboo stimuli. This expectation is abetted by evidence of differences between introverts and extraverts in the perception and recognition of threatening stimuli (cf. Gray, 1970), differences which are predicated on the thesis that introverts are more susceptible to fear and to warnings of punishment than extraverts and form conditioned fear reactions more readily.

In the present study, the pupillary response to negative valence stimulation was considered within the context of Eysenck's (1967) theory of extraversion. Auditory stimuli were employed to accommodate the frequently cited complaint (Woodmansee, 1966; Loewenfeld, 1966) that the pupillary responses to affective stimuli presented in the visual mode may be confounded with the effects of visual contrast on the pupillary light reflex.

Method

Subjects

The subjects were three groups of 11 introverts, 11 ambiverts, and 11 extraverts who were selected from a large pool of male university students on the basis of their scores on the EPI (Form A). The mean extraversion scores of the respective groups were 7.0, 12.9, and 18.2, with corresponding standard

Address requests for reprints to: Robert M. Stelmack, Faculty of Psychology, University of Ottawa, Ottawa, Ontario, Canada K1H 6K9.

TABLE 1

Affective, taboo, and neutral stimulus word pairs

Affective	Neutral	Taboo	Neutral
Vomit	Valley	Fuck	Fork
Pus	Purse	Prick	Prince
Mucous	Muffin	Balls	Bells
Parasite	Particle	Cunt	Corn
Scab	Scarf	Masturbation	Mosquito
Corpse	Coat	Fart	Farm
Slime	Sled	Shit	Shoe
Cripple	Cradle	Whore	Home
Infection	Inspection	Nipple	Noodle
Pimple	Pillar	Clitoris	Cloverleaf
Filth	Field	Penis	Penny
Guts	Goats	Bitch	Bench

deviations of 1.4, 1.0, and 1.7. The groups were equivalent for moderate neuroticism, having a mean neuroticism score of 10.8, SD=4.46. The mean age for the total group was 23.6 yrs, SD=4.1.

Stimuli

The stimuli, which are illustrated in Table 1, were 12 affective and 12 taboo words and 24 matched neutral words. The taboo and affective words were determined as the most unpleasant from lengthy lists by 10 raters prior to the experiment. The 24 neutral words had the same number of syllables as their affective and taboo partners. They were structurally similar in length, first letter, place of accent, and syllabular break. The stimulus words, spoken by a woman, were recorded on magnetic tape in a random order with the word "relax" presented between stimulus words. The interval between the onset of each word was 10 sec. Care was taken to ensure that the clarity and quality of enunciation was the same for all words. The tapes were recorded and played at a comfortable level of intensity, with a mean maximum intensity for all words of 60 dB and a range of 55 to 66 dB as determined with a Breul and Kjaer sound level meter, Type 2204.

Apparatus

The stimulus words, recorded and presented on a Sharp stereo tape recorder, were heard simultaneously by the subject and the experimenter via Pioneer stereo headphones. The pupillary response was recorded on a Polymetric Pupillometer system, which is a TV monitoring system. The right eye of the subject was illuminated by an infrared lamp. An infrared Vidicon tube and associated circuits converted the video image of the pupil into signals which were recorded on a Heathkit Servo Recorder, using a 10 in. pen sweep and a chart speed of 12.7 mm/sec.

Procedure

When the subject was comfortably seated at the pupillometer, the operation of the apparatus was explained to him. The headphones were properly placed and then the pupillometer was calibrated. The subject focused on a small circle on a 20 cm × 20 cm back-lighted opaque screen which was positioned 55 cm from the eye. The luminance of the screen was 2 ft-L as

determined with a Spectra Pritchard Photometer. In preliminary preparations, this luminance level was found to provide a pupil size approximately 4–5 mm in diameter, a range where initial pupil size presumably would not be biased toward either constriction or dilation. The taped instructions informed the subject that he would be hearing some words and requested him to picture the image suggested by the word and to try and maintain the image until he heard the word "relax." The 16 min stimulus presentation was interrupted at the halfway point to provide a 5 min rest period. The order of presentation of the first and second sections of the stimulus presentation was counterbalanced within groups. Although the random arrangements differed, an equal number of neutral, affective, and taboo words occurred in each section.

Results

The pupillometric data were analyzed second by second. For each word, the average pupil size was determined for (a) the 5 sec period prior to the onset of a stimulus word (prestimulus interval), (b) the first 5 sec period from the onset of a stimulus (stimulus interval), (c) the second 5 sec period after the onset of a stimulus word (poststimulus interval). A three factor analysis of variance (Extraversion × Words × Time Intervals) with repeated measures on the last two factors was applied to the pupil size data. The Newman-Keuls procedure was employed for *a posteriori* comparisons among means. The .05 level of confidence was adopted for all statistical tests.

Significant main effects due to extraversion were observed, $F(2/30)=5.061$, $MS_e=3.428$, with the introvert group showing larger mean pupil size than the extravert and middle groups. No significant main effects due to words were observed, $F(2/60)=2.083$, $MS_e=0.077$. The interaction of extraversion with words was not significant, $F<1$. Differences in pupil size between the observation time intervals were obtained, $F(2/60)=50.987$, $MS_e=0.034$, with pupil size during the stimulus and poststimulus intervals greater than during the prestimulus interval, an effect which indicates an increased pupillary response to the auditory stimulation. Significant interaction effects were observed between extraversion and time intervals, $F(4/60)=2.537$, $MS_e=0.034$, and between words and time intervals, $F(4/60)=5.931$, $MS_e=0.099$. Fig. 1 shows the mean pupil size of the extraversion groups for the neutral, affective, and taboo words during the prestimulus, stimulus, and poststimulus intervals.

Comparisons among individual means indicated that pupil size for the introvert group was significantly greater than for the middle and extravert groups at the prestimulus, stimulus, and poststimulus intervals. Although mean pupil size for the extravert group tended to be larger than for the

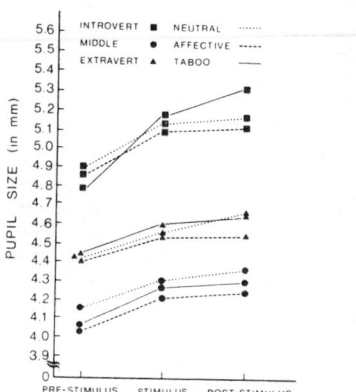

Fig. 1. Mean pupil size of extraversion groups to neutral, affective, and taboo words.

middle group, these differences were not significant at any time interval level. Comparisons among the means of the time intervals indicated that pupil size at both the stimulus and poststimulus intervals was significantly greater than at the prestimulus interval for all extraversion groups. No significant differences among the means of the stimulus and poststimulus intervals were noted for any of the extraversion groups.

Analysis of the simple main effects of words did not reveal any significant differences among the word conditions at any of the time interval levels. Comparisons among the means of the time intervals again indicated that pupil size was significantly greater at the stimulus and poststimulus intervals than at the prestimulus interval for all word conditions. No differences between the stimulus and poststimulus intervals were observed for any of the word conditions. It would seem that the significant interaction effects of time intervals with extraversion and time intervals with words are determined largely by the disparate differences in pupil size between the prestimulus and stimulus intervals which emerge for the introvert group under the taboo word condition.

Change in Pupil Size

Some individuals showed a decrease in pupil size from the prestimulus to the stimulus and poststimulus intervals, that is constriction responses, but only to certain words. Since these effects may have been cancelled out in the averaging of responses within each word condition, further analysis of pupil size change scores was warranted. Pupil size change was described in terms of the relative difference in pupil size (i.e. disregarding direction of change) between (a) the

prestimulus and stimulus intervals, (b) the prestimulus and poststimulus intervals, and (c) the stimulus and poststimulus intervals. In these terms, change in pupil size serves as an index of overall reactivity.

Significant main effects due to extraversion were observed, $F(2/30)=10.511$, $MS_e=0.073$, with the introverts showing significantly greater mean change in pupil size, 0.37 mm, than the middle, 0.26 mm, or the extravert group, 0.20 mm. Although differences between the middle and extravert groups were not significant under any word condition or time interval period, the middle group now falls in the central position; the cancelled effects of constriction responses seem to account for the extraversion group occupying the central position when the analysis was based on absolute pupil size. Significant effects due to word conditions were also observed, $F(2/60)=24.828$, $MS_e=0.006$, with changes in pupil size for the taboo words, 0.32 mm, significantly greater than for the affective, 0.26 mm, or the neutral words, 0.24 mm. Differences between neutral and affective words were not significant under any level of words or observation periods. A significant interaction between extraversion and words was noted, $F(4/60)=7.275$, $MS_e=0.047$. This interaction effect was determined largely by the relatively greater changes in pupil size under the taboo word condition, and in particular for the introvert group.

Differences in the amount of change in pupil size occurring between the observation periods were noted, $F(2/60)=63.614$, $MS_e=0.013$, with the largest magnitude of constriction occurring between the prestimulus and the poststimulus intervals. The amount of change occurring in the period between the stimulus and poststimulus intervals was significantly less than that occurring between the prestimulus and stimulus period and between the prestimulus and poststimulus period. Significant interactions were also noted between observation periods and extraversion, $F(4/60)=4.817$, $MS_e=0.013$, and between observation periods and words, $F(4/120)=5.887$, $MS_e=0.002$. These effects are determined largely by the relatively greater amount of change taking place between the prestimulus and poststimulus intervals for the introvert group under the taboo word condition.

Frequency and Magnitude of Pupillary Constriction

The mean frequency and magnitude of the negative difference scores, that is, constriction responses occurring in the three observation periods which defined pupillary change, were determined for each subject and for each word. Constriction responses were observed in 20% of all possible occasions. No significant differences in the frequency of constriction responses were observed between the extraversion groups, $F < 1$. The main effect of the words condition was significant, $F(4/60) = 5.58$, $MS_e = 2.91$, with the largest mean frequency of constriction responses occurring with the neutral words, followed by the affective and then the taboo words. Significant differences between the observation periods were also observed, $F(2/60) = 34.45$, $MS_e = 4.37$, with the largest number of constrictions occurring between the stimulus and the poststimulus intervals.

With regard to the magnitude of constriction, significant effects due to Extraversion were observed, $F(2/30) = 4.49$, $MS_e = 0.048$, with the introvert group showing the largest mean magnitude of constriction under all conditions. The main effect of the words condition was not significant, $F < 1$. Differences in the magnitude of constriction between the observation time intervals were obtained, $F(2/60) = 54.89$, $MS_e = 0.002$, with the largest magnitude of constriction occurring between the prestimulus and the poststimulus intervals. The interaction of observation intervals with extraversion was also significant, $F(4/60) = 52.41$, $MS_e = 0.002$, an effect which is due largely to the disparate increase in magnitude of constrictions for the introvert group observed between the prestimulus and poststimulus observation period.

Valence of the Stimuli

Since it could be argued that individual differences in the perceived unpleasantness of the stimuli could have prevailed in the experiment, all the subjects were asked to rate all the stimulus words on an 11 point scale, ranging from most pleasant imaginable to most unpleasant imaginable. There were no significant differences in the ratings applied by the extraversion groups, $F < 1$. Significant differences between the means of word groups were observed, $F(2/60) = 102.55$, $MS_e = 0.677$, with affective words being rated as more unpleasant (7.9) than the taboo (5.6) and neutral words (5.2).

Discussion

In addition to lending weight to the hypothesized relationship between extraversion and cortical arousal, with introverts characterized by higher levels of arousal (Eysenck, 1967), the present findings suggest that individual differences in degree of extraversion may be specified as a relevant source of variance in pupillometric studies. The greater magnitude of pupil size observed with the

introverts within all conditions, including the prestimulus interval, indicates that the introverts maintained a higher level of arousal throughout the entire experiment. The greater change in pupillary response under all word conditions further indicates that physiologically the introverts reacted to the words, and in particular the taboo words, more intensely. It is significant that changes in pupil size to sensory or emotional stimuli are understood in terms of changes in thalamo-hypothalamo-cortical activity (Lowenstein & Loewenfeld, 1969), since Eysenck (1967) and Gray (1970) propose that individual differences in this system constitute the biological basis for individual differences in degree of extraversion.

Allowing that taboo words are generally subject to aversive and punitive reactions in our society, the introverts' greater responsivity to the taboo words is consistent with Gray's (1970) notion that introverts form conditioned fear reactions more readily and that these fear reactions are stronger and more persistent than for the extraverts. These differences in pupillary reactivity prevailed despite the apparently equivalent valences of the word stimuli for the extraversion groups as determined by their ratings. The extraversion groups assigned essentially identical valences to the stimulus words; differences in their pupillary response to these stimuli, however, were clearly evident. Although the affective words had the highest unpleasant valences, the taboo words elicited the greatest change in pupil size. Within the terms of the present experiment, this seems to suggest that change in pupil size is more indicative of a response to arousing, or perhaps disturbing or threatening stimulation, than to unpleasant stimuli.

There is little evidence in the present data which supports the hypothesis that the pupil constricts to negative valence stimulation. When constriction is defined as a negative difference score from either prestimulus or stimulus levels, constrictions were observed in only 20% of the cases. Close inspection of these cases indicated that the largest mean frequency of constrictions occurred to neutral words and between the stimulus and poststimulus intervals, a situation which can best be interpreted as a relaxation effect. A similar interpretation seems to account for the fact that introverts displayed the largest magnitude of constriction, that is, introverts dilated more and then constricted (relaxed) more. The findings do not rule out the possibility of observing smaller pupil sizes during the presentation of dull or uninteresting stimuli as Hess (1972) suggests. However, saying that the pupil is smaller during the course of presentation of dull or uninteresting stimuli is vastly different from saying that the pupil constricts in response to those stimuli.

The conclusions concur with the results of a number of authors (cf. Libby, Lacey, & Lacey, 1973) that constriction seems to occur with a few stimuli and with a few individuals. Although individual differences in pupillary reactivity can be specified along the extraversion dimension, the pupillary constriction response could neither be specified in terms of individual differences in degree of extraversion nor valence of the stimulation. In view of the present findings, it seems appropriate to view pupillary constriction in terms of a relaxation or fatigue effect rather than as an idiosyncratic and specific response to specific stimuli.

REFERENCES

Coles, M. G. H., Gale A., & Kline, P. Personality and habituation of the orienting reaction: Tonic and response measures of electrodermal activity. *Psychophysiology,* 1971, *8,* 54–63.

Eysenck, H. J. *The biological basis of personality.* Springfield, Ill.: Charles C Thomas, 1967.

Goldwater, B. C. Psychological significance of pupillary movements. *Psychological Bulletin,* 1972, *77,* 340–355.

Gray, J. A. The physiological basis of introversion-extraversion. *Behavior Research & Therapy,* 1970, *8,* 249–266.

Hess, E. H. Pupillometrics: A method of studying mental, emotional, and sensory processes. In N. S. Greenfield & R. A. Sternbach (Eds.), *Handbook of psychophysiology.* New York: Holt, Rinehart, & Winston, 1972. Pp. 491–534.

Janisse, M. P. Pupil size and affect: A critical review of the literature since 1960. *Canadian Psychologist,* 1973, *14,* 311–329.

Libby, W. L., Lacey, B. C., & Lacey, J. I. Pupillary and cardiac activity during visual attention. *Psychophysiology,* 1973, *10,* 270–294.

Loewenfeld, I. E. Comment on Hess' findings. *Survey of Opthalmology,* 1966, *11,* 291–294.

Lowenstein, O., & Loewenfeld, I. E. The pupil. In H. Davson (Ed.), *The eye.* Vol. 3. 2nd ed. New York: Academic Press, 1969. Pp. 255–337.

Mangan, G. L., & O'Gorman, J. G. Initial amplitude and rate of habituation of orienting reaction in relation to extraversion and neuroticism. *Journal of Experimental Research in Personality,* 1969, *3,* 275–282.

Siddle, D. A. T., Moorish, R. B., White, K. D., & Mangan, G. L. Relation of visual sensitivity to extraversion. *Journal of Experimental Research in Personality,* 1969, *3,* 264–267.

Smith, S. L. Extraversion and sensory threshold. *Psychophysiology,* 1968, *5,* 296–297.

Stelmack, R. M., & Campbell, K. Extraversion and auditory sensitivity to high and low frequency. *Perceptual & Motor Skills,* 1974, *38,* 875–879.

Woodmansee, J. L. Methodological problems in pupillographic experiments. *Proceedings of the 74th American Psychological Association Convention,* 1966, 133–134.

(Manuscript received August 12, 1974; revision received December 26, 1974; accepted for publication December 30, 1974)

From K. O. Götz and K. Götz (1975). Perceptual and Motor Skills, *41*, 919–930, *by kind permission of the authors and Southern Universities Press*

COLOR PREFERENCES, EXTRAVERSION, AND NEUROTICISM
OF ART STUDENTS

KARL OTTO GÖTZ AND KARIN GÖTZ

Academy of Fine Arts Düsseldorf

Summary.—Color preferences of 190 art students (Götz & Götz, 1974, 1975) were compared with the corresponding scores on extraversion (E) and neuroticism (N). It was found that the preferences of a group of 27 highly gifted young artists were different from preferences of average and less gifted Ss who had little or no artistic practice. In the latter group extraverts and ambiverts mainly preferred primary and secondary colors (light clear and dark clear tones included), while introverts preferred tertiary colors (earth colors) and achromatics. However, in the group of highly gifted Ss no significant differences between positive and negative rankings in both color categories were found. Neuroticism had no effect on color preferences; this holds for introverts and extraverts and for each single color.

It is not a new idea that there may be a connection between aesthetic preference and personality. Such connection was found on experimental grounds by Burt (1939) who worked with reproductions of paintings and other test materials and who distinguished between four main temperamental types: the stable, the unstable, the introvert, and the extravert. Eysenck (1941a, 1941b) who continued the work of Burt, found that preferences for modern paintings with bright colors correlated with extraversion, while older paintings with subdued colors were more preferred by introverts; and in a following color-form test brightness of colors correlated with extraversion. In an experiment by Stephenson (1935) with 60 colors and with 20 Ss a bipolar factor became evident which divides those who prefer bright colors from those who prefer subdued colors, but he did not assess the personality of his Ss. In another experiment with 18 different hues with a corresponding tint and shade for each hue, and for 63 Ss, Barrett and Eaton (1947) found that preference for bright and pure colors was associated with extraversion, while preference for tints and shades was associated with introversion. Lynn and Butler (1962) replicating Eysenck's experiments with painting reproductions confirmed these findings and showed that subjects scoring introverted tended to prefer the less bright paintings. But the correlation between neuroticism and such preferences was not statistically significant.

Generally, less agreement can be found in studies on the relationship between color responses and neuroticism. Schachtel (1943) pointed out that persons showing color shock—stupor—are, according to Rorschach, always emotion-suppressors, neurotics of varying grades of severity. Wallen (1948) goes in the same direction when he claims that the data of his experiments provide some evidence on the Rorschach method, because they objectively demonstrate that unstable persons (mostly neurotics) show affective reactions different from those of stable persons. On the other hand, Keehn (1954b) is skeptical and writes: ". . . inasmuch as the Rorschach color responses are at best only indirectly affected by color, the use of the results of Rorschach studies either to support or to refute the color-emotionality hypothesis is invalid." In a study with a battery of nine color-form tests, and with three psychiatric groups, Keehn (1954a) showed that neurotics do not differ significantly from normals in their responses to color. However, tests of this sort are concerned more with the subject's attention to color in general than to his selectivity for specific colors. In an experiment with four psychiatric groups Warner (1949) used 30 colors which he divided in a hue series, a lightness series, and a saturation series. The results indicated that in the hue series anxiety neurotics preferred green to yellow more strongly than did any of the other three psychiatric groups. In the lightness series and a saturation series (Chap. II) the anxiety neurotics preferred the lighter colors more strongly than did any of the other groups. In the saturation series no significant differences between the psychiatric groups were noted in this area (Chap. IV, pp. 12-23).

It is the purpose of the present study to investigate the relationship between the results of two previous studies on color preferences of art students (Götz & Götz, 1974, 1975) and the personality dimensions extraversion and neuroticism of the same subjects.

METHOD

In both previous studies Ss were 190 art students from the Academy of Fine Arts Düsseldorf, 113 male and 77 female, mean age 23 yr., who had normal color vision and studied painting, sculpture, graphic-design, or art education. Ss were tested individually, and the Maudsley Personality Inventory (Eysenck, 1959) was administered before the beginning of the first color preference test. The test material of this test consisted of 14 colors: seven highly saturated primary and secondary colors, four tertiary colors (earth colors), and three achromatics (gray, white and black). In the second study 57 colors were used: 35 primary and secondary colors, light clear and dark clear tones included, 15 tertiary colors (earth colors), and 7 achromatics (5 grays, white and black). The Munsell notations of both color sets are indicated in the two studies (Götz & Götz, 1974, 1975).

In our investigation of a possible relationship between color preferences extraversion (E) and neuroticism (N) we started from the assumption that Ss who had ranked, for instance, yellow on the positive side of the preference scale would differ in their scores on Extraversion and/or Neuroticism from Ss who rejected this color. Perhaps such differences would arise with certain colors but not with all.

Therefore, in a preliminary study, by means of the results of the 14-color test (Götz & Götz, 1974), for each single color, the Extraversion scores of Ss who had ranked a color on the positive side of the preference scale were compared with the Extraversion scores of those who had rejected this color. Working with a 14-point scale, rankings covering the categories 1 to 6 were positive, and rankings over the categories 9 to 14 were negative, letting for the present the scores of the neutral categories 7 and 8 be separate. In the same way the Neuroticism scores of Ss who preferred a certain color were compared with those of Ss who rejected this color.

COLOR PREFERENCES, EXTRAVERSION, AND NEUROTICISM

The results were surprisingly disappointing. The means on Extraversion of the positive scorers did not differ significantly from the means of the negative scorers; in some cases they were even identical. This counts for all 14 colors. The same picture arose for all colors when the Neuroticism scores were compared. Here too, positive scorers had often the same means on Neuroticism as the negative scorers.

As a consequence, in a next step, the positive scores were now taken from the first four ranks (instead of the first six), and they were compared with the negative scores of the last four ranks of the 14-point scale. The results showed well some differences between the means on Extraversion for most colors, but none was statistically significant. On the other hand the differences between the means on Neuroticism were negligibly small or there were no differences at all. Therefore, in a next step the scores of the first three ranks (instead of the first four) were compared with those of the last three ranks of the scale. Herewith, only the extreme-scorers were recorded for each color, and their scores on Extraversion and Neuroticism compared.

RESULTS

Extreme-scorers

Considering the results with the 14-colors test, indicated in the upper part of Table 1, it can be seen that the means on Extraversion of extreme-scorers who prefer the primary and secondary colors red, blue, green, yellow, orange, etc., are significantly higher than the means of those who reject these colors. According to the standards of the Maudsley Personality Inventory and with a cut-off point on Extraversion at 25, among these extreme-scorers these colors are preferred by ambiverts and extraverts, and rejected by introverts.

The opposite is true for the tertiary earth colors brown, olive, ochre, beige, and for the achromatics. These colors are more preferred by introverted extreme-scorers than by ambiverts and extraverts. The differences are statistically significant for all 14 colors, and the scores in most samples are approximately normally distributed. Because of the relatively small Ns in some cases, these findings probably should be viewed as tentative.

On the other hand, neuroticism seems to have no effect on color preferences of extreme-scorers. The differences between positive and negative scorers on Neuroticism for all 14 colors were negligibly small and not statistically significant. These data are therefore omitted and not indicated.

In our next investigation we used the preference-data of the 57-colors test, obtained with a 7-point preference scale, and with five different reds, five blues, five greens, etc. (Götz & Götz, 1975). As mentioned above, this color set consisted of 35 primary and secondary colors, some highly saturated, and some corresponding light clear and dark clear tones, and 15 tertiary colors, i.e., the earth colors brown, olive, ochre, beige, and some variations, and finally 7 achromatics, i.e., 5 grays, white, and black.

It was decided that extreme-scorers were those Ss who had ranked at least four out of the five variations of a hue on either side of the preference scale and who had ranked at least one of them on rank 1 or 7, respectively. In the

K. O. GÖTZ & K. GÖTZ

TABLE 1

MEANS, STANDARD DEVIATIONS, AND t TESTS FOR COMPARISONS ON EXTRAVERSION OF
POSITIVE AND NEGATIVE EXTREME SCORERS ON TWO COLOR PREFERENCE TESTS

Color	Test 1 (14 colors)						t	p
	Positive			Negative				
	N	M	SD	N	M	SD		
Red	56	25.43	6.98	11	18.82	8.29	2.65	<.001
Blue	44	24.29	7.64	15	15.87	5.98	3.74	<.001
Green	16	27.00	8.62	19	18.68	8.67	2.74	<.01
Yellow	42	25.29	7.14	12	15.90	4.99	3.52	<.001
Orange	25	26.36	8.23	24	15.63	5.09	5.37	<.001
Violet	20	27.15	7.35	23	19.61	6.93	3.37	<.001
Pink	15	26.13	4.95	72	19.61	6.42	3.49	<.001
Brown	21	17.86	4.50	17	27.12	5.47	5.53	<.001
Olive	39	18.31	4.53	30	27.13	6.99	6.01	<.001
Ochre	32	18.88	6.01	20	28.35	5.14	5.70	<.001
Beige	25	16.92	5.39	36	28.05	7.19	6.49	<.001
Gray	22	15.73	6.42	39	26.62	6.69	6.02	<.001
Black	42	17.76	4.73	19	26.79	7.75	4.70	<.001
White	43	19.88	6.56	20	25.70	8.16	2.96	<.01
Test 2 (57 colors)								
5 Reds	45	25.42	7.56	23	18.30	6.29	3.85	<.001
5 Blues	22	31.50	5.09	14	17.07	4.31	8.50	<.001
5 Greens	21	26.90	7.83	32	17.97	7.08	4.20	<.001
5 Yellows	34	27.65	6.79	24	15.08	5.29	7.51	<.001
5 Oranges	28	27.82	8.13	21	15.76	4.96	5.94	<.001
5 Violets	21	28.48	6.74	53	17.32	5.78	7.12	<.001
5 Pinks	10	26.70	4.47	76	19.43	7.23	3.03	<.01
5 Browns	20	16.30	4.90	20	28.20	3.96	8.24	<.001
5 Olives	22	18.18	5.43	23	28.87	5.59	6.33	<.001
3 Ochres	43	17.05	5.32	31	30.61	4.56	11.38	<.001
2 Beiges	43	17.07	5.81	44	29.23	5.67	9.87	<.001
5 Grays	26	17.38	6.66	34	28.32	6.13	6.45	<.001
Black	64	18.75	5.85	20	27.05	4.95	5.51	<.001
White	42	18.78	7.02	18	24.00	7.11	2.54	<.02

case of the three ochres of our color set extreme-scorers were those Ss who had
ranked all three colors on either side of the scale, and at least one of them on
rank 1 or 7, respectively. Accordingly, the two beiges had to be either on the
first two or on the last two ranks; the same decision counted for white and
black. With this decision we tried to get an answer to the question if extraverted extreme-scorers prefer only the highly saturated primary and secondary
colors (as in our former test) or if they also prefer variations of these colors,
light clear and dark clear tones included. On the other hand, we wanted to
know if introverted extreme-scorers prefer only the very subdued earth colors

and the achromatics or if they probably would also prefer more saturated and bright earth colors, e.g., brown 5 (a broken but bright red-brown), olive 4 (a bright yellowish olive), ochre 1 (a warm gold-ochre) or beige 5 (a milky but very bright color), or if perhaps extraverted extreme-scorers would prefer these tones.

In the lower part of Table 1 the means on Extraversion of positive and negative extreme-scorers for 57 colors are indicated. As can be seen the results resemble those with 14 colors in the upper part of the table. The means on Extraversion of *S*s who prefer the primary and secondary colors are significantly higher than the means of *S*s who reject these colors, i.e., these 35 colors are more preferred by extraverts and ambiverts than by introverts. In other words, not only the highly saturated primaries and secondaries are preferred but also their corresponding light clear and dark clear variations. On the other hand, in the case of the earth colors, the browns, olives, ochres, beiges, and the achromatics, the opposite is true, i.e., introverted extreme-scorers prefer these colors while ambiverts and extraverts reject them. This counts likewise for the above mentioned more saturated or bright earth colors. The scores in nearly all samples are approximately normally distributed. So it seems not that saturation and/or value are the main dimensions which produce our results, but that it is the color category: primary and secondary colors and their variations on one side, and tertiary colors and their variations on the other side.

Again, neuroticism seems to have no effect on color preferences. The differences between the means on Neuroticism for all 57 colors were negligibly small and not statistically significant.

Color Preferences of Average and Less Gifted Versus Highly Gifted Ss

When we checked the individual data of the 57-colors test once more, we selected the color distributions of the few introverts who (against the majority of this group) had preferred primary and secondary colors and their variations, setting aside the data of extraverts and ambiverts. Among these introverts the names of some highly gifted art students—well known in the community of the Academy—were conspicuous. These names appeared again when we checked the color distributions of the few introverts who (against the majority of this group) had rejected the earth colors and some achromatics. If it were that color preferences of artists would eventually differ from those of average and less gifted art students, a comparison between both groups would be worth while. It must be said that most of the average and less gifted generally are more interested in theoretical lectures (art history, paedagogics, philosophy, sociology, etc.), and their practical work in the art studios is restricted to a necessary limit, i.e., they graduate in art education. On the other hand, among those who work continually in the art studios there are some highly gifted students whose works are exhibited once a year in the halls of the Academy.

K. O. GÖTZ & K. GÖTZ

In order to get the names of these highly gifted young artists we took advantage of such an art exhibition, and we recorded these names, 27 all together. We found out that they belonged to our 190 Ss, i.e., they had all taken the two color preference tests and the Maudsley Personality Inventory.

From the remaining 163 average and less gifted Ss 60 introverts ($M = 16.45, SD = 5.05$) and 60 extraverts ($M = 31.38, SD = 4.55$) were randomly chosen. Now the positive and negative scores of introverts for all primary and secondary colors of our set, taken together, were compared with the positive and negative scores of extraverts. In the same way for all tertiary colors (earth colors) and achromatics of our set the positive and negative scores of introverts were compared with those of extraverts. Table 2 shows the means, SDs, and t tests. As can be seen, in the case of primary and secondary colors, introverts have ranked fewer colors on the positive side of the preference scale than extraverts. Accordingly, introverts have ranked more of these colors on the negative side of the scale than extraverts, and the differences are statistically significant. With regard to the tertiary and achromatic colors the opposite is true, i.e., introverts have ranked more of these colors on the positive side of the scale than extraverts. Accordingly, on the negative side of the scale introverts have ranked fewer of these colors than extraverts, and the differences are also significant. These findings are in accordance with the results indicated in Table 1. The only difference is that in Table 1 the data of extreme-scorers were compared for each hue, while in Table 2 the scores of all positive and negative ranks were included in our comparisons. Moreover, this time comparisons were not made with the data of each single hue but of all primary and secondary colors taken together and of all tertiary colors and achromatics as a group. Again, neuroticism seems to have no effect on color preferences. The mean on Neuroticism for the group of introverts is 28.78 ($SD = 9.19$) and for the extraverts 26.68 ($SD = 8.17$; a nonsignificant difference).

These findings suggest strongly that in fact most introverted art students

TABLE 2

MEANS, STANDARD DEVIATIONS, AND t TESTS FOR COMPARISON ON COLOR PREFERENCES OF AVERAGE AND LESS GIFTED INTROVERTS AND EXTRAVERTS

	Introverts (N = 60)		Extraverts (N = 60)		t	p
	M	SD	M	SD		
Primary and Secondary Colors (light clear and dark clear)						
Positive	11.52	5.19	15.53	5.17	4.29	<.001
Negative	18.32	5.18	13.78	4.95	4.98	<.001
Tertiary (Earth Colors) and Achromatic Colors						
Positive	13.23	6.28	7.83	3.59	5.74	<.001
Negative	7.87	4.92	13.40	3.68	7.07	<.001

prefer the subdued earth colors and the achromatics of our set, and that most extraverts and ambiverts not only prefer the pure primaries and secondaries but also their light clear and dark clear tones.

But this is not the whole story if we look at the color preferences of the 27 highly gifted young artists, who were well among the extreme-scorers of Table 1 but whose data had obviously not falsified our results. Therefore, first, a comparison was made between positive and negative rankings of primary and secondary colors taken together (light clear and dark clear tones included), and secondly, between positive and negative rankings of tertiary and achromatic colors. As is apparent in Table 3, no significant differences between positive and negative rankings could be found in either color category. There are nearly equally many primary and secondary colors on both sides of the preference scale, and in the case of earth and achromatic colors the difference between positive and negative rankings is only 2.00. Because of the relatively small N, these findings probably should be viewed as tentative. But the result is nevertheless surprising if we compare it with the outcomes of the color preferences of the average and less gifted Ss. One may doubt the validity of a hypothesized relation between color preferences and extraversion, particularly because our 27 Ss are highly introverted ($M = 15.52$, $SD = 5.67$). That these Ss are also highly neurotic ($M = 33.74$, $SD = 6.35$) is less surprising, because in a recent study with another group of 15 highly gifted art students (Götz & Götz, 1973) we found the mean on Extraversion to be 16.40 ($SD = 3.70$) and the mean on Neuroticism 34.66 ($SD = 3.85$).

TABLE 3

MEANS, STANDARD DEVIATIONS, AND t TESTS FOR COMPARISON ON COLOR
PREFERENCES OF 27 HIGHLY GIFTED ART STUDENTS

	Positive		Negative		t
	M	SD	M	SD	
Primary and Secondary Colors (light clear and dark clear)	13.89	8.07	14.89	8.38	0.44
Tertiary (Earth Colors) and Achromatic Colors	11.78	5.14	9.33	4.24	1.87

DISCUSSION

According to a hypothesized relation between color preferences and extraversion, our results only partly agree with the findings of the above mentioned authors (Eysenck, 1941a; Barrett & Eaton, 1947; Lynn & Butler, 1962). If we compare their results with the data of Tables 1 and 2, we can state that our extraverted Ss preferred the bright and pure colors, as predicted by the above authors. However, we found that our extraverts preferred in addition certain subdued colors, i.e., the light clear and dark clear tones of the primaries and secondaries. This is in contrast to the hypothesis of the above authors who claim that, generally speaking, all subdued colors would be preferred by introverts. However, we cannot maintain the simple separation between bright and pure colors in connection with extraversion on one side, and subdued colors, tints and shades, in connection with introversion, on the other side. We rather propose a relation between two theoretically distinct color categories and Extraversion, i.e., primary and secondary colors (light clear and dark clear tones included) in connection with extraversion, and tertiary and achromatic colors in connection with introversion.

In our terminology we follow the norms of most color theorists and their descriptions of surface color systems (Birren, 1970; Frieling, 1968). Briefly, secondary surface colors are mixtures of primaries, and the light clear and dark clear tones belong to this color category. Tertiary surface colors are mixtures of secondary colors, and by the addition of black and/or white to such mixtures we get colors which belong to the scope of this category. In this sense the earth colors of our set form a subset of the tertiary color category. Most practical experts in surface colors stop here, but the system goes further. By mixture of neighboring tertiaries we get quartary colors, and by mixture of neighboring quartaries we get quintary colors. Yet, in our discussion on surface colors our theoretical interest concerns only the two main categories, the primaries and secondaries with their light clear and dark clear tones, and the tertiaries with the achromatics. Such a color system would be welcome with regard to our results which fit into the system (Tables 1 and 2). Moreover, we are forced to pose the question about the psychological and physiological bases for these results. And, here the structure of the color system should be taken into account.

As mentioned above we worked with a total of 190 Ss, and Table 1 shows the data of the extreme-scorers, while Table 2 summarizes the entire preferences of 60 extraverts and 60 introverts, randomly selected out of the total group, treating separately for the present the group of 27 highly gifted young artists apart. While our results are meaningful only within the limits of our sample of art students, and since predictions about other populations are in the meantime not possible, we nevertheless want to know more about the psychological and biological basis of our findings.

The Arousal Hypothesis

The stimulus characteristics which appear to affect the level of arousal are intensity, affect, and the collative variables complexity, incongruity, novelty, and ambiguity (Berlyne, 1960, Chap. 7, p. 174; 1963; 1967, p. 57). Although color cannot be considered to be a collative property, it must be noted that previous research has shown that color does affect the arousal level. Edwin, et al. (1961) investigated the effect of color on EEG desynchronization, and there were no significant differences between red, yellow, and blue. Desynchronization to green was significantly shorter than red or yellow, but not blue. Wilson (1966), using GSR as a measure of arousal, found that the magnitude to response was significantly larger for red than green. His prediction is that arousal values of various hues are related thus: $R>O>Y>G<B<I<V$. Jacobs and Hustmyer (1974) presented colored light patches for 1 min. each with GSR, heart rate, and respiration being recorded. They found a significant color effect on GSR but not on the other measures. Red was significantly more arousing than blue or yellow, and green more than blue. Sobol and Day (1967) who worked with red, yellow, green, and blue, noted that on the basis of their results alone, one could not substantiate the hypothesis that color, in itself, affects GSR, despite other findings which do substantiate this. But when the personal color preference, rather than fixed wavelength, was used as the independent variable, large significant effects on GSR were found. They suppose that a secondary intermediary, that of personal color preference, effects change in arousal. With regard to our problem these results are fairly meagre because only some highly saturated primaries and secondaries were used. The statement of Sobol and Day, that personal preference may effect change in arousal, throws us back to the question: what are the grounds of personal color preferences?

Psychophysiological Basis of Introversion-Extraversion

Eysenck (1957, 1967) postulates that due to greater inhibitory properties of their nervous systems and low level of cortical arousal, extraverts strive for relatively high amounts of stimulation. On the other hand, introverts, assumed to have weak inhibitory potential and high cortical arousal, require less stimulation from their environment. Color preferences and the presumed connection between GSR and the incentive value of colors would imply that extraverts mainly prefer vivid highly saturated colors, and that introverts mainly prefer subdued colors. Yet, this hypothesis would only partly be in accordance with our results indicated in the lower part of Table 1 and on Table 2, because extraverted Ss, in addition to the saturated primaries and secondaries, preferred also the light clear and dark clear tones of this category. This suggests strongly that saturation and value may not be the main dimensions of color preferences, but the crucial factor may be the category (of the color system) to which a color stimulus belongs. For comparison some examples from our data may be given: blue 1 is very dark and broken (5 PB 2.5/6), green 1 and 2 are also very dark and broken (5 G 3/4; 5 BG 4/6). As is apparent by the Munsell notations, these subdued colors are very low in saturation and value, and it could be assumed that, according to the arousal hypothesis, mainly introverts would prefer them. Nevertheless, they were preferred by extraverts, in addition to the highly saturated primaries and secondaries. If it were so that—according to the arousal hypothesis—saturation and value would be the main dimensions of color preferences, the following well saturated and bright colors should be preferred by extraverts: ochre 1, 2, 3 (5 YR 6/10; 7.5 YR 6/10; 10 YR 7/10), and olive 4 (2.5 GY 8/10). But these colors, on the contrary, were preferred by introverts; and for the present, we have no other explanation than this: these colors, in spite of their relatively high saturation and value, belong to the tertiary color category, and therefore are preferred by introverts.

The wavelengths of tertiary color mixtures, with or without black and/or white components, may represent much lower incentive values, so that introverts, according to the arousal hypothesis, respond in a positive way. Extraverts who strive for higher amounts of stimulation therefore reject these colors. With regard to the light clear and dark clear tones it may be assumed that the wavelengths of the primaries and secondaries, even in the case of changes to light clear or dark clear, still preserve their specific effect on the arousal system, i.e., their incentive value diminishes only unessentially when black and/or white components are added. Therefore, these colors are mainly preferred by extraverts. Such considerations remain speculative, especially with regard to the arousal hypothesis which is, experimentally, not well established. Until now our discussion concerned color preferences of average and less gifted art students. Yet, if we look at the data of the 27 highly gifted young artists (Table 3), it seems that our color-category hypothesis in relation to Extraversion does not work.

Color Preferences of 27 Highly Gifted Young Artists

As mentioned above, the data of Table 3 should be viewed as tentative, because this group is relatively small. Nevertheless, some considerations may be worthwhile. Applying the arousal hypothesis, the majority of these highly introverted *S*s should have rejected the primary and secondary colors. But these data show no significant differences between their positive and negative scores. The question arises: which factor may be responsible for this outcome which seems to contradict a relationship between extraversion and the arousal hypothesis. In the case of the highly gifted *S*s, a two-vectors model may illustrate a supposed mechanism where one vector represents an affective potential (explained by the arousal hypothesis) and where the other vector represents a 'cognitive set.' Then, the resultant would demonstrate the outcome of a color preference. In other words, if the high incentive value of primary and secondary colors elicits in these introverted *S*s a negative affective potential and if at the same time a positive cognitive set works in the opposite direction, then the data of Table 3 would take on meaning. With regard to a proposed cognitive set some comments may be given. The authors and two other experimenters, independently, interrogated the highly gifted *S*s about their color preferences. Those who worked predominantly with subdued colors were asked why they had ranked a lot of saturated colors on the positive side of the scale. The tenor of their answers was, briefly, the following: "... well, I work mainly with subdued colors, but I find no reason to make a negative judgment about some of these

COLOR PREFERENCES, EXTRAVERSION, AND NEUROTICISM

wonderful pure and vivid colors, no matter if they appear on the test cards or elsewhere." And, with regard to their preferences for subdued colors most of them answered spontaneously that they well prefer such colors, but that of course there are many, and that they like certain tones (in combination), while they dislike others. Ss who worked predominantly with vivid colors were asked why they had ranked a lot of subdued colors on the positive side of the scale. Instantaneously, some of them were startled, but then they said that they liked very well certain subdued colors, but that this fact had nothing to do with their present work in which they needed vivid colors.

If we disregard these statements, the question arises whether learning may play a part in color preferences of artists. Peters (1943) has verified in an experiment with color stimuli the relationship between learned reactions and affective judgments. He has demonstrated that positive and negative reactions established during learning are the determinants of the following changes in affective value. As we know, the creative work of highly gifted art students is a very stimulating and rewarding activity, even under uncomfortable circumstances. Therefore, the daily manipulation with a range of pure colors may be reinforced by the artistic activity, the creative emphasis, and the anticipation of the work in progress. If this is so, a positive cognitive set, concerning pure and vivid colors, may be conditioned and represent a performance effect. As mentioned above, such a cognitive set is one part of our two-vectors model where the other vector represents an affective potential elicited in a more direct way by the incentive value of colors. This model concerns the color preferences of the highly gifted young artists. These subjects are highly introverted and therefore are more susceptible to conditioning than extraverts or ambiverts. In the group of the average and less gifted Ss with little or no artistic practice, color preferences might be unconditioned, and may be tentatively explained by the arousal hypothesis.

Such highly speculative considerations are only prolific if they stimulate further experiments not only with creative artists as Ss but also with designers of several branches, photographers, house-painters, textile-clerks, etc. For comparison, other vocational groups, engaged in activities where no colors are manipulated, should be investigated, in order to find out if they show similar color preferences to those of our less gifted art students.

REFERENCES

BARRETT, D. M., & EATON, E. B. Preference for color or tint and some related personality data. J. Pers., 1947, 15, 222-232.
BERLYNE, D. E. Conflict, arousal and curiosity. New York: McGraw-Hill, 1960.
BERLYNE, D. E. Arousal and reinforcement. In D. Levine (Ed.), Nebraska Symposium on Motivation. Lincoln: Univer. of Nebraska Press, 1967. Pp. 1-110.
BERLYNE, D. E., & LEWIS, J. L. Effects of heightened arousal on human exploratory behavior. Canad. J. Psychol., 1963, 17, 398-411.
BIRREN, F. Creative color. New York: Reinhold, 1970.

K. O. GÖTZ & K. GÖTZ

BURT, C. The factorial analysis of emotional traits: Part II. *Charact. & Pers.*, 1939, 7, 285-299.

EDWIN, C. W., LERNER, M., WILSON, N. J., & WILSON, W. P. Some further observations on the photically elicited arousal response. *EEG clin. Neurophysiol.*, 1961, 13, 391-394.

EYSENCK, H. J. Personality factors and preference judgments. *Nature*, 1941, 148, 346. (a)

EYSENCK, H. J. 'Type'-factors in aesthetic judgments. *Brit. J. Psychol.*, 1941, 31, 262-270. (b)

EYSENCK, H. J. *The dynamics of anxiety and hysteria.* New York: Praeger, 1957.

EYSENCK, H. J. *Manual of the Maudsley Personality Inventory.* London: Univer. of London Press, 1959.

EYSENCK, H. J. *The biological basis of personality.* Springfield, Ill.: Thomas, 1967.

FRIELING, H. *Das Gesetz der Farbe.* Göttingen: Musterschmidt Verlag, 1968.

GÖTZ, K. O., & GÖTZ, K. Introversion-extraversion and neuroticism in gifted and ungifted art students. *Percept. mot. Skills*, 1973, 36, 675-678.

GÖTZ, K. O., & GÖTZ, K. Color preferences of art students: surface colors: I. *Percept. mot. Skills*, 1974, 39, 1103-1109.

GÖTZ, K. O., & GÖTZ, K. Color preferences of art students: surface colors: II. *Percept. mot. Skills*, 1975, 41, 271-278.

JACOBS, K. W., & HUSTMYER, F. E., JR. Effects of four psychological primary colors on GSR, heart rate and respiration rate. *Percept. mot. Skills*, 1974, 38, 763-766.

KEEHN, J. D. The color-form responses of normal, psychotic, and neurotic subjects. *J. abnorm. soc. Psychol.*, 1954, 49, 533-537. (a)

KEEHN, J. D. The response to color and ego functions: a critique in the light of recent experimental evidence. *Psychol. Bull.*, 1954, 51, 65-67. (b)

LYNN, R., & BUTLER, J. Introversion and the arousal jag. *Brit. J. soc. clin. Psychol.*, 1962, 1, 150-151.

PETERS, H. N. Experimental studies of the judgmental theory of feeling: V. The influence of set upon the affective value of colors. *J. exp. Psychol.*, 1943, 33, 285-298.

SCHACHTEL, E. G. On color and affect. *Psychiatry*, 1943, 6, 393-409.

SOBOL, M., & DAY, H. I. The effect of color on exploratory behaviour and arousal. Paper read at 28th Annual Meeting of the Canadian Psychological Association, Ottawa, June 1, 1967.

STEPHENSON, W. Correlating persons instead of tests. *Charact. & Pers.*, 1935, 4, 17-24.

WALLEN, R. The nature of color shock. *J. abnorm. soc. Psychol.*, 1948, 43, 346-356.

WARNER, S. J. The color preferences of psychiatric groups. *Psychol. Monogr.*, 1949, 63, 1-25 (Whole No. 301).

WILSON, G. Arousal properties of red versus green. *Percept. mot. Skills*, 1966, 23, 947-949.

Accepted September 23, 1975.

From C. R. Bartol and R. B. Martin (1974). Perceptual and Motor Skills, *38*, 1155–1160, *by kind permission of the authors and Southern Universities Press*

PREFERENCE OF COMPLEXITY AS A FUNCTION OF NEUROTICISM, EXTRAVERSION, AND AMPLITUDE OF ORIENTING RESPONSE

CURT R. BARTOL   AND   RANDALL B. MARTIN

Castleton State College   *Northern Illinois University*

Summary.—The study investigated personality variables of extraversion, neuroticism, magnitude of orienting response, and their relationship to stimulation preference using a continuous variable of complexity under diverse exploratory conditions. *S*s were asked to rank-order preferences for polygons differing in degrees of complexity. Data indicated extraverts preferred more complexity than introverts; there was a trend for low orienters to prefer more complexity than high orienters. Neuroticism was not a significant factor. The relationships between magnitude and habituation of orienting response and extraversion and neuroticism are discussed.

In theorizing about individual differences in degree of cortical arousal (extraversion) and in degree of peripheral, autonomic responsivity (neuroticism), Eysenck (1963, 1967) has proposed that the amount of stimulation an individual strives to receive from his environment is, in part, a function of his position on these two dimensions. Specifically, he postulates that due to the greater inhibitory properties of their nervous systems, and low level of cortical arousal, extraverts function under a kind of stimulus hunger, and, therefore, strive for relatively high amounts of stimulation. On the other hand, introverts, assumed to have weak inhibitory potential and high cortical arousal, require less stimulation from their environment.

While Eysenck emphasizes individual differences in stimulation preference, Berlyne (1960, 1971) has focused on certain external stimulus properties (complexity, novelty, ambiguity, incongruity, etc.) which are assumed to affect the cortical arousal of all individuals who encounter them. Specific to the present study, Berlyne has postulated that complex stimuli have the power to induce a specific type of conflict and a resultant state of cortical arousal. The level of cortical arousal generated corresponds roughly to the amount of conflict instigated by the complex stimulus pattern. The greater the complexity, the greater the potential for conflict. While Berlyne typically has employed a dichotomous variable of complexity, the present investigation used a continuous dimension of complexity. Moreover, Berlyne has emphasized the distinction between two exploratory paradigms in determining stimulus preference—specific and diverse. Specific exploration is principally concerned with an individual's "drive" to obtain information about his surroundings, whereas diverse exploration has an affective, arousing basis. The former would be illustrated by a brief exposure to a stimulus in which an organism received only partial or incomplete information about the stimulus; the latter would be implicated in preferential-choice measures under unlimited looking time.

C. R. BARTOL & R. B. MARTIN

The orienting response, assumed to represent a nonspecific, highly complex response to changes in stimulation, like extraversion, may be mediated by the ascending reticular activating system (Sokolov, 1963, pp. 289-291; Lykken, 1968). The orienting response produces an increase in the "discriminatory powers of the analyzers" (Sokolov, 1963), lowering sensory thresholds and increasing sensitivity to stimulation. The response is hypothesized by Sokolov to be an automatic, reflexive accompaniment to any perceptible stimulus change. This response in this experiment was operationally defined as the amplitude on the first skin conductance response to an innocuous visual stimulus following a 10-min. interval of relaxation. Since the response has been hypothesized to increase sensory sensitivity, individuals who gave a large orienting response (high orienters) should tend to show more sensitivity to stimulation than individuals who give a small one (low orienters). Correlations between the extraversion and neuroticism and amplitude of orienting response have in fact been reported (Mangan & O'Gorman, 1969; Sadler, Mefferd, & Houck, 1971; Siddle, 1971).

The purpose of the present study was to investigate the personality variables of extraversion, neuroticism, magnitude of orienting response, and their relationship to preference for stimulation, using complexity as a continuous variable under diversive exploratory conditions.

METHOD

Subjects

Forty male and 40 female Northern Illinois undergraduate students enrolled in an introductory psychology course were selected on the basis of their scores on the Eysenck Personality Inventory, Form B (Eysenck & Eysenck, 1968). Ss were contacted by phone and invited to participate. Students who volunteered to participate received extra credit on their final course grades.

Ss were drawn from a pool of 887 students, with a mean of 13.99 and SD of 3.96 on the Neuroticism scale, and a mean of 14.92 and SD of 3.79 on the Extraversion scale. The correlation between neuroticism and extraversion was —.077.

Ss scoring at least one SD above the mean on the Neuroticism scale were labeled as belonging to the neurotic group, those 1 SD below the mean as the stable group. Ss who obtained scores which were at least 1 SD above the mean on the Extraversion scale were categorized as extraverts, and Ss with a score at least 1 SD below the mean on the scale were regarded as introverts. These divisions resulted in classifying four groups ($N = 20$ for each group), viz., neurotic-extravert, neurotic-introvert, stable-extravert and stable-introvert. Ss who scored 4 or above on the Lie Scale were excluded.

Apparatus

Skin conductance response and tonic level of skin conductance were measured by a Beckman Dynograph Type R with Type 9842 Galvanic Skin Response

PREFERENCE FOR COMPLEXITY

Coupler, using a constant current of 10 μA. Amplifier sensitivity was set at 1.0 and pre-amplifier control remained at 100 mv/cm^2 for all Ss.

The orienting-response stimulus consisted of a 7.5-w orange-colored light approximately 3 ft. to the left of S and at table height. All Ss were run in the evening and the room was lit by an overhead 75-w light.

Stimulus Materials

Complexity in this study refers to the number of independent turns in randomly generated black polygons. A set of 12 random shapes, identical in shape to those used by Munsinger, Kessen, and Kessen (1964), was used. These asymmetrical random shapes varied in 12 steps from 3 to 40 independent turns. Each shape, approximately 3 in. square, was carefully reproduced on a 5- $\times$ 8-in. white index card.

Procedure

S was shown to a dim room and seated in a comfortable, semi-reclining padded chair. While electrodes were being taped to S's fingers, it was explained that one of the purposes of the study was to gain some measures of relaxation. Therefore, it was important for S to try to relax and made clear that he would receive no shock or anything aversive.

Two silver-silver chloride electrodes, 9 mm in diameter, were attached to the volar surfaces of the middle and index fingers of S's right hand. Electrodes and skin contact areas were cleansed with alcohol prior to each recording. Electrode cups were filled with Redux Electrode Gel and attached by medical adhesive tape. E then left the room. All equipment was located in an adjacent room.

After 10 min., without prior warning to S, the stimulus for the orienting response (orange light) was activated for 1 sec. and was repeated at 20-sec. intervals until S habituated. Habituation was defined as a response of less than 200Ω for three consecutive trials. E then returned to room, removed the electrodes, and requested S to place the random shapes on the index cards in the order of preference. S was asked to stack the cards in the order he liked them, the one on top being the most preferred, the second one from the top the one he liked second most, etc.

RESULTS

Ranking Data

Each polygon was assigned a $\log_{10}$ value based on its number of independent turns. In order to keep the increments of the complexity stimulus constant, the number of independent turns of each polygon was determined by approximately equal logarithmic steps. Then, $\log_{10}$ values were used for convenience and consistency in the analyses of the data. The sum of S's three most preferred was used as the dependent variable. A 2 (extraversion) $\times$ 2 (neuroticism) $\times$ 2 (sex) Ss analysis of variance indicated that extraverts preferred significantly

C. R. BARTOL & R. B. MARTIN

TABLE 1

MEAN LOG VALUES OF THREE MOST PREFERRED POLYGONS AS A
FUNCTION OF EXTRAVERSION, NEUROTICISM, AND SEX

| | Extraversion | | Introversion | |
	Neurotic	Stable	Neurotic	Stable
Male	3.67	3.68	3.09	3.07
Female	3.86	4.02	3.64	2.63

more complexity than introverts ($F = 12.92$, $df = 1/72$, $p < .001$; Table 1). Main effects for neuroticism and sex were not significant and the sex by extraversion interaction was only marginally significant ($F = 4.00$, $df = 1/72$, $p < .05$), with introverted females preferring less complexity than the other groups.

When preference of all 12 polygons was analyzed, using a 2 (extraversion) $\times$ 2 (neuroticism) $\times$ 2 (sex) $\times$ 12 (complexity) repeated measures, mixed design, a significant extraversion by complexity interaction was found ($F = 5.79$, $df = 11/792$, $p < .001$). Extraverts demonstrated a preference for increasing amounts of complexity, while introverts preferred lower amounts of complexity (Table 2).

TABLE 2

MEAN RANK OF POLYGONS AS A FUNCTION OF EXTRAVERSION,
NEUROTICISM, SEX, AND COMPLEXITY LEVEL*

| Independent Turns | Extraversion | | | | Introversion | | | |
| | Neurotic | | Stable | | Neurotic | | Stable | |
	M	F	M	F	M	F	M	F
3	4.2	2.9	3.7	3.9	7.0	6.6	4.9	8.8
4	4.8	4.0	4.4	3.9	6.6	6.0	6.1	8.3
5	3.2	3.0	3.3	2.7	3.2	3.4	2.7	3.7
6	5.0	5.3	5.2	5.2	8.4	7.8	4.0	5.7
8	8.3	6.8	6.3	5.5	7.0	8.2	7.7	7.2
10	8.0	7.5	8.3	7.4	7.6	8.9	7.5	8.4
13	6.6	7.0	7.7	7.6	7.1	6.5	6.4	5.5
16	7.5	7.2	8.4	7.2	7.2	7.7	7.4	7.3
20	6.7	8.4	8.5	8.0	5.8	6.8	8.0	6.5
25	6.4	8.5	8.0	8.5	7.1	5.6	7.4	6.2
31	8.9	9.5	7.7	9.1	6.3	6.0	7.7	5.5
40	8.4	8.3	6.5	9.4	4.8	4.5	8.2	5.3

*The higher the value, the higher the preference.

Orienting Response

Skin conductance level was measured by taking the recorded skin resistance just prior to the stimulus onset for the orienting response and transforming it into micromhos. The skin conductance response to the first light onset was measured

PREFERENCE FOR COMPLEXITY

as the maximum pen deflection which began within 1 to 4 sec. after stimulus onset. Both skin conductance level and skin conductance response were subjected to a square-root transformation as suggested by Woodworth and Schlosberg (1954) and Montague and Cole (1966).

Analysis of variance of magnitude of orienting response (skin conductance response) by extraversion, neuroticism, and sex showed that introverts gave slightly larger orienting responses than extraverts ($F = 3.91$, $df = 1/72$, $p <$ .10; Table 3). No other significant effects were found.

Surprisingly, analysis of variance of the number of trials to habituate to the light stimulus did not yield significant differences for extraversion, neuroticism and sex.

TABLE 3

MEAN MAGNITUDES OF ORIENTING RESPONSE AS A FUNCTION
OF EXTRAVERSION, NEUROTICISM, AND SEX

	Extraversion		Introversion	
	Neurotic	Stable	Neurotic	Stable
Male	.922	.801	1.193	.802
Female	.853	.405	.952	1.213

DISCUSSION

The results are consonant with the hypothesis that extraverts prefer more complexity than introverts. Extraverts demonstrated a monotonically increasing preference for the polygons as a function of complexity; while introverts tended toward a curvilinear function preferring the more simple polygons. This finding would indicate that extraverts and introverts do differ in their response to stimulus complexity, presumably due to differences in cortical excitation/inhibition factors and the levels of arousal potential inherent in stimulus complexity. Neuroticism did not emerge as a significant factor but this finding might stem from the lack of adequate stress generated by the experimental situation.

The orienting-response data suggest that extraverts tend to give smaller orienting responses than introverts and that there is no significant relationship between magnitude of orienting response and neuroticism. There was a non-significant trend for stable introverts to give the largest orienting response and for neurotic introverts to give the smallest. These findings are consistent with those reported by Sadler, Mefferd, and Houck (1971), who used visual trigrams for an orienting-response stimulus. In contrast, Siddle (1971) reported a significant correlation between neuroticism and magnitude of orienting response elicited by a tone, with Ss high on neuroticism giving high orienting responses, whereas extraversion and orienting response were unrelated. Mangan and O'Gorman (1969), who also used a tone for the orienting response stimulus, found high neuroticism scorers gave smaller orienting responses than stables. Mangan and O'Gorman also found a significant difference in magnitude of orienting response between stable extraverts and stable introverts, with extraverts giving larger orienting responses. Since in the Mangan and O'Gorman study magnitude of orienting response was reported in raw units (millimeters), these data remain open to question.

REFERENCES

BERLYNE, D. E. *Conflict, arousal, and curiosity.* New York: McGraw-Hill, 1960.

BERLYNE, D. E. *Aesthetics and psychobiology.* New York: Appleton-Century-Crofts, 1971.

EYSENCK, H. J. *Experiments with drugs.* New York: Pergamon, 1963.

EYSENCK, H. J. *The biological basis of personality.* Springfield, Ill.: Thomas, 1967.

EYSENCK, H. J., & EYSENCK, S. B. G. *Eysenck Personality Inventory: manual.* San Diego, Calif.: Educational & Industrial Testing Service, 1968.

LYKKEN, D. T. Neuropsychology and psychophysiology in personality research. In E. F. Borgatta & W. W. Lambert (Eds.), *Handbook of personality theory and research.* Chicago: Rand McNally, 1968. Pp. 413-509.

MANGAN, G. L., & O'GORMAN, J. G. Initial amplitude and rate of habituation of the orienting response in relation to extraversion and neuroticism. *Journal of Experimental Research in Personality,* 1969, 3, 275-282.

MONTAGUE, J. D., & COLE, E. N. Mechanism and measurement of the galvanic skin response. *Psychological Bulletin,* 1966, 65, 261-279.

MUNSINGER, H., KESSEN, W., & KESSEN, M. Age and uncertainty: developmental variation in preference for variability. *Journal of Experimental Child Psychology,* 1964, 1, 1-15.

SADLER, T. G., MEFFERD, R. B., & HOUCK, R. L. The interaction of extraversion and neuroticism in orienting response habituation. *Psychophysiology,* 1971, 8, 312-317.

SIDDLE, D. A. T. The orienting response and distraction. *Australian Journal of Psychology,* 1971, 23, 261-265.

SOKOLOV, E. N. *Perception and the conditioned reflex.* New York: Macmillan, 1963.

WOODWORTH, R. S., & SCHLOSBERG, H. *Experimental psychology.* (Rev. ed.) New York: Holt, Rinehart, & Winston, 1954.

Accepted March 12, 1974.

From C. R. Bartol (1975). Psychophysiology, *12*, 25–29, *by kind permission of the author and the Society for Psychophysiological Research*

The Effects of Chlorpromazine and Dextroamphetamine Sulfate On the Visual Stimulation Preference of Extraverts and Introverts

CURT R. BARTOL

Northern Illinois University

ABSTRACT

The study was designed to assess the hypothesis that preference for visual stimulation is at least in part determined by physiological mechanisms which can be modified by depressant and stimulant drugs. Thirty-six undergraduate females representing stable extraverts and stable introverts were used under diversive and specific exploration paradigms. While the specific exploration paradigm failed to reveal drug effects, the diversive exploration paradigm revealed that preference patterns of introverts were influenced by chlorpromazine, while dextroamphetamine sulfate had no significant effect on the preference patterns of extraverts. The relationship between the RAS, cortical arousal, and preferences for stimulation is discussed.

DESCRIPTORS: Extraversion, Introversion, Chlorpromazine, Dextroamphetamine sulfate, Complexity, Reticular activating system, Diversive exploration, Specific exploration, Eysenck, Berlyne.

Eysenck (1967, p. 230) has argued that individual differences of extraversion-introversion, as a personality dimension which is assumed to reflect the amount of external stimulation sought by an individual, is related to differential thresholds in certain portions of the reticular activating system (RAS). He has hypothesized that individuals high on the extraversion factor (extraverts) manifest relatively strong inhibitory and weak excitatory tendencies, the effect being a reduction in cortical "arousal" and efficiency. Individuals low on the extraversion factor (introverts) show the opposite tendency, weak inhibitory and strong excitatory tendencies, resulting in relatively high cortical arousal and excitation which facilitates learning, conditioning, and perception. This very general conceptualization of an inhibitory/excitatory ratio in an individual's central nervous system is hypothesized, in a rather vague and speculative way, to be a result of a complex interaction between the RAS and the cortex.

Eysenck further makes a very general hypothesis that the higher level of cortical arousal and excitation in introverts would be expected to lead to sensory sensitization, resulting in "stimulation avoidance"; whereas the higher level of cortical inhibition in ex-

Address requests for reprints to: Dr. Curt R. Bartol, Department of Psychology, Castleton State College, Castleton, Vermont 05735.

traverts would be responsible for sensory repression, resulting in "stimulation hunger." Some support for this hypothesis has been provided by Bakan and Leckart (1966), Day (1966), Farley and Farley (1967), Phillip and Wilde (1970), Skrzypek (1969), Bartol (1973), and several earlier studies cited by Eysenck (1963).

In a series of experiments by Bartol (1973) in which polygons or random shapes differing in levels of complexity (operationally defined by independent turns) were used as a quantifiable stimulation variable, introverts tended to allow all polygons, regardless of complexity level, to be flashed on a screen more often than extraverts. Although highly significant differences were not consistently found, these data tended to corroborate the hypothesis suggested by Berlyne (1960, 1971) that frequency of exposures reflects perceptual conflict and cortical arousal, which he refers to as "specific exploration." In a more convincing paradigm used in the experiments, subjects were asked to rate the polygons they had seen flashed on the screen in terms of how pleasing they found them, which Berlyne refers to as an example of "diversive exploration." Mean ratings of introverts depicted a negative monotonic function as the complexity level of the polygons increased. That is, introverts found simple polygons pleasing and complex polygons displeasing. Extraverts, on the other hand, consistently rated the polygons as neither pleasing nor displeasing (indifference), regardless of complexity level.

A strong case for the cortical arousal–stimulus preference relationship could be made if the exposure frequency and rating patterns of the extraverts and introverts could be reversed through manipulation of RAS and cortical arousal. Therefore, this study was designed to examine the possibility of preference reversal by attempting to modify states of cortical arousal temporarily by the use of so-called stimulant and depressant drugs. The hypothesis of this study rests with the postulate: "Depressant drugs increase cortical inhibition, decrease cortical excitation and thereby produce extraverted behavior patterns. Stimulant drugs decrease cortical inhibition, increase cortical excitation and thereby produce introverted behavior patterns [Eysenck, 1960, p. 106]."

Since the specific exploration paradigm (number of exposures) did not lend itself to significant and consistent personality differences, the diversive exploration (rating) paradigm will be the center of focus of this study. If Eysenck's postulate is correct and the extravert-introvert rating patterns are relatively consistent across similar situations, the predicted effect of a stimulant drug on the behavior of an extravert would be for him to find low levels of complexity pleasing and high levels of complexity displeasing. In other words the "stimulated" extravert (increased cortical arousal) will demonstrate a rating pattern akin to an introvert. On the other hand, it is expected that the "relaxed" introvert (decreased cortical arousal) will show a rating pattern similar to that of an undrugged extravert – indifference across all levels of complexity.

One of the stimulants commonly used to promote introverted behavior has been dextroamphetamine sulfate (Dexedrine), while a depressant frequently used to induce extraverted behavior has been chlorpromazine (Thorazine) (Eysenck, 1963; Eysenck, 1967, chpt.6). Although the site and mechanism of action of both Dexedrine and Thorazine are not completely understood, there are references in the literature that chlorpromazine (e.g., Smith, Kline, & French, 1968; Venning, 1963; Gray, 1964; Eysenck, 1967; Killam, 1962; Lynn, 1971, pp. 35–36) and dextroamphetamine sulfate (e.g., Eysenck, 1967; Aiba, 1963; Sylvester, 1963; Wilson & Schild, 1968) act principally on the RAS while having relatively little effect on the autonomic nervous system.

Method

Subjects

Thirty-six Northern Illinois University female students enrolled in undergraduate psychology courses during the summer session, 1972, were selected on the basis of their scores on the *Eysenck Personality Inventory, Form A*. Qualified Ss were contacted by phone and asked to volunteer. Ss who volunteered to participate in the experiment received extra credit toward their course grade.

Because the initial total S pool contained a far greater number of females than males, only females who scored as either stable extraverts (SEs) or stable introverts (SIs) were used. Ss who scored 1 SD above the mean on the extraversion scale and less than 1 SD above the mean on the neuroticism scale were designated SEs; whereas Ss who scored 1 SD below the mean on the extraversion scale and less than 1 SD above the mean on the neuroticism scale were classified as SIs. The two groups did not differ significantly in neuroticism. Ss scoring 4 or above on the lie scale were excluded.

Ss ranged in weight from 108 to 150, with SIs averaging 127.2 pounds and SEs averaging 118.3 pounds. The age range was 18 to 27 yrs, with SIs having a mean age of 21.4 and SEs having a mean age of 20.8. The groups did not differ significantly in age or weight.

Stimulus Materials

It was assumed in accordance with Berlyne (1960) that random shapes varying in some measure of operationally defined complexity would represent an appropriate index of stimulation levels. Moreover, it was also assumed in line with Berlyne's contention that the higher the stimulus complexity, the greater the potential for cortical arousal. A set of polygons or random shapes varying in 19 approximately logarithmic steps from 3 to 200 independent sides or turns were used as the complexity variable (see Attneave, 1957).

Twelve of the shapes of 3 to 40 independent turns were borrowed from the set constructed by Munsinger and Kessen (1964). Seven others, varying from 54 to 200 independent turns, were generated in accordance with Method 1 suggested by Attneave and Arnoult (1956). The 19 polygons were photographed and made into 35 mm slides, the shape being the black portion against a clear background.

Apparatus

Slides were shown by a carousel slide projector, forming approximately an 84×56 cm image on a beige-colored wall. A shutter and diaphragm, attached to the lens, controlled exposures, and was set at maximum aperture and at .25 sec duration.

Procedure

SEs were randomly divided into a Dexedrine or placebo group, while SIs were divided into a Thorazine or placebo group. E was unaware of S's personality or drug group before and during the experimental task. The drugs and placebo were prepared in similar capsular form and were placed in numbered envelopes by an assistant.

During initial phone contact potential Ss were screened for cardiovascular, liver, or respiratory problems, drug allergy, pregnancy, or medication regimen. They were again screened at the time of the experiment, and were also asked if they had taken any uppers, speed or stimulants, or downers, tranquilizers or depressants, within the past 4 weeks. Ss who exhibited the above-mentioned physical ailments or admitted drug usage within the past 4 weeks were excluded from the experiment. Four Ss were eliminated by phone screening and 1 S at the time of the experiment.

Participating Ss were asked not to take any form of medication except birth control pills at least 48 hrs prior to the experiment nor to eat anything at least 1 hr prior. At the beginning of the experiment, S was informed that she would receive one of three capsules. One would elicit a "pepped up" reaction, another would promote relaxation, and the third would be a sugar capsule with no effects. Possible side effects of the drugs were described to S.

Extraverts in the drug condition received 10 mg of Dexedrine orally, while introverts in the drug condition received 25 mg of Thorazine orally before testing. Personality and drug groups were counterbalanced in terms of the time of day they participated.

After ingestion of the capsule, S was left in a room by herself for 60 min and was encouraged to read or study, so as not to introduce a stimulus deprivation factor. No smoking was allowed. S was brought into the experimental room (at the end of 60 min) and she was informed that the experiment was concerned with her interest in designs and shapes, and was divided into two phases. In the first phase shapes would be flashed on the wall for an instant, but she could look at each shape as many times as she wished (specific exploration). It was emphasized to S that nothing would be asked about the shapes.

Following the specific exploration phase, S was told that she would see the shapes again but this time they would not be flashed. Rather they would be shown for a continued interval and S could look at them as long as she wished (diversive exploration). While each polygon was exposed S was requested to rate it on a 7-point scale, ranging from 7 (extremely pleasing) to 1 (extremely displeasing), with 4 representing a neutral point of neither pleasing nor displeasing. It was emphasized to S that E was interested in how pleasing she found each shape, not how interesting. In an attempt to neutralize context effects, slide order of the 19 stimuli was randomized for each S. The specific slide order used for the exposure phase was the same order employed in the rating phase. The shutter was operated manually by E, who was present throughout the exposure and rating phases.

Results

Specific Exploration

The dependent variable for the specific exploration paradigm was the number of times S allowed the polygon to be flashed on the screen. Analysis of variance ($2 \times 2 \times 19$ factorial design) revealed significant main effects for complexity, $F(18/576) = 8.60$, $p < .001$, indicating that frequency of exposures increased by both personality groups as complexity increased (Table 1). Also consistent with earlier findings (Bartol, 1973), there was a main effect for extraversion, $F(1/32) = 4.08$, $p < .05$, as SIs exposed the polygons more often than SEs in

TABLE 1

Mean exposure frequencies (specific exploration) of introverts and extraverts as a function of drug conditions and levels of complexity

Complexity Levels (Low to High)	Mean Exposure Frequencies			
	Introverts		Extraverts	
	Placebo	Thorazine	Placebo	Dexedrine
1	3.22	4.33	2.00	2.44
2	3.78	4.78	2.56	2.67
3	4.44	5.33	2.44	2.33
4	3.56	4.56	2.56	2.33
5	3.67	4.67	2.78	2.78
6	4.56	4.78	3.44	3.44
7	5.33	5.67	2.89	2.78
8	4.11	5.56	3.11	3.44
9	4.89	6.67	3.11	3.56
10	6.33	7.11	3.11	4.33
11	6.67	6.78	3.44	4.33
12	5.56	6.67	3.56	4.22
13	5.67	7.22	4.33	4.11
14	5.89	6.89	3.33	5.44
15	6.11	6.11	3.44	5.22
16	6.44	7.44	3.67	4.56
17	6.78	6.11	4.22	4.67
18	6.78	5.00	4.44	4.67
19	6.00	5.22	5.11	5.44

both drug and placebo conditions. Most pertinent to the present study, however, was the finding that the expected reversal of exposure patterns by the personality groups (placebo vs drugged) did not occur.

Diversive Exploration

The dependent variable for this paradigm was the numerical rating S gave the stimulus polygon on a 1–7 scale of pleasingness. The data in this paradigm become more explainable when the Thorazine/placebo groups of SIs and Dexedrine/placebo groups of SEs are treated in separate analyses of variance. Analysis of variance for the SI groups revealed a highly significant drug by complexity interaction, $F(18/288) = 3.48$, $p < .001$, clearly indicating that the drug conditions affected the ratings of SIs (Table 2). As reported in earlier findings, ratings by SIs in the placebo condition followed a negative monotonic function as complexity increased (average slope coefficient $= -.199$); whereas ratings by SIs in the Thorazine condition described a flat, extraverted pattern of indifference (average slope coefficient $= -.004$). On the other hand, the drug by complexity interaction for SEs was not significant, $F(18/288) = 0.70$, indicating that the drug conditions failed to affect the rating patterns of SEs. As found in previous studies, mean SE rating profiles were flat and

TABLE 2

Mean ratings (diversive exploration) of introverts and extra-
verts as a function of drug conditions and levels of complexity

Complexity Levels (Low to High)	Mean Ratings			
	Introverts		Extraverts	
	Placebo	Thorazine	Placebo	Dexedrine
1	5.78	4.67	3.00	4.00
2	5.00	4.44	3.33	4.00
3	4.22	4.00	2.89	4.00
4	4.22	4.11	3.33	3.33
5	5.11	5.33	4.44	3.11
6	5.11	4.33	4.22	4.00
7	4.33	3.22	4.00	2.78
8	4.44	3.33	3.78	3.55
9	4.11	3.44	4.00	3.88
10	3.55	4.00	3.67	3.33
11	3.78	3.78	4.67	3.33
12	3.00	4.33	3.22	2.77
13	3.55	4.56	3.89	4.22
14	3.33	3.56	3.89	3.67
15	2.66	3.33	4.22	4.33
16	2.78	4.78	4.11	4.33
17	2.11	3.89	4.11	5.22
18	1.88	4.33	4.44	4.66
19	1.33	5.00	4.44	4.78

indifferent for both the Dexedrine and placebo conditions (average slope coefficients
= .059 and .050, respectively). Analysis of
variance for SIs and SEs in only the placebo
condition revealed a highly significant complexity by extraversion interaction,
$F(18/288) = 5.44$, $p < .001$, which supports
earlier findings.

Discussion

The expected reversal involving exposure
frequencies of SEs and SIs was not found,
suggesting that the specific exploration paradigm is not easily modified. Because previous research (Bartol, 1973) has found this
paradigm to be a relatively insensitive and
inconsistent measure of individual differences, this finding came as no surprise. In
the diversive exploration paradigm, however. SIs in the placebo condition, theorized
to be functioning at high cortical arousal,
found the arousal-inducing complex stimuli
(see Berlyne, 1960) more displeasing than
SEs who are postulated to be operating at
relatively low levels of cortical arousal. It was
noted that as complexity (stimulus arousal)
increased the SI mean ratings of pleasingness decreased linearly. However, chlorpromazine, a depressant assumed to dampen
down RAS activity and cortical arousal, pro-

duced in the cortically aroused SIs the predicted effect of bringing their ratings of
pleasingness toward the neutral zone so
characteristic of SEs. Dextroamphetamine
sulfate, a stimulant believed to increase RAS
activity and cortical arousal, failed to produce the expected "introverted" rating pattern in the cortically underaroused SEs.

A constellation of possible explanations
immediately come to mind as to why Thorazine did have an effect on SIs, but why Dexedrine did not have appreciable effect on the
ratings of SEs. Obviously, the dosage parity
of 10 mg of Dexedrine vs 25 mg of Thorazine is certainly an important consideration.
Secondly, the specific effects of Thorazine on
the RAS and cortex may not be comparable
to the specific effects of Dexedrine. Thirdly,
Eysenck (1963) and Claridge (1967) cite substantial evidence which indicates introverts
have different sedation thresholds than extraverts, which would lead us to suspect personality differences in responsiveness to
drugs in general. In addition, the limitation
of using a small number of only female Ss in
an experiment controlled by a male E may
also be a crucial factor.

Despite methodological limitations and
molar conceptualizations about features of
the central nervous system, the study does
lend support to Eysenck's hypothesis that individual needs for stimulation may be determined, at least in part, by physiological
substrata, possibly the RAS. Quay (1965) and
more recently Hare (1970) have suggested
that psychopathic behavior (Eysenck's neurotic extraverts) might be classified as pathological stimulation seeking due to some malfunction or underactivity of the RAS. It
should be noted that Eysenck considered the
psychopath to be a *neurotic* extravert while
Hare argued that psychopaths are more likely *stable* extraverts since the research suggests
that they are "autonomically underreactive"
(Hare, 1970, p. 63). If the psychopath does
correspond to the stable extravert as suggested by Hare, the modification of RAS activity by some drug regimen may be a feasible first step in treatment as advocated by a
number of researchers. It would also be of
considerable interest to determine what
drugs (e.g., "uppers" or "downers") are typically preferred by extraverted and introverted personalities.

REFERENCES

Aiba, S. The suppression of the primary visual stimulus. In H. J. Eysenck (Ed.), *Experiments with drugs.* New York: Pergamon, 1963. Pp. 27-68.

Attneave, F. Physical determinants of the judged complexity of shapes. *Journal of Experimental Psychology,* 1957, *53,* 221-227.

Attneave, F., & Arnoult, M. D. The quantitative study of shape and pattern perception. *Psychological Bulletin,* 1956, *53,* 452-471.

Bakan, P., & Leckart, B. T. Attention, extraversion, and stimulus-personality congruence. *Perception & Psychophysics,* 1966, *4,* 355-357.

Bartol, C. R. Extraversion, neuroticism, the orienting response and preference for stimulation. (Doctoral dissertation, Northern Illinois University) Ann Arbor: University Microfilms, 1973, No. 73-20533.

Berlyne, D. E. *Conflict, arousal, and curiosity.* New York: McGraw-Hill, 1960.

Berlyne, D. E. *Aesthetics and psychobiology.* New York: Appleton-Century-Crofts, 1971.

Claridge, G. S. *Personality and arousal.* London: Pergamon, 1967.

Day, H. Looking time as a function of stimulus variables and individual differences. *Perceptual & Motor Skills,* 1966, *22,* 423-428.

Eysenck, H. J. (Ed.) *Experiments in personality.* New York: Praeger, 1960.

Eysenck, H. J. *Experiments with drugs.* New York: Pergamon, 1963.

Eysenck, H. J. *The biological basis of personality.* Springfield, Ill.: Thomas, 1967.

Farley, F., & Farley, S. V. Extraversion and stimulus-seeking motivation. *Journal of Consulting Psychology,* 1967, *31,* 215-216.

Gray, J. A. (Ed.) *Pavlov's typology.* New York: Macmillan, 1964.

Hare, R. D. *Psychopathy: Theory and research.* New York: John Wiley & Sons, 1970.

Killam, E. K. Drug action on the brain-stem reticular formation. *Pharmacological Review,* 1962, *14,* 175-224.

Lynn, R. *Personality and national character.* Oxford: Pergamon, 1971.

Munsinger, H., & Kessen, W. Uncertainty, structure and preference. *Psychological Monographs,* 1964, *78* (9, Whole No. 586).

Phillip, R. L., & Wilde, G. J. Stimulation seeking behavior and extraversion. *Acta Psychologica,* 1970, *32,* 269-280.

Quay, H. C. Psychopathic personality as pathological stimulus seeking. *American Journal of Psychiatry,* 1965, *122,* 180-183.

Skrzypek, G. J. Effect of perceptual isolation and arousal on anxiety, complexity preference, and novelty preference in psychopathic and neurotic delinquents. *Journal of Abnormal Psychology,* 1969, *74,* 321-329.

Smith, Kline, & French Laboratories. *Thorazine: Fundamental in psychiatry.* 1968.

Sylvester, J. Depressant, stimulant drugs, inhibition and the visual constancies. In H. J. Eysenck (Ed.). *Experiments with drugs.* New York: Pergamon, 1963. Pp. 284-312.

Venning, G. R. A hypothesis concerning a site of action of tranquilizing drugs and the significance of associated extrapyramidal motor phenomena. *Journal of New Drugs,* 1963, *2.* 351-353.

Wilson, A., & Schild, H. D. *Applied pharmacology.* New York: Little, Brown, 1968.

PART VI

PSYCHOMOTOR BEHAVIOUR

It is notoriously difficult to separate out perceptual and motoric elements in performance; clearly the two are closely intertwined, in that without perception there could be no co-ordinated movement, and without movement of some kind there could be no knowledge of someone else's perceptions. However, one side or the other is usually more prominent or important, or is singled out by theory, and it will be clear that the papers reprinted here differ considerably in their import from those contained in the previous section.

The paper by Corcoran restates the inverted-U relation between arousal and performance, and makes special predictions in relation to personality. Corcoran points out, quite rightly, that knowledge of level of performance is usually not sufficient to determine level of arousal for a given person or group, and that it is essential to *change* the level of arousal in order to determine whether a given subject is on the ascending or the descending limb of the inverted-U function. This is an important point, and it again emphasizes the importance of incorporating personality variables into the experiment if any proper predictions are to be made, or any theories to be tested. The Di Scipio experiment follows rather similar lines, but uses quite a different task.

Several papers deal with the concept of reminiscence in motor learning. The theory of reminiscence has a long and confused history, going right back to the close of the nineteenth century when Kraepelin and his students discovered the phenomenon, and elaborated a kind of inhibition theory which was very similar to that much later advanced by Hull. (Hull's ideas developed in complete ignorance of the earlier German work; like most English-speaking psychologists, he thought that reminiscence had been discovered more recently by English and American psychologists. The full story is told in detail by Eysenck and Frith, 1976.) Kraepelin already postulated an interaction between personality and reminiscence, but this association was not made in the later work which left personality out of account altogether.

In 1956, Eysenck published his first paper linking extraversion with reminiscence, suggesting, on the basis of Hull's inhibition theory, that extraverts would show more reminiscence than introverts. Several dozen papers have since verified this deduction, but unfortunately the theory itself was completely disproved in spite of its apparent success; as one of the reprinted papers makes clear, inhibition theory postulates that the cause of individual differences in reminiscence is the inhibition of pre-rest performance, leading to poor scores just pre-rest; what is actually observed is that extraverts do not show such poor pre-rest performance, but rather excel in post-rest performance! The best that can be said for Eysenck's original hypothesis is that it was specific enough to be disproved; the success of the deduction from a faulty hypothesis posed an entirely new problem, which was finally solved by having recourse to a consolidation, rather than an inhibition theory (Eysenck, 1965), thus going back to the conceptions of E. G. Müller, rather than E. Kraepelin. It is this change in theorizing that our reprinted articles take up; for a much more detailed account of the development of the new theory, the Eysenck and Frith book should be consulted.

REFERENCES

Eysenck, H. J. Reminiscence, drive and personality theory. *Journal of Abnormal and Social Psychology*, 1956, *53*, 328–333.

Eysenck, H. J. A three-factor theory of reminiscence. *British Journal of Psychology*, 1965, *56*, 163–181.

Eysenck, H. J. and Frith, C. D. *Reminiscence*. London: Academic Press, 1976.

From J. Stoudenmire (1972). Journal of Personality and Social Psychology, *24,* 273–275, *by kind permission of the author and the American Psychological Association*

EFFECTS OF MUSCLE RELAXATION TRAINING ON STATE AND TRAIT ANXIETY IN INTROVERTS AND EXTRAVERTS

JOHN STOUDENMIRE [1]

University of Southern Mississippi

Thirty-six anxious female undergraduate students served as the subjects in an experiment designed to test hypotheses regarding anxiety reduction following muscle relaxation training. The 18 introverted and 18 extraverted subjects were matched on pretreatment scores on two state anxiety (anxiety state) measures and three trait anxiety (anxiety trait) measures. Following three sessions in muscle relaxation training, they were readministered the anxiety measures. There were significant decreases in both the anxiety state measures for introverts but not for extraverts. There were no significant decreases in either group on anxiety trait measures. Results are interpreted as being consistent with Spielberger's state–trait anxiety theory and Eysenck's personality theory.

Spielberger's (1966) state–trait anxiety theory postulates two distinct anxiety constructs. State anxiety (anxiety state) is characterized by subjective, consciously felt periods of apprehension, tension, and autonomic nervous system activity. Trait anxiety (anxiety trait) is seen as the individual person's predisposition to manifest anxiety under any given stress situation. Muscle relaxation training can reliably reduce anxiety state but not anxiety trait (Johnson & Spielberger, 1968). The various parameters defining the optimal conditions under which relaxation training can reduce anxiety state have not been fully investigated, however. Paul (1969) has commented on this in terms of systematic desensitization, a therapeutic technique utilizing relaxation as a prelude. Paul noted, for example, that no systematic studies of client personality characteristics have been conducted to determine what personality variables are correlated with successful use of systematic desensitization. His review of the literature led him to conclude that most studies of systematic desensitization involve anxious introverts, but that anxious extraverts, hysterics, and sociopaths have also been used as subjects. He concluded that there is a need for more research in this area. It would

appear that the same need exists in regard to relaxation training when used in and of itself as an anxiety-reducing technique.

Paul's review suggested that introversion–extraversion may be a relevant variable to investigate. Eysenck's personality theory (Eysenck & Rachman, 1965) postulates extraversion as a personality variable affecting conditionability. Namely, extraverts condition poorly and need more time to learn new behavior due to their biologically determined tendency to rapidly develop reactive inhibitions. Introverts, on the other hand, condition rapidly, build up reactive inhibition slowly, and dissipate it quickly. Assuming that muscle relaxation training involves conditioning to some extent, then introverts should learn to relax better than extraverts. If one accepts the previously mentioned aspects of both Spielberger's and Eysenck's theories, then relaxation training should produce (*a*) more anxiety state reduction in introverts than in extraverts and (*b*) no significant anxiety trait reduction in either introverts or extraverts.

METHOD

Subjects

The subjects were 36 undergraduate female students at the University of Southern Mississippi. They were drawn from undergraduate psychology classes and received course credit for their participation. The average age was 20. All of the subjects were defined as anxious by virtue of falling at least one-half of one standard deviation above the trait

[1] Requests for reprints should be sent to John Stoudenmire, who is now at the Mental Health Complex, 830 South Gloster Street, Tupelo, Mississippi 38801.

JOHN A. STOUDENMIRE

TABLE 1

PRETREATMENT AND POSTTREATMENT RESULTS OF RELAXATION TRAINING IN INTROVERTS AND
EXTRAVERTS ON VARIOUS STATE AND TRAIT ANXIETY MEASURES

Anxiety measure	Group	Pretreatment		Posttreatment		t
		M	SD	M	SD	
STAI Anxiety State	Introverts	42.39	11.39	33.50	7.47	2.77*
	Extraverts	43.78	8.48	37.89	9.42	1.97
MAACL Anxiety (Today Form)	Introverts	8.33	4.10	5.46	3.85	2.16*
	Extraverts	7.50	5.69	4.36	4.72	1.80
STAI Anxiety Trait	Introverts	51.61	8.48	48.56	10.25	<1.00
	Extraverts	49.67	4.68	48.22	6.94	<1.00
TMAS	Introverts	25.94	9.45	24.89	9.61	<1.00
	Extraverts	27.06	7.01	28.17	6.88	<1.00
EPI Neuroticism	Introverts	14.39	4.75	13.17	4.48	<1.00
	Extraverts	15.50	3.79	15.33	4.27	<1.00

*$p < .05$.

anxiety mean of the State-Trait Anxiety Inventory (STAI) as published in the test manual (Spielberger & Gorsuch, 1966). Eighteen of the subjects were introverts, and 18 were extraverts as defined by the extraversion score on the Eysenck Personality Inventory (EPI; Eysenck & Eysenck, 1968).

Apparatus

Recording of instructions. To achieve uniformity in the presentation of verbal instructions in relaxation, a long playing phonograph record was used (Lazarus & Abramovitz, 1962). This recording has been used extensively by Lazarus (1964) in his own experimentation and private practice.

Measures of anxiety. The first measure of anxiety state was the Anxiety State scale of the STAI (Spielberger & Gorsuch, 1966). This scale consists of 20 statements that require people to indicate how they feel at the particular point in time. The subject indicates his answer on a 4-point rating scale ranging from "not at all" to "very much."

The second measure of anxiety state was the Anxiety scale of the Today form of the Multiple Affect Adjective Check List (MAACL; Zuckerman & Lubin, 1965). The MAACL contains 132 adjectives denoting affect, 21 of which relate to the presence or absence of anxiety. Others relate to depression or hostility. The subject is instructed to check off the adjectives that describe his feelings. In the Today form, the subject indicates how he feels "today" or "now." This measure is used as an anxiety state measure of anxiety. A general form is also available in which the subject indicates his general, day-in and day-out feelings. The general form is considered an anxiety trait measure.

The first anxiety trait measure was the anxiety trait scale of the STAI. This scale consists of 20 statements which ask people to indicate how they

feel in general. It also has a 4-point rating scale as has the Anxiety State scale.

The second anxiety trait measure was the Taylor Manifest Anxiety Scale (TMAS, Taylor, 1953). It contains 50 items selected from the MMPI which are answered true or false by the subject.

The third anxiety trait measure was the Neuroticism on the Eysenck Personality Inventory (Eysenck & Eysenck, 1968). It contains 57 items which the subject answers "yes" or "no." Twenty-four of the items relate to neuroticism, and 24 relate to introversion–extraversion.

Procedure

The 36 subjects were seen in groups of 6 subjects each. Within each group, there was an equal number of introverts and extraverts. The introverts and extraverts were matched on the pretreatment scores on each of the five above-mentioned anxiety state and anxiety trait measures of anxiety. The groups then received three sessions of muscle relaxation training. Each group received a different combination of length of session (15, 30, or 45 minutes) and schedule of session (three sessions spaced over 3 days, 9 days, or 15 days). An equal number of introverts and extraverts received each such combination. The above-mentioned anxiety measures were administered in counterbalanced orders at the pretreatment session and after the third treatment session.

RESULTS AND DISCUSSION

A comparison was made of the pretreatment and posttreatment scores for introverts and for extraverts on each of the anxiety measures, and the results are presented in

Table 1. The results indicate that the relaxation training produced no significant decrease in any of the three anxiety trait measures. There was, however, significant decrease in both of the anxiety state measures for introverts but not for extraverts. Although there was some anxiety state reduction in extraverts, it did not reach significance at the .05 level of confidence.

The results are seen as supporting Spielberger's theory which postulates anxiety state reduction following relaxation training but not anxiety trait reduction. Apparently, techniques of broader scope and/or longer duration are required to reduce anxiety trait.

The results also lend tentative support to Eysenck's theory of faster learning and conditioning in introverts than in extraverts. Muscle relaxation perhaps cannot be called "true" conditioning, but it does involve some learning and conditioning, and apparently it is affected by such personality variables as extraversion. Implications for therapy may be that introverts would respond better to systematic desensitization therapy, whereas other techniques would work better for extraverts. More research is needed, however, to replicate these findings and to explore other parameters of effective anxiety reduction.

REFERENCES

EYSENCK, H. J., & EYSENCK, S. B. G. *Eysenck Personality Inventory*. San Diego, Calif.: Educational and Industrial Testing Service, 1968.

EYSENCK, H. J., & RACHMAN, S. *Causes and cures of neurosis*. San Diego, Calif.: Knapp, 1965.

JOHNSON, D. T., & SPIELBERGER, C. D. The effects of relaxation training and the passage of time on measures of state- and trait-anxiety. *Journal of Clinical Psychology*, 1968, **24**, 20–23.

LAZARUS, A. A. Crucial procedural problems in desensitization therapy. *Behaviour Research and Therapy*, 1964, **2**, 65–70.

LAZARUS, A. A., & ABRAMOVITZ, A. *Learn to relax: A recorded course in muscular relaxation*. Troubadour Records, Wolhuter, Johannesburg, 1962.

PAUL, G. L. Outcome of systematic desensitization. II: Controlled investigation of individual treatment, technique variations, and current status. In C. M. Franks (Ed.), *Behavior therapy: Appraisal and status*. New York: McGraw-Hill, 1969.

SPIELBERGER, C. D. (Ed.) *Anxiety and behavior*. New York: Academic Press, 1966.

SPIELBERGER, C. D., & GORSUCH, R. *Mediating processes in verbal conditioning*. (Final rep. to the National Institutes of Mental Health and Child Care and Human Development, United States Public Health Service, Grants MH 7229 and 7446, and HD 947) Washington, D. C.: United States Public Health Service, 1966.

TAYLOR, J. A. A personality scale of manifest anxiety. *Journal of Abnormal and Social Psychology*, 1953, **48**, 285–290.

ZUCKERMAN, M., & LUBIN, B. *Manual for the Mulitple Affect Adjective Check List*. San Diego, Calif.: Educational and Industrial Testing Service, 1965.

(Received October 4, 1971)

From W. J. Di Scipio (1971). Perceptual and Motor Skills, *33*, 82, *by kind permission of the author and Southern Universities Press*

PSYCHOMOTOR PERFORMANCE AS A FUNCTION OF WHITE NOISE AND PERSONALITY VARIABLES

WILLIAM J. DI SCIPIO

Albert Einstein College of Medicine and Bronx State Hospital

The tendency of white noise to facilitate performance on certain vigilance and psychomotor tasks has been demonstrated under conditions of noise compared with silence (3, 4). In this respect, white noise is considered a useful experimental manipulation which increases cortical arousal. Eysenck (2) proposes that differential levels of arousal are related to personality type. Thus, the relation of level of arousal to psychomotor performance should vary as a function of both personality variables and external conditions such as white noise. It was hypothesized that, if introverts, characterized by high levels of arousal, are consequently at or near optimal performance levels initially, white noise would provide arousing properties only for the extraverts who are characterized by low levels of arousal. Also, if white noise becomes a distracting stimulus over successive trials, then noise would decrease efficiency of performance by extraverts before that by introverts because the former are more susceptible to distraction.

Ten men and 4 women of above average intelligence were divided into two groups of 7 Ss each on the basis of extreme scores of extraversion and introversion (E-I) on the Eysenck Personality Inventory, Form A. Ss were individually administered Ammons' version of the Tsai-Partington test (1) for 14 1-min. trials. Each trial required sequential connection of numbers which were distributed randomly on a sheet of paper. The first trial was accompanied by 80±5 db spl of white noise, alternating on each of the following trials with silence. Ammons' test was selected because of the minimal effects of learning associated with massed trials.

The significance of the difference in performance levels as a function of noise-silence, E-I, and trials was assessed by a repeated measures analysis of variance. The interaction of noise-silence by trials was significant ($F = 2.26$, $df = 6/156$, $p < .05$), indicating that performance under noise was better than silence initially for all Ss but this relationship reversed by the last trial. In accordance with hypothesis 1, on initial noise trials extraverts ($M = 15.0$, $SD = 5.3$) scored higher than introverts ($M = 13.0$, $SD = 2.0$), but this difference was nonsignificant. To assess the personality effect, difference scores were obtained for each group by subtracting the first noise trial from the last noise trial and handling first and last silent trials similarly. A 2×2 analysis of variance was applied to these data, with noise-silence and E-I as independent variables. The E-I effect was significant ($F = 4.44$, $df = 1/24$, $p < .05$). Performance for extraverts declined under noise ($M = -1.9$, $SD = 2.5$) and increased for introverts ($M = 2.3$, $SD = 3.7$).

White noise thus facilitated psychomotor performance as expected but only for a period of time after which performance was better for all groups under the silent condition. This finding suggests that increased arousal resulting from moderately loud white noise may become a distracting or aversive stimulus over time. As expected, extraverts were more susceptible than introverts to this effect.

REFERENCES

1. AMMONS, C. H. Temporary and permanent inhibitory effects associated with acquisition of a simple perceptual-motor skill. *Journal of General Psychology*, 1960, 62, 223-245.
2. EYSENCK, H. J. *The biological basis of personality.* Springfield, Ill.: Thomas, 1967.
3. KIRK, R. E., & HECHT, E. Maintenance of vigilance by programmed noise. *Perceptual and Motor Skills*, 1963, 16, 553-560.
4. OLTMAN, P. K. Field dependence and arousal. *Perceptual and Motor Skills*, 1964, 19, 441.

Accepted June 17, 1971.

From R. D. Savage and R. R. Stewart (1972). British Journal of Psychology, 63, 445–450, by kind permission of the authors and Cambridge University Press

PERSONALITY AND THE SUCCESS OF CARD-PUNCH OPERATORS IN TRAINING

By R. DOUGLASS SAVAGE AND RONALD R. STEWART*

*Department of Psychological Medicine,
University of Newcastle upon Tyne*

A short battery of tests consisting of the Eysenck Personality Inventory, a test of clerical aptitude and a coding test was given to a group of 100 young female card-punch operators during their first day in training. Test results were related to supervisors' ratings of output made at the end of each month of a three-month training period. There were significant negative correlations between extraversion and output ratings during the first two stages of training ($r = -0.29$, $P < 0.01$; $r = -0.33$, $P < 0.01$), but the relationship at the third stage fell short of significance. Neuroticism and coding scores were not related to training performance, but clerical aptitude became significant during the last month.

The report presents information on the relationship between the personality dimensions of Introversion–Extraversion and Neuroticism as measured by the Eysenck Personality Inventory (EPI) and the success achieved by young female card-punch operators in training. Klemmer & Lockhead (1962), in their analysis of productivity and error rates among IBM card-punch and bank proof machine operators, found a large gap between the performance of the best and poorest operators. Among experienced workers, the fastest tended to produce about twice as much as the slowest. They chose not to speculate on the factors involved in this discrepancy, but their results show that a need exists for further attempts to identify the range of factors involved in success or failure in these jobs. Although there exists a considerable literature on the aptitudes needed for success in clerical work, the number of studies utilizing quantitative personality measurements are limited. However, in the EPI Manual, Eysenck & Eysenck (1964a) present normative data on the personality characteristics of a mixed group of clerical workers which show them to be somewhat less extraverted (more introverted) than the average, but average with respect to neuroticism. This finding also has a certain amount of face validity in that one might expect clerical workers to be generally less socially driven and less impulsive than other work groups.

Theoretically, one could predict that on many clerical tests, particularly those of a routine nature, extraverts would do less well than introverts because of their tendency to build up relatively quickly higher levels of reaction and conditioned inhibition than introverts. Several laboratory studies have tended to support this prediction as far as simple motor tasks are concerned (Eysenck, 1959). In addition, Lynn (1960), using an inverted alphabet printing task, found that extraverts showed greater reminiscence than introverts, and gave some suggestion of greater work decrement under conditions of massed practice.

Tapping tasks also provide a convenient form of behaviour for studying the interaction of personality variables and simple motor skills. Jensen (1966) used Morse telegraph keys weighted by different amounts in studying reactive inhibition. His

---

* Now at the Department of Education, University of Liverpool.

R. Douglass Savage and R. R. Stewart

results were consistent with the view that the build up of reactive inhibition should be greater under massed than under distributed practice, greater under fast than under slow rates of tapping and least when tapping was self-paced. In the occupational field, card-punch operating may well be regarded as sufficiently related to tapping for a similar conceptual framework to apply. Work activity is sustained for periods long enough for inhibition effects to be expected to exert an influence on performance and, if Eysenck (1959) is right, the performance of extraverts will suffer most. Self-regulated punching will, of course, go on within the working period, and this will allow some reactive inhibition to dissipate. Overall output level should, however, be affected more in the case of the extraverts than introverts and show itself in reduced speed, if not in reduced accuracy, of performance.

Cooper & Payne (1967) have carried out a study among female packers in a tobacco factory which showed that extraversion, as measured by the EPI, was linked with several measures of job success. The more extraverted subjects had worse 'job adjustment' as rated by supervisors, shorter periods of service and a higher rate of absenteeism. A similar finding with respect to extraversion and absenteeism was reported by Taylor (1966).

The aim of the present study is to extend investigations into the field of training to see if similar relationships emerge. In addition to the EPI, scores on a clerical aptitude test and a visuo-motor coordination test were obtained and examined in relation to supervisors' ratings of a group of trainee card-punch operators. This information is considered as important for selection and may influence turnover and failure rates.

METHOD

Assessments

The measures used were the EPI (Eysenck & Eysenck, 1964a), tests of name and number checking taken from the Minnesota Clerical Test (Andrew & Paterson, 1959), and a coding test adapted from the Digit Substitution subtests of the Wechsler Adult Intelligence Scale (Wechsler, 1955).

The EPI is a self-administered questionnaire and consists of two parallel forms, A and B. Here, both forms, comprising 114 items, were used and total scores for both scales are reported. The test gives measures of Introversion–Extraversion (E scale), Neuroticism (N scale), and includes a measure of the subject's tendency to give socially desirable responses, called the Lie scale (L scale).

The names and number comparison tests were 5-min. timed versions of the Minnesota Clerical test, with a 3-min. rest-pause between them. A composite score (names plus numbers) was also obtained.

The coding test was used as a measure of visuo-motor coordination which also shows a moderately high correlation with general intelligence. The WAIS coding subtest was given by group administration.

Finally, the *criterion measures* of training success were made by supervisors at the end of each month of the three-month training period. The supervisors were asked to rate the efficiency of the trainee with respect to the speed and accuracy of her punching. Each set of ratings was made by the supervisors independently of any information previously obtained for the purpose of the study, such as initial test scores or earlier rating information. One exception to this was when termination of employment arose. Supervisors were then given access to previous ratings, but not to test scores. The operators were rated on a five-point scale, five being the best rating category, at the end of each month. Rating 1 was carried out by a single supervisor responsible for training all the girls to operate a conventional typewriter keyboard. The basis of judgement at this point was relatively objective, as speed and accuracy tests were given throughout the

Training of card-punch operators

Table 1. *Personality and the success of card-punch operators in training:*
means, standard deviations and ranges for all variables

Variable	Mean	S.D.	Range
Age	15·75	0·97	15–19
E scale	28·97	6·25	8–44
N scale	25·65	8·62	8–43
L scale	5·57	2·71	1–13
Coding	55·15	10·69	25–86
Names	41·20	10·51	16–66
Numbers	41·70	9·65	14–61
Total names and numbers	82·50	19·60	30–125
Rating 1	3·38	1·20	1–5
Rating 2	2·74	0·92	1–4
Rating 3	2·74	1·02	1–4

month. In the case of ratings 2 and 3, however, a uniform criterion of output was not available as the operators had split up to work on different types of machines. Their ratings were made by two different but highly experienced supervisors who shared the training responsibility.

Subjects

The subjects were the total group of trainee card-punch operators selected by officers of the Ministry of Health and Social Security for the clerical branch of the British Civil Service during 1966. They were recruited in groups of about 25 over a four-month period and were tested in groups during their first day in training. The selection requirements for entry were not stringent and no previous testing had taken place. The sample was not, therefore, likely to be biased as to intelligence and/or personality adjustment. A total of 100 girls was tested with an average age of 15·8 years, S.D. = 0·98 years.

Before testing began, the girls were reassured that the tests were not part of the selection process and that the people carrying them out were not Civil Service employees, but researchers from the local university. They were told that individual results would not be made known to their employers, although they would, in the course of events, be told how the group as a whole performed. On that basis, all the subjects were cooperative in the group testing.

RESULTS

The means and standard deviations for each of the measures employed are shown in Table 1. Table 2 presents the product-moment correlations between the psychological test measures and supervisors' ratings of output at each of the three stages of training. The hypothesis of a significant relationship between the EPI E scale and performance in training is confirmed at the 1 per cent level for the first two stages of training, but falls below an acceptable level at the third stage. Conversely, the measures of clerical aptitude do not show an association with success until the final month.

Neither the EPI N scale nor the coding test are correlated with the supervisor ratings. There is a correlation between the L scale and rating 2, which is significant at the 5 per cent level. This correlation does not yield to easy interpretation and, in the absence of additional evidence or theoretical position, may be regarded as a chance phenomenon.

An incidental, but interesting finding is that extraversion is not related to scores on the clerical or visuo-motor tests. This suggests that during these tests, at least within the time intervals given here, reactive inhibition has not built up sufficiently to handicap extraverts on these measures.

Table 2. *Personality and the success of card-punch operators in training: product-moment correlations between all main variables*

	E scale	N scale	L scale	Coding	Names	Numbers	Total names and numbers	Rating 1	Rating 2	Rating 3
E scale	—	+0·09	−0·30**	+0·02	+0·14	+0·11	+0·15	−0·29**	−0·34**	−0·14
N scale		—	−0·29**	−0·06	+0·14	+0·08	+0·10	−0·13	−0·06	−0·10
L scale			—	+0·16	−0·02	−0·01	−0·02	+0·15	+0·25**	+0·10
Coding				—	+0·23*	+0·17	+0·19*	−0·02	+0·10	+0·12
Names					—	+0·59**	+0·78**	+0·12	+0·08	+0·25**
Numbers						—	+0·93**	+0·02	+0·13	+0·27**
Total names and numbers							—	+0·05	+0·06	+0·27**
Rating 1								—	+0·50**	+0·45**
Rating 2									—	+0·68**
Rating 3										—

* P < 0·05. ** P < 0·01.

Training of card-punch operators

DISCUSSION

The means and standard deviations for the measures used are consistent with the previous reports of Andrew & Paterson (1959), Cooper & Payne (1967), Eysenck & Eysenck (1964*a*) and Klemmer & Lockhead (1962). The present results complement the findings of Cooper & Payne that extraversion is an important personality dimension in the performance of simple, repetitive skills, by identifying its influence during training. In the card-punch operating training described here, it seems that extraversion is more important in job success in the early stages of training and clerical aptitude less so, with the relative importance of these attributes being reversed at a later stage. This may well relate to the differential build-up of inhibition in learning between extraverts and introverts. The period of observation is, of course, very short and these trends in the data might not necessarily continue outside the period of training. The role of extraversion, however, may follow a fluctuating course and also relate to other job factors such as absenteeism and turnover at later stages. Within the training period, 12 out of the 100 trainees had their employment terminated because of poor work: their average E score is 32·00 compared to the average E of 28·56 for the 'survivors'. The t value does not reach the 5 per cent significance level, but is suggestive of a tendency for the extraverts to drop out from the job.

Eysenck & Eysenck (1964*b*) have pointed out that E and N scores are contaminated by social desirability bias, when obtained for personnel selection purposes. In spite of the fact that our subjects were given reassurances before testing that the results were 'off the record', distortion towards less neuroticism and less extraversion occurred. The tendency to play down extraverted characteristics is interesting and possibly resulted from a job stereotype that the girls shared. A liking for travel and social stimulation and excitement of various kinds was not likely to be satisfied by this job, and the girls gave more introverted responses than if they had been, say, trainee airline hostesses. Fortunately, the extent of the distortion has not been sufficient to mask the link between extraversion and rated output, which appears, in the circumstances, rather more impressive. A question one might ask is how much more social desirability and 'job' desirability bias will appear when the test is used under selection conditions and how this can best be controlled. One procedure would be to reject individuals whose lie scores were above a cut-off value. If the cut-off point were set on the basis of this investigation, it would, in any event, be a safety-first measure as respondents appear to under- rather than over-estimate their extraversion when their lie scores are high. A very high lie score in itself might also be regarded as a negative indicator for selection.

As the extraversion dimension seems to be important in the early training phase of card-punch operators, it suggests that training methods should reflect the current theoretical and practical views on speed versus massed practice.

We are grateful to The Training Section, Department of Health and Social Security, Longbenton, Newcastle upon Tyne, for their cooperation in this project.

R. Douglass Savage and R. R. Stewart

References

Andrew, D. M. & Paterson, D. G. (1959). *Manual of the Minnesota Clerical Test*. New York: Psychological Corporation.

Cooper, R. & Payne, R. (1967). Extraversion and some aspects of work behaviour. *Personnel Psychol.* **20**, 45–57.

Eysenck, H. J. (1959). *Manual of the Maudsley Personality Inventory*. London: University of London Press.

Eysenck, H. J. & Eysenck, S. B. G. (1964a). *Manual of the Eysenck Personality Inventory*. London: University of London Press.

Eysenck, S. B. G. & Eysenck, H. J. (1964b). 'Acquiescence' response set in personality inventory items. *Psychol. Rep.* **14**, 513–514.

Jensen, A. R. (1966). The measurement of reactive inhibition in humans. *J. gen. Psychol.* **75**, 85–93.

Klemmer, E. T. & Lockhead, G. R. (1962). Productivity and errors in two keying tasks: a field study. *J. appl. Psychol.* **46**, 401–408.

Lynn, R. (1960). Extraversion, reminiscence and satiation effects. *Br. J. Psychol.* **51**, 319–324.

Taylor, P. J. (1966). The distribution of sickness absence in an oil refinery and a clinical investigation of 194 men with different sickness experience. (Unpublished M.D. thesis, London University.)

Wechsler, D. (1955). *Manual of the Wechsler Adult Intelligence Scale*. New York: Psychological Corporation.

(Manuscript received 12 August 1971)

From P. W. Horn (1975). The Journal of Psychology, *90*, 41–44, *by kind permission of the author and*
The Journal Press

EVIDENCE FOR THE GENERALITY OF REMINISCENCE
AS A FUNCTION OF EXTRAVERSION
AND NEUROTICISM*

Indiana State University

PAUL W. HORN

SUMMARY

The study was conducted in order to determine whether magnitude of reminiscence would vary consistently across different motor tasks as a function of personality factors. Twenty-eight male and female college students were all given eight trials on both the inverted alphabet printing and pursuit rotor tasks. Personality measures of extraversion and neuroticism were obtained on all Ss by means of the Eysenck Personality Inventory. Results indicated that extraverts showed significantly more reminiscence than introverts on both tasks. Data argued against a "task-specific" account of reminiscence and suggested rather that reminiscence effects are characteristic of the individual.

A. INTRODUCTION

Studies by Eysenck (3) have shown that reminiscence is an increasing function of extraversion as measured by the Eysenck Personality Inventory (EPI). Eysenck concluded that reminiscence is highly task-specific, and that theoretical accounts of the phenomenon in terms of reactive inhibition or consolidation might vary according to the nature of the task.[1] An alternative conceptualization is that reminiscence effects are specific to the organism, and that individuals characteristically reflect the reminiscence phenomenon. Support for this argument derives from the research of Ritzler and Rosenbaum (5) who interpret their findings in bilateral reminiscence in terms of a *characteristic* proprioceptive deficit in schizophrenics involving central integrating mechanisms.

---

* Received in the Editorial Office on January 31, 1975, and published immediately at Provincetown, Massachusetts. Copyright by The Journal Press.

[1] It should be noted that Eysenck's argument depends upon an extremely broad definition of reminiscence. His inclusion of recovery from tapping decrement as a reminiscence phenomenon goes beyond conventional usage which has emphasized improvement in performance to new levels not yet manifested by the subject.

JOURNAL OF PSYCHOLOGY

In the present study, it was hypothesized that if reminiscence is a consistent phenomenon of the central nervous system, predictable from measurable personality factors, magnitude of reminiscence should be significantly correlated in different behavioral tasks. Specifically, individuals high on extraversion and neuroticism would be expected to show greater amounts of reminiscence across tasks than those who score low on these dimensions. The neuroticism factor is linked by Eysenck (4) after Spence (6) to a drive mechanism purportedly facilitating performance on less complex tasks.

B. Method

1. *Subjects and Apparatus*

Subjects were 28 introductory psychology students (14 male and 14 female). The apparatus was a standard Lafayette Instrument Co. pursuit rotor which rotated at 60 rpm. Inverted alphabet printing was done on prepared sheets with rows of ¼ inch squares.

2. *Procedure*

All Ss were tested individually and treated the same. Each had eight massed 30 second trials on two tasks known to produce reminiscence effects regularly: rotary pursuit (PR) and inverted alphabet printing (IA). All Ss were given three minutes rest between trials 6 and 7 on both tasks in order to generate reminiscence effects. All Ss were, finally, given the EPI to measure extraversion and neuroticism. To control order effects, half the Ss were given the PR task first, and half the IA first.

Reminiscence scores were obtained by subtracting each S's performance (time on target; number of letters printed) on the last two prerest trials from the two postrest trials. Analyses of variance were computed on the basis of the top 14 and bottom 14 scores on both extraversion and neuroticism.

C. Results

Results indicate that extraverts showed significantly more reminiscence than introverts on both PR [F (1, 24) = 8.50, $p < .05$] and IA [F (1, 24) = 14.51, $p < .01$]. Sex differences were partitioned in a 2 × 2 factorial design and found not to be significant. Interaction between sex and extraversion was significant, however [F (1, 24) = 5.81, $p < .05$]. The significant interaction was almost entirely due to the high reminiscence values for male extraverts ($\overline{X} = 24.42$) as compared with the significantly lower values ($\overline{X} = 13.54$) of male introverts. Females were undifferentiated on this dimension, with reminiscence means of 17.30 and 16.27 for extraversion and introversion, respectively. The correlation between extraversion and PR reminiscence was $r = +.56$, t (26) $= 3.45$, $p < .01$. The correlation between extraversion and IA reminiscence was $r = +.66$, t (26) $= 4.48$, $p < .01$.

Analysis of the data in terms of neuroticism yielded chance outcomes for PR reminiscence. On IA reminiscence however, neurotics showed significantly more reminiscence than those who scored low on neuroticism [F (1, 24) $= 4.31$, $p < .05$]. No other evaluations regarding neuroticism were significant.

D. Discussion

Results confirm that personality dimensions of extraversion and neuroticism were significantly related to reminiscence across two perceptual motor tasks. Of particular interest is the observation that the sex differences commonly noted in these two tasks (1, 2) did not appear when the data were ordered on either the extraversion or neuroticism continuum. It appears from this that those factors associated with these personality dimensions were more prepotent in these tasks than those associated with sex differences.

It is worth noting that extraversion was a strong controlling variable on PR reminiscence for males, and that neuroticism was the controlling factor especially for females on the IA task. Further examination of this issue seems warranted if one conjectures that PR and extraversion are "male" dimensions, and IA and neuroticism "female" factors. Evidence of male PR and female IA superiority noted above, taken with the findings of the present study, suggest potentially important relationships between reminiscence, sex, and personality.

References

1. Archer, E. J., & Bourne, L. E. Inverted alphabet printing as a function of intertrial rest and sex. *J. Exper. Psychol.*, 1956, **52**, 322-328.
2. Buxton, C. E., & Grant, D. A. Retroaction and gains in motor learning: II. Sex differences, and a further analysis of gains. *J. Exper. Psychol.*, 1939, **25**, 198-208.
3. Eysenck, H. J. A three-factor theory of reminiscence. *Brit. J. Psychol.*, 1965, **56**, 163-181.
4. —— Personality and learning. *Studia Psychologia*, 1973, **15**, 93-104.

JOURNAL OF PSYCHOLOGY

5. RITZLER, B., & ROSENBAUM, G. Bilateral transfer of inhibition in the motor learning of schizophrenics and normals. *J. Motor Behav.*, 1974, **6**, 205-215.
6. SPENCE, K. W. A theory of emotionally based drive (D) and its relation to performance in simple learning situations. *Amer. Psychol.*, 1958, **13**, 131-141.

Department of Psychology
Indiana State University
Reeve Hall
Terre Haute, Indiana 47809

From C. D. Frith (1971). British Journal of Psychology, *62*, 187–197, *by kind permission of the author and Cambridge University Press*

STRATEGIES IN ROTARY PURSUIT TRACKING

By C. D. FRITH

Department of Psychology, Institute of Psychiatry, University of London

Ten measures were derived describing different aspects of the pursuit rotor performance of 30 subjects. These included variables indicating the shapes of the distribution of hit and miss lengths and also variables indicating the amount of rhythmicity present in performance. The relationship between the various measures suggested that performance could be described in terms of two factors. The first represented the level of attainment (total time on target). The second was independent of the first and represented different strategies of performance. The measures defining these strategies suggested that at one extreme people were concerned only with velocity-matching, while at the other extreme they were concerned only with position-matching. There was a strong relationship between strategy and personality, extraverts adopting velocity-matching and introverts adopting position-matching. There was no evidence that these differences in response style were due to the greater production of rest pauses by the extraverts.

Most of the changes in performance which occur during massed practice on the pursuit rotor have been explained, at least in part, in terms of Hull's (1943) concept of reactive inhibition (I_R). It has been suggested (Kimble, 1949) that during massed practice the build-up of reactive inhibition eventually produces gaps in performance (rest pauses) resulting in an overall lowering of performance. During a programmed rest the I_R will dissipate, resulting in better performance immediately after the rest (reminiscence). Eysenck (1956) has suggested that extraverts, because of their greater proneness to the build-up of inhibition, should show more rest pauses, and therefore more reminiscence than introverts. (More recently (Eysenck, 1965) he has explained the differences in reminiscence between introverts and extraverts in terms of consolidation and conditionability.) However, no direct evidence for the existence of these rest pauses has yet been produced. Although much study has been made of performance decrement, i.e. post-rest down-swing, in relation to such variables as length of pre-rest practice, length of rest, drive, etc., few detailed investigations of the actual changes in performance involved have been carried out. This is because few studies have ever considered any measure of pursuit rotor performance other than total time on target. This is a measure of attainment which does not allow distinction between different styles, or strategies, of performance which result in the same level of attainment. Differences in strategy might be the crucial component of individual differences in performance. This has already been found to be the case with another very simple motor skill. Spielman (1963) demonstrated that in a tapping task extraverts produced more rest pauses than introverts, but that both types of people produced the same number of taps. In this case simple attainment level could not reveal an important dimension of individual difference, nor could it reveal the existence of rest pauses. These could only be demonstrated in the distribution of intertap intervals. For people producing rest pauses this distribution was bimodal, having a small secondary distribution of abnormally long intertap intervals. To demonstrate the existence of rest pauses in rotary pursuit tracking it would similarly be necessary

C. D. FRITH

to study the distribution of miss lengths (i.e. lengths of times off target). The experiment to be reported here involved precisely this.

However, a previous experiment (Frith, 1968) involving rather simpler measures had already revealed interesting features of pursuit rotor performance which could not have been found from the study of total time on target alone. In this experiment the number of times contact was made with the target (hits) was recorded in addition to the total time on target. From these two measures the average time of each unbroken contact (average hit length) and the average miss length could be estimated. Thus two independent measures of performance were available. The total time on target indicated the attainment level. The number of hits could indicate different strategies of performance for the same total time on target, i.e. either many short hits and misses or few long hits and misses. It was found that while extraverted and introverted people did not differ in attainment level, extraverted people tended to adopt the strategy involving long hits and misses. This finding would be consistent with the hypothesis mentioned earlier that extraverts produce more rest pauses than introverts, if long average miss lengths can be taken to indicate the presence of rest pauses. No definite conclusions can be reached until the distributions of hit and miss lengths have been studied. Rest pauses must be defined as abnormally long misses occurring during performance. Such abnormality can only be defined in terms of the total distribution of misses.

METHOD

A variable pattern polar tracker (Model PRI 15, Shaw Laboratories, N.Y.) was used. In this piece of apparatus the target is provided by a radial strip of light set in a revolving turntable. Above this is placed a sheet of glass, the undersurface of which is covered with light-proof paper. Tracks of any shape can be made by cutting away the appropriate parts of this paper. The target is then seen as a patch of light moving around the track. The stylus was a rigid L-shaped rod with a photo-electric cell at its tip which closed a relay whenever it was over the target patch of light. The maximum speed of revolution of the target was 37·5 r.p.m. The track consisted of a centrally placed equilateral triangle with sides 17·1 cm long and 1·2 cm wide.

Since all points on this track are not equidistant from the centre of revolution the target changes speed, moving faster along those parts of the tracks (the corners) which are farthest from the centre.

The photo-electric pursuit rotor was linked with an oscillator and tape-recorder so that whenever the person was on target a tone was recorded on the tape. The tape was then played back into a LINC 8 computer through a triggering device which caused the tones recorded on the tape to operate a relay. The main program used to analyse these data was called ROTMAP, which processed a 5 min. session of work on the pursuit rotor which it divided into ten 30 sec. periods. For each period the program provided histograms of hit and miss lengths from 50 to 5000 msec. in 50 msec. steps and also the total time on target and the total number of hits.

There were 30 subjects, male volunteers aged between 20 and 35. They worked at the pursuit rotor for three 5 min. sessions separated by 10 min. rest. The first 5 min. session was treated as practice and not recorded, since it was thought that any strategies of performance would take some time to develop and stabilize. All subjects were given the EPI (Eysenck & Eysenck, 1964). The distribution of scores was as follows: mean Extraversion score = 10·2; S.D. = 5·4; range = 2–23; mean Neuroticism score = 10·3; S.D. = 5·9; range = 2–22.

Instructions were kept to a minimum, all the subjects being told to 'keep the end of the stylus on top of the moving light'. A demonstration performance was then given by the experimenter. When the subject was on target a red light on the front of the pursuit rotor apparatus lit up and this was pointed out to all subjects, but they could not hear the tone being recorded on tape.

RESULTS

Description of performance

The following analysis is based on data from the whole of the second 5 min. session of work. The third 5 min. session gave essentially the same results.

The most obvious feature of the hit and miss distribution was the large positive skew. The position of the mode was remarkably constant for all subjects, being at 200 msec. for the hit distribution and at 100 msec. for the miss distribution. If only those parts of the curves to the right of the mode were considered they bore a strong resemblance to the Poisson distribution, this being particularly so with the distribution of miss lengths. The Poisson distribution is a particularly attractive curve with which to describe these data since it is completely defined by one parameter. Also,

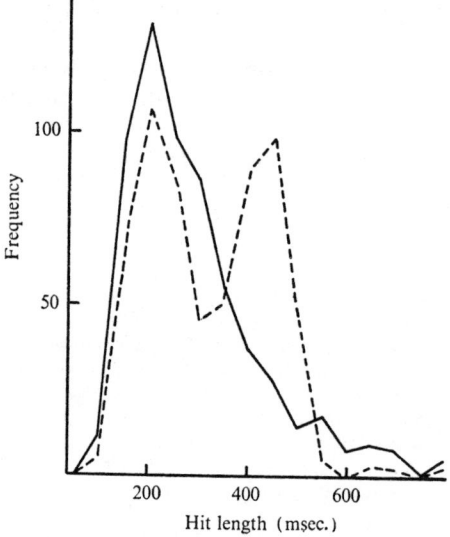

Fig. 1. Markedly different hit-length distributions for two subjects with the same level of performance in terms of total time on target. − − −, Subject H; ——, subject A.

the model itself has an intuitive appeal in the case of pursuit rotor performance, since the defining parameter would be the probability of coming off target in the case of the hit length distribution and the probability of coming on target in the case of the miss length distribution. The probabilities of coming on target and of coming off target should clearly be important components of pursuit rotor performance. They should be closely related to attainment, high attainment being associated with high probability of coming on target and low probability of coming off target. These two probabilities were estimated from the hit distributions. The probability of coming on target at 200 msec. after coming off it was given by the number of times this event occurred (i.e. number of miss lengths of 200 msec.) divided by the number of times the subject came back on target after this time interval or longer (i.e. number of miss lengths ⩾ 200 msec). The Poisson model requires that this probability should be the

Strategies in rotary pursuit tracking

C. D. Frith

same for all miss lengths and therefore only one estimate is needed for each subject. The most accurate estimation will be one involving the largest number of events. Probabilities were therefore calculated from the five classes of hit and miss lengths from 150 to 350 msec. and averaged.

The parts of the distributions to the left of the mode did not fit the Poisson model, there being too few short hit and miss lengths. Therefore a second parameter of the distributions was calculated for each subject which was the probability of coming back off or on target within 150 msec. or less.

There was another striking deviation from the Poisson distribution in that for many subjects the hit distribution was markedly bimodal. Fig. 1 shows the hit distribution for two subjects of the same performance level, one showing this bimodality and the other not. The mode of this secondary peak was also relatively constant across subjects, occurring at between 400 and 450 msec. Therefore a measure indicating the amount of bimodality in the hit distribution was calculated for each subject by subtracting the number of hits of length 300 and 350 msec. from the number of hits of length 400 and 450 msec., a high degree of bimodality giving a positive score and a lack of bimodality a negative score. It was considered that these five measures (Table 1) would sufficiently describe the hit and miss length distributions for each subject.

Five other measures were also derived to describe other aspects of performance. One was the total time on target during the 5 min. session. Another was derived from the curve relating hits and total time on target for each subject, being the number of hits at the maximum of the curve which was at 55 per cent time on target. This curve was derived by fitting a parabola to the 10 points given by the relation between total time on target and hits in each 30 sec. period of the 5 min. session. This procedure is exactly the same as the one used in the previous experiment (Frith, 1968) except that each curve is based on only 10 points from 30 sec. periods, whereas previously it was based on 30 points from 10 sec. periods.

Another measure was derived to indicate the frequency of occurrence of rest pauses. This was simply the number of miss lengths greater than 1000 msec. This cut-off point was chosen quite arbitrarily, the measure being supposed to provide information about particularly long misses.

The last two measures were concerned with the occurrence of rhythmicities in performance. The repetitive nature of the task and the shape of the track lead one to expect that rhythmicities should be present in performance. This would be especially likely if the subjects attempted to match their velocity with that of the target, since such subjects would try to make rhythmic movements. Thus it was hoped that the amount of rhythmicity present would indicate whether the subjects were paying attention to velocity errors rather than position errors. Such rhythmicities were investigated by calculating the spectral density function for pursuit rotor performance. This function was estimated with two LINC-8 programs written by the author. The first autocorrelated 30 sec. of pursuit-rotor performance and the second converted these autocorrelations into the spectral density function via a cosine transformation (Robinson, 1967). The data were 30 sec. taken from the middle of the 5 min. working session, i.e. from 2·5 to 3·0 min. For most subjects two peaks appeared in this function at 1·60 sec. per cycle and at 0·53 sec. per cycle, which

Strategies in rotary pursuit tracking

corresponded to the time for a complete revolution of the target and the time for the target to move down one side of the triangular track. The value of the spectral density function at each of these points for each subject was the last two measures used to describe performance.

Table 1 gives a list of all measures and their derivations.

Table 1. *Measures used to describe pursuit rotor performance*

1. Total time on target (TTT) in a 5 min. session.
2. Probability of a hit starting after 150 msec.
$$P(h) \geqslant 150 = \frac{\text{no. of misses between } 150\text{–}350 \text{ msec.}}{\text{no. of misses} \geqslant 150 \text{ msec.}}$$
3. Probability of a miss starting after 150 msec.
$$P(m) \geqslant 150 = \frac{\text{no. of hits between } 150\text{–}350 \text{ msec.}}{\text{no. of hits} \geqslant 150 \text{ msec.}}$$
4. Probability of a hit starting before 150 msec.
$$P(h) < 150 = \frac{\text{no. of misses} < 150}{\text{total no. of misses}}$$
5. Probability of a miss starting before 150 msec.
$$P(m) < 150 = \frac{\text{no. of hits} < 150 \text{ msec.}}{\text{total no. of hits.}}$$
6. Degree of bimodality of hit distribution.
   Bimod. = (no. of hits between 400 and 450 msec.)
   − (no. of hits between 300 and 350 msec.)
7. Estimated number of hits at 55 per cent total time on target.
   $h_{\max}$ is estimated from the best fit parabola relating hits and TTT in each 30 sec. period.
8. Rhythmicity with a period of 1600 msec. (1 rev.) from minutes $2\frac{1}{2}$–3 of the session.
9. Rhythmicity with a period of 533 msec. (1 side) from minutes $2\frac{1}{2}$–3 of the session.
10. Number of misses $\geqslant 1000$ msec.

Intercorrelations between the measures

Table 2 shows the correlation matrix for the 10 variables described and also the two personality measures of extraversion and neuroticism. In a principal component analysis of this matrix the first two factors accounted for about 60 per cent of the variance. Rotation in the plane defined by these two factors enabled one to define two alternative factors with about equal share of the variance, one of which loaded very highly on level of attainment (i.e. total time on target). The other variables loading most highly on this factor were $P(h) \geqslant 150$, $P(m) \geqslant 150$, and misses $\geqslant 1000$.

There is nothing surprising in this cluster of related measures. As expected, the probability of hits and misses starting related very strongly to total time on target. This gives some confirmation for the applicability of the Poisson model and shows that these measures based on the frequencies of hit and miss lengths from 150–350 msec. reflect a fundamental variable. It was also to be expected that subjects with large numbers of long misses should have a low level of attainment.

The second factor was chosen to be independent of total time on target and can therefore be represented by the correlation matrix in Table 3, from which total time on target has been partialled out. This table, since it shows relations independent of level of attainment, defines the strategies used by the subjects. The table reveals a

C. D. Frith

large cluster of related variables centred on the probabilities of hits and misses starting. Before total time on target was partialled out these correlated negatively (-0.542) but afterwards they correlated positively (0.583). The other variables loading most highly on this factor of strategy were h_{max}, rhythmicity (one rev.), bimodality and $P(h) < 150$.

Table 2. *Intercorrelations between measures of pursuit rotor performance for 30 subjects*

	TTT	Bimod.	$P(m) \geqslant 150$	$P(h) \geqslant 150$	$P(m) < 150$	$P(h) < 150$	h_{max}	One rev.	One side	Miss $\geqslant 1000$	E	N
TTT	.											
Bimod.	0·07	.										
$P(m) \geqslant 150$	−0·86	−0·22	.									
$P(h) \geqslant 150$	0·81	−0·14	−0·54	.								
$P(m) < 150$	−0·37	−0·12	0·45	−0·18	.							
$P(h) < 150$	0·86	0·46	−0·83	0·55	−0·36	.						
h_{max}	0·13	0·08	0·23	0·42	0·25	0·25	.					
One rev.	−0·33	−0·01	0·13	−0·54	0·09	−0·32	−0·30	.				
One side	−0·05	−0·03	−0·02	0·22	−0·26	−0·17	−0·06	−0·35	.			
Miss $\geqslant 1000$	−0·88	−0·15	0·67	−0·76	0·25	−0·73	−0·19	0·35	0·03	.		
E	0·14	0·45	−0·39	−0·15	−0·12	0·33	−0·32	0·01	0·18	−0·07	.	
N	−0·07	−0·16	0·07	−0·25	0·03	−0·00	−0·19	0·00	−0·26	0·16	−0·11	.

Table 3. *Intercorrelations between the measures of pursuit rotor performance, attainment level (TTT) partialled out*

	Bimod.	$P(m) \geqslant 150$	$P(h) \geqslant 150$	$P(m) < 150$	$P(h) < 150$	h_{max}	One rev.	One side	Miss $\geqslant 1000$	E	N
Bimod.	.										
$P(m) \geqslant 150$	−0·31	.									
$P(h) \geqslant 150$	−0·36	0·58	.								
$P(m) < 150$	−0·07	0·28	0·21	.							
$P(h) < 150$	0·68	−0·33	−0·51	−0·07	.						
h_{max}	0·07	0·69	0·54	0·31	0·02	.					
One rev.	0·01	−0·34	−0·50	−0·02	−0·10	−0·28	.				
One side	−0·03	−0·13	0·47	−0·30	−0·24	−0·05	−0·39	.			
Miss $\geqslant 1000$	−0·18	−0·38	−0·18	−0·16	0·13	−0·16	0·13	−0·01	.		
E	0·46	−0·54	−0·48	−0·08	0·45	−0·35	0·07	−0·17	0·12	.	
N	−0·15	0·01	−0·33	0·00	0·13	−0·19	−0·10	−0·24	0·20	−0·10	.

It can be seen from the partial correlation matrix (Table 3) that extraversion score also correlates highly with many of these measures. It is now necessary to consider the interpretation of this cluster of measures in terms of actual behaviour.

At least one of these relationships is a necessary result of the definitions of the measures. The finding that when total time on target is partialled out there is a positive correlation between the probability of a miss starting and the probability of a hit starting merely reflects the fact that for a given total time on target a subject who is more likely to come off target must be more likely to come on target (thus producing many short hits and misses). This aspect of performance is also measured by the variable h_{max} (the number of hits at 55 per cent time on target) which would therefore be expected to form part of the cluster. This measure was the one used to define strategy in the previous experiment and thus it seems that the cluster of variables defines the same strategy as was found in that experiment. However, with the additional measures taken it should now be possible to define these strategies more completely. It is not of course entirely necessary that $P(m)$ and $P(h)$ should be so closely related to the strategy defined in the first experiment since these measures are derived from hit and miss lengths between 150 and 350 msec. only. Thus the fact that these measures do relate so closely suggests that the strategies do concern these particular major sections of the hit and miss distributions and are not concerned merely with the occurrence of abnormally long misses or rest pauses. This is also suggested by the finding that the measure concerned with the frequency of long misses does not show either consistent or significant correlations with the various measures defining strategy.

There are three new and as yet unexplained aspects of strategy, which are bimodality, probability of hits starting in less than 150 msec., and rhythmicity with a period of one revolution of the target. The first two of these measures seem to be particularly highly related to each other (correlation 0·68). The probability of short misses loads in the opposite direction to the other hit and miss measures so that people characterized by long and therefore few hits and misses in the region above 150 msec. tend to show many of the very short misses.

DISCUSSION

It will be demonstrated later that there is an explanation for these effects by considering the particular tracking task used in greater detail. But first some remarks can be made concerning the rhythmicity measure. This measure is such that people showing in general relatively long and therefore few hits and misses (the low hit strategy of the previous experiment) show a high degree of rhythmicity with a period of one revolution of the target. It seems likely that this rhythmicity reflects concern with errors of velocity-matching. If a subject has matched velocity and is on target he will do very well. However, when he has matched velocity and is off target he will do very badly. Thus one might expect that his performance would be characterized by relatively long hits and misses resulting in the relation between measures that was found in the present study. A person who is concerned with position errors will correct such errors very quickly, thus showing short misses, but will fail to stay on target for long since he has not accurately matched velocity. Thus such a subject will show the high hit strategy of the previous experiment.

This detailed analysis of pursuit rotor performance has confirmed the results of the previous experiment demonstrating a strategy of pursuit rotor performance which is independent of level of attainment, and which relates significantly to the extraversion dimension of personality. However, the hypothesis that this dimension of individual differences would be related to the occurrence of rest pauses does not seem to be confirmed, since the dimension is concerned particularly with hit and miss lengths of 350 msec. and less. On the basis of the measures taken it is tentatively hypothesized that the differences in strategy reflect the subjects' concern with either errors of velocity or errors of position.

An estimate was made of the reliability of the two principal components of performance. Level of attainment (total time on target) showed a test–retest reliability of 0·700 (comparison of second and third 5 min. work sessions). A suitable measure of strategy was devised by adding together the principal measures that defined this

C. D. FRITH

dimension, i.e. $P(h)$ 150–350 and $P(m)$ 150–350. Since these two measures correlate equally with total time on target, but in opposite directions, adding them together effectively removes any relation to level of attainment. The correlation between this derived measure of strategy and total time on target was 0·032. The test–retest reliability of this strategy measure was 0·688. Thus both measures seem to be stable and characteristic of an individual's performance.

So far no attention has been paid to the particular nature of the task used in this experiment. The target that the subjects had to follow moved round a triangular track and therefore at the corners of the triangle the target abruptly changed direction. In addition, the target was produced by a radial band of light revolving underneath the track. It therefore moved much faster at the corners since these are farthest from the centre of revolution. Thus there were two factors making the target much more difficult to track at the corners of the triangle. It might be expected that these variations in task difficulty would affect the shape of the hit and miss distributions and might account for the bimodality shown by some subjects in the hit distribution. One noticeable feature of these distributions was that their modes occurred at the same points independent of both level of attainment and strategy. This suggests that the position of the modes is a function of the task itself. The target was revolving at 37·5 r.p.m. and so one revolution corresponded to 1600 msec. and one side of the triangle to 533·3 msec. Thus the two peaks of the bimodal hit distributions (250 and 450 msec.) corresponded to just under half a side and just under a side. Thus bimodality could be accounted for if the subjects' were particularly likely to come off in the middle of a side and at the end of a side. As has already been shown, subjects are particularly likely to come off at the end of a side when the corner occurs, but it seems very unlikely that they should come off at the middle of a side since at this point the target is moving more slowly than at any other time and in a straight line.

In order to investigate further the bimodality of the hit distribution two subjects were chosen from the original group who, while still available for testing, showed respectively extreme bimodality and extreme lack of bimodality. These subjects worked for another 5 min. with the triangular pursuit rotor, their performance on the last $2\frac{1}{2}$ min. being filmed with an 8 mm cine camera. When these films were viewed, differences in the subjects' performance were immediately apparent. There were two aspects of these differences. The first lay in the path followed by the subject's tracking stylus. Figs. 2 and 3 show the position of the end of the stylus in relation to the triangular track on successive frames of the film. The subject with the unimodal hit distribution (Fig. 2) shows a triangular course closely related to the track. The subject with the bimodal hit distribution (Fig. 3) follows a roughly circular course which thus necessarily cuts the corners of the triangle and sometimes swings out from the centre of the sides. The second aspect of the differences lay in the relationship between the end of the subject's tracking stylus and the position of the target. The subject whose stylus followed a circular course was nearly always radially in line with the target, even when he was not actually on the track. The subject following the triangular course, although nearly always on the track, was often in front of or behind the target. He showed a strong tendency to be behind the target immediately after rounding a corner and then to catch up with it rapidly to the extent of overshooting, especially since in terms of linear velocity the target was at this stage slowing down. Thus it is

Strategies in rotary pursuit tracking

clear, due perhaps to the paths the subjects choose to trace out, that one of them is concerned principally to match the angular velocity of the target, while the other is concerned with the spatial location of the target.

It is clear also that a bimodality of the hit distribution can result from the subject following a roughly circular path with his stylus. With such a path the subject will not only cut the corners of the triangle, but also will sometimes swing too far out at the centres of the sides. When this happens he will produce two hits with lengths equal to somewhat under half a side each. On those occasions when he does not swing too far out at the centre of a side he will produce one hit of approximately double the

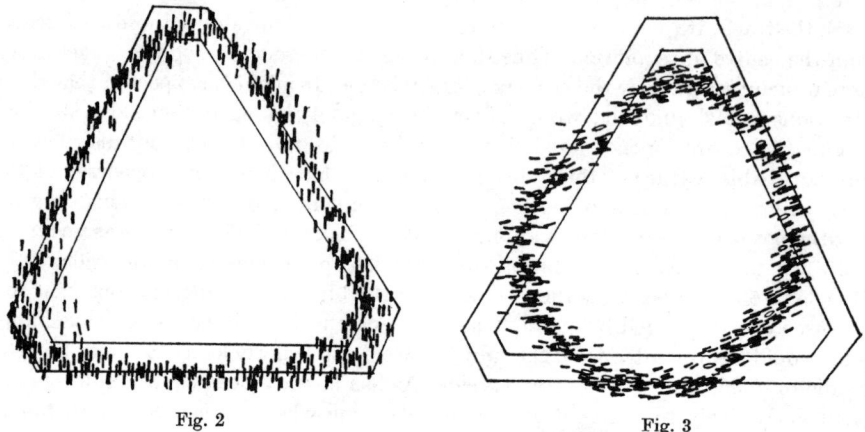

Fig. 2

Fig. 3

Fig. 2. Successive positions of the tracking stylus for a subject with a unimodal hit-length distribution.

Fig. 3. Successive positions of the tracking stylus for a subject with a bimodal hit-length distribution.

length. Intermediate values between these two will be much less frequent. This strategy of matching velocity will produce particularly short misses, since the subject, when returning to the track after cutting a corner or swinging too far out from the centre of a side, is automatically anticipating the position of the target, rather than having to catch up with it or take time for correcting movements. This will lead to a greater proportion of short misses and thus accounts for the high correlation between the probability of a hit starting in less than 150 msec. and bimodality.

This explanation of the bimodality of the hit distribution makes it fit in very well with the other measures of performance that were found to relate to bimodality, since these also suggested a dimension of strategy concerned with either velocity- or position-matching. However, it also shows that the shape of the track plays an important role in the determination of strategy. One way in which the photo-electric pursuit rotor differs from the one previously used is that the track the target follows is visible at all times, whereas with standard pursuit rotors only the target is visible. If, with the photo-electric pursuit rotor, subjects thought it an important part of the task to keep their stylus at all times in the right track even when not on target, they would be forced to adopt the position-matching strategy described above. It is entirely

C. D. Frith

consistent with the characteristics imputed to extraverts (risk-taking, not conscientious, etc.) who showed a significant tendency to bimodality that they should cut the corners of the triangle rather than stay rigidly in the tracks. Thus it might be that the differences between introverts and extraverts found in these experiments are specific to this kind of task in which the track is visible and not related to a more general favouring of velocity or position-matching.

It is clearly crucial to the hypothesis being put forward to study different track shapes and target velocities, since these variables should also influence the strategies adopted and their relation to personality. With regard to track shape it would be predicted that the farther removed this were from a circle in shape the more position-rather than velocity-matching would be adopted. Some evidence for this is provided by an earlier experiment (Frith, 1968) in which performance on the triangular track of the present study was compared with performance in a star-shaped track. Strategies of performance in terms of long or short hits were measured which in the light of the present results would be interpreted as velocity- and position-matching respectively. For both track shapes there was a significant relationship between strategy and personality, with extraverts tending to adopt velocity-matching. However, there was also a significant difference between tracks in the effects of practice on strategy. While practice on the star-shaped track had no effect on strategy, there was a general shift towards velocity-matching for the triangular track ($F = 26 \cdot 15$; d.f. $= 1, 18$; $P < 0 \cdot 001$) which was significantly greater for the introverted subjects ($F = 4 \cdot 56$; d.f. $= 1, 18$; $P < 0 \cdot 05$). These results support the hypothesis that the simpler triangular track induced velocity-matching and also that the introverts, since they tended to adopt position-matching, were more affected by this induction.

With regard to target speed it would be predicted that higher speeds would tend to induce velocity-matching since the fundamentally circular movement of the target would be more apparent and the position of the target at any instant would be more difficult to estimate. Performance of subjects in the present experiment has been compared with that of people practising on the same triangular track, but with a target speed of 50 r.p.m. instead of 37·5 r.p.m. I am indebted to Dr Gudrun Sartory for allowing me to use her data for this comparison. When groups were compared who had the same range of total time on target scores, the subjects tracking a target at 50 r.p.m. were significantly more likely to have long-hit strategies ($\chi^2 = 21 \cdot 08$; $P < 0 \cdot 001$). If long-hit strategies can be taken to indicate velocity-matching then this result confirms the hypothesis that high target speeds induce velocity-matching. For the group with the high target speed there was no relationship between strategy and extraversion. This would suggest that at this high speed all subjects rapidly adopt the strategy of matching velocity.

This experiment has confirmed the hypothesis that there are differences in the style of pursuit rotor performance between introverts and extraverts. However, this difference did not appear to result in extraverts producing more rest pauses than introverts. The cluster of measures defining the strategies rather suggested that the extraverts principally concerned themselves with errors of velocity-matching while the introverts principally concerned themselves with errors of position-matching. It is hoped that studies of pursuit rotor performance in terms of these strategies may be able to throw light on other phenomena such as the greater reminiscence shown by

Strategies in rotary pursuit tracking

extraverts as compared to introverts. It has been proposed that this difference between introverts and extraverts results from the greater proneness of the extraverts to the build-up of inhibition (Eysenck, 1956). This hypothesis could be reconciled with the present results if it is assumed that this inhibition build-up results, not in the production of rest pauses, but in a generally slower response rate. It is assumed that the responses in pursuit rotor performance consist of the detection and correction of errors and are therefore intermittent (Poulton, 1957). It seems probable that a slow rate of responding would favour velocity-matching whereas a fast rate of responding would favour position-matching. Estimation of velocity would require the integration of several successive positions of the target and would therefore take longer to estimate than position.

This study was supported by a grant from the Bethlem Royal and Maudsley Hospitals Research Fund. I am grateful to Professor H. J. Eysenck for his help and encouragement.

REFERENCES

EYSENCK, H. J. (1956). Reminiscence, drive and personality theory. *J. abnorm. soc. Psychol.* **53**, 328–333.

EYSENCK, H. J. (1965). A three-factor theory of reminiscence. *Br. J. Psychol.* **56**, 163–181.

EYSENCK, H. J. & EYSENCK, S. B. G. (1964). *Eysenck Personality Inventory.* London: University of London Press.

FRITH, C. D. (1968). Strategies in rotary pursuit tracking and their relation to inhibition and personality. *Life Sci.* **7**, 65–76.

HULL, C. L. (1943). *Principles of Behaviour.* New York: Appleton–Century–Crofts.

KIMBLE, G. A. (1949). An experimental test of a two-factor theory of inhibition. *J. exp. Psychol.* **39**, 15–23.

POULTON, E. C. (1957). On the stimulus and response in pursuit tracking. *J. exp. Psychol.* **53**, 189–194.

ROBINSON, E. A. (1967). *Multichannel Time Series Analysis with Digital Computer Programs.* London: Holden-Day.

SPIELMAN, I. (1963). The relation between personality and the frequency and duration of rest pauses during massed practice. (Unpublished Ph.D. thesis, University of London Library.)

(*Manuscript received* 17 *April* 1970)

From T. Fremont, G. H. Means, and R. S. Means (1970). Psychological Reports, *27, 455–458, by kind permission of the authors and Southern Universities Press*

ANXIETY AS A FUNCTION OF TASK PERFORMANCE FEEDBACK AND EXTRAVERSION-INTROVERSION

THEODORE FREMONT, GLADYS H. MEANS, AND ROBERT S. MEANS

Oklahoma State University

Summary.—200 volunteer Ss enrolled in a midwestern university were administered the Maudsley Personality Inventory (MPI). Those who scored in the top 15% and the bottom 15% of the population tested were identified as extraverts and introverts, respectively. These 2 groups, one composed of 30 extraverts and the other of 30 introverts, were administered the Digit Symbol test. Upon completion of the task, each S received one of three predetermined and randomly assigned types of feedback concerning his performance. Treatment I Ss were told that from the results of the Digit Symbol task, it appeared they had performed better than did most college students. Treatment II Ss were told that their task performance was lower than that of most college students. Treatment III Ss were given no information concerning their performances. A 2 ×3 multiple analysis of variance design was employed to analyze Ss' performances on the Multiple Affect Adjective Check List (MAACL), a standardized measure of anxiety, which was administered immediately after the feedback session. Significant differences were found on treatment and extravert-introvert dimension as well as an interactive effect.

Learning theory, in part supported by empirical evidence, suggests that knowledge of results following termination of performance is necessary for subsequent modification of the learning process and for future facilitation of appropriate task performance. Locke (1967) suggests that the positive influence of KR on learning and performance is one of the best established findings in the research literature. There have been limited systematic investigations, however, about the interactive influence that various types of feedback information and individual student characteristics might have on various dependent variables.

The intent of this investigation was to determine the effect that various types of feedback information interacting with selected personality traits might have on the dependent variable of anxiety level.

Individual students characterized as Introverts or Extraverts have been suggested as exhibiting unique patterns of academic performance in the classroom (Lynn & Gordon, 1961; Estrabrook & Sommer, 1966). Determining reactions to feedback given persons who differ significantly on this dimension might have implications for facilitating the learning process. In particular, this study was based upon the hypothesis that students characterized as Extraverts and those characterized as Introverts would react differentially to the type of feedback they received relative to prior task performance. It was also felt that the anxiety scores would be differentially influenced by the interaction of the extraversion-introversion dimension and the type of reinforcement administered.

T. FREMONT, *ET AL.*

METHOD

Two hundred volunteer Ss were solicited from those students enrolled in undergraduate educational psychology courses at a large midwestern university. Ss were administered the Maudsley Personality Inventory (Eysenck, 1962). The inventories were scored according to standardized procedures and the 15% ($N = 30$) with the lowest scores were identified as introverts. Similarly, the 15% ($N = 30$) with the highest scores were classified as extraverts. Students scoring between these extremes ($N = 140$) were dropped from the study. The remaining Ss ($N = 60$) were individually administered the Digit Symbol test (Wechsler, 1947). Upon completion of the test E scored the paper and proceeded to give one of the three predetermined types of feedback to S. The particular information given each S had been previously determined by separate random assignment of the two different groups under study. That is, each of the 30 extraverts was assigned to one of the three types of information by random procedure while each of the 30 introverts was randomly assigned in an identical but separate process. The first type of feedback consisted of telling S that his score was higher than that of the average college student. The second type involved communicating to S that his score was lower than that of the average college student. The third feedback situation simply centered around the statement that no comparison could be made of S's performance with college norms at that time.

Immediately after the statements were given, Ss were handed the Multiple Affect Adjective Check List (Zuckerman & Lubin, 1965), an anxiety scale, and asked to fill it out.

A 2×3 multiple analysis of variance design was employed to analyze performance on the anxiety scale. To ensure that the data could meet the basic assumptions of homogeneous variances, the F Max test was utilized. An F ratio of 4.74, a nonsignificant value, resulted.

RESULTS

An analysis of the differences in performance among the various treatment groups on the anxiety scale is summarized in Table 1. The following conclusions may be drawn. In this study the type of feedback given Ss significantly influenced their anxiety scores as measured on the MAACL. Duncan's multiple-range

TABLE 1

SUMMARY OF ANALYSIS OF VARIANCE

Source	SS	df	MS	F	P
Treatments (Feedback)	290.233	2	145.117	45.82	<.001
Levels (Introversion-Extraversion)	45.067	1	45.067	14.23	<.001
Interaction (F × I-E)	71.433	2	35.717	11.28	<.001
Error	171.000	54	3.167		
Total	577.733	59			

ANXIETY, FEEDBACK, AND EXTRAVERSION

TABLE 2

MEANS AND STANDARD DEVIATIONS FOR VARIOUS TREATMENT GROUPS ON MAACL

		Positive Information	Negative Information	No Information	Combined
Extraverts	M	5.70	8.60	6.90	7.06
	SD	1.57	2.01	1.52	2.04
Introverts	M	6.20	13.40	6.80	8.80
	SD	1.23	2.68	1.23	3.76
Combined	M	5.95	11.00	6.85	7.93
	SD	1.39	3.37	1.34	3.12

test ($p < .01$) showed that the negative feedback mean was significantly greater than the positive feedback mean and the no-feedback mean. There was no significant difference between the positive and no-feedback means.

In this study the particular orientation, extraversion or introversion, was significantly related to Ss' anxiety scores. The introverts had significantly higher anxiety scores than the extraverts ($p < .001$). Finally, the feedback given Ss significantly interacted with the type of orientation (extraversion or introversion) to help shape the scores made on the anxiety scale ($p < .001$). An analysis of simple interactive effects showed that the significant interaction with introversion-extraversion was between negative and positive feedback ($p < .001$) and between negative and no feedback ($p < .001$). Thus, the effect on

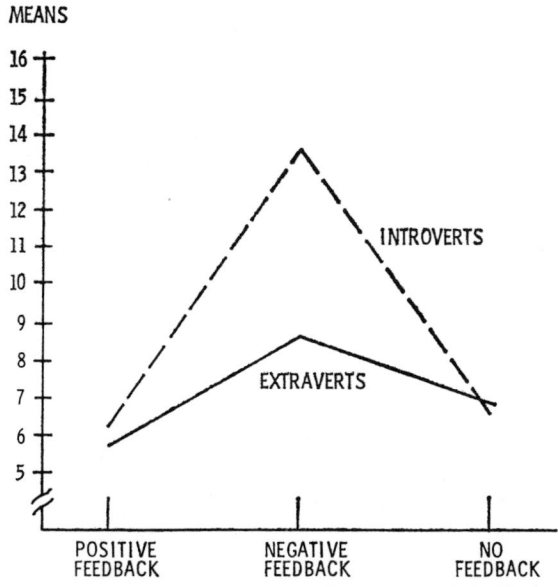

FIG. 1. Effect of Extraversion-Introversion dimension and feedback information on MAACL scores

the anxiety measure exerted by introverts and extraverts was dependent on the differences in the type of feedback given. More specifically, introverts given negative feedback demonstrated significantly higher anxiety than did extraverts given negative feedback ($p < .001$). No significant differences were found between extraverts and introverts on positive or no-feedback treatments. The interactive effect is graphically presented in Fig. 1.

These results present very limited implications for practical application at this time, but extensive research on types of feedback given students and their personality traits might be useful. Although the results yield no information concerning the lasting or long-term effects that type of feedback might have on level of anxiety, such a possibility should be explored.

REFERENCES

ESTRABROOK, M., & SOMMER, R. Study habits and introversion-extraversion. *Psychological Reports*, 1966, 19, 750.

EYSENCK, H. J. *Manual of the Maudsley Personality Inventory.* San Diego: Educational & Industrial Testing Service, 1962.

LOCKE, E. Motivational effects of knowledge of results: knowledge or goal-setting. *Journal of Applied Psychology*, 1967, 51, 324-329.

LYNN, R., & GORDON, E. I. The relationship of neuroticism and extraversion to intelligence and educational attainment. *British Journal of Educational Psychology*, 1961, 31, 194-203.

WECHSLER, D. *The Wechsler Adult Intelligence Scale manual.* New York: Psychological Corp., 1947.

ZUCKERMAN, M., & LUBIN, B. *Manual for the Multiple Affect Adjective Check List.* San Diego: Educational & Industrial Testing Service, 1965.

Accepted July 8, 1970.

PART VII

LEARNING AND CONDITIONING

Just as it is sometimes difficult to make a clear distinction between perception and motor movement, so it is not always easy to distinguish between learning and conditioning, on the one hand, and memory and retrieval, on the other. There can be no memory without learning, and no assessment of learning without measurement of what is remembered. At best, therefore, the distinction is a heuristic one, and it should certainly not be taken too seriously. Nevertheless, we can vary conditions which primarily affect learning (number of repetitions, spacing of repetitions, strength of UCS, etc.), or we can vary conditions which primarily affect reproduction (duration of learning–reproduction interval, induced level of arousal at reproduction, etc.); in this way it is possible to attempt at least to keep one variable constant while varying the other.

As pointed out in the first section, a great deal of work has been done on the Hull–Spence model of personality which postulates just one major variable, manifest anxiety, which is conceived as a drive variable. Eysenck (1973) has reviewed the evidence regarding this model at some length, and has come to the conclusion that the main weakness of this model is that the major concept of manifest anxiety is not univocal; in other words, the MAS of Janet Taylor measures both E (negatively) and N (positively.) Subjects selected on the basis of this scale as being high or low in anxiety respectively are either neurotic introverts or stable extraverts; as a consequence, it is impossible to make any specific predictions, or to interpret unambiguously the results from any experiments using the MAS. In so far as differences in drive are concerned, it would be predicted that it is differences in E which are important, particularly under experimental conditions which did not produce a high level of anxiety. The first two papers reprinted give some support for this view, particularly if we agree that the Thayer list measures arousal level (state arousal), as we have argued previously. Further evidence for this conception of the Thayer list is given in the next section.

Only one study of conditioning is included in this section. The reason is that while the concept of conditioning is a very important one in mediating physiological and social variables, there has been an enormous literature on this topic which could not realistically be compressed within the compass of a single section. It seemed better to present a single study, in which relevant experimental parameters were varied methodically and rely on this introduction to make clear the present position. Spence predicted (and found) that eyelid conditioning was positively correlated with high MAS scores. Eysenck predicted (and found) that eyelid conditioning was correlated with high introversion scores. For both, there were also negative findings; Kimble and others failed to find evidence in favour of Spence's hypothesis, and Spence and others failed to find evidence in favour of Eysenck's hypothesis. It now seems possible to reconcile all the available evidence in the following way. (1) Eysenck's hypothesis of greater conditionability in introverts applies only when testing conditions are non-arousing, i.e. when the UCS is not too strong, etc.; when conditions are highly arousing, they wash out differences in resting level of arousal, and may even (through transmarginal inhibition) lead to better conditioning in extraverts. This importance of parameter conditions for the proper testing of Eysenck's hypothesis has been well documented (Eysenck and Levey, 1972), and follows from the general theory of arousal. (2) Spence's hypothesis of greater conditionability of anxious subjects applies only when testing conditions are anxiety-arousing; when they are not, then the high- and low-anxiety subjects do not behave differently (Ominsky and Kimble, 1966).

(3) It follows that when conditions favouring Spence's hypothesis obtain (i.e. when conditions are anxiety-provoking) they are unfavourable for the testing of Eysenck's hypothesis, as producing a high degree of arousal. Thus on the whole it seems that we can reconcile the experimental literature on the basis of an arousal hypothesis; in line with this theory Spence's MAS

works because conditions productive of high anxiety also automatically produce high cortical arousal. This is not the way in which Spence would have formulated his particular theory, but it fits in with the rest of the data, and is the most parsimonious way of reconciling apparently contradictory results.

Another point concerning conditioning should be mentioned, as this is related to the very fundamental issue of scoring the record. The usual, and almost the only way of scoring eyeblink conditioning records currently employed is by noting the number of responses; as Martin and Levey (1969) have shown, this is a very rough-and-ready method which leaves out of account many important and valuable aspects of the record. In particular, they suggest the use of their "work-ratio" measure, which is defined as the ratio of CR amplitude at UCR onset over peak UCR amplitude, and is considered to be an estimate of the amount of "physiological work" taken over by the CR from the UCR. Another way of looking at it is that it measures the success of the person in avoiding the negative reinforcement produced by the UCR; looked at from this point of view one might suggest that frequency of CR is a measure of Pavlovian conditioning, work-ratio a measure of operant conditioning. The two types of measure are uncorrelated.

Our interest, of course, is in personality differences, and Jones (1975) has shown that extraverts are inferior to introverts with respect to *both* frequency and work-ratio of the conditioned eyeblink response. Using a group of 57 subjects, scored on the average of three successive sets of 25 trials, he found results shown in Figs. 3 and 4. below. It will be seen that for both frequency of response (Fig. 3) and for work-ratio (Fig. 4), introverts are significantly superior to extraverts. Put in the form of correlations, the relationship between extraversion and frequence for the third set of trials is −0.52; correlations for work-ratio are similar. Jones also compared the effectiveness of weak (1 p.s.i.) and strong (3 p.s.i.) UCS; strong stimuli were more effective in producing CS and in producing high work-ratios, and they were interacting with personality in the predicted direction, i.e. differences between introverts and extraverts were larger with the weak than with the strong stimuli. These results are in good accord with the results of Eysenck and Levey, reprinted below, and may serve as a replication, with the additional feature that they include work-ratio measurements.

The paradigm of conditioning can also be extended to verbal conditioning, and here also we might expect distinct personality differences to appear. The literature contains many reports of successful experiments, but also many reports of unsuccessful experiments; the reason for this difference in outcome may be in large measure due to the effects of awareness on the part of the experimental subject of the contingencies of the experiment. Gupta, in the study reprinted below, wisely excluded all aware subjects; clearly, when a sub-

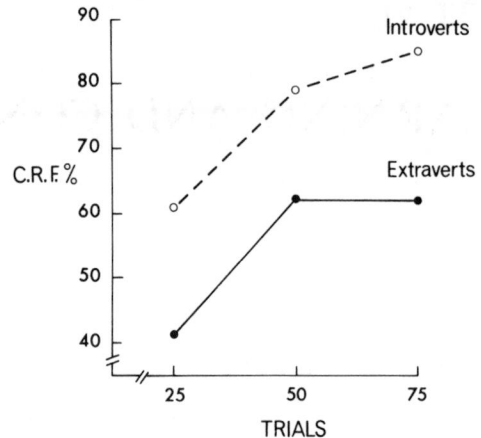

FIG. 3. Frequency of conditioned eyeblink responses for extraverts and introverts, averaged over three sets of 25 trials each. From Jones (1975)

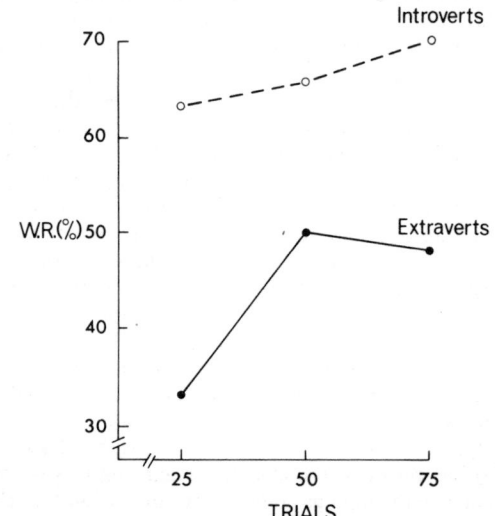

FIG. 4. Work-ratios calculated for eyeblink conditioning trials of extraverts and introverts respectively. From Jones (1975)

ject knows the purpose of the experiment his responses are not in any meaning of the term "conditioned"; they are determined by a variety of irrelevant attitudes, feelings and motivations. This was very clearly shown by Gidwani (1971) in a study of 14 extraverted and 14 introverted school children, given a test very similar to that used by Gupta, but using Smarties (sweets) as positive reinforcers. There was no overall difference between extraverts and introverts, but there was a highly significant ($p < 0.001$) interaction between personality and awareness. Unaware introverts conditioned significantly better than unaware extraverts; aware extraverts conditioned significantly better than aware introverts. Much of the confusion surrounding this area is undoubtedly due to failure to control the variable of awareness—no doubt due to lack of awareness on the part of many of the investigators of the importance of this variable!

REFERENCES

EYSENCK, H. J. Personality, learning and "anxiety". In: H. J. Eysenck (Ed.), *Handbook of abnormal psychology*. London: Pitman, 1973.

EYSENCK, H. J. and LEVEY, A. Conditioning, introversion–extraversion and the strength of the nervous system. In: V. D. Nebylitsyn and J. A. Gray (Eds.), *Biological bases of individual behaviour*. London: Academic Press, 1972.

GIDWANI, D. G. S. The effect of previously learned habits and personality variables in verbal conditioning. London: Unpublished Ph.D. thesis, University of London, 1971.

JONES, J. G. The relationship between U.C.S. intensity, rest, warning signal and personality in eyelid conditioning. London: Unpublished Ph.D. thesis, 1975.

MARTIN, I. and LEVEY, A. B. *The genesis of the classical conditioned response*. London: Pergamon Press, 1969.

OMINSKY, M. and KIMBLE, G. A. Anxiety and eyelid conditioning. *Journal of Experimental Psychology*, 1966, *71*, 471–472.

SPENCE, K. Anxiety, level and eyelid conditioning. *Psychological Bulletin*, 1964, *61*, 129–139.

From R. H. Willoughby (1967). Psychological Reports, *20,* 659–662, *by kind permission of the author and Southern Universities Press*

EMOTIONALITY AND PERFORMANCE ON COMPETITIONAL AND NONCOMPETITIONAL PAIRED-ASSOCIATES

ROBERT H. WILLOUGHBY

University of Minnesota[1]

Summary.—18 male college *Ss* scoring in the extreme quintiles on a unidimensional "emotionality" scale (Em) were tested on competitive and noncompetitive paired-associates. Results demonstrated that the low Em *Ss* made significantly fewer errors on both competitive and noncompetitive associates and required significantly fewer trials to reach criterion on the noncompetitive associates than did the high Em *Ss*. The results were compared to those of Spence, *et al.* (1963) for high- and low-"anxious" *Ss* on these same word pairs. Discrepant findings were interpreted as reflecting different operational measures of "anxiety" employed in the two studies.

Spence (1958) and Taylor (1963) have hypothesized that anxiety increases intratask competition. Thus, in situations where intratask competition is high, a high anxiety level should have a disruptive influence upon performance and low-anxious *Ss* should perform better than high-anxious *Ss*. Conversely, in learning situations where intratask competition is low, the greater drive (D) of the highly anxious *Ss* should facilitate their performance. Experimental investigations of the Spence hypothesis have centered about two learning paradigms, classical (defensive) conditioning and paired-associate learning. Classical conditioning is assumed to be relatively free from response interference and the hypothesis predicts that highly anxious *Ss* will condition more rapidly than those of low anxiety. Results from Spence's laboratory have reliably confirmed this predicton. [See Taylor (1963) for a review of this literature.] In paired-associate learning highly anxious *Ss* have been found to perform better than low-anxious *Ss* on noncompetitive word pairs whereas low-anxious *Ss* demonstrate superiority on competitive associates (Spence, Taylor, & Ketchel, 1956; Spence, Farber, & McFann, 1963).

In all of these studies, "anxiety" has been operationally defined as *S*'s score on the Manifest Anxiety Scale (MAS) (Taylor, 1953). The MAS has been criticized by some investigators on the grounds that it not only measures anxiety but also a number of other personality variables (Eysenck, 1953, 1961). Factor analyses of the MAS (O'Conner, Lorr, & Stafford, 1956; Bendig, 1957, 1958, 1960) suggest that it may contain as many as five different factors. Eysenck (1953) has stated that one of these factors ("introversion") accounts for the rather consistent superiority of highly anxious *Ss* in classical conditioning studies.

While Eysenck's contention that the MAS contains a "contaminating introversion component" has received some support from factor analytic investigations (Bendig, 1957, 1958), the effect of this "introversion" variable upon rate of

---

[1]This research was conducted while the author was at Alliance College.

R. H. WILLOUGHBY

learning is not at all clear. No study has replicated Spence's experimental procedures using a unidimensional measure of "anxiety" in the selection of experimental Ss. The present experiment replicated the verbal learning study by Spence, Farber, and McFann (1963) and used a unidimensional measure of "anxiety" rather than the MAS used by Spence and his associates.

METHOD

The Scale

The scale employed in the present investigation was the Em ("emotionality") scale of the Pittsburgh Temperament Inventory (Bendig, 1961). The Em scale consists of 30 items selected through factor analysis from the MAS, plus the N ("neuroticism") scale of the Maudsley Personality Inventory (MPI) and the T ("thoughtfulness") scale of the Guilford-Zimmerman Temperament Survey (GZTS). The relative item contributions to the Em scale include: MAS—11 items, N scale—12 items, and T scale—7 items. Each Em scale item has survived two factor analyses and has a high loading on a second-order "emotionality" factor. This factor correlates —.14 with another second-order factor termed "social extraversion-introversion" (SEI) (Bendig, 1961). The magnitude of this correlation may be compared with that obtained by Bendig (1957) between MAS scores and the "extraversion-introversion" dimension of the MPI (—.35), a comparison which suggests that the Em scale has a smaller "introversion" component than does the MAS.

Subjects

Ss were 18 undergraduate males from an introductory course in psychology. Nine of the Ss scored within the upper quintile of the distribution of the Em scale and nine scored within the lower quintile on the scale. Although both male and female Ss made up the original distribution of Em scale scores, only male Ss were used in the study. The decision to exclude females from the experimental sample was based upon the fact that in the Spence, et al. (1963) study only males were used as Ss.

Apparatus and Procedure

A Hull-type memory drum was used to present the test list. The test list consisted of 12 paired-associates, 4 competitive word pairs and 8 noncompetitive word pairs. The list used was identical to that used by Spence, et al. (1963, p. 236). The successive stimulus items of the test list were exposed every 4 sec. including a 1.67-sec. anticipation interval, with a 4-sec. rest between successive presentations of the list.

Immediately following the reading of instructions S received six trials on a practice list followed by a 2-min. rest period. After this interval S was run to a criterion of two successive errorless trials on the test list. An error consisted of making no response or an incorrect response during the anticipation interval.

EMOTIONALITY AND PERFORMANCE ON PAIRED-ASSOCIATES

RESULTS

Table 1 presents the mean number of errors made by the high- and low-Em *S*s on both the competitive and noncompetitive paired-associates. It may be seen in this table that the low-Em *S*s made fewer errors than the high Em *S*s on both of these kinds of word pairs. A Mann-Whitney test performed on the data for noncompetitive paired associates showed this difference to be statistically reliable ($U = 12.5, p < .01$). A similar analysis performed on the error data for the competitive word pairs showed that this difference was also statistically significant ($U = 21, p < .05$).

TABLE 1

MEANS AND *SD*s FOR ERRORS AND TRIALS TO CRITERION ON COMPETITIVE AND NONCOMPETITIVE PAIRED ASSOCIATES FOR HIGH- AND LOW-EMOTIONALITY GROUPS

Measure	Group	Competitive	Noncompetitive
Errors	High Emotionality	70.44±27.34	17.22±8.35
	Low Emotionality	44.55±11.15	8.33±5.08
Trials	High Emotionality	21.44± 6.38	15.44±5.64
	Low Emotionality	17.66± 4.22	10.56±4.69

Table 1 also presents the mean number of trials to criterion for both Em groups; it shows that the low-Em *S*s required fewer trials to attain the criterion of two successive errorless trials than did the high-Em *S*s on both competitive and noncompetitive associates. Statistical analyses performed on these data showed that the difference in trials to criterion was statistically significant for the noncompetitive pairs ($U = 19, p < .05$) but did not reach significance for the competitive paired associates ($U = 25, p > .05$).

DISCUSSION

The results of the present study partially support Spence's hypothesis by demonstrating the superiority of low-Em *S*s on the competitive paired-associates. On the other hand, the relatively poor performance of the high-Em *S*s on the noncompetitive paired associates is in contradiction to Spence's predictions. Since the procedures used in this study replicated those of Spence, *et al.*, including the use of *S*s drawn from a collegiate population, the differences between the present findings and those of Spence can be attributed to a difference in the operational measures of "anxiety" employed in the two experiments.

One possible basis for the discrepancy is that the "introversion" component is the main factor in the MAS producing a performance differential on the noncompetitive pairs. Bendig (1957) has noted that *S*s scoring in the upper regions of the MAS also have high scores on "introversion," and other investigators (Eysenck, 1953, 1957; Franks, 1956, 1961) have shown that *S*s with extreme scores on both "introversion" and "neuroticism" do better in noncompetitional learning situations than *S*s with high "neuroticism" scores but low "introversion" scores.

R. H. WILLOUGHBY

Such findings suggest that both the "introversion" and "anxiety" factors found within the MAS contribute to increased performance on noncompetitional learning tasks but that the "anxiety" factor alone is not sufficient to account for differences in performance on such tasks. The results of an unpublished study by Willoughby[2] support these notions. In that study *S*s scoring in the upper and lower quintiles of a unidimensional "anxiety" scale did not differ significantly in their rates of conditioning. These results were obtained despite the fact that the experimental procedures employed were similar to those used by Spence and associates in their conditioning studies. Such findings, taken in conjunction with those of the present study, indicate that Spence's results for noncompetitive paired-associates may be obtained only when measures of anxiety include an "introversion" component (as for example, in the MAS) but not when a more unidimensional emotionality scale is employed.

REFERENCES

BENDIG, A. W. Extraversion, neuroticism, and manifest anxiety. *J. consult. Psychol.*, 1957, 21, 398.

BENDIG, A. W. Identification of item factor patterns within the manifest anxiety scale. *J. consult. Psychol.*, 1958, 22, 158.

BENDIG, A. W. Factor analysis of anxiety and neuroticism questionnaires. *J. consult. Psychol.*, 1960, 24, 161-168.

BENDIG, A. W. The Pittsburgh Scales of social extraversion, introversion, and emotionality. *J. Psychol.*, 1962, 53, 199-209.

EYSENCK, H. J. *The structure of human personality.* London: Methuen, 1953.

EYSENCK, H. J. *The handbook of abnormal psychology.* New York: Basic Books, 1961.

FRANKS, C. M. Conditioning and personality. *J. abnorm. soc. Psychol.*, 1956, 52, 143-150.

FRANKS, C. M. Conditioning and abnormal behavior. In H. J. Eysenck (Ed.), *Handbook of abnormal psychology.* New York: Basic Books, 1961. Pp. 457-487.

O'CONNOR, J. P., LORR, M., & STAFFORD, J. W. Some patterns of manifest anxiety. *J. clin. Psychol.*, 1956, 12, 160-163.

SPENCE, K. W. A theory of emotionally based drive (*D*) and its relation to performance in simple learning situations. *Amer. Psychologist*, 1958, 32, 731-737.

SPENCE, K. W., FARBER, I. E., & McFANN, H. H. The relation of anxiety (drive) level to performance in competitional and noncompetitional paired-associates learning. In S. Mednick, & M. Mednick (Eds.), *Research in personality.* New York: Holt, Rinehart, & Winston, 1963. Pp. 232-242.

TAYLOR, J. A. A personality scale of manifest anxiety. *J. abnorm. soc. Psychol.*, 1953, 48, 285-290.

TAYLOR, J. A. Drive theory and manifest anxiety. In S. Mednick, & M. Mednick (Eds.), *Research in personality.* New York: Holt, Rinehart, & Winston, 1963. Pp. 205-222.

Accepted February 24, 1967.

[2]R. H. Willoughby. Extraversion, emotionality, and eyelid conditioning. (Unpublished manuscript, Alliance College, 1964)

From R. E. Thayer and S. J. Cox (1968). Journal of Experimental Psychology, *78*, 524–526, *by kind permission of the authors and The American Psychological Association*

ACTIVATION, MANIFEST ANXIETY, AND VERBAL LEARNING

ROBERT E. THAYER AND SHEILA J. COX

California State College at Long Beach

The Activation-Deactivation Adjective Check List (AD-ACL), a self-report test of transitory levels of activation, was hypothesized to have advantages over the Manifest Anxiety (MA) scale as an indicant of drive in tests of predictions drawn from Hull-Spence theory. 2 groups of Ss tested in a low-threat group procedure learned different lists of paired associates designed to elicit 2 levels of response competition. Groups differentiated by MA scale scores did not confirm predictions drawn from Hull-Spence theory, while predictions were confirmed by groups differentiated by AD-ACL scores.

Within the framework of Hull-Spence theory, the relationship between performance and level of emotionality as assessed by the Manifest Anxiety (MA) scale has been extensively investigated (Spence & Spence, 1966). Scores on the MA scale, which presumably denote the tendency to exhibit overt anxiety symptoms and thus emotionality, have been used as indicants of drive (D). Obvious alternatives to MA scale scores are physiological measures of emotionality which could be obtained within the experimental situation and would not have the limited generality of anxiety responses. The Activation-Deactivation Adjective Check List (AD-ACL) correlates substantially with composites of physiological variables and has advantages over individual physiological variables that are often poorly correlated (Thayer, 1967). Thus, this test can be used in situations in which physiological measures are difficult to obtain. The AD-ACL consists of a set of self-descriptive adjectives with which S reports his momentary perception of feelings of activation by rating each adjective on a 4-point scale. Four orthogonal activation dimensions have been factor analytically defined, and one dimension, General Activation (e.g., lively, active, full-of-pep, energetic), has been most sensitive in a wide variety of activation-inducing conditions. The present research was designed to test predictions drawn from Hull-Spence theory and to compare the AD-ACL and MA scale as indicants of D.

Experiment I.—Spence, Farber, and McFann (1956) constructed a paired-associates list to test a prediction drawn from Hull-Spence theory that high-D Ss would perform better than low-D Ss on tasks with dominant correct responses and few competing responses. Using the MA scale as an indicant of D, they found reliably superior performance by the high-D group. In the present research, which included the previouly constructed paired-associates task, superior performance by the high-D group was also predicted. In the original study the Iowa group employed an individual testing procedure and short stimulus presentation times; the present research used an anonymous group testing procedure and long stimulus presentation times in an attempt to reduce the arousal of emotionality among Ss. It was assumed that stress is a component of most psychology experiments and that the present low-threat group procedure, although somewhat stressful, would require maximum sensitivity of the two indicants of D because of the permissive conditions employed.

Method.—The Ss in Exp. I were 74 male introductory psychology college students. For analyses using the MA scale (Taylor, 1953), divisions were made into upper and lower 20% of all 160 Ss in Exp. I and II. Cutoff points were 23 and above and 8 below. Experiment I analysis involved 15 high and 20 low MA scale Ss. For analysis using the General Activation subscale of the

SUPPLEMENTARY REPORTS

AD-ACL (Thayer, 1967), all Ss in Exp. I and II were divided into upper and lower thirds. The rating scale for each self-descriptive adjective included: definitely do not feel, cannot decide, feel slightly, and definitely feel. The four alternatives were scored 1 through 4, respectively, and seven adjectives were used in the General Activation subscale. The cutoff points for upper and lower thirds for both groups were 19 and above and 12 and below (mean cutoff points, 2.7 and 1.7). Analysis for Exp. I involved 21 high and 33 low AD-ACL Ss.

A paired-associates list including 15 high intrapair association, low intralist association adjectives was used (Spence et al., 1956). The words were presented with a Kodak Carousel slide projector and a manual slide change control on a viewing screen in front of an average size classroom. The slide presentation time—10 sec. per stimulus, 5 sec. per pair, and 5 sec. between trials—was determined with a stopwatch. In the learning task, Ss recorded their responses in a small stapled booklet made of plain mimeograph paper cut into 45 numbered sheets.

The Ss were run in several groups ranging in number from 20 to 35. They were told their group was part of a large number of introductory students participating in this study. An E explained that a list of paired associates would be presented four times in different orders. Starting on the second presentation, as the stimulus word appeared, Ss would write the response word on one of the numbered sheets and fold the sheet back before the confirming pair appeared. The students were twice reminded of the anonymity of their recorded responses and asked to cooperate by stopping and folding the sheet back immediately upon the signal. During the experiment E observed Ss and noted that cooperation was excellent. After the instructions Ss filled out an AD-ACL, participated in the paired-associates task, and last filled out an MA scale.

Results.—The total number of correct words per trial was scored. Performance means based on MA scale and AD-ACL divisions are presented in Table 1. Performance means based on MA scale divisions were in the opposite direction to predictions drawn from Hull-Spence theory, and a between-groups analysis of variance indicated nonsignificant differences. The means based on AD-ACL divisions were in the expected direction, and an analysis of variance showed that the high-activation group performed reliably better than the low-activation group,

TABLE 1
MEAN PERCENTAGE OF CORRECT RESPONSES OF HIGH-ASSOCIATION PAIRED ASSOCIATES FOR ANXIETY AND ACTIVATION GROUPS

Groups	Percentage of Correct Responses		
	T_1	T_2	T_3
High Anxiety ($n = 15$)	61.3	77.8	87.5
Low Anxiety ($n = 20$)	69.7	87.3	94.3
High G-Act ($n = 21$)	72.4	89.2	94.3
Low G-Act ($n = 33$)	61.4	81.0	89.7

$F (1, 52) = 4.08, p < .05$. The within-groups interaction was not significant.

Experiment II.—Using MA scale scores as indicants of D and a second paired-associates list, Spence et al. (1956) tested a prediction drawn from Hull-Spence theory that low-D Ss would perform better than high-D Ss on tasks in which competing responses are initially stronger than correct responses. Results indicated that low-D Ss learned significantly faster than high-D Ss. The paired-associates list that was used included four high-association pairs from the list described in Exp. I and eight low-association pairs constructed in such a way that response tendencies were higher for the high-association response words than for the low-association response words. The Iowa group predicted superior initial performance by the high-D Ss on the high-association pairs; because of increasing interference among high- and low-association pairs they also predicted gradual superiority by low-D Ss as learning progressed. Some support was found for these predictions. In the present experiment the authors predicted superiority by low-D Ss on high- and low-association paired associates as well as the total list. It was assumed that using the low-threat group procedure described in Exp. I any initial superiority by the high-D Ss would be eliminated because of the probable rapid learning.

Method.—The Ss were 86 male introductory psychology college students. The cutoff points of the MA scale and AD-ACL were described in Exp. I. In the present experiment 16 and 15 Ss were in the upper and lower 20%, respectively, of the MA scale. And 31 and 22 Ss were in the respective upper and lower thirds of the AD-ACL. The 12 paired associates were taken from the study by Spence et al. (1956). The other apparatus and procedure were described in Exp. I.

Results.—The total number of correct

SUPPLEMENTARY REPORTS

TABLE 2

MEAN PERCENTAGE OF CORRECT RESPONSES ON HIGH- AND LOW-ASSOCIATION PAIRED ASSOCIATES
FOR ANXIETY AND ACTIVATION GROUPS

Paired Associates	High Anxiety ($n=16$)			Low Anxiety ($n=15$)			High G-Act ($n=31$)			Low G-Act ($n=22$)		
	T_1	T_2	T_3	T_1	T_2	T_3	T_1	T_2	T_3	T_1	T_2	T_3
High Association	68.8	67.2	82.8	58.2	65.0	78.2	48.5	58.0	73.5	61.2	76.2	83.0
Low Association	25.0	37.5	62.5	23.4	34.1	55.9	21.0	39.1	55.2	31.9	46.0	68.8
All	39.6	47.4	69.2	35.0	44.4	63.3	30.2	45.4	61.3	41.7	56.1	73.5

words per trial was scored. The means for performance trials of the individual sets of high- and low-association paired associates and the total set of words based on the MA scale divisions are presented in Table 2. The high MA scale Ss showed superior performance to lows on both sets and the total set. These differences when tested with analysis of variance were not statistically significant, however. The mean differences for the four pairs of high-association words are inconsistent with our predictions and the Iowa group's predictions of gradual superiority of low-D Ss. And differences for the eight low-association pairs are also inconsistent with predictions.

The performance means of Ss divided on the basis of AD-ACL scores are presented in Table 2 and are all consistent with predictions made in the present experiment. Differences for the eight pairs of low-association words were not statistically significant, though the means are in the expected direction, between-groups F (1, 51) = 3.05, $p <$ .10. On the four pairs of high-association words the low-activation group performed reliably better than the high, F (1, 51) = 5.35, $p < .05$. The interaction was not statistically significant in either analysis. Considering both sets of words together, the low-activation group performed reliably better than the high-activation group, F (1, 51) = 4.71, $p < .05$. The interaction was non-significant.

Previous experience with the AD-ACL had indicated one-third splits result in the most powerful discrimination. In order to more adequately compare the performance results based on the two indicants of D, several analyses were performed using comparable AD-ACL and MA scale cutoff points. The Ss in Exp. I and II were divided on the basis of one-third splits on the MA scale. For the noncompetitive list in Exp. I and the total competitive list in Exp. II, performance means were still in the opposite direction to our experimental predictions, and differences were not statis-

tically significant. The Ss in Exp. I and II were also divided into upper and lower 20% groups on the basis of AD-ACL scores. With these divisions, performance means for the noncompetitive list in Exp. I were in the expected direction but not significantly different. For the total competitive list in Exp. II, low AD-ACL Ss showed reliably superior performance to high Ss, F (1, 31) = 4.83, $p < .05$.

Discussion.—All predictions drawn from Hull-Spence theory were supported with AD-ACL scores used as indicants of D, but predictions were not supported with MA scale discriminations. The low-threat group procedure employed in this research required subtle discriminations of whatever reduced differences in emotionality existed. The lack of discrimination by the MA scale is not surprising in view of the mounting evidence that moderate psychological stress must be present for adequate MA scale discrimination (Spence & Spence, 1966).

The AD-ACL has at least two advantages over the MA scale as an indicant of D. Measures of emotionality can be obtained within the experimental situation instead of outside of it as is the case with the MA scale. This AD-ACL measurement property allows more direct monitoring of the effects of independent variables relevant to D. As an indicant of D the AD-ACL also has advantage over the MA scale since the former test is not limited to measurement of overt anxiety symptoms.

REFERENCES

SPENCE, K. W., FARBER, I. E., & McFANN, H. H. The relation of anxiety (drive) level to performance in competitional and noncompetitional paired-associates learning. *Journal of Experimental Psychology*, 1956, **52**, 296–305.

SPENCE, J. T., & SPENCE, K. W. The motivational components of manifest anxiety: Drive and drive stimuli. In C. D. Spielberger (Ed.), *Anxiety and behavior.* New York: Academic Press, 1966.

TAYLOR, J. A. A personality scale of manifest anxiety. *Journal of Abnormal and Social Psychology*, 1953, **48**, 285–290.

THAYER, R. E. Measurement of activation through self-report. *Psychological Reports*, 1967, **20**, 659–662.

(Received September 11, 1967)

From J. F. Allsopp and H. J. Eysenck (1975). British Journal of Psychology, *66*, 15–24, *by kind permission of the authors and Cambridge University Press*

EXTRAVERSION, NEUROTICISM, AND VERBAL REASONING ABILITY AS DETERMINANTS OF PAIRED-ASSOCIATES LEARNING

By J. F. ALLSOPP and H. J. EYSENCK

Institute of Psychiatry, University of London

Predictions based on theories of verbal learning proposed by Spence and Eysenck were compared by using a non-competitive list of paired-associates formed from seven synonym pairs, and a competitive list formed by pairing each of the seven S words with a R word with which it was not synonymous. Each list was presented in a $2 \times 2 \times 2$ design to groups of primary school children differing in extraversion, neuroticism, and verbal reasoning ability. Performance on both lists was related to ability level and extraversion, and these relationships did not interact with the stage of learning. It is concluded in support of Eysenck's theory that differences in extraversion are of importance in determining performance on such tasks.

Eysenck (1973) has reviewed the mass of verbal learning studies designed to test aspects of Spence's theory (Spence, 1956, 1958; Spence & Spence, 1966; Taylor, 1956) that performance is related to differences in drive level as measured by the Manifest Anxiety Scale (MAS) (Taylor, 1953). He concluded that an interpretation of these studies is extremely difficult because the MAS is a factorially complex measure correlating with two major orthogonal factors of personality, -0.3 to -0.4 with extraversion, and 0.6 to 0.7 with neuroticism. In his own theory (Eysenck, 1965, 1967, 1973), Eysenck separates MAS-type 'anxiety' into two components: cortical arousal, measured by personality differences in extraversion, and autonomic activation, measured by personality differences in neuroticism. It is hypothesized in a similar manner to Walker's theory of action decrement (Walker, 1968), that the greater cortical arousal of introverts than of extraverts will cause a stronger and more prolonged consolidation process resulting in better ultimate memory but a temporary interference with performance.

Jensen (1964) carried out a complex factor analytic study of various serial learning and short-term memory tasks which showed clearly that extraversion played a more prominent role than neuroticism. Extraversion was positively correlated with superior performance on most of the tasks in the battery, and had a loading of 0.41 on the general factor running through various short-term learning tasks. Jensen concluded that there is some common genotype underlying extraversion and learning ability, and suggested that extraversion is related to resistance to interference due to response competition.

Support for the hypotheses of Eysenck and Jensen has been obtained from a number of paired-associates learning experiments. Howarth & Eysenck (1968) used a paired-associates task of seven CVCs of medium association value, and found that extraverts learnt the list better and showed superior recall after intervals of up to 5 min., but that introverts were superior at longer intervals of 30 min. and 24 hr. McLaughlin (1968) used a list of 12 paired associates with three-letter words as stimuli and 40 per cent association value nonsense syllables as responses. He also found that extraverts performed better in learning the list, although he failed to

J. F. Allsopp and H. J. Eysenck

find support for the predicted interaction effect when comparing varying recall intervals of up to seven days. In a study comparing the effect of recall intervals of 2 min. and 24 hr. on paired-associates learning of single digits paired with nonsense syllables, McLean (1968) obtained psychophysiological measures of within-subject arousal, and imposed conditions of high or low arousal through the use of white noise in order to induce high arousal in the experimental group. The expected cross-over effect occurred when both methods of comparing arousal were considered, the high arousal group recalling more at the longer interval and the low arousal group more at the shorter interval. McLean compared the within-subject arousal measures with differences in arousal hypothetically measured by extraversion–introversion, in terms of the inverse-U curve relating arousal to performance. With increasing arousal, as measured psychophysiologically, performance decreased when the recall interval was 2 min. For the delayed recall interval, the optimal arousal category was the high arousal associates of the control group, while the same associates for the experimental group remained postoptimal for that recall period. On the other side of the inverted-U, low arousal associates for both noise conditions were suboptimal for the 24 hr. recall interval. The comparison between extraverts and introverts produced a remarkably similar pattern to this arousal–recall relationship found as a function of time. Introverts recalled fewer correct associates than extraverts when tested 2 min. after paired-associates presentation but recalled more a day later. From his extensive experiment, McLean concluded that the consistency and similarity with which personality derived arousal influences the magnitude of paired-associates recall as a function of time, compared to physiologically recorded arousal changes, adds considerable weight to the notion that introverts function at a higher state of cortical arousal than extraverts.

Howarth (1969) compared the susceptibility of extraverts and introverts to response interference by generating response competition within a five-pair word-list by twice changing the S-R combinations after the previous form of the list had been learnt. Extraverts performed slightly better on the first two list combinations, and much better on the third list in which response competition was hypothesized to be at a maximum. McLaughlin & Eysenck (1967) constructed an easy and difficult list of seven CVC pairs with identical stimuli but different responses, so that in the former list the responses were of low similarity to each other, but in the latter were of high similarity to each other. Extraversion was related to good performance on both lists, although the relationship was stronger in the difficult list where response competition was involved.

McLaughlin & Eysenck also showed a complex relationship between performance and extraversion and neuroticism considered in combination. According to Eysenck's physiological theory (Eysenck, 1967), a high level of arousal, in addition to being characteristic of introverts, is also automatically produced on the occurrence of strong emotion in the individual. From this McLaughlin & Eysenck hypothesized, in terms of the well-known inverse-U relationship between arousal and performance, that for the easy task stable extraverts (SEs) would be at suboptimal, and neurotic introverts (NIs) at superoptimal arousal levels, and that both groups would therefore perform less well than the intermediate groups of neurotic extraverts (NEs) and stable introverts (SIs). On the difficult task they predicted that a lower level of

Verbal learning and paired-associates learning

arousal would be optimal, and hence that a relative improvement in performance would be expected for the SEs and a relative decline for the NIs. The predictions concerning both lists were upheld. Very similar results were obtained by Allsopp & Eysenck (1974) who used a non-competitive and competitive list of paired associates taken from a study by Spence *et al.* (1956). On the non-competitive list the SEs and NIs were again inferior in performance to the NEs and SIs, and on the competitive list the hypothesized low arousal group of SEs showed the best performance. However, as was the case in the McLaughlin & Eysenck study, the NIs, who were assumed to be the group with highest arousal, and were predicted to provide the worst performance, did not in fact do so. In both studies the SIs showed the worst performance on the competitive list. Allsopp & Eysenck (1974) also obtained MAS scores for all subjects, and divided them into low, medium and high scorers. No support was obtained for the original findings of Spence *et al.* that high drive subjects, as measured by MAS scores, performed better on the non-competitive list, and worse on the competitive list, than low drive subjects. There was, however, a marked tendency for medium scoring subjects to perform worse on the competitive list than subjects with either high or low MAS scores.

In extending the Spence–Taylor theory of emotionally based drive, Spielberger (1966) has pointed to the importance of considering the interactive effect of anxiety and intelligence on performance. Katahn (1966) replicated the first complex serial learning study in which the differential effects of anxiety as a function of task difficulty were noted (Taylor & Spence, 1952). Katahn found that when subjects with high and low task ability, as measured by a test of mathematical aptitude which correlated with performance, were considered separately, high anxiety was facilitating for high ability subjects, but for those with low ability it made no difference. In Taylor & Spence's original study which had used subjects of still lower ability, the low anxiety subjects had provided the best performance. Katahn argues that there are certain tasks in which high ability may operate to lower the effective difficulty, so that high anxiety may facilitate the learning of an assumed difficult task.

In studies which have considered both extraversion and neuroticism, the former dimension has more consistently been shown to correlate with differences in remembering and learning. A similar finding has been obtained with respect to the effect of personality on the academic achievement of primary schoolchildren (Eysenck & Cookson, 1969). Extraverts were found to do better scholastically and on verbal reasoning tests than introverted children. Further, stable children did better than neurotic ones, but here the relationship was far less strong. These studies, in conjunction with those showing the effect of anxiety to be dependent on ability level (Katahn, 1966; Spielberger, 1966), suggest that future work should consider individual differences on at least three dimensions. Thus the present study was designed to consider simultaneously the effects of extraversion, neuroticism and ability level on non-competitive and competitive paired-associates learning tasks..

J. F. ALLSOPP AND H. J. EYSENCK

Table 1. *S-R pairs of non-competitive and competitive word lists*

Non-competitive list		Competitive list	
S	R	S	R
Broad	Wide	Broad	Hard
Difficult	Hard	Difficult	Strong
Powerful	Strong	Powerful	Quick
Mad	Insane	Mad	Old
Ancient	Old	Ancient	Wide
Rapid	Quick	Rapid	Gigantic
Enormous	Gigantic	Enormous	Insane

METHOD

Subjects

The subjects were third- and fourth-year primary school children aged 9 to 11 years, who were selected following preliminary testing on a new personality questionnaire for children, the JPQ (Eysenck & Eysenck, 1973) from which scores for E and N were obtained, and on Verbal Test D, a verbal reasoning test produced by the National Foundation for Educational Research. The latter test was chosen as probably the most suitable of the commonly used mental ability tests to predict performance on the lists of paired associates. Different schools were used to select subjects for the two word lists. Subjects with scores of 18 on E or 10 or 11 on N were not selected for testing. According to whether they scored above or below these cut-off points on E and N, the remaining subjects were categorized as stable extraverts (SEs), neurotic extraverts (NEs), stable introverts (SIs) or neurotic introverts (NIs). Each personality group was further divided into high and low ability levels, so that each paired-associates list was presented to eight groups of subjects in a $2 \times 2 \times 2$ design (two levels of extraversion, two levels of neuroticism and two levels of ability, eight subjects per group). For the non-competitive list, subjects were categorized to be of high ability if their verbal reasoning score was 35 or above, but for the competitive list were so categorized if their score was 25 or above. While this difference in cut-off point, which approximately reflects the difference in the mean verbal reasoning scores of the samples from which subjects for the two lists were selected, probably indicates an overall difference in ability, it is also partly due to the children in the school from which the first sample was drawn having had regular experience on similar tests.

Word-lists

Seven pairs of synonyms were chosen as being of suitable difficulty for children of the age range under consideration. The non-competitive list was formed from the synonym pairs, and the competitive list by pairing each S word with a R word from one of the other synonym pairs. These lists, which were presented in three different random orders to prevent serial learning, are shown in Table 1.

The lists were set up in block capitals on 16 mm. film and presented on a screen by back projection from a 'Specto' projector. A digit timer was used to control the rate of presentation, each S word being presented for a 1·67 sec. anticipation interval, and each R word for 2·33 sec. There was a 4 sec. inter-trial interval.

Testing

The subjects were tested individually in a small, semi-darkened room. The children were told that there would be a prize for the child in each class who made the most successful anticipations of the R word. They were encouraged to guess if they were not sure as no credit would be lost for incorrect responses. The subjects were first tested on a practice list consisting of three orders of the pairs cat–dog, table–chair and salt–pepper, until they were performing perfectly and it was clear to the experimenter that they fully understood what was required of them. The subjects were then given either 10 trials on the non-competitive, or 19 trials on the

Verbal learning and paired-associates learning

Table 2. *Analysis of variance on total error scores in the non-competitive list*

Source	D.F.	M.S.	F
Ability	1	2704·00	24·87***
E	1	1660·56	15·27***
N	1	52·56	< 1
Ability × E	1	52·56	< 1
Ability × N	1	855·56	7·87**
E × N	1	6·25	< 1
Ability × E × N	1	729·01	6·70*
Residual	56	108·74	

$* P < 0.05.$ $** P < 0.01.$ $*** P < 0.001.$

Table 3. *Analysis of variance on total error scores in the competitive list*

Source	D.F.	M.S.	F
Ability	1	1580·06	3·50
E	1	2025·00	4·49*
N	1	132·25	< 1
Ability × E	1	68·07	< 1
Ability × N	1	689·07	1·53
E × N	1	1369·00	3·04
Ability × E × N	1	95·05	< 1
Residual	56	451·02	

$* P < 0.05.$

competitive list. At the completion of testing each child was told that he had done well, and was encouraged not to talk about the experiment to his classmates as this would spoil his own chance of winning the prize.

RESULTS

The first trial was not scored as any success on this was due to guessing. Hence error scores were obtained for nine trials on the non-competitive and 18 trials on the competitive list. For each list a $2 \times 2 \times 2$ analysis of variance was undertaken on the total error scores to compare the eight groups formed from the two levels each of ability, E and N. These analyses are presented in Tables 2 and 3. To help interpret the results of the analyses, the performance on both lists of the four personality groups at each level of ability is shown in Fig. 1.

Table 2 shows that on the non-competitive list both verbal reasoning ability and extraversion are strongly related to good performance. The analysis of variance term for the interaction between ability level and neuroticism shows that for high ability subjects a high level of neuroticism improves performance, but that for low ability subjects it worsens performance. However, the significance of the ability × E × N interaction term, and the differences between the personality groups shown in Fig. 1, show that more complex relationships held in the present experiment. The superiority of high N over low N scorers in the high ability group was due to the markedly poor performance of the SIs, while the inferiority of high N scorers in the low ability group was due to the exceptionally poor performance of the NIs. Table 3 shows that for the competitive list extraversion is the only factor to reach significance. The variability in performance between subjects was so high

J. F. Allsopp and H. J. Eysenck

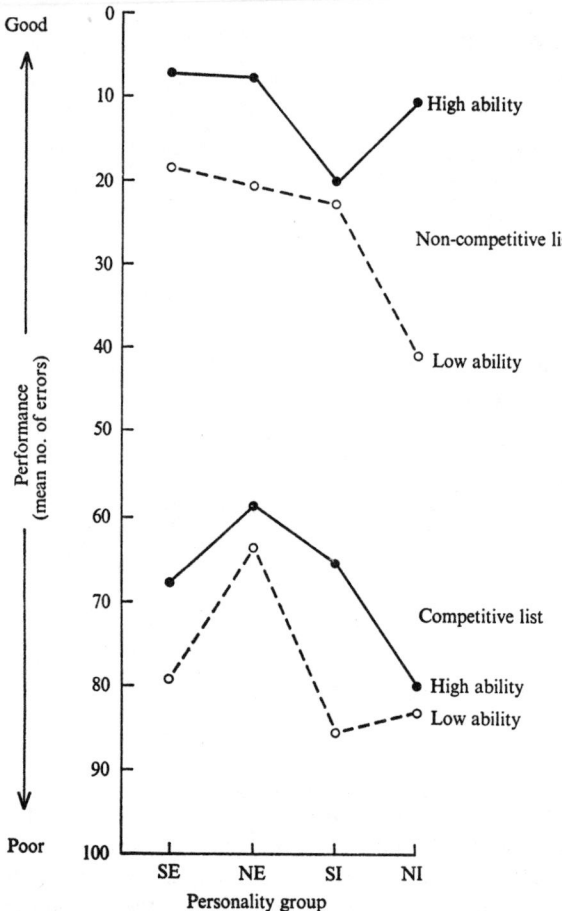

Fig. 1. Performance on paired-associates lists of four personality groups at two levels of ability.

that the two levels of ability, the differences between which are certainly not due to chance, are not shown to be significantly different by the analysis of variance.

As the subjects were selected for testing merely according to their scores in relationship to the cut-off points, the groups were not perfectly matched on the independent variables used in the analyses of variance. It is debatable whether any further matching is required to accurately interpret the results, for any differences between the groups on the independent variables will reflect differences holding in the population; however, it could be questioned whether the significant personality effects are artifacts due to group differences in ability level. For each list a 2 × 2 analysis of covariance was undertaken to compare the four EN groups (16 subjects per group) taking verbal reasoning score as the covariate. Significant effects were found for E ($P < 0.005$) on the non-competitive list, and borderline significant effects for E ($P < 0.1$) and for the E × N interaction ($P < 0.1$) on the competitive

Verbal learning and paired-associates learning

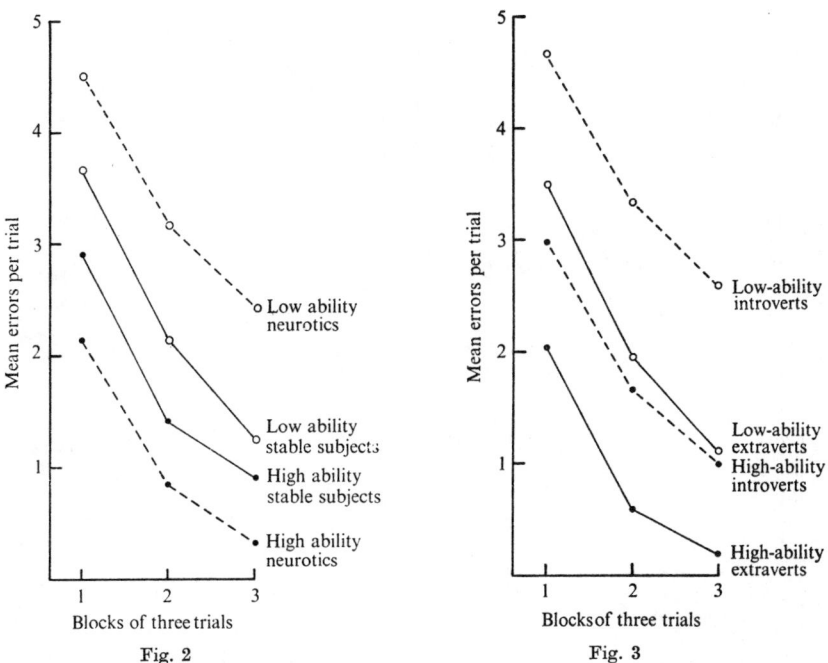

Fig. 2

Fig. 3

Fig. 2. Non-competitive list: performance over blocks of three trials for high and low ability stable and neurotic subjects.

Fig. 3. Non-competitive list: performance over blocks of three trials for high and low ability extraverts and introverts.

list. A comparison of these results with those shown in Tables 2 and 3 suggests that partialing out ability level slightly reduces the strength of the extraversion effect. This would be expected on the basis of the established relationship between extraversion and verbal reasoning (Eysenck & Cookson, 1969).

To check for possible interaction effects between individual differences and the stage of learning, error scores for each task were calculated separately for three successive blocks of trials. Fig. 2 shows changes in performance over blocks of three trials for high and low ability stable and neurotic subjects on the non-competitive list, and Fig. 3 shows the changes for high and low ability extraverts and introverts. Figs. 2 and 3 show that the effects found in the analysis on the overall performance (see Table 2) do not vary with the stage of learning. This was confirmed by an analysis of variance in which the total error score was subdivided into the errors made on each block of three trials. None of the terms for interactions with the Trials effect reached significance. Figs. 4 and 5 show the changes in performance on the competitive list over blocks of six trials for high and low ability stable and neurotic subjects, and for high and low ability introverts and extraverts. Figs. 4 and 5 show that the only change in relative performance over trials is between ability levels. Again this was confirmed by an analysis of variance in which the total error score was subdivided into the errors made on successive blocks of three trials. The only

J. F. Allsopp and H. J. Eysenck

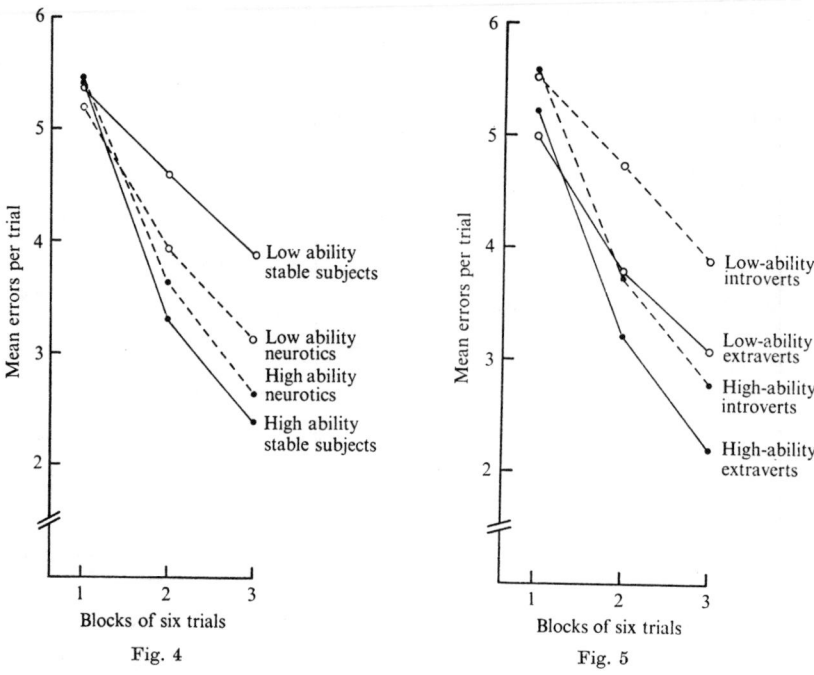

Fig. 4. Competitive list: performance over blocks of six trials for high and low ability stable and neurotic subjects.

Fig. 5. Competitive list: performance over blocks of six trials for high and low ability extraverts and introverts.

significant interaction with the trials effect was ability $\times$ trials ($P < 0.05$). The low ability subjects perform as well as those with high ability during the early stages of learning, but this effect is the same for all personality groups.

Discussion

The analyses of variance show that in addition to ability, extraversion is related to good performance on both the non-competitive and competitive lists. The clearer relationship between errors and extraversion for the non-competitive than for the competitive list casts doubt on Jensen's suggestion that extraverts are particularly at an advantage when response competition is involved (Jensen, 1964). On the competitive list, there is no evidence for the effect of neuroticism considered either independently or in interaction with ability level. The results for the non-competitive list provide some support for Spence's theory when Katahn's suggestion is followed and task difficulty is considered as a function of ability (Katahn, 1966). Whereas Katahn's results suggested that in a complex situation high ability lowers the effective difficulty so that high anxiety will facilitate performance, it could be argued on the basis of the present results that low ability increases the effective difficulty of the non-competitive list so that a high level of neuroticism worsens performance.

Verbal learning and paired-associates learning

These findings are difficult to interpret, however, for at both levels of ability three of the personality groups performed about equally as well, the differential effect of neuroticism at the two levels being due to the exceptionally poor performance of the SIs at the high ability level, and of the NIs at the low ability level.

The data provide little support for the suggestion that performance in non-competitive and competitive paired-associates tasks can be explained in terms of the inverse-U relationship between arousal and performance. Fig. 1, and the border-line significant E × N interaction effect, suggests the possibility of such a relationship for the competitive list, with neurotic extraverts being at an optimal level of arousal, and arousal being hypothesized on the basis of Eysenck's theory to increase through the personality groups from SEs to NIs. However, for this to be a compelling explanation it would be necessary to have found an optimum level of performance on the non-competitive list for a personality group hypothesized to be at a higher level of arousal than the NEs, and this is clearly not indicated by the results.

The only evidence for interaction effects between personality types and the stage of learning is the finding that in the early stages of learning the competitive list low ability subjects perform as well as high ability subjects. It is possible that the minor role of neuroticism in determining performance is due to the 4 sec. S-R cycle used in the present testing situation being too long to differentially affect the neurotic and stable subjects. Jensen (1962), with a serial rote learning task presented at either a 2 sec. or a 4 sec. rate, found that low N subjects were not affected by the difference in length of interval but high N subjects did much worse at the shorter interval. Young school children probably do not find such a testing situation, which they tend to view as a competition, as stressful as do students who are usually used as subjects, and who see their performance as reflecting on their intellectual ability. In retrospect, a shorter S-R cycle could usefully have been used with these subjects in order to create additional stress. Thus the failure to replicate with neuroticism earlier findings using the MAS as a measure of anxiety cannot be taken to cast doubt on the replicability of the mass of studies supporting Spence's theory, or some later studies showing the interactive effect of anxiety and intelligence on both overall performance and different stages of learning (Gaudry & Spielberger, 1970; Katahn, 1966; Spielberger, 1966).

It can be concluded from the relationships between extraversion and good performance on both word-lists, in conjunction with the absence of any interaction between extraversion and ability level, that extraversion is of importance in determining performance in both non-competitive and competitive learning situations for subjects varying considerably in ability. It is hoped that these results, which extend to subjects of a far wider range of ability than is generally considered, the findings of earlier studies in support of Eysenck's theoretical arguments concerning the effect of extraversion on verbal learning tasks, will encourage experimentalists to take into account this important personality dimension.

We are indebted to the Colonial Research Fund for the support of this investigation.

J. F. Allsopp and H. J. Eysenck

References

Allsopp, J. F. & Eysenck, H. J. (1974). Personality as a determinant of paired-associates learning. *Percept. mot. Skills* **39**, 315–324.

Eysenck, H. J. (1965). A three-factor theory of reminiscence. *Br. J. Psychol.* **56**, 163–181.

Eysenck, H. J. (1967). *The Biological Basis of Personality.* Springfield, Ill.: Thomas.

Eysenck, H. J. (1973). Personality, learning and 'anxiety'. In H. J. Eysenck (ed.), *Handbook of Abnormal Psychology*, 2nd ed. London: Pitman.

Eysenck, H. J. & Cookson, D. (1969). Personality in primary school children. 1. Ability and achievement. *Br. J. educ. Psychol.* **39**, 109–122.

Eysenck, S. B. G. & Eysenck, H. J. (1973). Test–retest reliabilities of a new personality questionnaire for children. *Br. J. educ. Psychol.* **43**, 126–130.

Gaudry, E. & Spielberger, C. D. (1970). Anxiety and intelligence in paired-associate learning. *J. educ. Psychol.* **61**, 386–391.

Howarth, E. (1969). Extraversion and increased interference in paired-associate learning. *Percept. mot. Skills* **29**, 403–406.

Howarth, E. & Eysenck, H. J. (1968). Extraversion, arousal, and paired-associate recall. *J. exp. Res. Person.* **3**, 114–116.

Jensen, A. (1962). Extraversion, neuroticism and serial learning. *Acta psychol.* **20**, 69–77.

Jensen, A. (1964). *Individual Differences in Learning: Interference Factor.* Washington: U.S. Department of Health, Education and Welfare, Project Report no. 1867.

Katahn, M. (1966). Interaction of anxiety and ability in complex learning situations. *J. Person. soc. Psychol.* **3**, 475–479.

McLaughlin, R. J. (1968). Retention in paired-associate learning related to extraversion and neuroticism. (Paper presented at Midwestern Psychological Association Convention, Chicago.)

McLaughlin, R. J. & Eysenck, H. J. (1967). Extraversion, neuroticism and paired-associates learning. *J. exp. Res. Person.* **2**, 128–132.

McLean, P. D. (1968). Paired-associate learning as a function of recall interval, personality and arousal. (Unpublished Ph.D. thesis, University of London.)

Spence, J. T. & Spence, K. W. (1966). The motivational components of manifest anxiety: drive and drive stimuli. In C. D. Spielberger (ed.), *Anxiety and Behaviour.* London: Academic Press.

Spence, K. W. (1956). *Behaviour Theory and Conditioning.* New Haven: Yale University Press.

Spence, K. W. (1958). A theory of emotionally based drive (D) and its relation to performance in simple learning situations. *Am. Psychol.* **13**, 131–141.

Spence, K. W., Farber, I. E. & McFann, H. H. (1956). The relation of anxiety (drive) level to performance in competitional and non-competitional paired-associates learning. *J. exp. Psychol.* **52**, 296–305.

Spielberger, C. D. (1966). The effects of anxiety on complex learning and academic achievement. In C. D. Spielberger, (ed.), *Anxiety and Behaviour.* London: Academic Press.

Taylor, J. A. (1953). A personality scale of manifest anxiety. *J. abnorm. soc. Psychol.* **48**, 285–290.

Taylor, J. A. (1956). Drive theory and manifest anxiety. *Psychol. Bull.* **53**, 303–320.

Taylor, J. A. & Spence, K. W. (1952). The relationship of anxiety level to performance in serial learning. *J. exp. Psychol.* **44**, 61–64.

Walker, E. L. (1968). Action decrement and its relation to learning. *Psychol. Rev.* **65**, 129–142.

(Manuscript received 18 December 1973; revised manuscript received 23 May 1974)

From E. Howarth (1969). Perceptual and Motor Skills, *29*, 403–406, *by kind permission of the author and Southern Universities Press*

EXTRAVERSION AND INCREASED INTERFERENCE IN PAIRED-ASSOCIATE LEARNING[1]

EDGAR HOWARTH

University of Alberta

Summary.—A previous study had shown that extraverts were superior in serial learning under distraction by competing responses from previously learned material. The present study introduced an incremental interference technique applied to paired-associate learning and verified the previous finding that personality differences can systematically affect standard learning tasks. The learning performance of 11 extraverts, 11 controls and 11 introverts was compared on a task consisting of five pairings of a color and a short animal name, e.g., Black-pig. After *S* had mastered the first series, the animal names were differently assigned among the colors so *S* had to learn in the face of competing responses. Finally, the pairings were changed in a third series, at which time the extraverts significantly outperformed (trials to criterion) the introverts, control *S*s occupying an intermediate position.

A number of recent studies have been concerned with personality differences in learning (Howarth & Eysenck, 1968; Howarth, 1968). It appears from these studies that extraverts are superior to introverts in short-term recall, a finding which confirms an earlier finding of Howarth (1963) who used a modified Wechsler digit-repetition task. Both Jensen (1964) and Shanmugan and Santhanam (1964) have provided correlational evidence for the superiority of extraverts in short-term recall tasks.

The present study introduced a method for increased interference in which, after a series of S-R pairs had been learned, the responses were differently assigned among the stimuli. Thus, as the experiment progressed, *S* acquired several alternative responses to a given stimuli, and this provided for response competition. The question is whether extraverts would outperform introverts under these conditions, and if this is the case the experiment would support the suggestion of Jensen (1964) that extraverts are resistant to interference from competing responses.

METHOD

The experiment was designed to increase interference through three series of trials in a paired-associate learning task. The task was simple, for example, if the first series used Red (color)—PIG (word) as one of the five pairs to be learned, the second series might use Red—HORSE. The original response having been learned and overlearned, should interfere with learning the correct response in succeeding series. As the experiment progressed through further series there would be several competing responses to the stimulus, and *S* should, therefore, have greater difficulty in overcoming response competition. The five

[1]Based on a paper presented to the XIX International Congress of Psychology, London, England, August, 1969.

pairs were selected from five colors (red, black, blue, yellow, green) and five animal names (horse, cow, cat, dog, pig). In Series 1 S learned the five pairs to a criterion of once through correct, then had three overlearning trials. In Series 2 S learned five pairs with responses differently allocated among the five stimuli, then had three over-learning trials. In Series 3 S learned five pairs with responses differently allocated to a criterion of once through correct.

Ss ($n = 33$) were selected from a large introductory psychology class by means of the Eysenck Personality Inventory (Eysenck & Eysenck, 1964) and were within the stable range on neuroticism; extraverts had E scores greater than 17, controls had E scores between 8 and 17, and introverts had E scores less than 8. Thus, 11 Ss in each of the three groups were compared on performance of the learning task.

The slide material was cycled at 2.5-sec. exposure using a Carousel AV-900 projector and Hunter timers (Models 115D, 116D) in tandem. Ss were instructed to call out the stimulus (name the color) and the response word and to try to anticipate the response word. A correction procedure was used. Number naming for 10 sec. was used between the complete presentations of the five pairs, i.e., to separate the trials within a series; a letter cancellation task for 2 min. was used in the interseries interval.

RESULTS

The results are shown in Table 1 and Fig. 1. In the first series all groups learned the five-pair series in the region of 7½ to 8½ trials, the total time for this being on the order of 2.5 min. Differences among the three groups (extraverts, controls, introverts) were not significant ($p > .05$) although the intro-

TABLE 1
TRIALS TO CRITERION

Group		N	Series 1	Series 2	Series 3
Extraverts	M	11	7.9	6.7	6.2
	SD		3.1	3.8	2.6
Controls	M	11	8.0	6.8	7.3
	SD		2.6	2.4	3.0
Introverts	M	11	8.7	6.9	8.1
	SD		2.9	2.3	1.9

verts showed a tendency toward slower learning under these conditions. In the second series, the performances of all groups improved and again the differences were not significant. In the third, and final series, the extraverts outperformed the introverts, the difference being significant at the 5% level ($t = 1.96$). The controls occupied an intermediate position.

These results are sufficiently clear to obviate extended discussion but some aspects of the technique should be noted for any further investigation. Minimi-

EXTRAVERSION AND INTERFERENCE IN P-A LEARNING

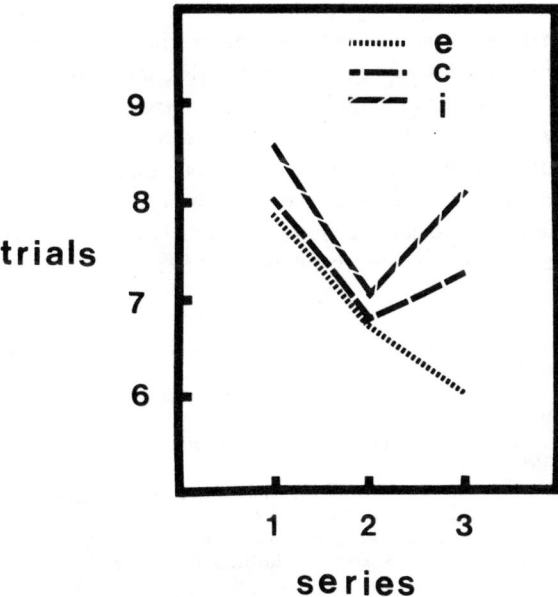

FIG. 1. Mean trials to criterion in paired-associate learning of five color-name pairs. Once the criterion has been attained in Series 1, S—after a 2-min. interval—learns a new set of responses in Series 2 and so on.

zation of response interference *per se* within a series may be accomplished by using a relatively short and well defined series of stimuli and responses. Use of overlearning trials should terminate each series of learning trials. A possible improvement in technique would be the shortening of the interseries interval but it is felt that some short-term consolidation should be permitted. It will be recalled that the Howarth and Eysenck (1968) study pointed to 5 min. as a boundary beween short- and long-term memory, using conventional CVC paired associates and a somewhat longer list. Therefore, the 2-min. interseries interval should have favored the extravert. It is possible that a shorter interval (or a more rapid presentation rate *within* series) *between* series would earlier have produced differences which appeared during the second series.

However, Fig. 1 clearly shows a deterioration in recall (mean trials to criterion) for both the controls and introverts, while the extraverts continue to improve under the conditions of increased interference. It is possible that between Series 1 and 2 there may be a "learning to learn" effect, but certainly this is overcome by the increased difficulty in the majority of Ss by the third series. As in a previous article (Howarth, 1968) we can state that "this empirical result is not a direct confirmation of the theory of response competition" because, in the present instance, although we have arranged for response competition we cannot guarantee that the data are produced by it. The findings may be due to basic differences in trace registration involved in learning, possibly comprising, as Jensen (1964) pointed out, (a) initial strength of the stimulus (meaning by this the stimulus aspects of the material, including the response to be learned) and (b) speed of consolidation of the trace. More work needs to be done on these fundamental aspects of learning as related to personality and specifically to introversion-extraversion. It is hoped that the present article, along with the others quoted, will encourage research on the individual differences in learning because for too long a period research has been concentrated on "average performance" and allocated individual differences to an error term.

REFERENCES

EYSENCK, H. J., & EYSENCK, S. B. G. *Manual of the Eysenck Personality Inventory.* San Diego: Knapp, 1964.

HOWARTH, E. Some laboratory measures of extraversion. *Percept. mot. Skills,* 1963, 17, 55-60.

HOWARTH, E. Personality differences in serial learning under distraction. *Percept. mot. Skills,* 1968, 28, 379-382.

HOWARTH, E., & EYSENCK, H. J. Extraversion, arousal and paired-associate recall. *J. exp. Res. Pers.,* 1968, 3, 114-116.

JENSEN, A. R. *Individual differences in learning: interference factor.* Washington, D. C.: Office of Education, U. S. Dept of Health, Education and Welfare, 1967. (Project No. 1867)

SHANMUGAN, T. E., & SANTHANAM, M. L. Personality differences in serial learning when interference is presented at the marginal visual level. *J. Indian Acad. Appl. Psychol.,* 1964, 1, 25-28.

Accepted July 23, 1969.

From R. N. Bone (1971). British Journal of Social and Clinical Psychology, *10*, 284–285, *by kind permission of the author and Cambridge University Press*

Interference, Extraversion and Paired-Associate Learning

By RONALD N. BONE

West Virginia Wesleyan College

Recently, McLaughlin & Eysenck (1967) found extraverts superior to introverts on both easy and difficult paired-associate tasks. These data were interpreted by assuming that introverts possess higher cortical arousal which interferes with the integration on the lists. This inference is supported by Jensen's (1964) finding of introverts being less resistant to response competition in a serial-learning task.

If these findings have generality, similar effects should be obtained using other verbal learning tasks, especially those containing built-in interference. Such a task has been utilized by Spence (1963) involving a paired-associate list of stimulus and response members having strong associative strength. These pairs were scrambled, however, so that practically no associative connexion existed between pairs, though each stimulus had a strong association among the response members elsewhere in the list. Such a list was viewed as comparable to the A–B, A–B$_r$ transfer paradigm (stimuli and responses of the first list are re-paired to form a second list), assuming that the first list (A–B) is composed of strongly associated word pairs brought into the laboratory via natural language habits. The second list (A–B$_r$) was composed of a scrambled version of the first list. When compared to a control list consisting of no cross-associates, she found performance to be significantly inferior. Presumably this effect is due to both forward (S–R) and backward (R–S) interference (McGovern, 1964).

Using Spence's (1963) version of the A–B$_r$ paradigm, it was predicted that introverts would display more errors than extraverts on a list containing re-paired primary associates. An equal number were predicted for introverts and extraverts on a list containing unrelated words.

The subjects were introductory psychology students participating as part of a class requirement. Two weeks prior to the experiment 127 students were given the Maudsley Personality Inventory (Eysenck, 1959). Twenty subjects scoring in the introverted direction and 20 in the extraverted direction were chosen to represent extreme groups. These groups were, in turn, randomly divided into two groups of 10 each to learn either interference or control lists. Mean extraversion scores were 40·37 and 14·28 for interference lists; 39·08 and 15·21 for control lists. While neuroticism was not investigated as a variable in this study, it may be pointed out that mean neuroticism scores did not differ in the four treatments.

The paired-associate lists consisted of 10 pairs, the stimuli being the same in both interference and control lists. The mean cross-associate strength for the interference list was 0·60; for the control list 0·00. Association values were obtained from Bilodeau & Howell's (1966) norms for discrete associations. Associative strength between individual stimulus members, response members and S–R pairs was kept to a minimum. All of the stimulus words were of high frequency.

Each was given standard paired-associate instructions using the anticipation method. The lists were presented in four random orders to prevent serial learning. The intertrial interval was 6 sec. Learning was taken to a criterion of one errorless trial.

The results are shown in Tables 1–3 and lend strong support to the hypothesis that introverts are more prone to interference than extraverts on tasks containing built-in interference, but not on tasks where interference is absent or at a minimum.

These findings are for the most part consistent with the study by McLaughlin & Eysenck (1967), the only difference being that they found the performance of extraverts superior on both difficult and easy lists. Possibly the difference between these two studies is more apparent than real and lies in the definition of easy and difficult tasks. McLaughlin & Eysenck (1967) defined difficulty in terms of formal response similarity, with difficult and easy lists containing formal high and low response similarity respectively. The easy list could still be difficult since nonsense syllables of low formal similarity may place considerable demands on the response learning phase of paired-associate learning (Underwood *et al.*, 1959).

Interference, Extraversion and Paired-Associate Learning

Table 1. *Mean trials to criterion and mean number of errors*

Treatments	Trials to criterion	Errors
Extravert		
Interference	15·20	55·00
Control	8·90	21·90
Introvert		
Interference	18·20	77·90
Control	8·40	20·50

Table 2. *Analysis of variance for the trials to criterion*

Source of variation	D.F.	M.S.	F	P
Extraversion	1	15·62	1·69	
List (B)	1	648·02	69·98	<0·001
A × B interaction	1	30·63	3·31	
Error	36	9·26		

Table 3. *Analysis of variance for the number of errors*

Source of variation	D.F.	M.S.	F	P
Extraversion (A)	1	1152·62	4·72	<0·05
List (B)	1	20475·62	83·80	<0·001
A × B interaction	1	1476·23	6·04	<0·05
Error	36	244·34		

In conclusion, it is suggested that verbal learning tasks are ideally suited for the investigation of personality variables. However, anyone attempting to work in this area should pay particular attention to an excellent article by Goulet (1968) concerning methodology.

REFERENCES

BILODEAU, E. A. & HOWELL, D. C. (1966). Free association norms: discrete and continuous methods. (Office of Naval Research Department of the Navy, Washington, D.C. Tulane University. Technical Report no. 1 for contract Nonr-475 (10).)

EYSENCK, H. J. (1959). *Manual of the Maudsley Personality Inventory.* London: University of London Press.

GOULET, L. R. (1968). Anxiety (drive) and verbal learning: implications for research and some methodological considerations. *Psychol. Bull.* **69**, 235–247.

JENSEN, A. R. (1964). Individual differences in learning: interference factor. (Co-operative Research Project no. 1867. Office of Education, U.S. Department of Health, Education and Welfare.)

MCGOVERN, J. B. (1964). Extinction of associations in four transfer paradigms. *Psychol. Monogr.* **78**, no. 16. (Whole no. 593.)

MCLAUGHLIN, R. J. & EYSENCK, H. J. (1967). Extraversion, neuroticism and paired associate learning. *J. exp. Res. Person.* **2**, 128–132.

SPENCE, J. T. (1963). Associative interference on paired-associate lists from extra-experimental learning. *J. verb. Learn. verb. Behav.* **2**, 329–338.

UNDERWOOD, B. J., RUNQUIST, W. N. & SCHULZ, R. W. (1959). Response learning in paired-associate lists as a function of intra-list similarity. *J. exp. Psychol.* **58**, 70–78.

Manuscript received 28 May 1970

Revised manuscript received 5 October 1970

From M. A. Wallach and R. C. Gahm (1960). Psychological Reports, 7, 387–398, *by kind permission of the authors and Southern Universities Press*

EFFECTS OF ANXIETY LEVEL AND EXTRAVERSION-INTROVERSION ON PROBABILITY LEARNING[1]

MICHAEL A. WALLACH AND RUTHELLEN C. GAHM

Massachusetts Institute of Technology and The Age Center of New England, Inc.

Suppose an individual has to predict which of two events will occur on each of a series of tries, and one of these events is more likely than the other although both in fact occur in a random sequence. How often will the rare event be predicted? Two factors might conceivably make for a high rate of predicting the rare event. It is the purpose of this study to separate them and examine their possible relationships to aspects of personality in an older sample.

A high rate of predicting the rare event will result if the person assumes there is some pattern to the rare event's occurrence, and tries to solve the problem of accurately predicting when the rare event will occur (the "problem" approach). For such a person, trying to "catch" the rare event's occurrence is a challenge which he accepts: being correct in predicting the rare event is more important to him than being correct in predicting the frequent event. On the other hand, a high rate of predicting the rare event also will result if the person simply isn't sensitive to the infrequency of the rare event and hence treats it as if it occurs more often than it does (the "50:50" approach).

Although both "problem" and "50:50" approaches lead to more frequent prediction of the rare alternative, the former is a much more "thoughtful" approach to the task than the latter. Can we distinguish the two in terms of some additional response measure? Latency of predicting the rare alternative seems to provide a method. If high frequency of choosing the rare alternative is due to the "problem" approach, then choice of the rare alternative should be preceded by a longer latency than choice of the frequent alternative: S should be especially thoughtful before predicting the rare event since its accurate prediction is the challenge for him; it is the rare event with which his hypotheses specifically are concerned. Predicting the frequent event, on the other hand, is more likely to be correct and hence poses less of a problem. If, on the other hand, high choice frequency for the rare event is due to the "50:50" approach, then S should be about as fast in predicting the rare alternative as he is in predicting the frequent one since he is insensitive to the difference between them. Although a frequency measure alone, then, is not sufficient to distinguish the "problem" and "50:50" approaches, measuring latencies as well as frequencies seems to provide a way of making this discrimination. We hence may

[1]This investigation was supported by a research grant (M-2269) from the National Institute of Mental Health, Public Health Service, conducted under the auspices of The Age Center of New England, Inc. Grateful thanks are due Marguerite Braun, Leonard R. Green, and Lynne Hamilton, for aid in data analysis.

operationally define the "problem" approach in terms of high choice frequency for the rare event, and also a longer latency of choice for the rare event than for the frequent one. The "50:50" approach, on the other hand, may be defined in terms of high choice frequency for the rare event, and also as short a latency of choice for the rare event as for the frequent one.

While clear relationships have been found between probability learning performance and stimulus condition independent variables (such as the degree of deviation from 50:50 in the relative frequencies of the two events),[2] little understanding has been obtained of how probability learning performance may vary with personality when stimulus conditions are held constant. Fillenbaum (1959), for instance, using young adult males, found no correlations beyond what might be expected by chance between scores on MMPI scales and individual differences in choice frequency for a rare alternative occurring in a random sequence with 67:33 as the actual relative frequencies. However, variability for young adults in cognitive performances of the kind just cited typically is not large. It may be especially difficult to obtain relationships between personality and probability learning among younger Ss, therefore, because of an insufficient range of individual differences in the probability learning measures.

The impetus to the present research was the view that work with an older male sample well might cast light on these apparently elusive relationships between personality and probability learning. The greater variability in cognitive performances found, on the average, among older as compared with younger Ss, might reveal relationships between probability learning and personality that remain concealed in younger individuals.

In particular, it was desired to investigate two aspects of personality which might be expected to influence the use of the more deliberative "problem" approach to probability learning versus the more thoughtless "50:50" approach. These aspects are manifest anxiety level and extraversion-introversion. A high level of anxiety has been found to disrupt attempts at rational, deliberative solving of complex problems (see, e.g., Easterbrook, 1959). So also we well might expect extraverts to be more impulsive and less contemplative than introverts. In sum, the presence for older Ss both of high anxiety and of extraversion might be expected to favor the occurrence of the thoughtless "50:50" approach. On the other hand, the presence for older Ss both of low anxiety and of introversion might be expected to favor the occurrence of the thoughtful, deliberative "problem" approach.

The hypotheses under examination in the present research, then, are that (a) *high anxiety extraverts in an older male sample will be most likely to show*

---

[2]See Feather (1959) for a review of such stimulus condition variables, and see Bruner, Goodnow, and Austin (1956) for some relevant experiments.

ANXIETY, EXTRAVERSION, AND PROBABILITY LEARNING

a "50:50" approach to probability learning, while (b) low anxiety introverts in an older male sample will be most likely to show a "problem" approach.[3]

METHOD

The Experimental Situation

A simple binary choice situation was arranged, analogous to ones used with young adult males by Goodnow (1955) and others. On each of 100 trials, S had to predict which of two lights would appear. He made his prediction by pressing the button under the light on which he was betting. After each prediction, the left- or right-hand light immediately went on for one second, thus informing S which side was correct on that trial.

In actuality the left-hand light was correct on 70 trials and the right-hand light on 30, with this 70:30 probability being present and order randomized within each block of 10 trials. Which button S pushed on a trial, and which light was illuminated on that trial from the automatic program sequence, were recorded by pen marks on the channels of an Esterline-Angus moving tape. Later reading of the tape permitted us to count the number of times the right-hand button was pushed within a series of trials, and to measure, in terms of length of tape, the latency between a light's going off and S's next push of the left- or right-hand button. Because an initial period of familiarization with the payoff schedule was necessary before scores would become meaningful, it was decided beforehand to consider frequency and latency measures for the last 20 trials: that is, Trials 81-100.

The latency score used was a ratio consisting of the mean of an S's latencies for right-hand choices, divided by the mean of that S's latencies for left-hand choices. Mean latency for right-hand choices indicated S's reaction speed when predicting the rare alternative, while mean latency for left-hand choices indicated the same S's reaction speed when predicting the frequent alternative. Dividing the former mean by the latter mean hence provided an index of S's latency in predicting the rare alternative compared to his latency in predicting the frequent one.

Instructions to S directed him to predict which of the two lights would go on for each trial. S knew that the machine was programmed, so he couldn't alter or control the lights in any way. His only job was to predict, by pushing the appropriate button, which light would come on next. The main object of the test, S was told, was to predict correctly as often as possible.

Personality Variables of Manifest Anxiety and Extraversion-Introversion

The group form of the MMPI (Hathaway & McKinley, 1940) was in-

---

[3]Examples of analyzing the personality variables of manifest anxiety and extraversion-introversion in combination may be seen in research by Wallach and Gahm (1960) and Wallach and Greenberg (1960).

dividually administered to each S some time before he went through the probability-learning task. Scale scores then were obtained for each of the MMPI scales listed by Kassebaum, Couch, and Slater (1959, p. 228), plus certain others which are of too specialized interest to report here but are described by Slater in 1958.[4,5] Scores for these MMPI scales were intercorrelated for a sample of 129 older males, including Ss in the present study plus additional Ss from the same population. The correlation matrix was factor analyzed by Thurstone's complete centroid method (Thurstone, 1947), and orthogonal rotations carried out with the aim of maximizing the similarity of the two largest factors to the comparable two largest factors in the parallel MMPI study by Kassebaum, Couch, and Slater (1959) using male college students.

The two factors, each accounting for more of the total variance than any other factor, had to do with manifest anxiety and extraversion-introversion. It is of interest that the two largest factors emerging in the present older sample closely matched the two largest factors that emerged from the study of college students just cited. This finding provides evidence that these aspects of personality structure do not change with increasing age.

On the first factor, which accounted for about 32% of the total variance, those scales that were highest loading (.74 or better) were "admission of weaknesses" (Slater[5]), "anxiety" (Welsh & Dahlstrom, 1956, pp. 264-281), "caudality" (Williams, 1952), "dependency" (Navran, 1954), "hypertension correction scale" (described by Slater[5]), "neuroticism" (Winne, 1951), "parietal" scale (Friedman, 1950), "psychasthenia," and "schizophrenia" (Hathaway & McKinley, 1943), with negative loadings for "ego functioning" (Hathaway & McKinley, 1943) and "leadership" (Oettel, 1952). The "admission of weaknesses" scale, developed by Slater[5], contains those items from the MMPI for which a "yes" response means that S admits there is something psychologically or physically wrong with him. The presence of this scale, the Welsh "anxiety" scale, and Winne's "neuroticism" scale, plus the fact that most of the other scales noted above also are indicative of manifest feelings of "disturbance," seemed to make "manifest anxiety" the most appropriate label for this first factor.[6]

On the second factor, which accounted for about 10% of the total variance, those scales that were highest loading (.60 or better) were "agreement with general assertions" (Slater[5]), an "extraversion index" consisting of hypomania

[4]All statistical treatment of these MMPI data, the factor analysis, and computation of factor scores, were carried out by Philip E. Slater, to whom we are greatly indebted for aid in facilitating the present research. These data were processed at the MIT Computation Center.
[5]"Preliminary report of progress on 'correlates of anxiety' project," unpublished manuscript by P. E. Slater, 1958.
[6]It might also be called "neuroticism" (see Eysenck, 1956) or "ego weakness" (see Kassebaum, Couch, & Slater, 1959).

score minus depression score (Slater[5]), "hypomania" (Hathaway & McKinley, 1943), and "sociability" (Gough, 1957), with negative loadings for "repression, denial" (Welsh & Dahlstrom, 1956, pp. 264-281), and "social introversion" (Hathaway & McKinley, 1943). Slater's 1958 scale[5] for "agreement with general assertions" contains those items from the MMPI for which agreement means adherence to generally held preferences, interests, and beliefs about people and things. The nature of the various scales loading highly on this second factor seemed to make "extraversion-introversion" the most appropriate label for it.

Ss' anxiety and extraversion-introversion scores were based on these respective factors rather than on single scales, in order to enhance the reliability of the measures employed. Individual factor scores were obtained by a method described in detail by Kassebaum, Couch, and Slater (1959). In brief, the variables included for computation of factor scores on each of the two factors were so selected as to satisfy the following double criterion: (a) maximizing the communality of the factor measure in question, and (b) minimizing the saturation on the remaining factors by equalizing the positive and negative loadings of these variables on each of the remaining factors. When the set of variables was found which satisfied this double criterion for a factor measure, the individual scores for each variable (i.e., scale) in the set were converted into standard scores so that score distributions on the variables in question could be treated as equivalent. An individual's factor score for anxiety or extraversion then consisted of the algebraic sum of his standard scores for the variables included in the factor measure in question. The correlation between anxiety factor scores and extraversion factor scores was — .09 for the 52 older males in the present study, thus indicating the orthogonality of these two score dimensions.

Ss were separated into extraverts and introverts by dichotomizing the distribution of extraversion factor scores as close to the median as possible. Similarly, Ss were separated into high and low anxiety groups by dichotomizing the distribution of anxiety factor scores as close to the median as possible.[7] Four groups of Ss resulted from these dichotomizations: high anxiety extraverts, high anxiety introverts, low anxiety extraverts, and low anxiety introverts. As expected from the orthogonality of these two factors, a similar, although not identical, number of Ss fell into each of these four groups. These groups contained not the extremes of the anxiety and extraversion-introversion factor score distributions, but rather all of the cases.

---

[7]Splits could not occur exactly at the median because, for each of the two distributions of factor scores, a score for which several Ss were tied overlapped the median, with a majority of the tied Ss falling on one side of it. Each split was made by assigning all tied Ss to this majority side.

These two dichotomized personality dimensions constituted our treatment variables. Their effects on the dependent variables of frequency and latency of choice were investigated by 2-by-2 analyses of variance. Because of some inequalities in the cell sizes for each analysis, Snedecor's Method of Unweighted Means (Snedecor, 1956, pp. 385-388; Gosslee, 1959) was used in the computation. Since none of the bases of classification involved random sampling, the fixed constants model (McNemar, 1955, pp. 304-306) provided the suitable method for selecting the error term in computation of F ratios.

Control Variables

It was desirable to insure that any frequency and latency differences among the personality groups were not artifacts of intelligence, education, or age differences among these same groups. The intelligence measure used was the vocabulary subtest from the Wechsler intelligence test for adults (Wechsler, 1944). A vocabulary index was chosen to assess intelligence for two reasons. First of all, the vocabulary subtest of the Wechsler group has a very high correlation with the score based on the complete Wechsler battery of 11 subtests. Secondly, vocabulary scores have been reported to show the least decrement with age of any intelligence test measure (see, for instance, Doppelt & Wallace, 1955; Strother, Schaie, & Horst, 1957). Since our Ss were of an older age group and we wished to determine their intellectual comparability to young adults, vocabulary score seemed to be the most appropriate way of doing so.

The vocabulary test was administered individually after S went through the probability-learning task. Vocabulary scoring was done according to Wechsler's manual of instructions by each of two independent judges. The score used was the sum numerical value of S's vocabulary credits. Reliability of the two judges' sum scores, as determined by an intraclass correlation coefficient (Robinson, 1957; 1959) was .95 for a larger sample of older males and females including the 52 older males of the present study. Disagreements were resolved by taking the average of the two discrepant sum scores in question.

Highest attained level of education and date of birth also were known for all Ss. Education level was measured in terms of years of schooling. Age was determined to the nearest year by taking an arbitrary current date (the same date for all Ss) and subtracting from it each S's date of birth.

Subjects

The participants in the present study were 52 older males.[8] Their high

---

[8]While the work cited by Fillenbaum, Goodnow, and other researchers on probability learning has focussed on young adult males, the present research thus utilizes a sample of older males. That research on probability learning has focussed on males probably reflects the difficulty of inducing females to understand the nature of the probability learning task. Indeed, attempts by the present investigators to use older females proved infeasible for just this reason: interviews indicated that older females were unable to understand the nature of the experimental task.

ANXIETY, EXTRAVERSION, AND PROBABILITY LEARNING

intellectual and educational status made them comparable in these respects to male college students. Mean age was 70.6 ($SD = 7.0$). With regard to Wechsler vocabulary test score, the mean was 34.8 ($SD = 5.0$).[9] Finally, mean level of education was 13.6 years of schooling ($SD = 3.0$), or an average of 1.6 years of college.

RESULTS AND DISCUSSION

Table 1 presents the means and Table 2 the analysis of variance for frequency of choice of the rare alternative during the last 20 trials, i.e., Trials 81-

TABLE 1

MEAN FREQUENCIES OF CHOICE OF RARE ALTERNATIVE DURING THE LAST 20 TRIALS FOR PERSONALITY GROUPS ($N = 52$) *

Groups	Extraversion	Introversion
High anxiety	8.07	4.67
Low anxiety	6.33	8.14

*Group sizes in this and all following tables are 12, 14, 14, and 12, for high anxiety introverts, high anxiety extraverts, low anxiety introverts, and low anxiety extraverts, respectively.

100, for the four personality groups. Scores are approximately normally distributed and variances are homogeneous by Bartlett's test (Walker & Lev, 1953, pp. 193-194). The only significant F value is for the interaction of anxiety and extraversion. Frequency of choice of the rare alternative is higher for anxious extraverts and nonanxious introverts than the frequency of the rare alternative's actual occurrence. For the remaining two personality groups, however, frequency of choice of the rare alternative matches or is lower than the frequency of its actual occurrence. With 1 and 48 degrees of freedom, the F for this interaction is 5.92 ($p < .03$).

TABLE 2

ANALYSIS OF VARIANCE, FREQUENCIES OF CHOICE OF RARE ALTERNATIVE DURING THE LAST 20 TRIALS FOR PERSONALITY GROUPS ($N = 52$)

Source	df	Mean square	F	p
Extraversion	1	8.02	0.54	n.s.
Anxiety	1	9.83	0.66	n.s.
Interaction	1	87.79	5.92	$< .03$
Within cells	48	14.83		

[9]Data on college students reported by Dana (1957) and others indicate that our older Ss' scores tend, if anything, to exceed those of young adult college students.

M. A. WALLACH & R. C. GAHM

The latency ratio score means and analysis of variance are presented in Tables 3 and 4, respectively, for the four personality groups during the last

TABLE 3

MEAN LATENCY RATIO SCORES FOR SPEED OF CHOICE OF THE ALTERNATIVES DURING THE LAST 20 TRIALS FOR PERSONALITY GROUPS ($N = 52$) *

Groups	Extraversion	Introversion
High anxiety	1.01	1.27
Low anxiety	1.08	1.53

*Each S's ratio score consists of the mean latency of his right-hand responses divided by the mean latency of his left-hand responses during these 20 trials.

20 trials. An S's latency ratio score is the mean latency of his right-hand responses during those 20 trials divided by the mean latency of his left-hand responses during the same series of 20 trials.[10] The more a latency ratio score exceeds one, the greater is S's latency in predicting the rare in contrast to the frequent alternative. We find a significant effect for the extraversion-introversion dimension, introverts being slower in predictions of the rare in contrast to the frequent alternative than extraverts. As variances proved heterogeneous by Bartlett's test, a square root transformation was applied and led to homo-

TABLE 4

ANALYSIS OF VARIANCE, LATENCY RATIO SCORES FOR SPEED OF CHOICE OF THE ALTERNATIVES DURING THE LAST 20 TRIALS FOR PERSONALITY GROUPS ($N = 52$) *

Source	df	Mean square	F	p
Extraversion	1	2.70	6.21	< .03
Anxiety	1	0.69	1.58	n.s.
Interaction	1	0.24	0.54	n.s.
Within cells	48	0.43		

*While the means in Table 3 are raw scores, a square root transformation was applied for the analysis of variance in order to avoid heterogeneity of variances. Before the transformation, decimal points were moved one digit to the right and scores carried out to two figures beyond the new decimal point.

geneous variances by that test. The analysis of variance on transformed scores, which were approximately normally distributed, yielded an F of 6.21 (1 and 48 df, $p < .03$) for extraversion-introversion, with no other effect significant. The finding of larger latency ratio scores for introverts is heavily contributed to by the low-anxiety introverts, who show the largest latency ratios of all four groups. High-anxiety extraverts, on the other hand, show the smallest latency ratios of all the groups.

[10] In the case of two Ss (one in each of two groups), no right-hand responses were given during Trials 81 to 100. The mean right-hand latency term for their latency ratio score was estimated as the grand mean of the mean right-hand latency scores for all Ss during Trials 81 to 100. Such a procedure provides the most conservative estimate one could make.

ANXIETY, EXTRAVERSION, AND PROBABILITY LEARNING

These frequency and latency results constitute our main findings. What light do they shed on our initial questions of separating "problem" and "50:50" approaches to the probability-learning task and finding hypothesized personality correlates of each? From the means of Table 1, we note that high anxiety extraverts and low anxiety introverts both predict the rare alternative more frequently than it occurs, and more often than the other groups. Turning now to the means of Table 3, we find that a sizeable difference in latency ratio scores discriminates high-anxiety extraverts from low-anxiety introverts, even though both predict the rare event very often. High-anxiety extraverts have the smallest latency ratio scores of all four groups; indeed, they predict the rare alternative just about as quickly as they predict the frequent alternative. Low-anxiety introverts, on the other hand, have the largest latency ratio scores of all four groups, taking about 50% longer in predicting the rare alternative than they do in predicting the frequent one.

The probability-learning behaviors of high-anxiety extraverts and low-anxiety introverts thus meet our operational definitions for the "50:50" and "problem" approaches, respectively. While high anxiety extraverts predict the rare event with high frequency, their latency in predicting it is short—no longer than when they predict the frequent event. This is the behavior in terms of which we defined the "50:50" approach. According to this approach, S simply isn't sensitive to the infrequency of the rare event, and treats it as if it occurs more often than it does because, in effect, he doesn't really know any better. On the other hand, while low-anxiety introverts also predict the rare event with just as high a frequency, their latency in predicting it is long—half again longer than when they predict the frequent event. This is the behavior in terms of which we defined the "problem" approach, according to which S assumes the rare event occurs in some pattern and tries to solve the problem of accurately predicting when the rare event will occur.

Our expectations were confirmed, furthermore, with regard to which personality group would exhibit each approach. High anxiety should disrupt attempts at problem-solving, and extraversion should represent a relatively impulsive, non-contemplative attitude also inimical to problem-solving. Ss for whom both high anxiety and extraversion are present hence should be most likely to exhibit the impulsive, thoughtless behavior of the "50:50" approach, and this was the case. On the other hand, low anxiety should provide a supportive context for attempts at problem-solving, and introversion should represent an attitude of deliberation and contemplation also favorable to problem-solving. Ss who are low in anxiety and introverted hence should be most likely to show the deliberative, thoughtful behavior of the "problem" approach, and this too was the case.

In order to determine whether the relationships we have reported were influenced by intelligence, education, or age differences, analyses of variance were performed using the same four personality groups. The dependent variables tested were vocabulary score, education, and age, respectively, in three separate two-way analyses of variance. In none of the analyses did the F for interaction, rows, or columns even approach significance. We therefore may conclude that no vocabulary score, education, or age differences are influencing the relationships obtained.

SUMMARY AND CONCLUSIONS

The purpose of the present research was to use older males as Ss in an attempt to determine relationships between personality and approaches to a probability-learning situation. While attempts to obtain such relationships with young adult males have met with little success, it was felt that the wider range of individual differences in cognitive performances typically found in older as compared with younger Ss might reveal relationships between personality and probability learning that remain concealed in younger adults.

The probability-learning situation required S to predict which of two alternatives would occur on each of many tries, one of these alternatives occurring less frequently than the other but in a random sequence. Two approaches which involved a high rate of predicting the rare event were isolated as dependent variables whose relations with personality were to be assessed. In one approach, S supposes that there is some pattern to the rare alternative's occurrence and tries to solve the problem of accurately predicting when the rare event will occur (the "problem" approach); while in the other, S simply fails to discriminate just how infrequently the rare event occurs (the "50:50" approach). Although both approaches should lead to high frequency of predicting the rare event, we reasoned that the "problem" approach should result in longer latencies for predicting the rare event than for predicting the frequent event (since accurate prediction of the rare event is perceived as the main challenge), while the "50:50" approach should result in about the same latencies for predicting the rare as for predicting the frequent event (since S is insensitive to the difference between them).

High manifest anxiety was expected to disrupt, and low manifest anxiety to facilitate, attempts at deliberative problem-solving. So also extraverts were expected to be more impulsive and thoughtless, introverts more contemplative and thoughtful. Presence both of high anxiety and extraversion hence was expected to favor the occurrence of the thoughtless "50:50" approach to the probability learning task, while presence both of low anxiety and introversion was expected to favor the occurrence of the more thoughtful "problem" approach. These expectations were confirmed in an experiment with 52 older males.

ANXIETY, EXTRAVERSION, AND PROBABILITY LEARNING

Our main conclusions are as follows: (a) Light can be shed on relationships between personality and probability learning by using an age sample whose probability-learning performances provide a wider range of individual differences than typically is the case with young adults. (b) It is of importance to use combined rather than single procedures for the assessment of probability learning and of personality. In the present study, frequency and latency of choice were jointly used as probability learning indices; and manifest anxiety and extraversion-introversion were jointly used as personality indices.

REFERENCES

BRUNER, J. S., GOODNOW, J. J., & AUSTIN, G. A. *A study of thinking.* New York: Wiley, 1956.

DANA, R. H. A comparison of four verbal subtests on the Wechsler-Bellevue, Form I, and the WAIS. *J. clin. Psychol.,* 1957, 13, 70-71.

DOPPELT, J. E., & WALLACE, W. L. Standardization of the Wechsler Adult Intelligence Scale for older persons. *J. abnorm. soc. Psychol.,* 1955, 51, 312-330.

EASTERBROOK, J. A. The effect of emotion on cue utilization and the organization of behavior. *Psychol. Rev.,* 1959, 66, 183-201.

EYSENCK, H. J. The questionnaire measurement of neuroticism and extraversion. *Rivista di Psicologia,* 1956, 54, 113-140.

FEATHER, F. T. Subjective probability and decision under uncertainty. *Psychol. Rev.,* 1959, 66, 150-164.

FILLENBAUM, S. Some stylistic aspects of categorizing behavior. *J. Pers.,* 1959, 27, 187-195.

FRIEDMAN, S. H. Psychometric effects of frontal and parietal lobe brain damage. Unpublished doctoral dissertation, Univer. of Minnesota, 1950.

GOODNOW, J. J. Determinants of choice-distribution in two choice situations. *Amer. J. Psychol.,* 1955, 58, 106-117.

GOSSLEE, D. G. Level of significance and power of the unweighted means test. Paper read at Amer. Statist. Assn, Chicago, 1959.

GOUGH, H. G. *Manual for the California Psychological Inventory.* Palo Alto, Calif.: Consulting Psychology Press, 1957.

HATHAWAY, S. R., & MCKINLEY, J. C. A multiphasic personality schedule (Minnesota): I. Construction of the schedule. *J. Psychol.,* 1940, 10, 249-254.

HATHAWAY, S. R., & MCKINLEY, J. C. *Manual for the Minnesota Multiphasic Personality Inventory.* (Rev. ed.) New York: Psychological Corp., 1943.

KASSEBAUM, G. G., COUCH, A. S., & SLATER, P. E. The factorial dimensions of the MMPI. *J. consult. Psychol.,* 1959, 23, 226-236.

MCNEMAR, Q. *Psychological statistics.* (Rev. ed.) New York: Wiley, 1955.

NAVRAN, L. A rationally derived MMPI scale to measure dependence. *J. consult. Psychol.,* 1954, 18, 192.

OETTEL, A. Leadership: a psychological analysis. Unpublished doctoral dissertation, Univer. of California, 1952.

ROBINSON, W. S. The statistical measurement of agreement. *Amer. sociol. Rev.,* 1957, 22, 17-25.

ROBINSON, W. S. The geometric interpretation of agreement. *Amer. sociol. Rev.,* 1959, 24, 338-345.

SNEDECOR, G. W. *Statistical methods.* (5th ed.) Ames, Iowa: Iowa State Coll. Press, 1956.

STROTHER, C. R., SCHAIE, K. W., & HORST, P. The relationship between advanced age and mental abilities. *J. abnorm. soc. Psychol.,* 1957, 55, 166-170.

M. A. WALLACH & R. C. GAHM

THURSTONE, L. L. *Multiple factor analysis.* Chicago: Univer. of Chicago Press, 1947.

WALKER, H. M., & LEV, J. *Statistical inference.* New York: Holt, 1953.

WALLACH, M. A., & GAHM, R. C. Personality functions of graphic constriction and expansiveness. *J. Pers.,* 1960, 28, 73-88.

WALLACH, M. A., & GREENBERG, C. Personality functions of symbolic sexual arousal to music. *Psychol. Monogr.,* 1960, 74, No. 7 (Whole No. 494).

WECHSLER, D. *The measurement of adult intelligence.* Baltimore: Williams & Wilkins, 1944.

WELSH, G. S., & DAHLSTROM, W. G. *Basic readings on the MMPI in psychology and medicine.* Minneapolis: Univer. of Minnesota Press, 1956.

WILLIAMS, H. L. The development of a caudality scale for the MMPI. *J. clin. Psychol.,* 1952, 8, 293-297.

WINNE, J. F. A scale of neuroticism: an adaptation of the MMPI. *J. clin. Psychol.,* 1951, 7, 117-122.

Accepted August 31, 1960.

From G. O. M. Leith and E. A. Trown (1970). Programmed Learning, 7, 181–188, *by kind permission of the authors and Sweet and Maxwell*

PROGRAMMED

LEARNING

Vol. 7	July 1970	No. 3

THE INFLUENCE OF PERSONALITY AND TASK CONDITIONS ON LEARNING AND TRANSFER

G. O. M. LEITH and E. ANNE TROWN
*Sussex University and Memorial University of Newfoundland
City of Leicester College of Education*

Abstract: To test hypotheses about the optimal place of rules in school learning tasks 124 12-year-old children from a single campus were categorised by ability, sex and two personality traits—extraversion/introversion and general anxiety. The learning task was a program on vectors from which rules were abstracted and given either before or after sections of the program containing practice examples.

Further evidence for the superiority of rules following practice was obtained. Significant interactions of treatments and extraversion on post- and transfer-tests showed, however, that this occurred because the "rules before" was significantly poorer than the "rules after" condition for extraverts of both above and below average ability. There was no significant difference between the treatments for introverts. Anxiety level differences were not significant, but anxious children were slightly better than non-anxious.

INTRODUCTION

THIS experiment was undertaken as a further exploration of two areas of study. One of these is a series of investigations of the role of reviews and previews in overcoming conflict and interference between successive parts of a learning task. The other concerns the influence of two personality variables—anxiety and introversion/extraversion—on learning.

One of the authors has found that losses in recall and transfer from meaningful learning tasks may be accounted for by the occurrence of large amounts of inter-section interference between parts of a task, but that such conflict can be overcome by including summaries at the end of each section. Also effective is the provision of an overall final summary, though previews, whether given as a whole or distributed throughout the learning material, are ineffective (Leith and McHugh, 1967; Leith and Blake, 1967; Leith and Webb, 1968; Leith, Biran and Opollot, 1969). The present report takes up the same theme, while varying the breadth of summaries and the subject-matter. Single or double rules were employed rather than the much more extended summary passages of three of the experiments (*e.g.* ten propositions, a half-hour lesson, 1,000 words) though one other study used relatively short abstractions. Previous work was concerned with Social Anthropology, English, Geography and Physics. Modern Mathematics was chosen to extend the scope of the experiments.

The other aspect of the research is an inquiry into the extent to which anxiety and extraversion are influential in determining achievement. In refining our knowledge of psychology, there is a growing rapprochement between the psychology of individual differences and the psychology of learning. Not merely are questions being asked about the ways in which children and adults may differ from each other in abilities, attainments and personality or about the general principles of learning which apply to all organisms. There is a growing tendency to ask: " What significance have individual differences for *how* particular people learn and *what* they achieve? " The implication is that individuals may well differ in their manner of approaching learning tasks, that some methods of instruction may be suitable for a proportion but not for *all* pupils and that ideally we should match methods, media and order of presentation, in teaching, to particular students' strategies and modes of learning, their previously acquired knowledge, skills and aptitudes and their experience of success and failure.

This is the eventual aim of those teachers and psychologists who are endeavouring to establish principles for genuinely individual instruction and is a prime motive for research into computer-aided instruction. There has, however, been little success, as yet, in arriving at settled conclusions—indeed most of the work has been carried out in the tradition of individual differences only. Thus research has largely been directed at questions like: " is anxiety correlated with achievement in school? "; " which personality type is most or least successful in school and university? " Again, there have been inquiries into the validity of theoretical points of view, *e.g.* that anxiety hinders complex learning at extremes of the scale (too much, too little), though moderate amounts may be helpful.

Research on these points tends to be conflicting (Warburton, 1962; Lavin, 1967; Rushton, 1966). Several reasons may be put forward for the conflicts. Thus, there may be changes with age in the personality structures which most readily meet with success. The different conditions of primary, secondary and university education give prima facie grounds for expecting that independence and submissiveness may find fulfilment at different times or in different places. Another reason may be a fundamental instability in personality assessments in contrast with the *relative* consistency of cognitive measures. A third reason might be that conditions of learning, teaching and testing have different effects on different people so that, if these differences are neglected in a study, they will tend to cancel each other out or become revealed, now in one direction, now in another, depending on the predominance of unreported features of the situation or the sample.

That personality assessment is less consistent than attainment or intelligence measurement need not be argued.

Evidence for the first and third of the above points is beginning to accumulate. Some of this evidence has been summarised elsewhere (Leith, 1969; Amaria and Leith, 1969). A brief outline is given below.

Ten-year-old children in an experiment on the influence of several degrees of guidance on learning and applying concepts showed that, though there were no overall differences, this was because absence of structure and guidance favoured non-anxious but not anxious children, while a great amount of structuring and prompting was helpful to anxious but not to non-anxious children (Leith and Bosett, 1967). In comparing children of different personality types, the most successful were anxious introverts—a finding which was repeated with 12-year-olds in a study of social reinforcement and achievement (Leith and Davis, 1969). The learning materials of the first study were used again with students in a further education college where the finding was, once more, that the methods of guidance made no overall difference but that, within methods, opposite types benefited or were unsuccessful. This time, however, the maximum amount of prompting and guidance led to poor performance on the part of the extraverts and good performance by introverts. There was also a very great difference between anxious and non-anxious halves of the sample—the latter having the clear advantage.

A further study employed two carefully validated forms of a programmed text which were prepared and tested so as to give equivalent results. One form was highly structured, the other required a much greater tolerance of uncertainty in searching for explanatory principles.

Over 200 college of education students worked through the programs and were given transfer tests which required application and re-organisation of principles. Extraverts were more successful than introverts with the discovery type of program. Introverts were good with the clearly structured well-guided one though extraverts were significantly poorer with this type of learning. Overall, and cutting across this finding, non-anxious (below the median) subjects were better than anxious ones (Shadbolt and Leith, 1967).

One further study may be cited which brings in another dimension. Adults (aged around 40) were given training in the new decimal currency system and exchange, and conversion from the present coinage. One method was a succinct set of rules followed by a self-correctional test (together with a set of simulated coins). This may be considered to involve less structuring and guidance than the other methods which were: a linear programmed text with explicit practice in conversion, etc. and with directed coin handling; and the same material presented simultaneously (*i.e.* group paced) on sound tape. The unstructured method showed a significant positive relationship with extraversion (*i.e.* extraverts got higher scores than introverts) and a significant negative relationship with neuroticism (general anxiety)—in other words the greater the degree of anxiety, the lower the test score. On the other hand, the linear programmed text group showed zero relationships between personality and scores and the tape group larger but also non-significant correlations (Leith *et al.*, 1968). A small-step linear program on spelling given to secondary school children also showed no relationships between personality and achievement. The possibility thus arises that when the stress of difficulty is avoided, as in small-step programs, personality differences do not emerge but, when the mental effort is great, as in the studies cited earlier, personality factors have some influence on achievement.

THE EXPERIMENT

The entire project, of which this is one part, was carried out in two Leicestershire junior high schools which are situated on the same campus, children being allocated to one school or the other alphabetically. From a pool of 371 boys and girls aged between 11 years 8 months and 13 years 4 months in the second-year classes, 160 children of each sex were randomly chosen. After being dichotomised within schools and sexes at the median scores for general ability (Raven's Matrices) anxiety and extraversion/introversion (H.B. Personality Inventory, Hallworth, 1962), they were assigned randomly to one of ten groups. Thus each group contained 32 children, a boy and a girl from each school above the median intelligence, of more than average anxiety and of greater than average extraversion, and so on, completing all combinations of ability, anxiety and extraversion. Four of these groups were assigned to treatment conditions in which, in addition to working through a programmed text on modern mathematics, children were given verbally formulated rules either one at a time or two at a time and either before the section(s) they applied to or after them. In other words, a learner would read a rule, and a short section of program, then a second rule and another section of program, or he would be given

the two rules together followed by the two sections. Alternatively, he got the rules after sections.

The programmed texts were based on the approach of the Midlands Mathematics Experiment, chapter 12, Book I. This was considered particularly suitable since it was completely new work and yet required no particular background in order to enter it. They were validated in four schools different from the experimental schools.

Sixteen rules were identified, each of which was given expression in a sequence of frames containing exemplification in exercises and problems. Each of the frames in sequences embodying the rules required a response by the pupil, upon completion of which he was given immediate feedback in the form of knowledge of correct result. The total number of frames was 246.

In one of the schools the program was administered twice a week in lessons of 45 minutes duration for four weeks. The other school had some lessons of 35 minutes only. It was intended that two sections should be completed in each lesson but since lesson time was too short in one of the schools, these pupils were not strictly scheduled but nevertheless completed the task within the same total period. The tests were given immediately after completion of the program (*i.e.* in the fifth week). One of these tests assessed knowledge of the material of the program by means of test items on addition of vectors. The transfer test was made up of items not taught, *viz.* subtraction of vectors.

For the purpose of this analysis the groups reading rules one or two at a time were pooled. The treatments compared are thus reading rules before or

INFLUENCE OF PERSONALITY AND TASK CONDITIONS ON LEARNING

after practice examples. This design gives a total of 128 children with eight in each sub-group (categorised by treatments, ability, anxiety and extraversion). Four subjects were " lost " during the course of the experiment, two from one cell and one each from two of the others. To compensate for this, the missing scores were filled in by inserting the mean score of the original cell (*i.e.* group of four subjects) and four degrees of freedom were subtracted from the total number. This is essentially equivalent to carrying out an analysis on the means of the sub-groups and makes computation easier.

It was expected that the children reading rules after practice would achieve higher mean scores than those receiving rules first. The more anxious children were expected, at this stage, to score higher than the non-anxious. The most difficult prediction to make was that of the interaction of personality and attainment. Learning from the rules-first condition was expected to benefit pupils who welcome clear guidance and precisely outlined structure but to handicap those who react against the imposition of structure. From previous evidence and from observation there seems to be a class of individuals whose preferred method of learning is to plunge into an initially confused situation, manipulate and test correspondences and connections, and try hypotheses until a structure emerges. They are perhaps those people who resist being told how to get to places in a locality but prefer to keep trying alternative routes until they can get from anywhere to any other place without always knowing how they did so or being able to explain. This class of pupils was thought likely to get lower scores when reading rules before practising, even

though the opportunity for engaging in a search strategy was limited, since they are probably impatient of initial attempts to define structure. Which categories of personality fit pupils with these different strategies or styles are less certain. In older subjects the strategies go along with extraversion and introversion, whereas there is some evidence for expecting anxious and non-anxious junior school age children to react in these ways. The possibility is open, too, that 12-year-olds are at a transition point in development.

RESULTS

The post-test and transfer test scores were each given a $2 \times 2 \times 2 \times 2$ factorial analysis of variance. The post-test data showed two significant effects. An ability levels difference accounted for more than a third of the total variance, the more intelligent children having very significantly higher scores than those below average in I.Q. The second finding was a significant treatments $\times$ extraversion interaction ($p < 0.05$) which is shown in Table I.

Follow-up tests were made at each level of personality. There was no difference between the two groups of introverts, but the Rules After condition was superior to the Rules Before in the case of extraverts, ($t = 2.46$; $p < 0.02$, two-tailed). In fact, the rules before practice debilitated extraverts whose performance under this condition was clearly different from that of the other three groups.

Analysis of the transfer test scores revealed a similar pattern. Over one-third of the total variance was taken up by the difference between ability levels. There was also a treatments $\times$ extraversion interaction which was significant at

PROGRAMMED LEARNING

TABLE I

MEAN POST-TEST SCORES OF INTROVERTS AND EXTRAVERTS
UNDER TWO CONDITIONS OF LEARNING

Personality		Position of Rules	
	Before Practice	After Practice	Overall
Introverts	54·75	52·56	53·66
Extraverts	42·72	55·06	48·88
Overall	48·74	53·81	51·27

$$\sigma_{X_1 - X_2} = 5\cdot02; \quad df \ 108$$

TABLE II

MEAN TRANSFER TEST SCORES OF INTROVERTS AND EXTRAVERTS
UNDER TWO CONDITIONS OF LEARNING

Personality		Position of Rules	
	Before Practice	After Practice	Overall
Introverts	39·75	36·88	38·31
Extraverts	25·16	42·88	34·02
Overall	32·45	39·88	36·17

$$\sigma_{X_1 - X_2} = 6\cdot33; \quad df \ 108$$

less than the 0·05 level. Table II summarises the results.

Introverts, though again better if they were given their rules before practice, were not significantly so. Extraverts, however, were much lower in transfer when given rules first. A t-test (two-tailed) showed that the difference was significant at less than the 0·01 level (t = 2·80).

Two further points were of interest in the analysis. The non-significant Anxiety levels effect appeared both in the post-test and transfer test data and all interactions of anxiety with the other factors had F ratios of less than 2·00. Subjects above the median anxiety level were, in fact, slightly higher in post-test and in transfer test scores.

The other question under investigation was whether the provision of rules before or after practice gives better achievement —in conformity with four previous investigations.

In the present case this has been established for extraverts, though not for introverts. Since, however, the rules-after condition was expected to give better results, one-tailed t-tests were carried out to compare the means of those receiving rules before and rules after practice. The results are tabulated below in Table III. Though results were in the expected direction, they achieved significance overall between the two conditions of learning only in the test of transfer.

A further aspect of the results should be noted. The pattern in which rules after was better than rules before, for extraverts (but not for introverts) was repeated at both levels of ability.

INFLUENCE OF PERSONALITY AND TASK CONDITIONS ON LEARNING

TABLE III

ONE-TAILED COMPARISONS OF GROUPS LEARNING RULES BEFORE AND
RULES AFTER PRACTICE

	Rules Before	Rules After	Difference	t	p
Post-test	48·74	39·88	5·07	1·43	N.S.
Transfer test	32·55	53·81	7·43	1·66	0·05

DISCUSSION

Many previous studies have discussed relationships between personality and achievement. Almost all of them, however, have failed both to inquire into the nature of the teaching given and to consider the possibility that individuals of different temperaments may be helped or hindered in their learning by differences in teaching method. The present research is based on findings in two series of experiments. In one it has been shown that interference between the sections of verbal learning tasks may be overcome by means of reviews or summaries given at the end of sections, though the same material given in advance is of no value in enhancing learning. One question which arises is how small or large each section should be for optimum effectiveness. The sections in this experiment were short and the rules were somewhat difficult and abstract.

The second series of experiments which suggested the hypotheses tested, obtained results in which children of 10 to 11 years and students of over 16 years learned to solve problems under varying conditions of ambiguity and structure. Thus one condition contained sets of problems which had been given a random sequence, whereas another arranged them in sets and gave structuring prompts such as statements of rule and correct answers. With younger children, an interaction of anxiety with method was found, whereas the older students showed an interaction of extraversion and learning condition, anxious subjects being poorer than non-anxious.

This gave rise to the hypothesis that teaching materials constructed so as to induce errors and to arouse ambiguity and uncertainty would favour extraverts, while carefully structured, clearly defined sequences of teaching material would give better results with introverts, the anxious having lower scores than non-anxious subjects. These predictions were confirmed with college of education students who were given carefully prepared self-instructional programs on genetics which were constructed to implement these conditions.

Further work was clearly demanded which sought to find if the effects of anxiety, and extraversion, could be replicated with children of 12–13 years and if the proposed explanation of the interaction in terms of tolerance for structure could be confirmed. It was considered that giving rules which explain or cover the logic of practice examples would be likely to impose a greater degree of structuring than giving the same rules after practice examples. Thus, some learners would react unfavourably to the rules-first condition, and hence, achieve a poorer performance than when the results of their mode of attack are confirmed by means of a formulated rule. On the other hand, other pupils—those having a greater tolerance for formal guidance—would not be put off by the initial position of the rules though their status with rules after practice in a programmed learning sequence might not be seriously lowered.

The results of the experiment support the notion that individuals have different approaches to these learning tasks. Furthermore, at the age of 12–13 years, these differences in methods of learning can be categorised as belonging to children who are more or less introverted or extraverted (above and below the median score on a personality inventory).

The writer's previous work with children of about this age has indicated that, if anything, greater anxiety (scores above the median) results in higher achievement. In the present case this is in fact so, though no significant differences were revealed.

It may be stressed that the findings were obtained under regular school conditions (save that self-instructional programs were used to avoid teacher variance). Children from two different schools and both sexes were equally distributed across the experimental conditions but no attempt was made to reduce these sources of variance in the analysis. These measures were taken in order to overcome the objection that experimental results obtained in controlled conditions are unlikely to show up in the " noisy " conditions of the school situation.

REFERENCES

AMARIA, RODA P. and LEITH, G. O. M. (1969) " Individual versus co-operative learning II: the influence of personality," *Educational Research* **11**, 193–199.

HALLWORTH, H. J. (1962) *The H.B. Personality Inventory* (unpub.). University of Birmingham.

LAVIN, D. E. (1967) *The Prediction of Academic Performance*. New York: John Wiley.

LEITH, G. O. M. (1969) " Learning and personality " in W. R. Dunn and C. Holroyd (eds.), *Aspects of Educational Technology II*. London: Methuen.

LEITH, G. O. M., BIRAN, L. A. and OPOLLOT, J.A. (1969) " The place of review in meaningful verbal learning sequences," *Canadian Journal of Behavioural Science* **1**, 113–118.

LEITH, G. O. M. and BLAKE, I. H. (1967) *Teaching the Formulation of Definitions; a further study of the place of integrating rules.* Research Reports on Programmed Learning No. 16. University of Birmingham.

LEITH, G. O. M. and BOSETT, R. (1967) *Mode of Learning and Personality.* Research Reports on Programmed Learning No. 14. University of Birmingham.

LEITH, G. O. M. and DAVIS, T. N. (1969) " The influence of social reinforcement on achievement," *Educational Research* **11**, 132–137.

LEITH, G., LISTER, A., TEALL, C. and BELLINGHAM, J. (1968) " Teaching the new decimal currency by programmed instruction," *Industrial Training International* **3**, 424–427.

LEITH, G. O. M. and McHUGH, G. A. R. (1967) " The place of theory in learning consecutive conceptual tasks," *Education Review* **19**, 110–117.

LEITH, G. O. M. and WEBB, C. C. (1968) " A comparison of four methods of programmed instruction with and without teacher intervention," *Education Review* **21**, 25–31.

LEITH, G. O. M. and WISDOM, B. (1969) *An Investigation of the Effects of Error-making and Personality on Learning.* Unpublished report, University of Birmingham.

RUSHTON, J. (1966) " The relationships between personality characteristics and scholastic success in eleven-year-old children," *British Journal of Educational Psychology* **36**, 178–184.

SHADBOLT, D. R. and LEITH, G. O. M. (1967) *Mode of Learning and Personality II.* University of Birmingham.

WARBURTON, F. W. (1962) " The measurement of personality III," *Educational Research* **4**, 193–206.

From B. S. Gupta (1973). British Journal of Psychology, *64*, 553–557, *by kind permission of the author and Cambridge University Press*

THE EFFECTS OF STIMULANT AND DEPRESSANT DRUGS ON VERBAL CONDITIONING

By B. S. GUPTA

Department of Psychology, Guru Nanak University, Amritsar, India

The effect of stimulant and depressant drugs, affecting primarily either the CNS or the ANS, on verbal conditioning was examined. The subjects were allocated to three levels of the extraversion dimension of personality. A 5×3 randomized block design was replicated ten times. The sentence-completion technique was used. The study supports the following conclusions: (1) introverted subjects are more easily conditioned than extraverted subjects; (2) dexedrine facilitates, and phenobarbitone and chlorpromazine inhibit, the conditioning process; (3) dexedrine does not improve the conditioning level of introverted subjects; (4) ephedrine does not affect the process of conditioning; (5) variability (standard deviation) tends to increase under the influence of drugs primarily affecting the CNS.

This study was carried out within the framework of Eysenck's (1957, 1960*a*, 1967*a*) drug postulates that stimulant drugs increase introverted behaviour patterns and depressant drugs increase extraverted behaviour patterns, and that the susceptibility to the action of drugs is determined by the individual's temperamental characteristics. Similarly, stimulant drugs increase and depressant drugs decrease neuroticism (Eysenck, 1960*b*). However, in normal subjects the neuroticism dimension of personality probably does not exert its effect unless the situation is perceived as anxiety-producing (Eysenck, 1967*a*, *b*). In a recent study on verbal conditioning by Gupta & Singh (1971) the results indicate that neuroticism exerts little influence.

Pharmacologically the drugs primarily affecting the higher central nervous system (CNS) are termed central stimulants and depressants, and those affecting the autonomic nervous system (ANS) are known as autonomic stimulants and depressants. But such a classification seems arbitrary because the site of action of a drug is frequently not well established. Some researches (Broadhurst, 1957; Broadhurst *et al.*, 1959; Jawanda, 1965), however, have used such a classification for investigating the effects of drugs on various psychological phenomena.

The present study was designed to evaluate the comparative effects of central and autonomic stimulant and depressant drugs on verbal conditioning in subjects at three different levels (high, medium and low) on the extraversion (E) dimension of personality. The main objectives of the present investigation were: (i) to study the relationship between verbal conditioning and chemical agents, and (ii) to study the interaction of chemical agents and extraversion in verbal conditioning.

METHOD

Subjects

The subjects were graduate and postgraduate male students of different colleges and university departments. Their age range was 20–25 years. Ten subjects, selected on a random basis, were assigned to each of the five drug conditions at each level of extraversion. The Hindi translation (Das, 1961) of Eysenck's (1959) Maudsley Personality Inventory (MPI) was used for determining the level of extraversion. The number of subjects was 150. They were selected out of a sample of 1500 students to whom the MPI was administered. The distribution of E scores

B. S. Gupta

of the selected subjects was: E+, 39+ ; E, 26–28; E−, 15−. The selection of the extreme groups was done on the basis of mean ± 1·5 s.D. of E scores (E mean = 26·8; E s.D. = 7·9). The scores of the average group ranged between mean ± 0·1 s.D. The mean and s.D. of 1500 students were used for grouping the subjects. All the subjects ranged between mean ± 1 s.D. on the neuroticism dimension.

Drugs. The nature of each drug, its dose and the latency period are given below:

Drug	Nature of the drug	Dose (mg)	Latency period (min.)
Dexedrine	CNS stimulant	10	60
Phenobarbitone	CNS depressant	100	60
Ephedrine	ANS stimulant	30	35
Chlorpromazine	ANS depressant	100	90

The latency period of the drugs was determined on the basis of the pilot observations regarding the time of peak effect of the drugs. The latency periods are also in agreement with those suggested by Goodman & Gilman (1965) and the Pharmaceutical Society of Great Britain (1968). Calcium tablets were used as placebo.

Stimulus material

Taffell's (1955) sentence-completion technique was used. The stimulus material was 100 white unlined index cards (3 × 5 in.). A neutrally toned verb, in past tense, was typed in block letters in the centre of each card. Five pronouns, I, WE, YOU, HE and THEY, were inserted in one line in block letters below the verb. The sequence of pronouns on each card differed randomly.

Procedure

The subjects were tested individually after the oral administration of the drug or placebo. The drug or placebo was given, in a powdered form with water, by the experimenter's assistant to ensure a blind effect. The time between the treatment and the commencement of the experiment was in accordance with the drug schedule given above.

The subject's task was to construct, for each card, a sentence containing the verb and beginning with one of the pronouns. The first 20 cards were used to establish the operant level (initial score). The experimenter simply noted the subject's response whenever he began a sentence either with I or WE. For the next 60 cards the experimenter praised the subject by saying 'Good' in a flat unemotional tone whenever he used I or WE at the beginning of a sentence. This was the conditioning stage. Finally, for the last 20 cards no reinforcement was given and the procedure was similar to that adopted for the first 20 cards. The score obtained in this way was named the 'test score'. The cards were exposed on a slightly slanting board which held the entire stack of cards. The cards were presented, one by one, by simply removing the card on the top of the stack. Subject's choice of the pronoun was recorded verbatim on a record sheet and the frequency of the response, i.e. the desired pronoun, was used as a quantitative measure of the conditioned response. The order in which the cards were arranged was randomized from subject to subject by shuffling them before the commencement of each conditioning session. Immediately after the experiment, each subject, tested individually, was carefully interviewed with a view to eliciting information regarding his awareness of the correct contingency between his behaviour and experimenter's reinforcer. The sentence-completion technique of verbal conditioning is prone to be susceptible to cognitive awareness (Ingling, 1968; Miller, 1967, 1968; Miller & Babcock, 1970; Miller & Knoll, 1971); hence, during the course of the experiment, 24 subjects showing awareness were eliminated and replaced by others not showing awareness.

The subjects were requested, through personal communication, to avoid alcohol and other strong drinks during the 12 hr. prior to the experiment.

Effects of drugs on verbal conditioning

Table 1. *Results of analysis of variance*

Source of variance	D.F.	M.S.	F	P
Drug treatments (T)	4	2·59	12·33	0·01
Extraversion (E)	2	0·71	3·38	0·05
T × E	8	0·87	4·14	0·01
Within	135	0·21		

Table 2. *Means and S.D.s of drug treatments within each of the extraversion groups*

Extraversion		Dexedrine	Pheno-barbitone	Ephedrine	Chlor-promazine	Placebo
E+	Mean	1·25	0·34	0·70	0·35	0·62
	S.D.	0·36	0·25	0·12	0·11	0·06
E	Mean	1·86	0·41	0·94	0·63	0·88
	S.D.	0·39	0·30	0·14	0·12	0·07
E−	Mean	1·20	0·56	1·01	0·73	0·93
	S.D.	0·45	0·31	0·13	0·14	0·07

The differences between the means of phenobarbitone and placebo, and chlorpromazine and placebo conditions, are significant at the 0·01 level for each level of extraversion. The differences between the means of dexedrine and placebo conditions are significant at the 0·01 level for E+ and E groups.

The differences between the S.D.s of dexedrine and placebo, and phenobarbitone and placebo conditions, are significant at the 0·01 level for each level of extraversion.

RESULTS

The test scores of the subjects were evaluated against their respective operant scores. This was done by transforming the scores into inflexion ratios by the following formula:

$$\text{inflexion ratio} = (B-A)/A$$

(A and B represent a subject's operant and test scores, respectively). The positive and negative values of the ratio indicate an increase or decrease in the level of conditioning. Inflexion ratios, thus obtained, were subjected to two-way analysis of variance, the results of which are given in Table 1.

Table 2 shows the means and S.D.s of various drug treatments within each of the extraversion groups.

DISCUSSION

The results of analysis of variance (Table 1) reveal that extraversion, drugs and their interaction are significant variables in verbal conditioning. The variance due to extraversion was evaluated by a t test. The results afford good support for Eysenck's (1967a) theory by revealing that subjects scoring low on the E scale (introverts) are more conditioned, in a situation like Taffell's (1955) verbal conditioning, than their counterparts scoring high on this scale (extraverts). Similar analysis of the variance, due to drug treatments, indicates that both phenobarbitone and chlorpromazine inhibit conditioning ($P < 0.01$), and dexedrine facilitates this tendency ($P < 0.01$). Ephedrine, a stimulant drug primarily affecting the ANS, also tends to facilitate conditioning, but the results are non-significant statistically.

The results also support our previous findings that individuals differ in their

B. S. GUPTA

susceptibility to drug effects (Gupta, 1970; Gupta & Singh, 1971) as significant interaction of extraversion and drug treatments has been obtained (F ratio significant at 0·01 level – Table 1). In order to ascertain which drug treatment reactions of various groups were more pronounced, the t test was applied to evaluate the significance of differences among the various means (Table 2) of drug and E groups. The results reveal that neither dexedrine (CNS stimulant) nor ephedrine (ANS stimulant) facilitate conditioning in introverted subjects. Introverted subjects, who possess a high basic level of cortical excitation (Eysenck, 1967a), are known as highly aroused people (Claridge, 1967; Davies & Tune, 1970; Gray, 1964, 1967, 1968, 1970; Nebylitsyn & Gray, 1972; Passingham, 1970; White & Mangan, 1972). Probably such persons are already at the optimal level of performance (Eysenck, 1967b). Further increase in their excitation or arousability level, with stimulant drugs, activates the neural inhibitory centres (Davies & Tune, 1970) and either this leads to impairment in performance or the facilitating effect of the drugs gets masked. This seems to be the case with our introverted subjects who do not show expected trends in verbal conditioning under the influence of stimulant drugs.

Table 2 indicates that the variability (standard deviation) tends to increase under the influence of both stimulant and depressant drugs primarily affecting the CNS ($P < 0·01$). A similar trend is also discernible in the case of drugs primarily affecting the ANS, but the results are non-significant.

The data were collected when the author was at Government College, Kurukshetra, India. The author's thanks are due to Dr K. C. Sharma, Principal, Government College, Kurukshetra, for providing the necessary facilities for data collection.

REFERENCES

BROADHURST, P. L. (1957). Determinants of emotionality in the rat. 1. Situational factors. *Br. J. Psychol.* **48**, 1–12.

BROADHURST, P. L., SINHA, S. N. & SINGH, S. D. (1959). The effect of stimulant and depressant drugs on a measure of emotional reactivity in the rat. *J. genet. Psychol.* **95**, 217–226.

CLARIDGE, G. S. (1967). *Personality and Arousal.* London: Pergamon Press.

DAS, G. (1961). Standardization of Maudsley Personality Inventory (MPI) on an Indian population. *J. psychol. Res.* **5**, 7–9.

DAVIES, D. R. & TUNE, G. S. (1970). *Human Vigilance Performance.* London: Staples Press.

EYSENCK, H. J. (1957). *The Dynamics of Anxiety and Hysteria.* London: Routledge & Kegan Paul.

EYSENCK, H. J. (1959). *Manual of the Maudsley Personality Inventory.* London: University of London Press.

EYSENCK, H. J. (ed.) (1960a). *Experiments in Personality*, 2 vols. London: Routledge & Kegan Paul.

EYSENCK, H. J. (1960b). Drug postulates, theoretical deductions, and methodological considerations. In L. Uhr & J. G. Miller (eds.), *Drugs and Behaviour.* New York: Wiley.

EYSENCK, H. J. (1967a). *The Biological Basis of Personality.* Springfield, Ill.: Thomas.

EYSENCK, H. J. (1967b). Intelligence assessment: a theoretical and experimental approach. *Br. J. educ. Psychol.* **37**, 81–98.

GOODMAN, L. S. & GILMAN, A. (1965). *The Pharmacological Bases of Therapeutics.* New York: Macmillan.

GRAY, J. A. (1964). *Pavlov's Typology.* London: Pergamon Press.

GRAY, J. A. (1967). Strength of the nervous system, introversion–extraversion, conditionability and arousal. *Behav. Res. Ther.* **5**, 151–169.

GRAY, J. A. (1968). The physiological basis of personality. *Adv. Sci.* **24**, 293–305.

Effects of drugs on verbal conditioning

GRAY, J. A. (1970). The psychophysiological basis of introversion–extraversion. *Behav. Res. Ther.* **8**, 249–266.

GUPTA, B. S. (1970). The effect of extraversion and stimulant and depressant drugs on verbal conditioning. *Acta psychol.* **34**, 505–510.

GUPTA, B. S. & SINGH, S. D. (1971). The effect of extraversion, neuroticism and a depressant drug on verbal conditioning. *Ind. J. exp. Psychol.* **5**, 15–17.

INGLING, J. (1968). The effects of factors associated with the Taffell presentation technique in the operant conditioning of verbal behaviour. *Diss. Abstr.* **29**, IB, 259.

JAWANDA, J. S. (1965). Age, sex and personality variables in verbal conditioning and its modification by drugs. (Unpublished Ph.D. thesis, Punjab University.)

MILLER, A. (1967). Awareness, verbal conditioning and meaning conditioning. *Psychol. Rep.* **21**, 681–691.

MILLER, A. (1968). The dimensionality of awareness in verbal conditioning. *J. Psychol.* **70**, 99–111.

MILLER, A. & BABCOCK, B. (1970). The operant conditioning of awareness. *J. gen. Psychol.* **83**, 169–177.

MILLER, A. & KNOLL, C. (1971). Meaning conditioning and awareness among children. *J. genet. Psychol.* **119**, 187–194.

NEBYLITSYN, V. D. & GRAY, J. A. (eds.) (1972). *Biological Bases of Individual Behaviour.* New York: Academic Press.

PASSINGHAM, R. E. (1970). The neurological basis of introversion–extraversion: Gray's theory. *Behav. Res. Ther.* **8**, 353–366.

PHARMACEUTICAL SOCIETY OF GREAT BRITAIN (1968). *British Pharmaceutical Codex.* London: Pharmaceutical Press.

TAFFELL, C. (1955). Anxiety and the conditioning of verbal behaviour. *J. abnorm. soc. Psychol.* **51**, 496–501.

WHITE, K. D. & MANGAN, G. L. (1972). Strength of the nervous system as a function of personality type and level of arousal. *Behav. Res. Ther.* **10**, 139–146.

(Manuscript received 24 *October* 1972)

From H. J. Eysenck and A. Levey (1972). In: V. D. Nebylitsyn and J. A. Gray (Eds.), "Biological bases of individual behaviour," pp. 206–220, *by kind permission of the authors and Academic Press*

Chapter 13

Conditioning, Introversion–Extraversion and the Strength of the Nervous System*

H. J. EYSENCK and A. LEVEY

Institute of Psychiatry, University of London, England

Teplov's main contribution to psychology consisted of the systematic working out of the relations obtaining between personality, on the one hand, and the concepts of excitation and inhibition, on the other (Gray, 1964). The work carried out in our laboratories, too, has concerned itself very much with these relations (Eysenck, 1957), and in spite of obvious differences in approach there have also been certain interesting similarities. In particular, it would seem that the Pavlovian notion of "strong" and "weak" nervous systems, which has formed the basis for most of Teplov's experimental work, bears a striking similarity to the notions of extraverted and introverted personality types, as they emerge from our own. The "weak" personality type appears to resemble the introvert, the "strong" personality type the extravert. Even if it is admitted that similarity does not imply identity, it is certainly striking that two quite independent approaches should issue in such closely related concepts (Eysenck, 1967).

This similarity becomes even more apparent when we consider these personality types in terms of physiological and neurological concepts. Gray (1964) has translated the concepts used by Pavlov and Teplov into the language of modern neurophysiology, and has shown that different degrees of arousal of the reticular formation can mediate all or most of the experimentally ascertained differences between "weak" and "strong' nervous systems. In a similar manner, Eysenck (1967) has suggested a close relationship between reticular formation arousal thresholds and introversion–extraversion. According to these theories, low thresholds of the ascending reticular activating system would be characteristic of the "weak" nervous system and the introvert, high thresholds of the

* Thanks are due to the M.R.C. for the support of this investigation.

"strong" nervous system and the extravert. Again, the synchronizing part of the reticular formation exerts an inhibitory influence on cortical activity, and it may be supposed that low thresholds of this system characterize the extravert and the "strong" nervous system. Unfortunately, little direct evidence is available relating to these theories, but work on the EEG (Savage, 1964), on critical flicker fusion (Gray, 1964) and in particular on drugs known to affect the reticular formation (Killam, 1962) has on the whole borne out the general theory in a rather striking manner (Eysenck, 1963b).

Among the similarities resulting from experimental work perhaps the most impressive is that relating to sensory thresholds. The lower thresholds found in persons possessing a "weak" nervous system constitute one of the most important proofs of the Teplov school for the correctness of their theories. As a direct consequence of their work, and the hypothesis relating introversion to a "weak" nervous system, several studies have recently been carried out in England to study sensory thresholds in introverts and extraverts. Using the Maudsley Personality Inventory (Eysenck, 1959) as the measure of personality, Haslam (this volume) has several times found a significantly lower pain threshold in introverts as compared with extraverts, and Smith (1968) has similarly discovered lower auditory thresholds in introverts using the usual psychophysical methods as well as a forced-choice technique. These and other experiments, too numerous to mention, make it likely that the conceptions of our two schools are in fact closely related, and that empirical work directly devoted to a verification of this hypothesis would be of considerable value.

One interesting contrast between the Russian and the English work has been the comparative neglect of direct measures of conditioning by Teplov, as compared with the large body of work reported on this topic by the Maudsley group (Eysenck, 1965b). We have used in the main the eyeblink conditioning experiment, in which a puff of air to the eye is the unconditioned stimulus (UCS), and a tone delivered over ear-phones the conditioned stimulus (CS). A summary of the work on this test and on GSR conditioning, carried out by us and also by various other experimenters, has shown that different investigators have reported very divergent results, some producing the predicted positive correlation between introversion and conditionability, others failing to find such a correlation. The failure of so many experiments to duplicate the results of our early studies, which gave very positive results, would appear to be due to their failure to duplicate the exact conditions of the tests carried out; as will be shown below, the general theory linking introversion with greater cortical arousal ("excitation") predicts in some

H. J. EYSENCK AND A. LEVEY

detail the exact choice of parameters which alone would be expected to generate positive correlations between introversion and conditioning. In particular, it is proposed that the following three parameters are crucial, and must be carefully selected and controlled in order to obtain positive results. (1) Partial reinforcement favours introverts; 100% reinforcement does not. (2) Weak unconditioned stimuli favour introverts; strong UCS do not. (3) Small CS–UCS intervals favour introverts; large US–UCS intervals do not.

Partial reinforcement. Pavlov has already pointed out that unreinforced trials produced inhibition, and if we link the growth of inhibition with extraversion in particular, then clearly partial reinforcement will impede conditioning more in extraverts than in introverts (Eysenck, 1957). Furthermore, there is direct evidence to link partial reinforcement with cortical inhibition along neurophysiological lines; as Magoun (1963) has pointed out, "in each of the several categories of conditioned reflex performance in which Pavlov found internal inhibition to occur . . . recent electrophysiological studies have revealed features of hyper-synchronization and/or spindle bursting in the EEG".

UCS strength. It is well known that conditioning is in part a function of the strength of the UCS (and possibly of the CS also—Kimble, 1961). Given that introverts have lower sensory thresholds (and probably smaller difference thresholds as well) than extraverts, then objectively identical UCS would be subjectively stronger for introverts, and should therefore produce stronger conditioned responses. UCS of too great strength, on the other hand, should produce "protective inhibition" much earlier in introverts than in extraverts. It may further be surmised that UCS of low strength adapt quickly, and thus produce inhibition; this growth of inhibition again should be stronger in extraverts than in introverts. There is direct experimental backing for the inhibitory action of weak UCS and of partial reinforcement in the work of Ross and Spence (1960) who conclude that "inhibition of performance is more readily accomplished under conditions of low puff strengths . . . The differences between the 100% and 50% reinforcement groups at high levels of puff strength require that considerable 'inhibition' still be present with such puffs".

CS–UCS interval. It is well known that optimal CS–UCS intervals in eye-blink conditioning centre around 500 msec, but no work appears to have been done on individual differences in this respect. The concept of reaction time is clearly relevant here; Gray has summarized the work of the Teplov school by saying that "at stimulus intensities below that at which asymptotic reaction time is reached, the weaker the nervous system, the faster the reaction time". By going below the 500 msec mark, we can ensure that we go below the asymptotic value for conditioning, and under those conditions, particularly when allied with weak UCS, we would expect introverts to react better to short CS–UCS intervals than extraverts. Gray (1964) has reviewed the whole literature on these relations quite exhaustively, including the work of Fuster (1958) and of Isaac (1960) on the association with the reticular formation, and there seems little doubt that the experimental findings mediate a relationship such as that proposed.

It follows from what has been said that the very divergent findings with respect to the proposed relationship between introversion and eyeblink conditioning which form such a prominent feature of the literature, including the Russian, are only to be expected, considering that many different variations of type of reinforcement, CS–UCS interval and strength of UCS and CS have been employed. The experiment to be reported here, which was carried out by Levey in the Maudsley laboratory, was specially designed to throw light on the hypotheses outlined above, relating to the change in the relation between conditioning and introversion with change in the conditions of the experiment. Subjects were tested under all possible combinations of two conditions of reinforcement, two CS–UCS intervals, and two UCS strengths; for each pair of conditions a prediction was made (this has already been outlined) as to which condition would favour the introverts as compared with the extraverts. The detailed conditions of testing were as follows: *Reinforcement schedule*—100% reinforcement against 67% reinforcement. *CS–UCS interval*: 400 msec vs. 800 msec. *UCS strength*: 6 lb/in^2 vs. 3 lb/in^2.

Subjects were selected on the basis of the Maudsley Personality Inventory, and categorized as extraverted, introverted, or intermediate (ambivert); they were also categorized as high, low or average on neuroticism. Equal numbers were then chosen from each of these categories, until 18 subjects had been included in each of the eight experimental groups (combinations of reinforcement schedule, CS–UCS interval, and UCS strength), making a total of 144 subjects in all; all of these were male. Figure 1 shows the growth, over 48 acquisition trials, of conditioned habit strength for the extraverted, introverted and ambivert groups; there is a slight superiority of the introvert group over the extravert group in this overall comparison, amounting to some 20% on the last few trials; the ambivert group is situated in between the other two groups most of the time, although it overlaps with both other groups on occasion. The differences are not significant on an analysis of variance, largely because of the tremendous size of the variances; this of course is not unexpected because of the variations in testing conditions imposed by

H. J. EYSENCK AND A. LEVEY

our general scheme. Figures 2a and 2b show the results for weak and strong UCS respectively; as expected the weak UCS shows introverts much more conditionable, while the strong UCS shows extraverts more conditionable. Ambiverts are intermediate between the two extreme groups. This reversal is quite dramatic and supports the prediction.

The results for the 400 and 800 msec CS–UCS interval show, as expected, that the short interval favours the introverts; for the long interval there is very little difference between the groups (Figs. 3a, b). The results for partial and continuous reinforcement show that there is a slight tendency for partial reinforcement to favour the introverts, but

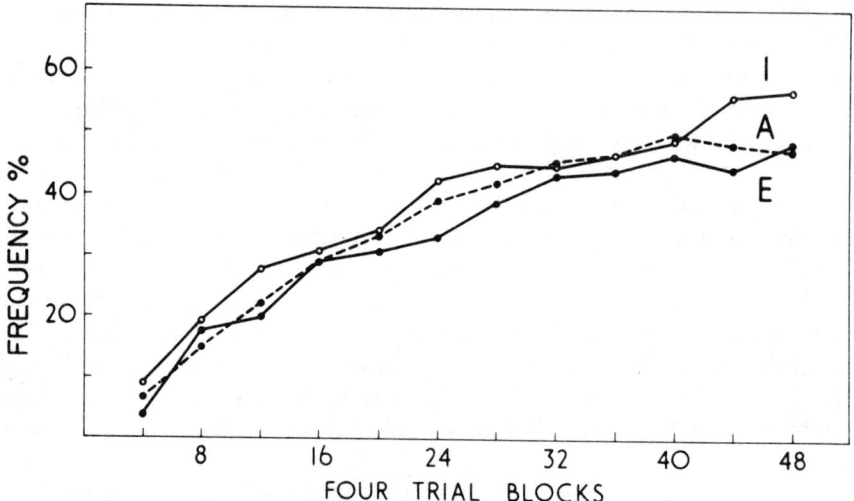

FIG. 1. Rate of eyelid conditioning in extraverts, introverts and ambiverts under combination of all parameters.

this tendency is not strong enough to give much support to our hypothesis (Figs. 4a, b). If the results of this experiment can be taken as representative, we might conclude that strength of UCS was the most important parameter, followed by CS–UCS interval, with reinforcement schedule last. However, any such generalization would of course be restricted to the values of UCS strength, interval duration, and reinforcement schedule adopted in this experiment; there is no reason to suppose that these are in any sense optimal. It seems very likely that much greater differences between introverts and extraverts could be demonstrated with better choice of parameter values. In particular, pressures of less than 3 lb/in^2 as UCS strength, and intervals even shorter than 400 msec, present good prospects of improving discrimination.

13. CONDITIONABILITY AND EXTRAVERSION

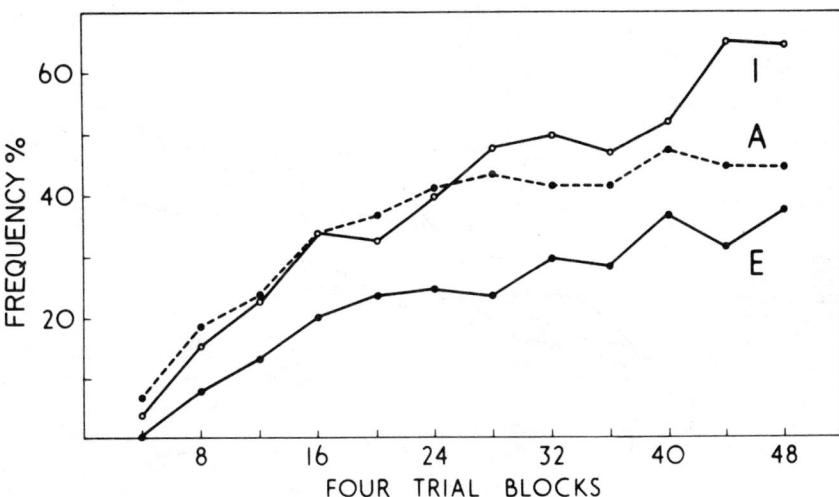

FIG. 2a. Rate of eyelid conditioning for introverts, ambiverts and extraverts under weak UCS conditions.

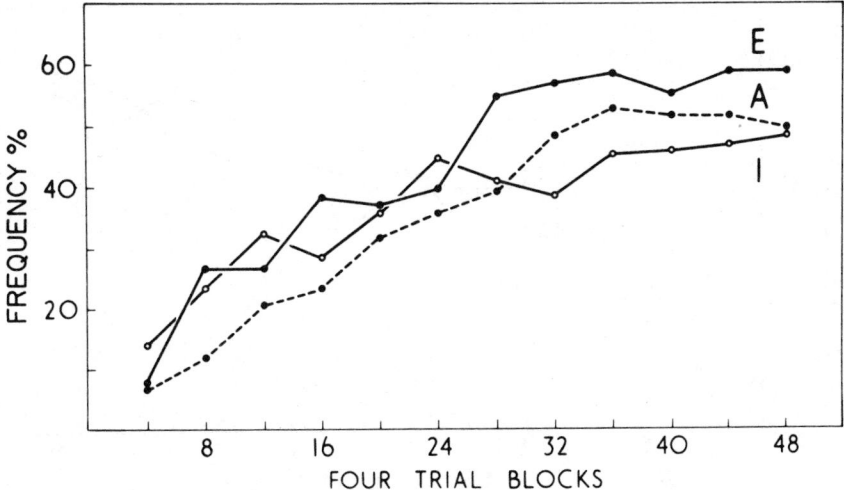

FIG. 2b. Rate of eyelid conditioning for extraverts, ambiverts and introverts under strong UCS conditions.

Figures 5a and 5b present results for optimal and worst combinations of conditions respectively, i.e., weak UCS, short CS–UCS interval, and partial reinforcement (Fig. 5a) as against strong UCS, long CS–UCS interval, and continuous reinforcement (Fig. 5b). The difference is

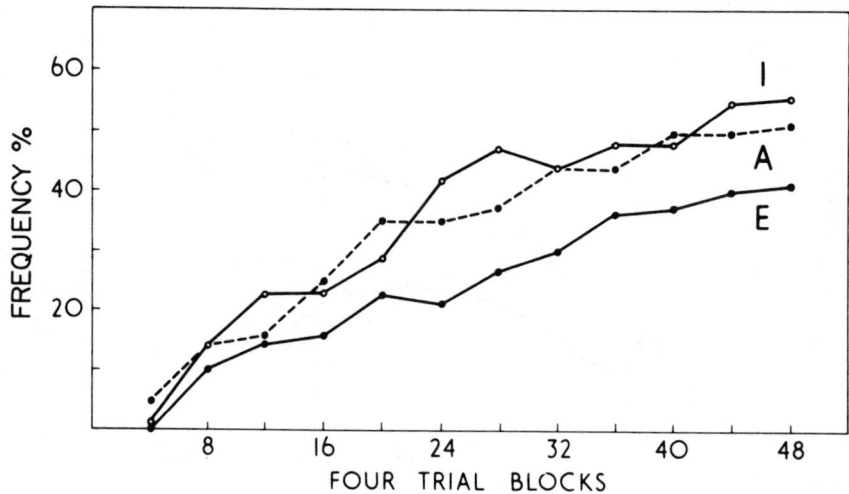

FIG. 3a. Rate of eyelid conditioning for introverts, ambiverts and extraverts under short CS–UCS interval conditions.

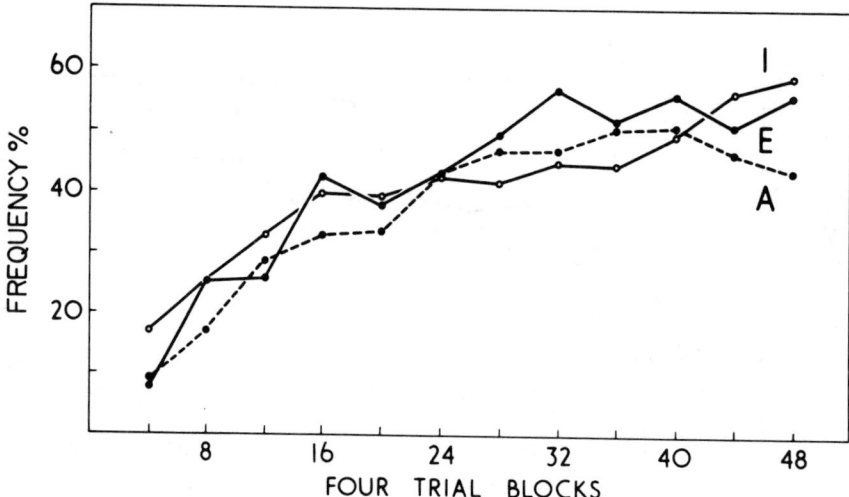

FIG. 3b. Rate of eyelid conditioning for extraverts, ambiverts and introverts under long CS–UCS interval conditions.

obvious, and may be summed up in the intra-group correlations. For the optimal conditions, the correlation between introversion and conditioning is +0·40, while for the worst conditions it is −0·31; this difference is significant at the 1 % level on a one-tail test. In the combination of

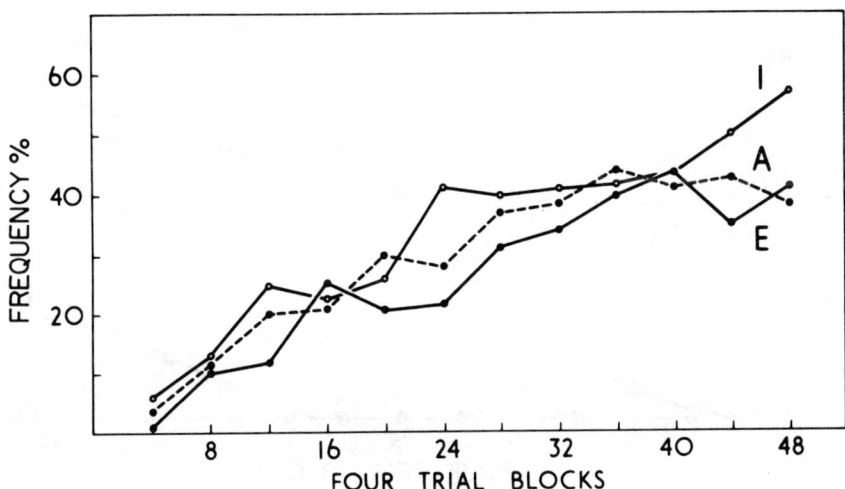

FIG. 4a. Rate of eyelid conditioning for introverts, ambiverts and extraverts under partial reinforcement conditions.

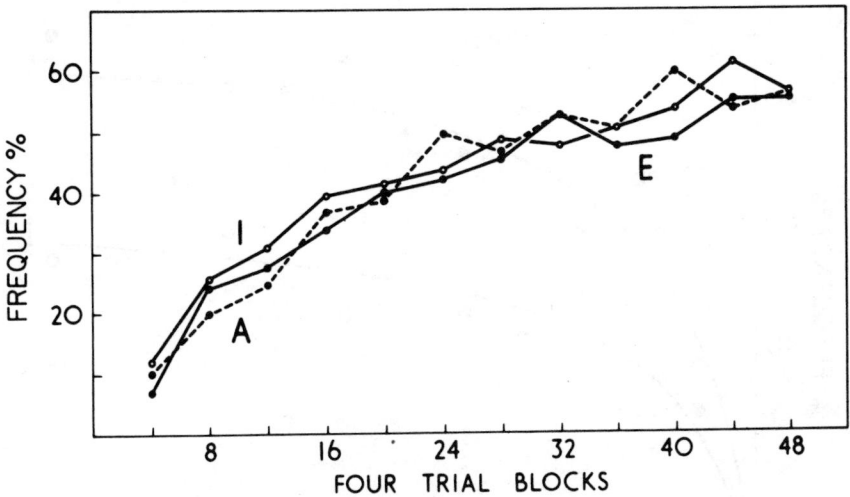

FIG. 4b. Rate of eyelid conditioning for extraverts, ambiverts and introverts under 100% reinforcement conditions.

conditions favourable, according to theory, to the introverts, we find that after 30 trials the extraverts show no evidence of any conditioning at all, while the introverts have reached a level of conditioning at which 46% of responses are in fact conditioned. Conversely, under conditions

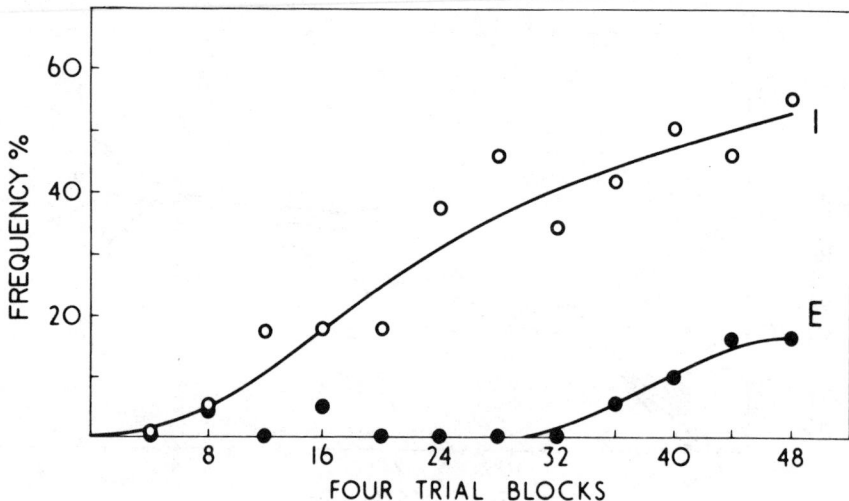

FIG. 5a. Rate of eyelid conditioning for introverts and extraverts under conditions of partial reinforcement, weak UCS, and short CS–UCS interval.

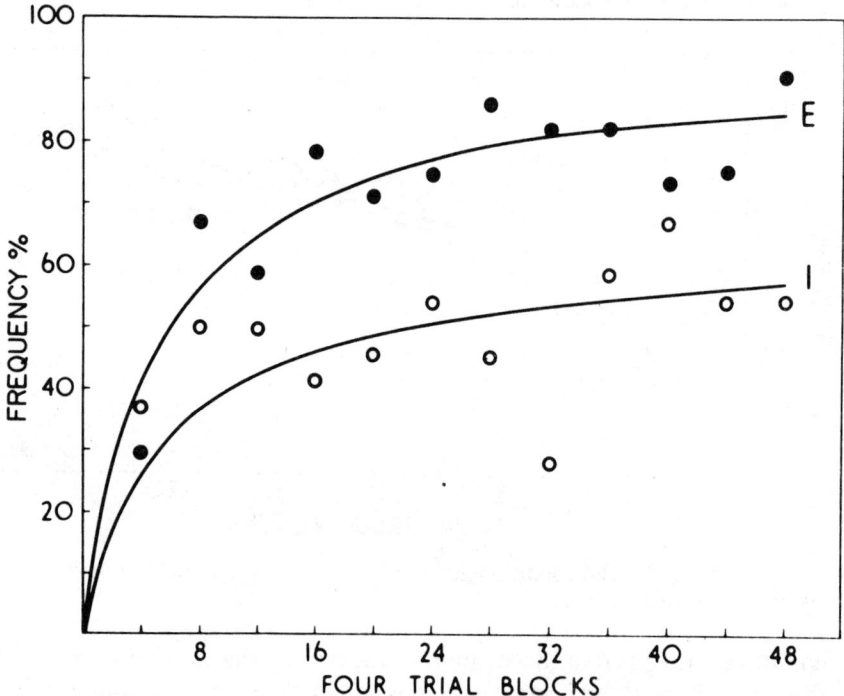

FIG. 5b. Rate of eyelid conditioning for extraverts and introverts under conditions of 100% reinforcement, strong UCS, and long CS–UCS interval.

favouring the extraverts, these produce after 30 trials almost twice as many conditioned responses as do the introverts.

When we say that conditions are favourable to the introverted or the extraverted group, we are of course speaking in terms of comparison of the one group with the other. In actual fact there are many interesting comparisons to be made taking into account absolute levels of conditioning. Thus introverts achieve identical levels of conditioning at the end of the experiment (54%), but they reach this end along quite different paths (Fig. 6a). The introverts working under unfavourable conditions (as compared with extraverts) achieve a high level of conditioning very early (after four trials only) and do not change much after that; under favourable conditions (as compared to extraverts) they show a regular increase which gradually brings them up to the same level. Extraverts under favourable and unfavourable conditions behave quite differently, as shown by the fact that the terminal values reached by them after 48 trials differ sharply; under unfavourable conditions, only 12% condition, under favourable conditions, 92% (Fig. 6b). If these data can be assumed to be generally valid, then it would seem that extraverts are much more at the mercy of conditions, while introverts ultimately reach reasonable levels of conditioning regardless of conditions. Replication of these results would seem to be desirable before too much effort is spent on explanations along theoretical lines. [It is interesting to note that the ambivert group shows very similar growth patterns under both conditions, namely the usual gradual increment in number of conditioned responses (Fig. 6c). As might have been expected the strong UCS–continuous reinforcement conditions result in better conditioning, but there is no dramatic difference in the shape of the curves; all that is apparent is a lower starting point and a less marked slope for the weak UCS–partial reinforcement conditions.]

In this case conditions may be said to be *overall* favourable or unfavourable according to the total amount of conditioning that takes place under these conditions for the total population tested. Thus strong UCS intensity produces quicker conditioning than does weak UCS intensity; 800 msec CS–UCS intervals are somewhat better than 400 msec intervals; continuous reinforcement is better than partial reinforcement. The results clearly show that the conditions which are favourable for the formation of conditioned responses *on the whole* are, in this experiment at least, also those which are favourable to extraverts and unfavourable to introverts, respectively. One might be tempted to argue from these facts towards some general law of the following kind: introverts form conditioned responses even under objectively unfavourable conditions, whereas extraverts only form conditioned responses

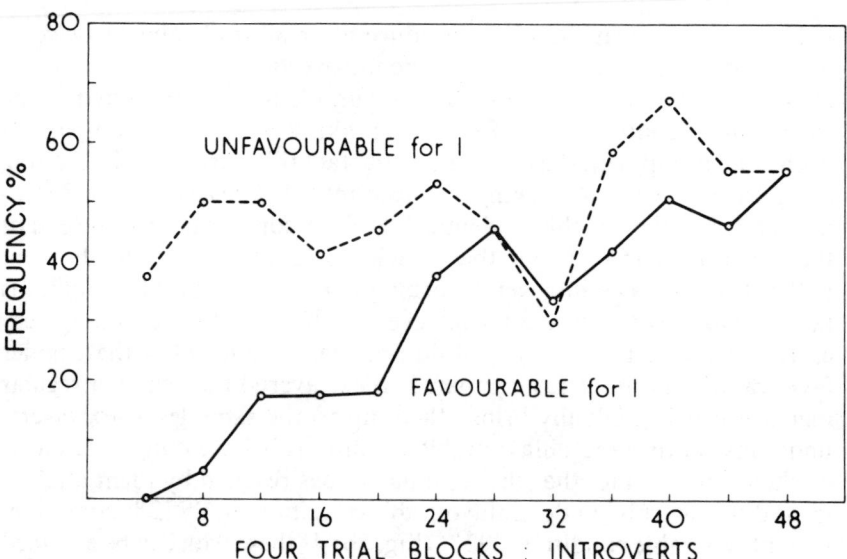

FIG. 6a. Rate of eyelid conditioning for introverts under conditions favourable and unfavourable for introverts.

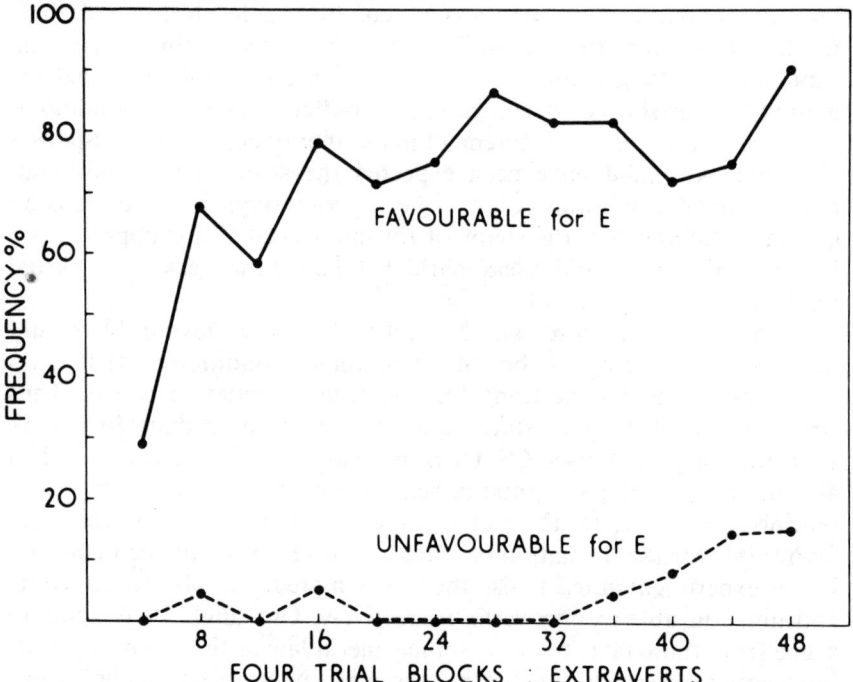

FIG. 6b. Rate of eyelid conditioning for extraverts under conditions favourable and unfavourable for extraverts.

13. CONDITIONABILITY AND EXTRAVERSION

when conditions are optimal. Such a statement is in agreement with our results, but much more work along these lines will be required before we can regard it as well supported; clearly the particular selection of conditions of this one experiment, and the inevitably small number of subjects tested, restrict the generality of our findings. Nevertheless, it may be useful to restate our major finding in this form, if only to suggest a possible link with clinical, penological and other applied fields (Eysenck, 1957, 1964).

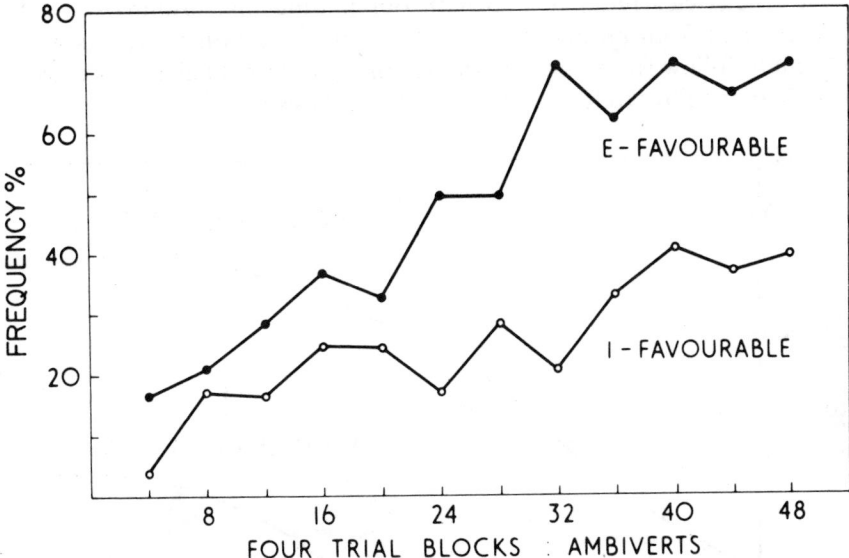

FIG. 6c. Rate of eyelid conditioning for ambiverts under conditions favourable for introverts and extraverts, respectively.

One last point requires investigation. Eysenck and Eysenck (1969) have shown that extraversion is made up of several primary factors, themselves of course intercorrelated, of which Sociability and Impulsiveness are the main ones. The possibility exists that the correlation between eyeblink conditioning and extraversion is mediated by only one of these factors, and it seemed likely to us that the Imp. factor would reflect more directly than the Soc. factor the intensity of ongoing cortical activation; we might expect, therefore, that subjects differing in Impulsivity would show more clearly the differences in conditioning performance owing to the strength of the nervous system than would subjects differing in Sociability. The subjects' questionnaires were therefore re-scored for Imp. and Soc., and divided into high and low respectively on these two sub-factors. Conditioning scores for the weak UCS, short CS–UCS

H. J. EYSENCK AND A. LEVEY

interval and partial reinforcement condition were calculated for high- and low-scorers on these two factors, and are plotted in Figs 7 and 8; Fig. 7 shows the comparison between extraverts and introverts when scored only for Imp., and Fig. 8 shows the comparison between extraverts and introverts when scored only for Soc. It will be clear that any differentiation between extraverts and introverts on eyeblink conditioning is due entirely to Imp., and not at all to Soc. The data are only suggestive, and the original experiment was not planned with this analysis in mind, but the results clearly agree well with our finding that criminals are differentiated from normals only on Imp., not at all on Soc.; this would seem to follow from our hypothesis linking criminal behaviour causally with an inability to form conditioned responses readily.

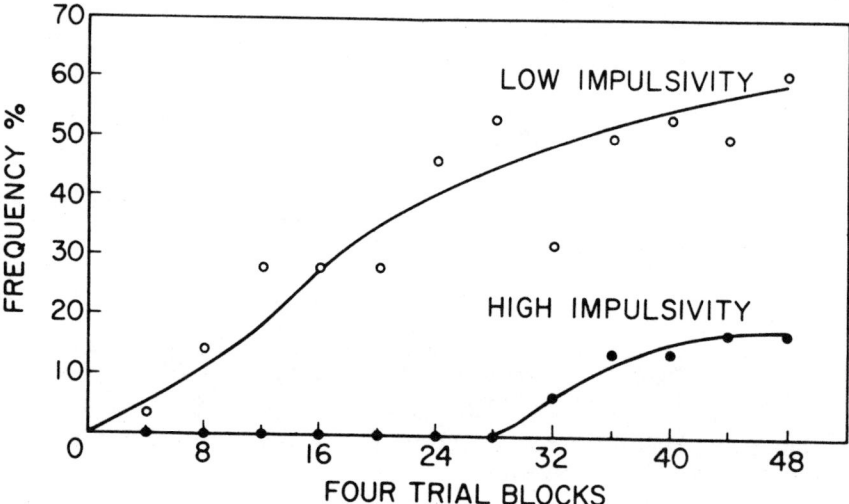

FIG. 7. Rate of eyelid conditioning for high impulsive and low impulsive subjects.

It is now time to summarize the results obtained. As has been stressed before (Eysenck, 1962), it is meaningless to compare groups of persons on a test of conditioning unless parameters are precisely specified, and if individual differences are the subject matter of the experiment, then such parameters must be chosen in accordance with a specific theory. The fact that the literature is full of contradictory results, achieved with apparently random selection of parameters, reinforces this point. Our data show that it is possible to choose conditions which give results favouring introverted subjects or extraverted subjects; what is interesting and important is that these conditions could be formulated and stated on theoretical grounds, so that the experimental results serve to support

13. CONDITIONABILITY AND EXTRAVERSION

and verify the theory. The overall failure of the experiment to show differences between introverts and extraverts at a reasonable level of significance is also in line with the hypothesis: when conditions are evenly balanced between favouring one group or the other, then averaging results over all conditions should not give results strikingly favouring one side. It should be noted that the conditions chosen were by no means extreme; it will be interesting to continue experimentation with more extreme conditions, and thus render the differentiation of introverts and extraverts even more clear-cut and obvious than has been possible in the present experiment. It should also be interesting to continue work

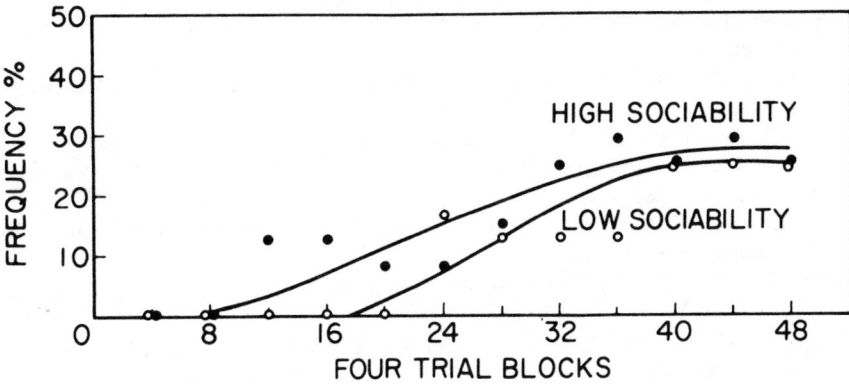

FIG. 8. Rate of eyelid conditioning for sociable and unsociable subjects.

on eyeblink conditioning by linking it up with experimental measures of the Pavlov–Teplov dimension of weak–strong nervous system; predictions here are in general very similar to those made in connection with introversion–extraversion. Altogether it is believed that Pavlov was right in pointing out the fact that individual differences in conditioning are extremely prominent in work in this field, and that these differences hold much promise in mediating predictions and explanations of human conduct, neurosis and crime. Efforts to do so (Eysenck, 1957, 1965b; Eysenck and Rachman, 1965) can only benefit from more intensive study of the relation between personality and different parameters of eyeblink conditioning.

REFERENCES

Eysenck, H. J. (1957). "The Dynamics of Anxiety and Hysteria." Routledge and Kegan Paul, London.
Eysenck, H. J. (1959). "The Maudsley Personality Inventory". University of London Press.

Eysenck, H. J. (1962). Conditioning and personality. *Br. J. Pyschol.*, **53**, 299.

Eysenck, H. J. (1963a). The biological basis of personality. *Nature*, **199**, 1031.

Eysenck, H. J. (Ed.) (1963b). "Experiments with Drugs". Pergamon, Oxford.

Eysenck, H. J. (1964). "Biological factors in neurosis and crime." *Scientia*, **1**.

Eysenck, H. J. (1965a). Extraversion and the acquisition of eyeblink and GSR conditioned responses. *Psychol. Bull.*, **63**, 258.

Eysenck, H. J. (1965b). "Crime and Personality". Routledge and Kegan Paul, London.

Eysenck, H. J. (1967). "The Biological Basis of Personality". C. C. Thomas, Springfield, Ill.

Eysenck, H. J., and Eysenck, S. B. J. (1969). "Personality Structure and Measurement". Routledge and Kegan Paul, London.

Eysenck, H. J. and Rachman, S. (1965). "The Causes and Cures of Neurosis". London.

Fuster, J. M. (1958). Effects of stimulation of brain stem on tachistoscopic perception. *Science, Lond.* **127**, 150.

Gray, J. A. (1964). "Pavlov's Typology". Pergamon, Oxford.

Isaac, W. (1960). Arousal and reaction times in cats. *J. comp. physiol. Psychol.*, **53**, 234.

Killam, E. K. (1962). Drug action on the brain stem reticular formation. *Pharmacol. Rev.*, **14**, 175.

Kimble, C. A. (1961). "Conditioning and Learning." Appleton, Century Croft, New York.

Magoun, D. W. (1963). Central Neural Inhibition. *In* Jones, M. R. (Ed.), "Nebraska Symposium on Motivation 1963." Lincoln, Nebraska.

Ross, L. E. and K. W. Spence, (1960). Eyelid conditioning performance under partial reinforcement as a function of UCS intensity. *J. exp. Psychol.*, **59**, 379.

Savage, R. D. (1964). Electro-cerebral activity, extraversion and neuroticism. *Br. J. Psychiat.* **110**, 98.

PART VIII

MEMORY AND RECALL

Recent years have seen a proliferation of experimental studies in the field of memory (particularly short-term memory), and at first sight it might seem that this field would not be a good one for studies of personality determinants. Where so much is already known, and where research methodology is so sophisticated, it might be argued, surely there is no room for new and untried variables such as personality. In actual fact exactly the opposite is true; there are few fields in which personality determinants are more important than in that of memory, and furthermore it is precisely because of the methodological sophistication in this field, and the fairly exact knowledge we have of other determinants, that researches involving personality can be planned with such precision, and that predictions can be made with such confidence. Beginning with the well-planned studies of Spence already referred to in the previous section, work on personality as related to memory has progressed considerably in the past few years; an excellent account of this work, relating it to the general body of theoretical knowledge in the whole field, is given by M. W. Eysenck (1976). It seems a pity that only a few of the many outstanding articles in this field can be reprinted here, but a book such as this must seek to cover many different fields rather than cover just one or two in depth.

The different theoretical approaches adopted by the various writers are explicated sufficiently in their contributions. Of particular interest and importance is the introduction into this field of the distinction between state- and trait-arousal; the prediction that state-arousal would improve performance of extraverts, but lower that of introverts, is another way of manipulating the arousal variable, and one which seems of considerable importance. The fact that predictions such as this can be verified lends more credence to the inverted-U hypothesis on which so much of the work described in this book has been based.

Of equal importance has been the introduction of the Walker hypothesis linking high arousal with strong consolidation and also with action decrement, i.e. the incompatibility of consolidation and recall. Two studies deriving from this hypothesis are reprinted here, but others are available, and have been reviewed in detail elsewhere (Eysenck, 1973). Walker's hypothesis was only very weakly supported when he put it forward originally (Walker, 1958), but these studies of short-term memory lend it considerable support. Further work along these lines should clarify not only the dynamics of personality structure, but also the action of consolidation itself. In this way can personality study repay the debit it owes to experimental and theoretical psychology.

There are some interesting links between this work and some of the studies considered in a later section, dealing with social interaction with personality. It will be argued that social interaction is arousing (hence that extraverts seek it out more than do introverts); if this were so, then social interaction should produce precisely the "action decrement" effect predicted by Walker, i.e. recall should be better after a lengthy period (when consolidation has been completed) than after a short period (when consolidation was still going on). Geen (1973, 1974) has shown that this is indeed so. However, it is interesting to note that his findings are not novel; as long ago as 1933, Perrin found that social stimulation hindered immediate recall but facilitated recall after three days—a reminder that there are many forgotten results in the literature which only acquire meaning in terms of later theories!

REFERENCES

EYSENCK, H. J. Personality, learning and "anxiety". In: H. J. Eysenck (Ed.), *Handbook of abnormal psychology*. London: Pitman, 1973.

EYSENCK, M. W. *Human memory*. London: Pergamon Press, 1976.

EYSENCK, M. W. Extraversion, verbal learning and memory. *Psychological Bulletin*, 1976, *83*, 75–90.

GEEN, R. G. Effects of being observed on short- and long-term recall. *Journal of Experimental Psychology*, 1973, *100*, 395–398.

GEEN, R. G. Effects of evaluation apprehension on memory over intervals of varying length. *Journal of Experimental Psychology*, 1974, *102*, 908–910.

PERRIN, J. The comparative effects of social and mechanical stimulation on memorizing. *American Journal of Psychology*, 1933, *45*, 203–270.

WALKER, E. L. Action decrement and its relation to learning. *Psychological Review*, 1958, *65*, 129–142.

From E. Howarth and H. J. Eysenck (1968). Journal of Experimental Research in Personality, *3*, 114–116, *by kind permission of the authors and Academic Press*

Extraversion, Arousal, and Paired-Associate Recall

E. HOWARTH[1] AND H. J. EYSENCK

Institute of Psychiatry, University of London

From a total of over 600 female Ss, 110 were selected with extreme extraversion scores. Fifty-five extraverts and 55 introverts were allocated among five recall intervals: 0, 1, 5, 30 min, 24 hrs in a 10-cell design. The subjects were first trained to a criterion of once through correct on seven CVC pairs, then were tested for recall of the material after the appropriate time interval. The results showed that extraverts were superior at the short-term intervals but inferior at the long-term intervals. These findings were interpreted in accord with Eysenck's theory that lower arousal in extraverts produces weaker consolidation processes which interfere less at short-term intervals but which do not facilitate long-term recall.

Kleinsmith and Kaplan (1963, 1964) have demonstrated that associations learned in the presence of low arousal, as measured by skin resistance change, showed high immediate recall which fell over the course of several days, whereas items learned under high arousal showed poor immediate recall which improved with the passage of time. Walker and Tarte (1963) compared high arousal and low arousal stimuli and found a similar effect. It has been suggested, in connection with these findings, that high arousal produces strong consolidation which interferes with immediate recall in some way, but which facilitates later recall. Eysenck (1967) has proposed that extraverts have higher arousal thresholds in the brain-stem reticular system leading to lower arousal in the cortex. If this is correct they may be less affected by strong interfering consolidation in short-term recall and perform better, whereas introverts might perform poorly at short-term intervals but show good long-term recall. While there is little previous relevant work on paired-associates learning, Eysenck (1967) has used this theoretical formulation as a possible explanation of the higher reminiscence scores of extraverts in pursuitrotor learning after relatively short rest intervals and several

other facets of the formulation have been confirmed by Farley (1966). Also, Howarth (1963) found that the short-term recall of extraverts was superior in a modified Wechsler digit-repetition task. The present study compares extraverts and introverts in a paired-associates recall task at time intervals up to and including 24 hr. On the basis of the theory it was predicted that extraverts would show greater recall at the short-term intervals and less recall at the long-term intervals, but it was impossible to define *a priori* the terms long and short term or to anticipate the kind of data which would emerge. For example, the arousal differences postulated in the theory might be far less marked, and therefore less effective, than those in the Kleinsmith and Kaplan study. Moreover, the differences observed by Walker at the shorter intervals were minimal.

METHOD

Subjects. In order to obtain extreme extraverts and introverts over 600 students were given the Eysenck Personality Inventory (Eysenck and Eysenck, 1964) and 110 Ss were selected as being outside the range of ±1 SD, on the E dimension at the same time those with neuroticism (N) scores greater than 17 were rejected in order to attenuate the possible effect of neuroticism. All Ss were female (except three) in the age range 18–22.

Material. Seven pairs of CVCs of medium association value (Noble, 1961) were used in four

[1] Now at the University of Alberta, Edmonton, Canada.

orders of presentation. *One of the four orders was as follows:* SIP-WOL; VIL-MUF; GOP-FER; MEV-LAR; SEL-PON; MOT-PED; NOR-BEV. This material was presented by a Carousel projector cycled at 3 sec. The intertrial interval of 18 sec was occupied by color-naming.

Instructions to S. "This is an experiment on the relation of learning and personality. You have already taken a personality test, we will now test your learning ability. The test consists of learning to associate word pairs. In each case pronounce each word at it appears, and as the trials progress show that you have learned the association by anticipating the response word. There are seven word pairs (example shown, but not from the series) but these will be in a different order on each trial, although the pairs will always remain the same. Between each series colors will be

Intervening task. The *S* was instructed to make words of any length out of a longer word containing letters from which none of the CVC words could be made.

This method worked well up to the 30-min recall interval but could not be sustained at the 24-hr interval.

Experimental design. This comprised ten cells (a) Two personality extremes (E vs. I) being randomly allocated among the five recall intervals (b) 0, 1, 5, 30 min, 24 hr.

RESULTS

As the results of the experiment were quite clear (Fig. 1) the results section merely explains that; (a) initial differences in learning rates were lacking, (b) the

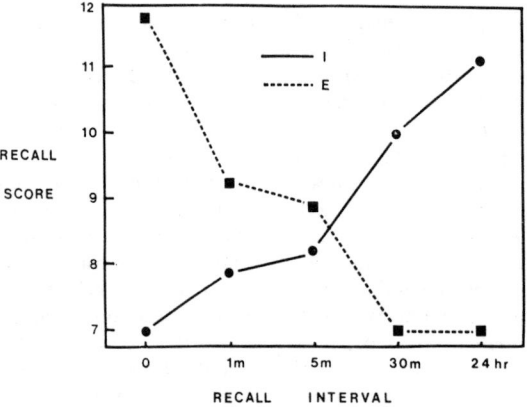

FIG. 1. Mean recall scores of extraverts and introverts at the recall interval stated. Maximum recall score possible was 14. Each point is the mean score of 11 *S*s.

shown, do not learn the colors, simply name them as they appear."

Learning and recall measures. (1) Learning of the list was to a criterion of once through correct. (2) Recall of the material was carried out as follows: *S* was asked to "print all the stimulus words, you can remember on the left-hand side of this line in any order you like, you have one minute." Then *S* was asked to "Now, print all the associated response words on the right-hand side of this line, pairing the correct response word to each stimulus word, you have one minute." The recall score consisted of a combination (sum) of (a) all stimulus words correctly recalled (written down by *S*), and (b) all response words correctly reproduced by *S*, with the proviso that these should be correctly paired with the appropriate stimulus word.

overall effect in the recall scores was significant. In initial learning the mean trials to criterion for the extraverts was 15.85, that for the introverts 18.29. This overall difference was not significant nor were the several group differences significant when a series of t tests was applied. Analysis of variance of the recall scores revealed a significant interaction effect between recall intervals and the E-I parameter ($F = 229$, $df = 4$, df for the error term = 100).

Mean recall scores are shown in Fig. 1.

DISCUSSION

According to Eysenck (1967) we could expect extraverts to be better at short term intervals; "conversely, we would expect intraverts to show better serial learning, paired-associate learning and digit-span memory when the interval between learning and testing was relatively long."

The results of this experiment are consistent with an expectation derived from the theoretical supposition of differences in arousal thresholds between extraverts and introverts. The general picture resembles that presented by the results of Kleinsmith and Kaplan except that their crossing point occurs at about 20 min, whereas that in the present experiment occurs at about 5 min, therefore for the purpose of the present study it appears convenient to define short-term recall as less than 5 min, and long-term recall as greater than this interval.

These findings, therefore, offer strong support for Eysenck's latest theoretical position regarding higher thresholds of arousal in extraverts. Combining this hypothesis with that of Walker's, that retention is a function of consolidation of traces and that high arousal results in slower but more permanent consolidation, it follows that high arousal *S*s should have poorer immediate recall but superior delayed recall. We have shown that, in this respect, extraverts behave as though they have lower arousal.

Although there is no previous evidence to support Eysenck's contention that long-term memory will be superior in introverts, there is some evidence (e.g., Howarth, 1963), to show that the short-term recall of extraverts is superior. However, there has been no previous study which compares extraverts and introverts in both short and long recall performance.

REFERENCES

EYSENCK, H. J., AND EYSENCK, S. B. G. "Manual of the Eysenck Personality Inventory." R. R. Knapp, P. O. Box 7234, San Diego, California.

EYSENCK, H. J. *The Biological basis of Personality.* Springfield: Thomas, 1967.

FARLEY, F. H. Reminiscence and post-rest performance as a function of length of rest, drive and personality. University of London Doctoral thesis, 1966.

HOWARTH, E. Some laboratory measures of extraversion-introversion. *Perceptual and Motor Skills,* 1963, 17, 55–60.

KLEINSMITH, L. J., AND KAPLAN, S. Paired-associate learning as a function of arousal and interpolated interval. *Journal of Experimental Psychology,* 1963, 65, 190–193.

KLEINSMITH, L. J., AND KAPLAN, S. Interaction of arousal and recall interval in nonsense syllable and paired-associate learning. *Journal of Experimental Psychology,* 1964, 67, 124–126.

NOBLE, C. E. Measurements of association value, rated association and scaled meaningfulness for the 2100 CVC combinations of the English alphabet. *Psychological Reports,* 1961, 8, 487–521.

WALKER, E. L., AND TARTE, R. D. Memory storage as a function of arousal and time with homogeneous and heterogeneous lists. *Journal of Verbal Learning and Verbal Behavior,* 1963, 2, 113–119.

From J. W. Osborne (1972). Perceptual and Motor Skills, *34*, 587–593, *by kind permission of the author and Southern Universities Press*

SHORT- AND LONG-TERM MEMORY AS A FUNCTION OF INDIVIDUAL DIFFERENCES IN AROUSAL[1,2]

JOHN W. OSBORNE

University of Alberta

Summary.—In a paired-associate learning experiment employing 40 university students as *S*s, the contribution of individual differences in arousal to short- and long-term retention was investigated using individual differences in salivary response to lemon juice stimulation as an index of arousal. Experimental *S*s were pre-selected from 99 *S*s on the basis of extreme arousal scores. The hypotheses were confirmed; low-arousal recall is greater than high-arousal recall on a test of short-term retention ($p < .08$) and high-arousal recall is greater than low-arousal recall on a test of long-term retention ($p < .04$).

Studies by Michigan researchers (Kleinsmith & Kaplan, 1963, 1964; Walker & Tarte, 1963) have demonstrated a significant relationship between level of arousal during learning and subsequent recall over short and long retention intervals. A high-arousal state during learning resulted in superior recall over the long-term while a low-arousal state resulted in superior recall over the short period. These findings were explained in terms of neural consolidation theory (Hebb, 1958).

The level of arousal measured in these studies for each *S* was that induced by the stimulus materials during learning. Stimuli (nonsense syllable paired associates and differentially arousing words) were classified as effecting high arousal if they resulted in sizeable GSR deflections while the remaining stimuli were classified as effecting low arousal. The purpose of this study was to determine the feasibility of employing a measure of individual differences in pre-experimental arousal as a predictor of recall. In this study arousal was operationally defined as an individual's reaction to a standard stimulus measured in terms of specified effector output.

There is some reason to believe that salivation can be an index of arousal. Sternbach (1966) has suggested that salivation is an index of the balance between the sympathetic nervous system and the parasympathetic nervous system which he believes to be synonymous with level of arousal. More saliva indicates apparent parasympathetic system dominance (high arousal), while less saliva indicates apparent dominance by the sympathetic nervous system (low arousal). If,

[1]This paper was submitted in partial fulfillment of the requirements for the degree of Master of Science in Educational Psychology at the University of Wisconsin. The author is indebted to Frank H. Farley, who served as advisor for this thesis.
[2]This study was supported in part by funds from the United States Office of Education, Department of Health, Education and Welfare. The opinions expressed herein do not necessarily reflect the position or policy of the Office of Education and no official endorsement by the Office of Education should be expressed. Center No. C-03/Contract OE 5-10-154.

J. W. OSBORNE

as Bremer (1954) postulates, a neurophysiological correlate of a high level of arousal is a state of high cortical facilitation, the effector output of a highly aroused organism can be expected to be greater than that of a less aroused organism.

Support for this hypothesis has come from the work of Corcoran (1964) and Eysenck and Eysenck (1967) which has shown a strong relationship between extraversion and salivation to lemon juice. Extraverts salivate less while introverts salivate more to the stimulus of four drops of lemon juice. Previous studies using EEG (Savage, 1964; Marton & Urban, 1966) have supported Eysenck's (1967) hypothesis that introverts are characterized by a state of higher arousal as a result of parasympathetic nervous system dominance while extraverts are characterized by a state of low arousal as a result of sympathetic nervous system dominance. Consequently, it appears that salivation might be used as an index of personality or arousal or both.

Support for the reliability and validity of salivation as an arousal measure has come from the work of Farley and Osborne.[3] They have obtained stability estimates over 24 hr. of .81 for basal salivation, .78 for gross salivation to lemon juice, and .78 for net salivation to lemon juice ($ps < .01$). As regards the validity of salivation as a measure of arousal, Farley and Osborne have reported a correlation of $-.57$ ($p < .02$) between salivation and the threshold of fusion of paired light flashes, or two-flash threshold, which has been shown through correlations with skin conductance (Maley, 1967) and EEG alpha amplitude (Venables & Warwick-Evans, 1967) to be a measure of arousal. The relationship between salivation, as measured, and two-flash threshold is not an exceptionally strong one in absolute magnitude; however, where arousal is concerned, it is an encouraging one in an area not noted for significant relationships among measures (Sternbach, 1966).

The intention of the present study was to perform a modified replication of the study of Kleinsmith and Kaplan (1964), treating arousal as an individual difference variable, measured in terms of salivary output to lemon juice rather than measured during learning trials in the form of GSRs to each consonant-vowel-consonant (CVC) nonsense syllable. The hypotheses tested were that (a) low-arousal Ss have significantly higher recall scores than high-arousal Ss over a short period (2.5 min.); (b) high-arousal Ss have significantly higher recall scores than low-arousal Ss over the longer term (24 hr.).

METHOD

Subjects

Ss were obtained from an undergraduate course in educational psychology at the University of Wisconsin; there were 75 females and 24 males. Participa-

---

[3]F. H. Farley & J. W. Osborne. Reliability and validity of salivation as a measure of individual differences in arousal. (Unpublished study, 1969)

tion in departmental research for up to 3 hr. was a course requirement that was strongly urged though not rigidly enforced.

Materials

Fresh lemon juice was squeezed into a glass beaker after being strained through a fine wire gauze. Standard cotton dental swabs were used in conjunction with 50 (16 $\times$ 150 mm.) test tubes and stoppers (size "0") to obtain from each S a measure of salivary output to lemon juice which was placed on the tongue by means of a 1-cc. glass syringe. Stainless steel forceps were used for the deposition and removal of the swabs. The forceps were sterilized for each S in an American Sundries Co. Renewal Electric Sterilizer Model No. 5. The weighing of swabs and test tubes was done with a Right-a-Weigh electronic balance. A stopwatch was used for timing while a 9-in. $\times$ 6-in. mirror was available for rehearsal of mouth movements. Forceps were removed from the sterilizer by means of tongs and dried with clean tissues. The equipment was arrayed on a covered aluminum tray.

The visual stimuli (6 paired-associate slides, 12 slides each with a different stimulus word only and 28 slides of colored spots) were presented by means of a Kodak Carousel AV900 projector, screen, and Cousino Syncro-Repeater (Model SR-7341). A Hunter GSR amplifier was also used as part of the rationale to divert Ss' awareness from the main purpose of the study.

Procedure

A measure of salivary response to lemon juice was taken from each S by means of the absorbent technique (Razran, 1935). Standard cotton dental swabs were used throughout while equipment coming into contact with S's mouth was sterilized. Each S was told that this measure was one of a series of physiological measures being taken in a study of individual differences.

Basal salivation was first measured by placing a cotton dental swab upon S's sublingual salivary gland for 20 sec. Following its removal, the moistened swab was placed in a sealed test tube to be weighed. In measuring gross salivation the procedure was repeated 1 min. and 40 sec. later with the addition of four drops of lemon juice (mean weight .176 gm.) placed on the lateral margins of the tongue. In both cases the difference between the previously determined dry weight on the swab and its wet weight constituted the measure of interest. The difference between basal and gross salivary responses yielded the net salivary output for each S.

From the distribution of the salivary responses of 99 Ss, the 20 highest scoring Ss (salivation $>$ .35 gm.) and 20 lowest Ss (salivation $<$ .025 gm.) were selected for the second stage of the experiment which was patterned after that of Kleinsmith and Kaplan (1964). The 20 high-arousal Ss and 20 low-arousal Ss were given a single learning trial with a list of six nonsense syllable-number pairs. The following six 0% association value CVC nonsense syllables (Hil-

J. W. OSBORNE

gard, 1951) were used: CEF, QAP, TOV, JEX, LAJ, DAX. The response items were respectively the single digits from 2 to 7. As a result of a pilot study the time for learning and recall trials was increased from 4 sec. to 6 sec. to alleviate the possibility of a "floor effect" upon performance (Runquist, 1966).

Prior to learning and recall trials, Ss were attached to a disconnected GSR amplifier and told that a physiological measure would be taken while they were "doing a task." During learning and recall trials, E pretended carefully to watch the GSR amplifier which was placed behind Ss. This procedure was used in an attempt to disguise the actual interest in learning and retention. During the training trial, S first saw the nonsense syllable alone, then repeated with a single-digit response term. To separate the arousal effects of the stimuli from one pairing to the next, two slides containing four differently colored spots in a horizontal line were inserted before and after each paired associate. S was instructed to name the colors (red, green, yellow, orange, black, and blue were used randomly on these slides). Two color slides were presented prior to the first paired associate so that S could "settle down" before the paired associates were presented. S was instructed to "concentrate carefully on both colors and nonsense syllable-number pairs" and to call them out loud, but to avoid rehearsal S was not specifically told that he would be tested for recall.

During the recall session, S was instructed to recall the correct number of each nonsense syllable as it appeared for 6 sec. and to guess if uncertain. The correct numbers were not repeated. Colors were used as an interpolated task as before.

Ten high-arousal Ss and 10 low-arousal Ss were tested for immediate recall (2.5 min. as measured from presentation of the first slide) while 10 high-arousal and 10 low-arousal Ss were tested for long-term recall (24 hr.). Ss within arousal levels were randomly assigned to retention intervals.

To correct for serial order effects, 10 different training lists were used, each list given to one S in each group. Two 6 × 6 balanced Latin squares were used to derive the lists after randomly omitting one row (Cochran & Cox, 1957). The order of the recall lists was varied in the same manner.

RESULTS

In Fig. 1 is presented the distribution of salivary responses to lemon juice by 99 Ss. The cut-off points for the 20 highest and 20 lowest salivators were .35 gm. and .025 gm., respectively.

Table 1 shows the differential recall of high- and low-arousal Ss as a function of time. At the immediate test, greater recall was demonstrated by the low-arousal Ss than the high-arousal Ss, whereas on the long-term (24-hr.) test, the reverse was true.

An analysis of serial position effects in the recall scores for all conditions showed slight signs of primacy and recency effects; however, performance was so low that no trends were clearly identifiable.

MEMORY AND AROUSAL

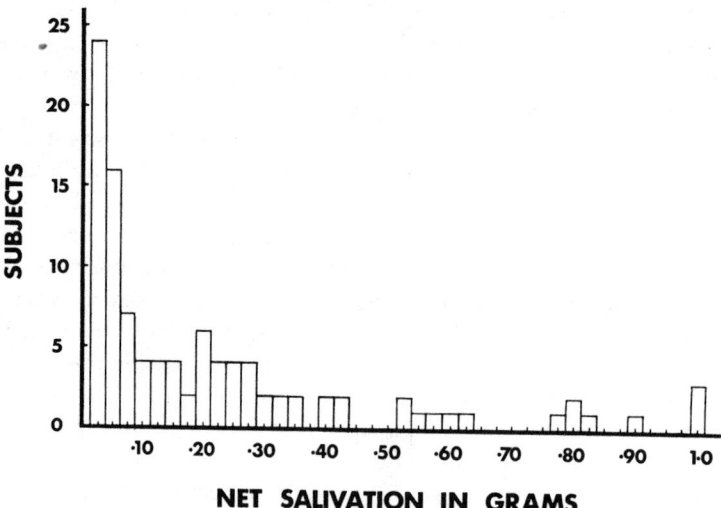

NET SALIVATION IN GRAMS

FIG. 1.   Distribution of net salivation to lemon juice

Because of the frequency of low recall scores across all conditions the assumption of normality of distribution for the analysis of variance model was checked by application of the Shapiro-Wilks (1965) test. The assumption was not met. However, the application of the Mann-Whitney U test showed a statistically significant difference between high- and low-arousal recall at short ($Z = 1.3, p < .08$) and longer-term ($Z = 1.7, p < .04$) retention intervals. The differences were in the hypothesized directions.

TABLE 1

TOTAL RECALL SCORES OF PAIRED ASSOCIATES AS A FUNCTION OF
AROUSAL AND RECALL INTERVAL

Arousal Level	N	Short-term Recall	Long-term Recall
High	10	7	13
Low	10	13	7
Mann-Whitney		$Z = 1.4, p = .08$	$Z = 1.7, p = .04$

DISCUSSION

The present study was an attempt to see whether the results of Kleinsmith and Kaplan (1964) could be reproduced when Ss were preselected on the basis of a response to a standard stimulus measured prior to the learning phase of the experiment. In spite of the procedural difficulties with the measures used, the "cross-over" effect associated with arousal appeared here as it did in the work of Kleinsmith and Kaplan; however, it was not as large as that found by those Es. The present study indicates the feasibility of an alternative measure of arousal in experiments concerned with arousal and recall.

J. W. OSBORNE

The distribution of salivary responses to lemon juice had a marked positive skew. With most of the scores tightly clustered around a small part of the range, it is apparent that individual differences in salivation are going to be reflected in very slight differences in weight, making the measurement procedure critical. The absorbent technique is subject to difficulties in this regard which when combined with the difficulty of temporal fluctuation of salivary secretion within Ss, makes reliable measurement of salivation a problem (Feather, 1967). In spite of this the present author has demonstrated that the procedure used in this study has good temporal stability, cited earlier.

If salivation approximates an index of intrinsic arousal the positively skewed distribution of salivary responses suggests that a sample of undergraduates is going to contain a preponderance of Ss with a low level of intrinsic arousal. This suggests the importance of considering the possible contribution of intrinsic arousal in earlier studies such as those of Kleinsmith and Kaplan where two sources of arousal were confounded.

The range of scores for paired associates correctly recalled was low in spite of the extension of the exposure times originally used by Kleinsmith and Kaplan. No S recalled more than two. It seems desirable to design the learning task to permit a wider range of recall scores while at the same time maintaining control over associative characteristics or other features peculiar to the stimuli. It would be useful to take a random sample of Ss unselected with respect to level of arousal and run them through the learning and recall trials. This may help determine whether the low scores are more a function of the present method of selecting Ss or the stimuli.

The low recall scores may also have been partially a function of instability resulting from measurement of recall after only one learning trial. However, this may have been offset by the fairly long exposure time (4 sec.) for each slide during learning. Increasing the number of trials would have made a possible increase in reliability difficult to assess because of the repetition bias predicted by consolidation theory.

A criticism of the design used in this study and that of Kleinsmith and Kaplan has been that arousal-inducing stimuli (nonsense syllables) were presented on both learning and recall trials. This meant that, at the time of recall, Ss were exposed to the same words whose initial arousal-inducing function was the object of investigation. This raised the possibility of arousal during recall trials being more relevant to performance than arousal prior to and during learning. In answering this criticism, Kaplan and Kaplan (1968) reanalyzed the data of the Kleinsmith and Kaplan study (1964) to find that GSRs on recall did not correlate with recall performance. They concluded that recall GSRs did not predict recall performance while the GSRs during learning did.

The evidence from this study indicates a relationship between arousal and recall like that found by Kleinsmith and Kaplan. In spite of methodological problems, salivation appears to be a feasible means of determining individual differences in arousal level. A unique feature of the present research has been the attempt to measure arousal and use it as a predictor of performance rather than examine the relationship between arousal, measured during learning, and performance on a *post hoc* basis.

REFERENCES

BREMER, F. The neurophysiological problem of sleep. In J. F. Delafresnaye (Ed.), *Brain mechanisms and consciousness: a symposium.* Oxford: Blackwell Scientific Publications, 1954. Pp. 137-162.

COCHRAN, W. G., & COX, G. M. *Experimental designs.* New York: Wiley, 1957.

CORCORAN, D. W. J. The relation between introversion and salivation. *American Journal of Psychology,* 1964, 77, 298-300.

EYSENCK, H. J. *Biological basis of personality.* Springfield, Ill.: Thomas, 1967.

EYSENCK, S. B. G., & EYSENCK, H. J. Salivary response to lemon juice as a measure of introversion. *Perceptual and Motor Skills,* 1967, 24, 1047-1053.

FEATHER, B. W. Human salivary conditioning: a methodological study. In G. A. Kimble (Ed.), *Foundations of conditioning and learning.* New York: Appleton-Century-Crofts, 1967. Pp. 117-143.

HEBB, D. O. *A textbook of psychology.* Philadelphia: Saunders, 1958.

HILGARD, E. R. Methods and procedures in the study of learning. In S. S. Stevens (Ed.), *Handbook of experimental psychology.* New York: Wiley, 1951. Pp. 517-567.

KAPLAN, S., & KAPLAN, R. Arousal and memory: a comment. *Psychonomic Science,* 1968, 10, 291-292.

KLEINSMITH, L. J., & KAPLAN, S. Paired-associate learning as a function of arousal and interpolated interval. *Journal of Experimental Psychology,* 1963, 65, 190-193.

KLEINSMITH, L. J., & KAPLAN, S. Interaction of arousal and recall interval in nonsense syllable paired-associate learning. *Journal of Experimental Psychology,* 1964, 67, 124-126.

MALEY, M. J. Two-flash threshold, skin conductance and skin potential. *Psychonomic Science,* 1967, 9, 361-362.

MARTON, M., & URBAN, I. An electroencephalographic investigation of individual differences in the process of conditioning. In *Proceedings of the 18th International Congress of Psychology.* Amsterdam: North Holland, 1966. Pp. 106-109.

RAZRAN, G. Conditioned responses: an experimental study and a theoretical analysis. *Archives of Psychology, New York,* 1935, 28, 1-124.

RUNQUIST, W. N. Verbal behavior. In J. B. Sidowski (Ed.), *Experimental methods and instrumentation in psychology.* New York: McGraw-Hill, 1966. Pp. 487-540.

SAVAGE, R. D. Electro-cerebral activity, extraversion and neuroticism. *British Journal of Psychiatry,* 1964, 110, 98-100.

SHAPIRO, S. S., & WILKS, M. B. An analysis of variance test for normality (complete samples). *Biometrika,* 1965, 52, 591-611.

STERNBACH, R. A. *Principles of psychophysiology: an introductory text and readings.* New York: Academic Press, 1966.

VENABLES, P. H., & WARWICK-EVANS, L. A. Cortical arousal and two-flash threshold. *Psychonomic Science,* 1967, 8, 231-232.

WALKER, E. L., & TARTE, R. D. Memory storage as a function of arousal and time with homogeneous and heterogeneous lists. *Journal of Verbal Learning and Verbal Behavior,* 1963, 2, 113-119.

Accepted January 21, 1972.

From D. W. Forrest (1963). Psychological Reports, 13, 564, by kind permission of the author and Southern Universities Press

RELATIONSHIP BETWEEN SHARPENING AND EXTRAVERSION

D. W. FORREST

Trinity College, Dublin

During the course of a recent investigation (2) Ss were asked to recall a series of 10 drawings depicting "stick men" engaged in various activities representative of certain of the needs in Murray's system. It was noticed, *en passant,* that the ways in which Ss described these drawings in their efforts at recall seemed to be related to a personality characteristic which might be termed "social extraversion." Those Ss who were lively and sociable in the testing situation appeared to exaggerate their descriptions of the activities portrayed in the drawings, e.g., in recalling a drawing designed to represent n Aggression, which was usually described as "Two men fighting a duel," such Ss might say, "One man running his sword through and killing his opponent." This type of exaggeration in which the activity is expressed in a stronger or more violent form than usual resembles the "sharpening" found by Allport and Postman (1) in their study of rumor, and we followed their usage in terming such descriptions "sharpened."

The object of the present experiment was to put this incidental observation to a more exact test by noting the number of sharpened descriptions given to the recalled pictures by a group of 40 Ss drawn from the same population of British undergraduate women, and by subsequently obtaining their extraversion (E) scores from the Maudsley Personality Inventory (MPI).

Ss were classified as "extreme sharpeners" if they gave four or more sharpened responses out of the 10 possible, while those who gave none were termed "levelers." This procedure led to 12 Ss falling in each of these categories, the remaining 16 Ss with 1, 2, or 3 sharpened responses being termed "average sharpeners."

The extreme sharpeners had a mean E score of 33.1; the average sharpeners, 31.3; and the levelers, 18.9. An analysis of variance gives an F of 20 ($p < .05$) and t tests run between the three pairs of means reveal that the levelers differ significantly from both groups of sharpeners at $p < .001$, there being no significant difference between the extreme and average sharpeners.

Thus the original observation seems to have been supported: those who gave sharpened descriptions of these pictures in a recall situation were more extraverted than those who were unable or unwilling to provide such redundancy. Such a finding needs to be further generalized before any definite rationale can be offered. It is tentatively suggested that the extraverts' tendency to sharpen is an aspect of their greater verbal fluency in a test situation (cf. 3).

REFERENCES

1. ALLPORT, G. W., & POSTMAN, L. *The psychology of rumor.* New York: Holt, 1947.
2. FORREST, D. W., & LEE, S. G. Sensitization and defense in perception and recall. *Psychol. Monogr.,* 1962, 76, No. 4 (Whole No. 523).
3. FOULDS, G. A. A method of scoring the TAT applied to psychoneurotics. *J. ment. Sci.,* 1953, 99, 235-246.

Accepted September 4, 1963.

From M. W. Eysenck (1974). Journal of Research in Personality, *8,* 307–323, *by kind permission of the author and Academic Press*

Individual Differences in Speed of Retrieval from Semantic Memory[1]

Michael W. Eysenck

University of London

In the first of two experiments, the stimulus items consisted of category names followed by a single letter (e.g., fruit–P). The subjects (half introverted, half extraverted) were required to respond as quickly as possible with a member of the specified category starting with the letter. Extraverts responded significantly faster than introverts, and more so when the most likely response was of low frequency than when it was of high frequency. In the second experiment, subjects were assigned to one of four groups representing the four combinations of high and low Extraversion and high and low General Activation. The speed-of-recall task from the first experiment was used on some trials; on the remaining trials, a speed-of-recognition task was used. Extraverts had greater response speed than introverts for recall, but not for recognition. That finding, plus interactions between Extraversion and General Activation, suggested an interpretation of the results in terms of the Yerkes–Dodson Law.

Several studies have reported a positive relationship between verbal fluency and tests of extraversion or surgency (Cattell, 1934; Gewirtz, 1948; White, 1968; Di Scipio, 1971; M. W. Eysenck, 1974). In these studies, the assessment of fluency was frequently based on the number of appropriate items written down by the subject within a fixed interval of time when required to generate words from some specified category. M. W. Eysenck (1974) has suggested that such tests of verbal fluency involve retrieval from semantic memory, which Tulving (1972, p. 368) defines as "a mental thesaurus, organized knowledge a person possesses about words and other verbal symbols." Thus, the superior performance of extraverted subjects may indicate greater speed of retrieval from semantic memory. However, Cattell (1934) obtained a correlation of $+0.30$ ($n = 62$) between a speed-of-writing test and surgency, which suggests that at least some of the positive correlation between fluency and extraversion may be artifactual. Additionally, it is likely that, par-

[1] Requests for reprints should be made to Michael W. Eysenck, Department of Psychology, Birkbeck College, University of London, Malet Street, London, WC1E 7HX, England.

MICHAEL W. EYSENCK

ticularly towards the end of the recall period, subjects search through their previous emissions in order to avoid the repetition of responses. The greater cautiousness of introverts (Cameron & Myers, 1966) may mean that they perform more rechecks than extraverts, and thus have less effective time available for retrieval from semantic memory.

A methodologically superior way of investigating the hypothesis that extraverts retrieve information from semantic memory faster than introverts is to be found in recent work by Freedman and Loftus (Loftus, Freedman & Loftus, 1970; Freedman & Loftus, 1971; Loftus & Suppes, 1972). These investigators presented their subjects with a category name followed by a single letter (for example, fruit–P). The task for the subject was to respond as quickly as possible with the name of a member of the designated category, the name to begin with the specified letter. Thus, in the above example, "pear," "peach" and "plum" would all be acceptable responses. This research paradigm not only avoids some of the problems associated with multiple-response emission, but also allows fuller study of the variables that affect retrieval time from semantic memory. In the first experiment, three of the more consequential of such variables investigated by Loftus and Freedman were considered: dominance, response frequency, and pool size. Any instance which is given frequently by subjects has high dominance. Response frequency was defined as the frequency of occurrence in the English language of the most dominant appropriate response to each category–letter pair. Pool size was defined as the number of different words from the Battig and Montague (1969) norms satisfying the requirements of each category–letter pair.

A plausible assumption concerning the subject's strategy in this situation is that he searches through a serial list of category instances, with the latency of response depending upon how far down the list he must search before encountering an appropriate instance (Anderson & Bower, 1973). If one assumes that the position in the list of this instance is a function of its dominance and frequency in the language, then reaction time should be negatively related to both dominance and response frequency. Freedman and Loftus (1971), and Loftus and Suppes (1972) have found this to be the case. Pool size has also been found to be an important determinant of reaction time (Loftus & Suppes, 1972), suggesting that fewer items need to be searched in order to locate an appropriate response where the potential number of responses is large. If extraverts retrieve information faster from semantic memory than do introverts, and if the extent of the memory search required varies inversely with dominance, response frequency, and pool size, then the following hypothesis suggests itself. Extraversion will interact with each of the variables of dominance, response frequency, and pool size, so that extraverts will have faster response speeds than introverts particularly where considerable memory search is required (i.e., with low dominance, low response frequency, or small pool size), but less so where only a limited search is needed (i.e., with high dominance, high response frequency, or large pool size).

In sum, there are three major aims of this experiment: (1) to investigate the hypothesis that extraverts retrieve information from semantic memory with greater speed than introverts; (2) to replicate previous findings indicating the importance of the structural variables of dominance, response frequency, and pool size to speed of retrieval; and (3) to look for predicted interactions between Extraversion and the structural variables.

EXPERIMENT I

Method

Subjects. The subjects were 57 college students under the age of 30 who participated in the experiment in return for course credit or modest payment. On the basis of scores on Form A of the Eysenck Personality Inventory (Eysenck & Eysenck, 1964), subjects scoring 12 or more on the Extraversion scale were designated as extraverts, while those scoring 10 or fewer were classified as introverts. Those scoring 11 on the Extraversion scale (an intermediate score), or obtaining a Lie scale score of 4 or more were excluded. Further subjects were randomly excluded, in order that there would be an equal number of subjects (23) in each of the personality groups. The two personality groups did not differ significantly in mean Neuroticism score on the Eysenck Personality Inventory or in mean vocabulary score on the Mill Hill Vocabulary.

Materials. The category names and single letters were printed on slides by means of Letraset. There was a total of 56 category–letter pairs, consisting of two different pairs from each of 28 categories selected from the Battig and Montague (1969) norms. The pairs were selected in such a way that they fell into eight different equal-sized groups representing all the possible combinations of high and low dominance, high and low response frequency, and large and small pool size. The dominance associated with any category–letter combination was determined by reference to the Battig and Montague (1969) norms, in which subjects were asked to name words that belonged to a particular category. The relative frequency of the most commonly given word in a category that satisfies a category–letter pair defines the dominance rating of that category–letter pair. For example, in the Battig and Montague (1969) norms of responses to the category label "fruit," the most frequently given word satisfying the pair "fruit–P" is "pear," which is the third most frequent word given to the category. Thus, "pear" has a dominance rating of three. For "fruit–L," "lemon" was the most frequently given appropriate response; it was the tenth most frequent word given to the category "fruit." It thus has a dominance rating of ten.

An attempt was made to manipulate the three variables of dominance, response frequency, and pool size in a rigorous way: The mean of high and low dominance pairs was 2.64 and 14.21; of high and low response frequency, 87.57 and 5.32 (from Kučera & Francis (1967)); of large and small pool size, 10.50 and 3.10 alternative responses. Each pair was always presented with the category name first, and with an interval of 2.0 sec between the onset of the category and the onset of the letter. The pairs were presented in a random order, except that at least 12 trials always intervened between successive presentations of the same category.

Procedure. The subjects were informed that they would be presented with a category name followed by a single letter, and that they were to respond with a word belonging to that category starting with that letter. They were given an example of this, and told to respond as quickly as possible, but at the same time to avoid error.

Each subject was tested individually. He sat in a semidarkened room 5 ft in front of a screen. He had a throat microphone around his throat, and the need for avoidance of unintentional use of the throat musculature was explained to him. The experimenter initiated each trial by saying, "Ready," followed within 1 sec by the projection of the category slide. The subsequent onset of the letter slide was coincident with the starting of an electric timer. The subject's overt verbal response activated the voice key that stopped the electric timer. A warm-up period of 18 trials preceded the experimental trials.

Results

Errors and omissions accounted for 8.97% of all responses. The remaining data were reciprocally transformed prior to analysis; the transformed mean response speeds are given in Table 1. These data were analysed by means of a 2 (Extraversion) by 2 (dominance) by 2 (pool size) by 2 (response frequency) analysis of variance in which the first factor was between-subjects and the other three factors were within-subjects. The main effect of Extraversion was highly significant $(F(1,44) = 10.23, \ p < .005)$, with extraverts consistently producing shorter reaction times than introverts. The main effect of dominance was also highly significant $(F(1,44) = 59.43, \ p < .001)$, as was the main effect of response frequency $(F(1,44) = 16.93, \ p < .001)$. High-dominance pairs were associated with faster response speeds than low-dominance pairs, and pairs with high response frequency produced faster responses than those with low response frequency. The final main effect, that of pool size, was unrelated to performance $(F < 1)$.

Of the interactions involving Extraversion, the two-way interaction between response frequency and Extraversion was significant $(F(1,44) = 11.03, \ p < .005)$. In this interaction, the superiority of extraverts was rather greater with low response frequency items than with high response frequency items. The further two-way interactions between Extraversion and dominance $(F(1,44) = 2.99)$, and between Extraversion and pool size $(F(1,44) = 3.39)$ were both statistically nonsignificant.

There was a highly significant interaction between dominance and frequency $(F(1,44) = 18.67, \ p < .001)$, in which the effect of the fre-

TABLE 1

MEAN RECALL RESPONSE SPEEDS IN EXPT. I (RECIPROCALLY TRANSFORMED DATA)
AS A FUNCTION OF EXTRAVERSION, DOMINANCE,
RESPONSE FREQUENCY, AND POOL SIZE

	Extraverts							
Dominance	High	High	High	High	Low	Low	Low	Low
Frequency	High	High	Low	Low	High	High	Low	Low
Pool size	High	Low	High	Low	High	Low	High	Low
Mean	0.87	0.78	0.68	0.77	0.66	0.50	0.64	0.66
SD	0.21	0.16	0.14	0.16	0.18	0.19	0.16	0.21
	Introverts							
Dominance	High	High	High	High	Low	Low	Low	Low
Frequency	High	High	Low	Low	High	High	Low	Low
Pool size	High	Low	High	Low	High	Low	High	Low
Mean	0.76	0.72	0.49	0.63	0.60	0.55	0.47	0.53
SD	0.18	0.17	0.20	0.19	0.21	0.18	0.14	0.20

quency variable was more apparent with high- than low-dominance items. Finally, the two-way interaction between response frequency and pool size was highly significant ($F(1,44) = 31.47$, $p < .001$). In this interaction, large pool size facilitated performance when associated with high response frequency but not when associated with low response frequency. None of the remaining two-way, three-way, or four-way interactions even approached the conventional 5% level of statistical significance, except for the interaction between dominance and pool size ($F(1,44) = 3.38$, n.s.).

Further analyses were conducted on the error and omission data. While extraverts on average produced more incorrect responses than introverts (1.83 and 1.09, respectively), the two personality groups did not differ significantly ($t(44) = 1.54$). The introverted subjects had more mean omissions than the extraverted subjects (4.74 and 2.39, respectively), and this difference was highly significant ($t(44) = 3.26$, $p < .01$).

DISCUSSION

Many of the findings serve to confirm the results of the study by Loftus and Suppes (1972), in which dominance, response frequency, and pool size emerged as important determinants of response latency. Such findings are clearly consistent with the notion of a serial scan through categorical instances, in which the serial position of the first-scanned appropriate response is contingent upon its dominance and frequency. However, while this hypothesis, proposed by Anderson and Bower (1973), is attractively simple, the general problem of distinguishing between parallel and serial processes is exceedingly complex (Townsend, 1971). Furthermore, the existence of interactions among these structural variables complicates the interpretive problem.

The interaction between response frequency and pool size was due to large pool size leading to an increase in response speed when combined with high response frequency, but not when combined with low response frequency. A relevant consideration may be that subjects were rather more likely to give the most dominant appropriate response (as given in the Battig and Montague norms) with low response-frequency items than with high response-frequency items (65.2 and 60.7%, respectively). The pool-size variable is likely to be ineffective when the most dominant of the range of possible responses is consistently selected. While clarification of this interaction, and the further interaction between dominance and frequency, obviously requires additional experimentation, it seems highly desirable for subsequent investigators to be alive to the possibility of interactive effects among the various structural variables.

The findings with respect to the personality variable provided confirmation of the hypothesis that extraverts can retrieve at least certain kinds of information more rapidly from semantic memory than can introverts. That this same result has also been obtained with a verbal fluency task (M. W. Eysenck, 1974) suggests that the finding has a certain generality. However, alternative interpretations of the data are clearly tenable. For instance, Cameron and Myers (1966) have obtained evidence indicating that introverts are more cautious than extraverts, and McLaughlin (1968) and McLaughlin and Kary (1972) in experiments on memory have found that extraverts were apparently more willing than introverts to "guess" when they thought they might possibly be correct. If the slower response speed of the introverted subjects were due to their cautiousness in responding, one might anticipate that they would be less liable than extraverts to produce error responses. While the difference between the two personality groups was in the direction predicted by a caution hypothesis, this difference was not significant. Moreover, it would require an elaborated version of this caution hypothesis to explain the significant interaction between Extraversion and response frequency. This interaction appears to substantiate the favored interpretation of the data, in that it would be expected that differences in response speed between introverts and extraverts would be reduced under conditions (such as high response frequency) in which a relatively short search process was involved. The nonsignificance of the Extraversion-by-dominance interaction is puzzling; it is unclear as to which of the various theoretical assumptions underlying the prediction of a significant interaction requires amendment.

EXPERIMENT II

The first experiment clearly showed that Extraversion is a strong determinant of response speed from semantic memory, but more clarification of the processes involved would be desirable. In order to investigate more thoroughly the hypothesis that differences in response latency between introverts and extraverts are due to greater retrieval efficiency in extraverts, it was decided to utilize both speed-of-recall and speed-of-recognition indices in the second experiment. Although retrieval processes may be of importance to some recognition situations (Tulving & Thomson, 1971), the evidence seems generally favorable to Kintsch's (1970) theory, in which it is postulated that recall involves a considerably larger retrieval component than recognition. If one makes that initial assumption, then the prediction follows that extraverts should outperform introverts in speed of recall, but not in speed of recognition.

The second main focus of this experiment was upon the relationship between arousal and speed of retrieval from semantic memory. The concept of "arousal" has received several different operational definitions and does not appear to constitute a unidimensional concept (Lacey, 1967). However, as Uehling (1972) has pointed out, it is commonly supposed that arousal is noninformational, represents a nonspecific increment in physiological activity, and refers to some elevated state of bodily function. We shall use "arousal" in this sense. While several studies have investigated the relationship between arousal and verbal learning (for a review, see Uehling (1972)), relatively few studies have considered the effects of arousal on retrieval processes (Bourne, 1955; Uehling & Sprinkle, 1968; Berlyne, Borsa, Craw, Gelman & Mandell, 1965; M. W. Eysenck, 1974). Both Bourne (1955), and Uehling and Sprinkle (1968) found facilitatory effects of arousal on retrieval; Berlyne *et al.* (1965) did not. M. W. Eysenck (1974), in an experiment comparing the number of words from five different categories which could be spontaneously produced by introverts and by extraverts, also administered Thayer's Activation–Deactivation Adjective Check List. This test, which is an objective self-report measure of transient levels of activation, was investigated in several experiments by Thayer (1967). Thayer's main finding was that the General Activation scale derived from the Check List correlated substantially with physiological measures of arousal in each of three separate experiments. M. W. Eysenck found that high levels of arousal (as indicated by the General Activation scale) appeared to increase the number of words recalled by extraverts, but to reduce the recall of introverts. In fact, the interaction between Extraversion and General Activation was significant at the .005 level. This interaction indicates that Extraversion and General Activation are affecting the same mechanism. Since some evidence indicates that introverts are character-ized by higher cortical arousal than extraverts (Eysenck, 1967; Savage, 1964; Gale, Coles & Blaydon, 1969), it was tentatively concluded that the arousal mechanism was implicated, and that the results thus conformed to the curvilinear relationship between arousal and performance pro-posed by Hebb (1955).

The Activation–Deactivation Adjective Check List was administered to all subjects in the second experiment in order to evaluate further the relationship between arousal and retrieval. Further predictions follow from a consideration of the Yerkes–Dodson Law (Broadhurst, 1959), interpreting this to mean that the optimal level of arousal decreases with increasing task difficulty. Arousal will be lowest for low General Activa-tion extraverts and highest for high General Activation introverts. Task difficulty (if indexed in terms of the mean response latencies obtained in other studies) runs from high-dominance recognition items, to low-dominance recognition items (Wilkins, 1971), to high-dominance recall items, to low-dominance recall items (Loftus & Suppes, 1972). The Yerkes–Dodson Law predicts that there should be a significant Task-Difficulty-by-Arousal interaction in which the high-arousal groups will be at an advantage with the easier tasks, but at a disadvantage with the harder tasks.

Method

Subjects. The subjects were divided into four groups on the basis of scores on the Extraversion scale of the Eysenck Personality Inventory (Form A), and the Gen-eral Activation scale of the Activation–Deactivation Adjective Check List. All those scoring 11 on the extraversion scale (an intermediate value), 4 or more on the Lie scale, or 18 on the General Activation scale (also an intermediate value) were excluded. Further random exclusion of subjects was required in order that each group should comprise 13 subjects.

Materials. For the recall part of the experiment, category names and single letters were printed on slides using Letraset. A pool of 48 category–letter pairs was formed by pairing each of 12 categories with 4 different letters, two of the pairs within each category being high dominance (mean dominance rank = 2.50) and two being low dominance (mean rank = 9.96). Each subject, however, only received 24 category–letter pairs, one high-dominance and one low-dominance pair from each of the 12 categories. The mean response frequency (from Kučera & Francis, 1967) was 39.79 for the high-dominance pairs, and 40.46 for the low-dominance pairs.

For the recognition part of the experiment, category names and category in-stances were printed on slides. The same pool of 48 category–letter pairs was used, except that, instead of a single letter, that instance of highest dominance appro-priate to the category–letter combination was presented. Thus, for example, where the pool pair might be "fruit–A," the recognition pair would be "fruit–apple." Dur-ing the recognition trials, each subject received 24 category-instance pairs, one high-dominance and one low-dominance pair from each of the 12 categories. Any particular item from the pool was used only once for each subject, in either a recall or a recognition trial, depending upon random allocation of items to recall or recognition. An additional 24 category–word distractor pairs were formed by pairing each of the 12 category names with two different distractor words. These distractor words were selected so as to be of equal word frequency to the instances (41.17 vs 40.13, according to Kučera & Francis (1967)) and quite unrelated to any of the categories (in the opinion of two independent judges).

Altogether each subject received a total of 24 recall trials and 48 recognition trials. On recall trials, the subject was required to produce a word from the specified category beginning with the specified letter; on recognition trials, the subject was to respond "yes" if the category name was followed by an instance of that category, and "no" otherwise. Three blocks of recall trials (8 trials per block) and three blocks of recognition trials (16 trials per block) were formed randomly for each subject, the subject alternating between recall and recognition blocks, with a rest of approximately 1.5 min between blocks. Half the subjects started with a recall block, and half with a recognition block.

Procedure. The subject was informed of the alternating sequence of recall and recognition blocks, and was reminded immediately prior to each block about the nature of the forthcoming trials. Particular emphasis was placed upon speed of response. In other respects, the procedure closely resembled that of the first experiment, except that the time between onset of the category slide and onset of the second pair-member was 3.0 sec in this experiment. Twenty practice trials (ten recall, ten recognition) preceded the experimental trials.

Results

As in the first experiment, all the latency data were reciprocally transformed prior to analysis. Errors and omissions were excluded from all analyses; they accounted for 6.92% of all recall trials and 2.40% of all recognition trials. The means for the various conditions are to be found in Table 2. A 4 (Arousal) by 4 (Task Difficulty) analysis of variance, with the first factor between-subjects and the second factor within-subjects was performed on these data. The main effect of Arousal was significant $(F(3,48) = 4.72, p < .01)$, as was the main effect of Task Difficulty $(F(1,48) = 471.75, p < .001)$ on a Geisser–Greenhouse conservative F test. Finally, the critical Arousal-by-Task-Difficulty interaction was highly significant $(F(3,48) = 5.40, p < .005)$ on a conservative F test. Inspection of Fig. 1 indicates that the shape of the arousal-performance function changes from a positive, to an inverted-U, to a negative function as task difficulty increases, i.e., the optimal level of arousal is reduced as task difficulty increases.

Several further analyses were subsequently performed. The recall data were submitted to a 2 (Extraversion) by 2 (General Activation) by 2 (dominance) analysis of variance, with the first two factors between-subjects and the last factor within-subjects. As expected, there was a highly significant effect of Extraversion $(F(1,49) = 16.42, p < .001)$,

MICHAEL W. EYSENCK

TABLE 2
MEAN RESPONSE SPEEDS IN EXPT II
(RECIPROCALLY TRANSFORMED DATA)
FOR RECALL AND RECOGNITION

				Recall				
Extraversion	High	High	High	High	Low	Low	Low	Low
General Activation	High	High	Low	Low	High	High	Low	Low
Dominance	High	Low	High	Low	High	Low	High	Low
Mean	1.05	0.75	0.89	0.81	0.78	0.60	0.89	0.72
SD	0.16	0.14	0.14	0.16	0.14	0.14	0.13	0.13
			Recognition (positive responses)					
Extraversion	High	High	High	High	Low	Low	Low	Low
General Activation	High	High	Low	Low	High	High	Low	Low
Dominance	High	Low	High	Low	High	Low	High	Low
Mean	1.69	1.62	1.61	1.52	1.70	1.64	1.45	1.39
SD	0.16	0.14	0.14	0.16	0.13	0.14	0.13	0.13
			Recognition (negative responses)					
Extraversion	High	High	Low	Low				
General Activation	High	Low	High	Low				
Mean	1.59	1.39	1.57	1.42				
SD	0.20	0.20	0.13	0.15				

extraverts responding much faster than introverts. The main effect of dominance was also highly significant ($F(1,48) = 59.35$, $p < .001$), with high dominance leading to faster response speeds than low dominance. The main effect of General Activation was not significant ($F(1,48) = 1.12$).

The critical Extraversion-by-General-Activation interaction was significant ($F(1,48) = 6.82$, $p < .025$). Extraverts responded more quickly under high General Activation than under low General Activation, whereas the reverse was the case for introverted subjects. Further analysis of the simple main effects indicated that extraverts with high General Activation were significantly faster than introverts with high General Activation ($F(1,48) = 22.19$, $p < .001$), but that, under low General Activation, introverts and extraverts did not differ significantly ($F(1,48) = 1.04$). Furthermore, introverts with high General Activation responded more slowly than introverts with low General Activation ($F(1,48) = 6.75$, $p < .025$), but extraverts with high General Activation

SPEED OF MEMORY RETRIEVAL

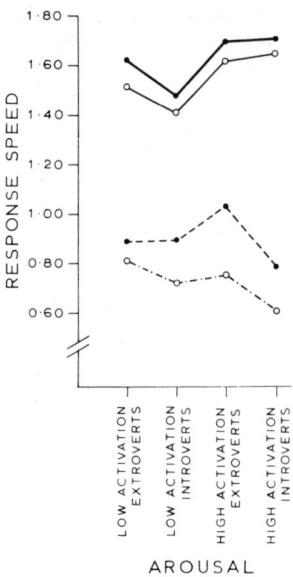

Fig. 1. Mean response speeds for each condition (reciprocally transformed data). Recognition (●—● Hi Dom; ○—○ Lo Dom). Recall (● ---- ● Hi Dom; ○—·—·—○ Lo Dom).

did not differ from extraverts with low General Activation ($F(1,48) = 1.20$).

The General-Activation-by-dominance interaction was also significant ($F(1,48) = 5.77$, $p < .025$). High General Activation slightly improved with performance with high-dominance pairs, but slowed performance with low-dominance pairs. Analysis of the simple main effects indicated that low General Activation subjects responded faster than high General Activation subjects with the low-dominance pairs ($F(1,48) = 5.29$, $p < .05$), but not with the high-dominance pairs ($F < 1$). High-dominance pairs were responded to much quicker than low-dominance pairs both by high-General Activation ($F(1,48) = 51.05$, $p < .001$) and by low-General Activation subjects ($F(1,48) = 14.06$, $p < .001$).

The remaining two-way interaction between Extraversion and dominance was not significant ($F < 1$). However, the three-way interaction of Extraversion, General Activation, and dominance was significant ($F(1,48) = 4.87$, $p < .05$). This interaction indicates that the two-way interaction between Extraversion and General Activation is qualified by the level of dominance. With high-dominance pairs, extraverts with high General Activation responded faster than extraverts with low General

MICHAEL W. EYSENCK

Activation, whereas introverts with high General Activation responded slower than introverts with low General Activation. With low-dominance pairs, on the other hand, high General Activation was associated with slow responding for both introverts and extraverts.

For recognition, a 2 (Extraversion) by 2 (General Activation) by 2 (dominance) analysis of variance, with the first two factors between-subjects and the last factor within-subjects was done on the category–instance data (i.e., positive responses only). The main effect of General Activation was highly significant ($F(1,48) = 15.70$, $p < .001$), with high General Activation associated with faster responding than was low General Activation. The main effect of dominance was also significant ($F(1,48) = 4.44$, $p < .05$), high dominance leading to the faster responses. The main effect of Extraversion was not significant, but, for the Extraversion-by-General-Activation interaction ($F(1,48) = 3.31$; $.10 > p > .05$). All the remaining interactions had $F < 1$.

A 2 (Extraversion) by 2 (General Activation) analysis of variance on the distractor items (i.e., negative responses) produced a nonsignificant effect of Extraversion ($F < 1$), and a nonsignificant interaction ($F < 1$). However, the main effect of General Activation was significant ($F(1,48) = 13.00$, $p < .001$), high General Activation being associated with quicker responding than low General Activation.

In order to explore more closely the differential effects of the personality and dominance variables on recall and recognition, a 2 (Extraversion) by 2 (General Activation) by 2 (recall–recognition) by 2 (dominance) analysis of variance was done, with the first two factors between-subjects and the second two factors within-subjects. The reciprocally transformed recall and category–instance data were used in the analysis. The main effects of Extraversion ($F(1,48) = 9.25$, $p < .005$) and General Activation ($F(1,48) = 4.92$, $p < .05$) were significant. The other main effects were also significant (for recall–recognition, $F(1,48) = 1,302.95$, $p < .001$, and for dominance, $F(1,48) = 37.69$, $p < .001$).

There was a significant interaction between General Activation and recall–recognition ($F(1,48) = 22.88$, $p < .001$), in which recall performance was faster under low than high General Activation, but the opposite was the case for recognition performance. The interaction between dominance and recall–recognition was highly significant ($F(1,48) = 7.85$, $p < .01$), the dominance variable producing greater effects on recall than on recognition. Additionally, there was a highly significant three-way interaction among Extraversion, recall–recognition, and General Activation ($F(1,48) = 14.09$, $p < .001$). This interaction indicated that extraverts performed faster under high General Activation for both recall and recognition, whereas introverts performed faster under high

General Activation for recognition, but slower for recall. None of the other two-way, three-way, or four-way interactions attained the .05 level of statistical significance.

Separate analyses were performed on the recall and recognition error and omission data. None of the main effects or interactions was significant. For the recall error data, extraverts produced nonsignificantly more errors than introverts ($F(1,48) = 1.38$), there was no effect of General Activation ($F < 1$), and the interaction between Extraversion and General Activation was nonsignificant ($F < 1$). For the recall omission data, high General Activation was associated with a greater number of omissions than was low General Activation ($F(1,48) = 3.18$, n.s.), but there was no effect of Extraversion ($F < 1$), and there was no interaction between General Activation and Extraversion ($F < 1$). For the recognition error data, all Fs were less than one, and the same was the case for the recognition omission data.

DISCUSSION

The major finding of the second experiment was the highly significant interaction between Arousal and Task Difficulty. Speed of retrieval from semantic memory is thus conjointly determined by the task difficulty and the subject's level of arousal. This result conforms to the Yerkes–Dodson Law. It has sometimes been suggested (e.g., Uehling (1972)) that a major problem with any study attempting to test the adequacy of the inverted U-shape for describing the relationship between arousal and performance is that other functions (e.g., positive or negative) can be "explained" on a post hoc basis by assuming that insufficient points along the arousal continuum were utilized. In this experiment, however, we have 16 data points, and the shape of the arousal–performance functions changes from a positive, to an inverted-U, to a negative function as anticipated from the Yerkes–Dodson Law. Nevertheless, it is clear that this "Law" merely provides a descriptive statement of the relationship between two variables. It does not provide an explanation for that interaction. Broadbent (1971) reviewed the relevant literature and concluded that a crucial characteristic of the aroused system was that it devoted a higher proportion of its time to the intake of information from dominant sources and less from nondominant ones.

For recognition, the storage locations to be accessed are directly given to the subject, and thus constitute dominant sources of information. The subject appears to evaluate the degree of feature overlap between an instance and its category (Rips, Shoben & Smith, 1973). Since high-dominance sources of information are involved, high levels of arousal should be associated with faster response latencies. The results indicated

MICHAEL W. EYSENCK

that, for both introverts and extraverts, high levels of General Activation were associated with significantly better performance than low levels of General Activation.

For recall, the appropriate storage locations to be accessed are not given to the subject. The subject must perform a serial search through the category instances until an appropriate one is encountered (Anderson & Bower, 1973). If the highly aroused subject devotes a higher proportion of his time to searching through the most dominant category instances, then the response speed for relatively nondominant instances will be reduced. The detrimental effects of a high level of arousal on response speed were revealed in several of the findings. For example, introverts performed significantly more slowly than extraverts on the recall task. This main effect was qualified by a significant interaction between Extraversion and General Activation which indicated that the most aroused group (the high General Activation introverts) had the slowest retrieval times of any group. Exactly in line with Broadbent's hypothesis was the General-Activation-by-dominance interaction, which indicated that low General Activation subjects with the low-dominance pairs responded faster than high General Activation subjects, but this superiority was not maintained with the high-dominance pairs. Further confirmation of the proposed interpretation of the results is available in the three-way interaction of Extraversion, General Activation, and dominance. With high-dominance items, high General Activation facilitated the retrieval of extraverts, but slowed retrieval for introverts. With low-dominance items, involving the intake of information from less dominant sources, high General Activation was associated with slow responding for both introverts and extraverts.

While the above explanation of the data appears to account for most of the major findings from the second experiment, other possibilities should be considered. For example, it is likely that a subject's degree of caution is a determinant of his speed of response. However, several analyses of the error data from both experiments indicated that the error rate was not significantly affected by Extraversion, General Activation, or their interaction. Furthermore, a simple caution hypothesis could not readily account for the several interactions obtained in the studies reported here. Nevertheless, it seems that an adequate appraisal of the caution hypothesis would require either a task producing a greater number of errors than the task used here or instructional manipulation of the subjects' degree of caution.

The dominance variable seemed to be a more potent determinant of performance in the recall than in the recognition situation, as evidenced by the significant dominance by recall–recognition interaction. If the dominance variable is an index of the serial position in which items are accessed during serial search, then it should be a more powerful variable in recall, where search processes are involved, than in recognition, where minimal retrieval is required.

In sum, the findings of this study indicate that retrieval speed from semantic memory is conjointly influenced by the amount of retrieval necessitated by the task (theoretically, the extent to which dominant sources of information are sufficient for successful task performance) and by the arousal level of the subject. These two variables interacted with each other in ways largely predictable from the Yerkes–Dodson Law. A theoretical assumption which provides a substantial underpinning for the Yerkes–Dodson Law is Broadbent's (1971) hypothesis, which appears to provide a satisfactory explanation for the results.

The findings appear to have clear relevance to the examination situation, where it would be predicted that high levels of arousal would greatly increase the difficulty of retrieval of the nondominant items of information commonly required for examination success. The findings may also be relevant to some work by Ramsay (1968) on patterns of speech, in which he found that introverts tended to have longer silences between utterances than extraverts. One interpretation of that result is that introverts, due to their high level of arousal, take longer to retrieve each successive phrase from semantic memory than do extraverts.

Finally, it may be noted that tasks involving recall from semantic memory represent reasonably pure measures of information retrieval. In previous work investigating relationships between personality and memory, it has not been obvious whether obtained differences among personality groups were attributable to individual differences in storage or retrieval, or to a combination of both. It should also be noted that some of the more important findings of this study derive from interactions between Extraversion and General Activation. It appears likely that both the subject's relatively permanent personality characteristics and his transient state or mood are powerful determinants of performance.

REFERENCES

ANDERSON, J. R., & BOWER, G. H. *Human associative memory*. Washington, DC: V. H. Winston & Sons, 1973.

BATTIG, W. F., & MONTAGUE, W. E. Category norms for verbal items in 56 categories: A replication and extension of the Connecticut Category Norms. *Journal of Experimental Psychology Monographs*, 1969, **80** (3, Pt. 2).

BERLYNE, D. E., BORSA, D. M., CRAW, M. A., GELMAN, R. S., & MANDELL, E. E. Effects of stimulus complexity and induced arousal on paired-associate learning. *Journal of Verbal Learning and Verbal Behavior*, 1965, **4**, 291–299.

BOURNE, L. E., JR. An evaluation of the effect of induced tension on performance. *Journal of Experimental Psychology*, 1955, **49**, 418–422.

MICHAEL W. EYSENCK

BROADBENT, D. E. *Decision and stress.* London: Academic Press, 1971.

BROADHURST, P. L. The interaction of task difficulty and motivation: the Yerkes–Dodson Law revived. *Acta Psychologica,* 1959, **16**, 321–338.

CAMERON, B., & MYERS, J. L. Some personality correlates of risk taking. *Journal of General Psychology,* 1966, **74**, 51–60.

CATTELL, R. B. Temperament tests: II. Tests. *British Journal of Psychology,* 1934, **24**, 20–49.

DI SCIPIO, W. J. Divergent thinking: a complex function of interacting dimensions of extraversion–introversion and neuroticism–stability. *British Journal of Psychology,* 1971, **62**, 545–550.

EYSENCK, H. J. *The biological basis of personality.* Springfield, IL: Thomas, 1967.

EYSENCK, H. J., & EYSENCK, S. B. G. *Manual of the Eysenck Personality Inventory.* London: University of London Press, 1964.

EYSENCK, M. W. Extraversion, arousal, and retrieval from semantic memory. *Journal of Personality,* 1974, **42**, 319–331.

FREEDMAN, J. L., & LOFTUS, E. F. The retrieval of words from long-term memory. *Journal of Verbal Learning and Verbal Behavior,* 1971, **10**, 107–115.

GALE, A., COLES, M., & BLAYDON, J. Extraversion-introversion and the EEG. *British Journal of Psychology,* 1969, **60**, 209–223.

GEWIRTZ, J. L. Studies in word-fluency. II. Its relation to eleven items of child behavior. *Journal of Genetic Psychology,* 1948, **72**, 177–184.

HEBB, D. O. Drives and the C. N. S. (conceptual nervous system). *Psychological Review,* 1955, **62**, 243–254.

KINTSCH, W. Models for free recall and recognition. *In* D. A. Norman (Ed.), *Models of human memory.* London: Academic Press, 1970.

KUČERA, H., & FRANCIS, W. N. *Computational analysis of present-day American English.* Providence, RI: Brown University Press, 1967.

LACEY, J. I. Somatic response patterning and stress: Some revisions of activation theory. *In* M. H. Appley & R. Trumbull (Eds.), *Psychological stress.* New York: Appleton–Century–Crofts, 1967.

LOFTUS, E. F., FREEDMAN, J. L., & LOFTUS, G. R. Retrieval of words from subordinate and superordinate categories in semantic hierarchies. *Psychonomic Science,* 1970, **21**, 235–236.

LOFTUS, E. F., & SUPPES, P. Structural variables that determine the speed of retrieving words from long-term memory. *Journal of Verbal Learning and Verbal Behavior,* 1972, **11**, 770–777.

McLAUGHLIN, R. J. Retention in paired-associate learning related to extraversion and neuroticism. *Psychonomic Science,* 1968, **13**, 333–334.

McLAUGHLIN, R. J., & KARY, S. K. Amnesic effects in free recall with introverts and extroverts. *Psychonomic Science,* 1972, **29**, 250–252.

RAMSAY, R. W. Speech patterns and personality. *Language and Speech,* 1968, **11**, 54–63.

RIPS, L. J., SHOBEN, E. J., & SMITH, E. E. Semantic distance and the verification of semantic relations. *Journal of Verbal Learning and Verbal Behavior,* 1973, **12**, 1–20.

SAVAGE, R. D. Electro-cerebral activity, extraversion and neuroticism. *British Journal of Psychiatry,* 1964, **110**, 98–100.

THAYER, R. E. Measurement of activation through self-report. *Psychological Reports,* 1967, **20**, 663–678.

SPEED OF MEMORY RETRIEVAL

TOWNSEND, J. T. A note on the identifiability of parallel and serial processes. *Perception & Psychophysics,* 1971, **10,** 161–163.

TULVING, E. Episodic and semantic memory. *In* E. Tulving & W. Donaldson (Eds.), *Organization of memory.* London: Academic Press, 1972.

TULVING, E., & THOMSON, D. Retrieval processes in recognition memory: Effects of associative context. *Journal of Experimental Psychology,* 1971, **87,** 116–124.

UEHLING, B. S. Arousal in verbal learning. *In, Human memory: festschrift in honor of Benton J. Underwood.* New York: Appleton–Century–Crofts, 1972.

UEHLING, B., & SPRINKLE, R. Recall of a serial list as a function of arousal and retention interval. *Journal of Experimental Psychology,* 1968, **78,** 103–106.

WHITE, K. Anxiety, extraversion–introversion, and divergent thinking ability. *Journal of Creative Behavior,* 1968, **2,** 119–127.

WILKINS, A. T. Conjoint frequency, category size, and categorization time. *Journal of Verbal Learning and Verbal Behavior,* 1971, **10,** 382–385.

From M. W. Eysenck (1975). British Journal of Social and Clinical Psychology, *14*, 269–277, *by kind permission of the author and Cambridge University Press*

Arousal and Speed of Recall

BY MICHAEL W. EYSENCK

Department of Psychology, Birkbeck College,
University of London

Subjects were divided into four groups based upon the possible combinations of high or low Extraversion and high or low General Activation. They learned two lists of paired associates in an A–B, A–Br paradigm, with a record being kept of the number of errors and the latency of correct responses. The groups were found to differ considerably more in terms of response latency than in terms of the probability of responding correctly. A number of the analyses indicated an interactive effect of Extraversion and General Activation on retrieval performance, in which high General Activation led to reduced response latencies for extraverts, but to slower latencies for introverts. This finding was interpreted with reference to arousal theory. Additional findings suggested that the poor performance of high arousal subjects was partially due to their tendency to take in information from dominant sources, a hypothesis suggested by Broadbent (1971).

Jensen (1964) carried out a number of experiments in which he investigated the relationship between personality and performance on serial-learning and digit-span tasks. One of his main findings was that introverts were less resistant than extraverts to response competition in a serial-learning task. Subsequent attempts have been made to extend the generality of this finding to paired-associate learning (Howarth, 1969; Bone, 1971). They both used variations on the A–B, A–Br transfer paradigm, in which the stimuli and responses of the first list are re-paired to form the second list. In both studies, inferior performance by the introverted subjects was only apparent on the re-paired, or transfer, list, which would presumably involve response competition. Additional work with paired associates by McLaughlin & Eysenck (1967) provided more support for Jensen's (1964) finding.

Interpretations of the above findings have used the concept of arousal. McLaughlin & Eysenck (1967) argued that introverts were characterized by higher levels of arousal than extraverts, a conclusion for which some evidence exists (Eysenck, 1967; Savage, 1964; Gale *et al.*, 1969). They obtained a significant personality by list difficulty interaction, with the optimal level of arousal varying inversely with task difficulty; this interaction clearly conforms to the Yerkes–Dodson Law (Broadhurst, 1959). McLaughlin & Eysenck (1967) also found an overall superiority of extraverted subjects, which was explained with reference to Walker's action-decrement theory. This theory assumes that high arousal leads to the setting up of a strong perseverative trace, resulting in greater long-term memory, but greater temporary inhibition against recall ('action decrement') during the process of consolidation. Several studies have obtained evidence supporting this theory (e.g. Kleinsmith & Kaplan, 1963, 1964). It can be predicted from the theory that extraverts, being characterized by low arousal, should show superior recall to introverts at short retention intervals (as McLaughlin & Eysenck found), but inferior recall at long retention intervals (subsequently found by

Howarth & Eysenck, 1968). However, Berlyne & Carey (1968) obtained superior retention for extraverts after 24 hr., which appears contrary to the theory.

A number of other studies have indicated effects of arousal on recall probability which do not appear to be due to consolidation processes. For example, Pascal (1949) found that brief relaxation instructions given immediately prior to recall significantly improved recall performance, subsequently, both Bourne (1955) and Uehling & Sprinkle (1968) obtained facilitatory effects of arousal on retrieval; Berlyne *et al.* (1965) did not. M. W. Eysenck (1974) required spontaneous retrieval without prior presentation of items from each of five categories. He administered Thayer's Activation–Deactivation Adjective Check List. This test, which is an objective self-report measure of transient levels of activation, was investigated in several experiments by Thayer (1967). Thayer's main finding was that the General Activation scale derived from the check list correlated substantially with physiological measures of arousal in each of three separate experiments. A highly significant interaction between Extraversion and General Activation was obtained, in which high levels of arousal (as indexed by the General Activation scale) increased the number of words recalled by extraverts, but reduced the recall of introverts.

Further studies have looked at effects of arousal on speed of retrieval rather than probability of recall. Straughan & Dufort (1969) found that relaxation instructions reduced the response latencies of anxious subjects, but increased the latencies of non-anxious subjects. M. W. Eysenck (in preparation) has found in studies of the speed of retrieval from semantic memory that extraverts retrieve information from semantic memory considerably faster than introverts. Speed of retrieval from semantic memory was found to be conjointly determined by task difficulty and the subject's level of arousal. In conformity with the Yerkes–Dodson Law, the optimal level of arousal (as determined by the General Activation scale and the degree of introversion) decreased as task difficulty increased. This interaction was interpreted by assuming, firstly, that difficult tasks require the emission of non-dominant responses, and, secondly, that Broadbent (1971) was correct in concluding that a crucial characteristic of the aroused system is that it devotes a higher proportion of its time to the intake of information from dominant sources and less from non-dominant ones.

In sum, this study has three main aims. The first is to investigate further the effects of arousal on the probability and the latency of correct responses by obtaining both measures in the same experimental situation. Secondly, in view of previous findings, this study also considers personality differences as they are affected by transient levels of activation. Finally, in an attempt to assess the tenability of Broadbent's (1971) hypothesis, dominance of the correct response was experimentally manipulated.

METHOD

Subjects

The subjects were divided into four groups on the basis of scores on the Extraversion scale of the Eysenck Personality Inventory (Form A), and the General Activation scale of the Activation-Deactivation Adjective Check List. All those scoring 11 on the Extraversion scale, 4 or more on the Lie scale, or 18 on the General Activation scale were excluded. Further random exclusion of subjects was required in order that each group should comprise

Arousal and Speed of Recall

13 subjects. On the Neuroticism scale of the Eysenck Personality Inventory, the groups of low General Activation introverts and extraverts had higher mean Neuroticism scores than the groups of high General Activation introverts and extraverts. However, an analysis of variance indicated that the four groups did not differ in mean Neuroticism scores ($F = 1·39$; d.f. $= 3, 48$). The Pearsonian correlation coefficient between General Activation and Neuroticism was $-0·15$, which is non-significant.

Materials

Sixteen paired-associates were obtained by reference to Palermo & Jenkins (1964). One of the three strongest associates to each of sixteen nouns from their norms was selected, with the constraint that only nouns were selected and associative strength between each response and the remaining fifteen stimuli was kept to a minimum. These strongly associated word pairs constituted the first list. The second list consisted of a random re-pairing of these stimuli and responses. Thus the A–B, A–Br transfer paradigm was used.

Procedure

Each subject was informed that he would receive an alternating sequence of study and test trials. On each study trial, the 16 stimulus-response pairs would be presented at a rate of 3·2 sec. per pair. Ten seconds after each study trial, the subject would be given a test trial, on which the stimulus members of each pair would be presented. The subject would be allowed up to 10 sec. to say the appropriate response aloud, and he was encouraged to guess in the case of uncertainty. A different random order was used on each study and test trial.

Each subject was tested individually. He had a throat microphone around his throat, and the need for avoidance of unintentional use of the throat musculature was explained to him. The experimenter preceded presentation of each stimulus word by saying, 'Right', followed within 2 sec. by the presentation of the next stimulus word. The onset of the letter slide was coincident with the starting of an electric timer. The subject's overt response activated the voice key that stopped the electric timer. The study and test trials on each list were continued until two criteria were reached: firstly, all the responses on the final test trial had to be correct and with latencies of less than 1·5 sec.; secondly, all stimuli must have been correctly responded to at least three times in succession.

RESULTS

List 1

Error data (i.e. omissions and intrusions) for the first list are presented in Table 1. In order to assess the importance of the retrieval time available in determining performance, two error scores were calculated for each subject. The first simply comprised the total number of failures to respond correctly within the 10 sec. interval. The second, based upon the latency data, comprised the total number of failures to respond correctly within 1·5 sec. of stimulus onset. These scores will be referred to as long and short retrieval period error scores, respectively.

The data were analysed by means of a 2 (Extraversion) by 2 (General Activation) by 2 (Retrieval Period) three-way analysis of variance, with the first two factors between subjects and the last factor within subjects. Of the main effects, those of Extraversion ($F = 1·16$; d.f. $= 1, 48$) and General Activation ($F < 1$) were not significant, but that of Retrieval Period was highly significant ($F = 98·78$; d.f. $= 1, 48$; $P < 0·001$). As anticipated, considerably more correct responses were produced in the long than the short retrieval period. None of the interactions even approached the 0·05 level of statistical significance.

MICHAEL W. EYSENCK

A second analysis was performed on the mean latencies of correct responses, on the first three trials on which any particular response was correctly given. The data are presented in summary form in Table 2. A 2 (Extraversion) by 2 (General Activation) by 3 (Trials) analysis of variance, with the last factor within subjects, was performed on these data. The main effect of Extraversion was highly significant ($F = 9\cdot63$; d.f. = 1, 48; $P < 0\cdot005$), with introverts responding faster than extraverts. The main effect of Trials was also highly significant ($F = 133\cdot84$; d.f. = 2, 96; $P < 0\cdot001$), subjects tending to respond faster over successive trials. The main effect of General Activation was non-significant ($F = 1\cdot48$; d.f. = 1, 48). The interaction between General Activation and Extraversion was highly signifi-

Table 1. *Mean errors with short and long retrieval periods (list 1)*

Extraversion ...	High	High	High	High	Low	Low	Low	Low
General Activation ...	High	High	Low	Low	High	High	Low	Low
Retrieval period ...	Long	Short	Long	Short	Long	Short	Long	Short
Mean	1·31	3·08	1·62	3·46	1·15	3·00	1·23	2·38
S.D.	1·25	1·80	1·04	2·22	1·07	1·47	1·24	1·85

Table 2. *Mean latencies of correct responses over trials for list 1 (in sec.)*

Extraversion ...		High	High	Low	Low
General Activation ...		High	Low	High	Low
Trial 1	Mean	1·02	1·13	1·12	0·99
	S.D.	0·13	0·17	0·12	0·11
Trial 2	Mean	0·89	0·98	0·89	0·82
	S.D.	0·10	0·12	0·09	0·07
Trial 3	Mean	0·80	0·96	0·76	0·78
	S.D.	0·06	0·08	0·08	0·06

cant ($F = 15\cdot52$; d.f. = 1, 48; $P < 0\cdot001$). In this interaction, extraverts responded faster under high General Activation than they did under low General Activation, whereas introverts responded faster under low General Activation, than under high General Activation. There was a further significant interaction between Extraversion and Trials ($F = 4\cdot85$; d.f. = 2, 96; $P < 0\cdot025$). In this interaction, there was a non-significant difference between introverts and extraverts on trial 1 ($F < 1$), with introverts showing a latency advantage on trials 2 and 3 ($F = 8\cdot96$; d.f. = 1, 144; $P < 0\cdot005$, and $F = 14\cdot28$; d.f. = 1, 144; $P < 0\cdot001$, respectively). Finally, there was a significant interaction between General Activation and Trials ($F = 5\cdot58$; d.f. = 2, 96; $P < 0\cdot01$), in which high levels of General Activation became progressively more associated with relatively fast responding over trials. Analysis of the simple main effects indicated that there was no effect of General Activation on either trial 1 ($F < 1$) or trial 2 ($F < 1$), but that high General Activation led to faster responding than low General Activation on trial 3 ($F = 8\cdot72$; d.f. = 1, 144; $P < 0\cdot005$).

Arousal and Speed of Recall

List 2

Short and long retrieval period error scores derived from the second list are presented in Table 3. These data were analysed by a 2 (General Activation) by 2 (Extraversion) by 2 (Retrieval Period) analysis of variance, with the first two factors between subjects and the last factor within subjects. The main effect of Extraversion was significant ($F = 4.12$; d.f. $= 1, 48$; $P < 0.05$), as was the main effect of Retrieval Period ($F = 699.92$; d.f. $= 1, 48$; $P < 0.001$). Introverts had significantly fewer errors than extraverts, and more errors occurred with the short than the long retrieval period. The remaining main effect, that of General Activation, was not statistically significant ($F = 3.51$; d.f. $= 1, 48$).

Table 3. *Mean errors with short and long retrieval periods (list 2)*

Extraversion	High	High	High	High	Low	Low	Low	Low
General Activation ...	High	High	Low	Low	High	High	Low	Low
Retrieval period ...	Long	Short	Long	Short	Long	Short	Long	Short
Mean	24·69	63·08	25·85	76·15	27·85	73·46	18·85	51·46
S.D.	7·02	12·06	4·51	11·84	8·01	11·98	5·39	13·70

Of the interactions, Retrieval Period did not interact significantly with either Extraversion or with General Activation ($F = 2.75$; d.f. $= 1, 48$, and $F < 1$, respectively). However, there was a highly significant interaction between Extraversion and General Activation ($F = 25.55$; d.f. $= 1, 48$; $P < 0.001$). In this interaction, high General Activation extraverts produced fewer errors than low General Activation extraverts, whereas high General Activation introverts produced more errors than low General Activation introverts. Finally, there was a highly significant three-way interaction involving General Activation, Extraversion and Retrieval Period ($F = 15.60$; d.f. $= 1, 48$; $P < 0.001$). Tests of simple main effects were made, adopting a conservative error rate. The interaction between Extraversion and General Activation was not significant at the long retrieval period ($F = 3.44$; d.f. $= 1, 96$), but was highly significant at the short retrieval period ($F = 41.05$; d.f. $= 1, 96$; $P < 0.001$). At the long retrieval period, high General Activation introverts and extraverts performed equivalently ($F < 1$), as did low General Activation introverts and extraverts ($F = 3.27$; d.f. $= 1, 96$). Furthermore, high and low General Activation extraverts did not differ ($F < 1$), nor did high and low General Activation introverts ($F = 5.40$; d.f. $= 1, 96$). At the short retrieval period, however, extraverts had fewer errors than introverts under high General Activation ($F = 7.20$; d.f. $= 1, 96$; $P < 0.05$), and introverts had fewer errors than extraverts under low General Activation ($F = 40.68$; d.f. $= 1, 96$; $P < 0.001$). Additionally, high General Activation extraverts had fewer errors than low General Activation extraverts ($F = 11.41$; d.f. $= 1, 96$; $P < 0.005$), whereas high General Activation introverts had more errors than low General Activation introverts ($F = 32.29$; d.f. $= 1, 96$; $P < 0.001$). Thus the significant two-way interaction between General Activation and Extraversion is due largely to performance with the short retrieval period.

MICHAEL W. EYSENCK

A further analysis was performed on the mean latencies of correct responses on the first three trials on which each response was correctly given. These data, which are given in summary form in Table 4, were cast into a 2 (General Activation) by 2 (Extraversion) by 3 (Trials) analysis of variance. The main effect of trials was highly significant ($F = 65·41$; d.f. $= 2, 96$; $P < 0·001$), but the effects of main General Activation and Extraversion were not ($F < 1$, and $F = 1·81$; d.f. $= 1,48$). The critical interaction between General Activation and Extraversion was highly significant ($F = 6·24$; d.f. $= 1, 48$; $P < 0·025$). In this interaction, extraverts responded faster under high General Activation than under low General Activation, whereas the reverse was the case for introverts.

Table 4. *Mean latencies of correct responses over trials for list 2 (in sec.)*

Extraversion		High	High	Low	Low
General Activation ...		High	Low	High	Low
Trial 1	Mean	2·67	3·11	2·83	2·24
	S.D.	0·75	0·82	0·59	0·60
Trial 2	Mean	2·07	2·20	2·23	1·84
	S.D.	0·35	0·74	0·54	0·47
Trial 3	Mean	1·77	2·04	1·93	1·67
	S.D.	0·34	0·69	0·45	0·32

DISCUSSION

A major implication of the analyses of the first list data is the importance of considering separately the probability of correct recall and the latencies of correct responses. Neither General Activation nor Extraversion was significantly related to recall probability on list 1, probably due to ceiling effects. However, several interesting findings emerged from an analysis of the latency data. There was a highly significant interaction between General Activation and Extraversion. If one assumes that arousal level may be indexed by scales of Extraversion and of General Activation, then the groups of intermediate arousal level (high General Activation extraverts and low General Activation introverts) responded faster than those characterized by low General Activation extraverts) or high (high General Activation introverts) levels of arousal. This result is compatible with arousal theory.

The further interactions involving trials may be interpreted in the light of Broadbent's (1971) assumption that the highly aroused system will take in information from highly dominant sources. The first list consisted of dominant responses to the respective stimulus words, and the functional dominance would increase over a series of trials. Thus the relative superiority of high-arousal subjects should increase over trials. This prediction was confirmed by the significant interaction between General Activation and Trials, in which high General Activation subjects had shorter latencies than low General Activation subjects only on the third of three trials. It was further confirmed by the Extraversion × Trials interaction, in which the latency advantage of introverts over extraverts increased progressively over trials. A similar result was obtained by Standish & Champion (1960).

The major finding with the second list was the highly significant three-way interaction among General Activation, Extraversion, and Retrieval Period. In this interaction, neither Extraversion, nor General Activation, nor their interaction was related to the number of errors made with the long retrieval period. At the short retrieval period, however, a highly significant interaction between General Activation and Extraversion was obtained. High General Activation reduced the number of errors obtained by extraverts, and increased the number of errors made by introverts. The poor performance of high-arousal subjects (the high General Activation introverts) may be explained by reference to Broadbent's (1971) dominance hypothesis. The second list clearly involved non-dominant responses, both because of the existence of other, stronger, pre-experimentally acquired associations to the stimulus words and because of the dominant associations formed during first list learning. Furthermore, the tendency of high-arousal subjects to sample dominant sources of information would seem to suggest that high arousal would lengthen retrieval time for non-dominant responses, but would not necessarily affect retrieval probability if sufficient time for retrieval were available. The results clearly accord with that prediction.

Further support for the curvilinear relationship between arousal and retrieval speed comes from an analysis of the latencies of correct responses. The highly significant interaction between General Activation and Extraversion was consistent with arousal theory, in that high General Activation reduced the response latencies of extraverts, but increased those of introverts.

The several significant interactions between General Activation and Extraversion indicate the value of a simultaneous consideration of two (or more) individual-difference measures. This type of analysis has been designated 'zone analysis' by Furneaux (1961) and 'moderator variable' analysis by Ghiselli (1963). Such an analysis is particularly relevant where theory predicts an interactive relationship. While zone analysis has been applied successfully to Extraversion and Neuroticism considered conjointly (Eysenck, 1967), it should be noted that these are both trait measures. If one is interested in the effects of arousal on performance, it seems preferable to use both trait and state indices of arousal (cf. Spielberger, 1966).

The major explanation for effects of arousal on paired-associate learning has been Walker's (1958) action decrement theory, which predicts that low arousal should lead to better performance than high arousal at short retention intervals. While this theory has a considerable amount of supporting evidence (e.g. Kleinsmith & Kaplan, 1963, 1964), it does not appear to explain the non-effectiveness of arousal as a variable in determining errors on the first list, the non-significant effects of arousal with long retrieval periods in the second list, or the curvilinear relationship between arousal and performance with short retrieval periods in the second list (the low arousal group should have performed better).

In sum, arousal affects speed of retrieval rather than probability of retrieval, and its effects are dependent upon the functional dominance of the appropriate response. The results broadly accord with arousal theory, and, more particularly, with Broadbent's (1971) assumption that high arousal leads to decreased sampling from non-dominant sources. Furthermore, the several interactions between Extraversion and General Activation indicate that the subject's relatively permanent

MICHAEL W. EYSENCK

personality characteristics and his transient mood or state are powerful determinants of performance, and should be considered together. Finally, the finding that arousal affect retrieval speed has important methodological implications for studies in this area. As the comparison between a short and a long retrieval period with the second list indicated, a totally different relationship between arousal level and recall can be obtained with different retrieval periods. Accordingly, the experimental situation used in previous studies, involving the use of a single length of retrieval period, cannot be recommended.

REFERENCES

BERLYNE, D. E., BORSA, D. M., CRAW, M. A., GELMAN, R. S. & MANDELL, E. E. (1965). Effects of stimulus complexity and induced arousal on paired-associate learning. *J. verb. Learn. verb. Behav.* **4**, 291–299.

BERLYNE, D. E. & CAREY, S. T. (1968). Incidental learning and the timing of arousal. *Psychon. Sci.* **13**, 103–104.

BONE, R. N. (1971). Interference, extraversion and paired-associate learning. *Br. J. soc. clin. Psychol.* **10**, 284–285.

BOURNE, L. E., Jr. (1955). An evaluation of the effect of induced tension on performance. *J. exp. Psychol.* **49**, 418–422.

BROADBENT, D. E. (1971). *Decision and Stress.* London: Academic Press.

BROADHURST, P. L. (1959). The interaction of task difficulty and motivation: the Yerkes–Dodson Law revived. *Acta psychol.* **16**, 321–338.

EYSENCK, H. J. (1967). *The Biological Basis of Personality.* Springfield: Thomas.

EYSENCK, M. W. (1974). Extraversion, arousal, and retrieval from semantic memory. *J. Personality* **42**, 319–331.

FURNEAUX, W. D. (1961). Neuroticism, extraversion, drive and suggestibility. *Int. J. clin. exp. Hypn.* **9**, 195–214.

GALE, A., COLES, M. & BLAYDON, J. (1969). Extraversion–introversion and the EEG. *Br. J. Psychol.* **60**, 209–223.

GHISELLI, E. E. (1963). Moderating effects and differential reliability and validity. *J. appl. Psychol.* **47**, 81–86.

HOWARTH, E. (1969). Extraversion and increased interference in paired-associate learning. *Percept. mot. Skills* **29**, 403–406.

HOWARTH, E. & EYSENCK, H. J. (1968). Extraversion, arousal, and paired-associated recall. *J. exp. Res. Person.* **3**, 114–116.

JENSEN, A. (1964). Individual differences in learning: interference factor. (Cooperative Research Project no. 1867 Office of Education, U.S. Department of Health, Education and Welfare.)

KLEINSMITH, L. J. & KAPLAN, S. (1963). Paired-associate learning as a function of arousal and interpolated interval. *J. exp. Psychol.* **65**, 190–193.

KLEINSMITH, L. J. & KAPLAN, S. (1964). Interaction of arousal and recall interval in nonsense syllable paired-associate learning. *J. exp. Psychol.* **67**, 124–126.

McLAUGHLIN, R. J. & EYSENCK, H. J. (1967). Extraversion, neuroticism and paired associate learning. *J. exp. Res. Person.* **2**, 128–132.

PALERMO, D. S. & JENKINS, J. J. (1964). *Word Association Norms: Grade School through College.* Minneapolis: University of Minnesota Press.

PASCAL, G. R. (1949). The effect of relaxation upon recall. *Am. J. Psychol.* **62**, 33–47.

SAVAGE, R. D. (1964). Electro-cerebral activity, extraversion and neuroticism. *Br. J. Psychiat.* **110**, 98–100.

SPIELBERGER, C. D. (1966). Theory and research on anxiety. In C. D. Spielberger (ed.), *Anxiety and Behaviour.* London: Academic Press.

STANDISH, R. R. & CHAMPION, R. A. (1960). Task difficulty and drive in verbal learning. *J. exp. Psychol.* **59**, 361–365.

STRAUGHAN, J. H. & DUFORT, W. H. (1969). Task difficulty, relaxation, and anxiety level during verbal learning and recall. *J. abnorm. Psychol.* **74**, 621–624.

Arousal and Speed of Recall

THAYER, R. E. (1967). Measurement of activation through self-report. *Psychol. Rep.* **20**, 663–678.

UEHLING, B. & SPRINKLE, R. (1968). Recall of a serial list as a function of arousal and retention interval. *J. exp. Psychol.* **78**, 103–106.

WALKER, E. L. (1958). Action decrement and its relation to learning. *Psychol. Rev.* **65**, 129–142.

Manuscript received 10 *April* 1974

Revised manuscript received 30 *May* 1974

From S. Schwartz (1975). Journal of Research in Personality, *9*, 217–225, *by kind permission of the author and Academic Press*

Individual Differences in Cognition: Some Relationships Between Personality and Memory

STEVEN SCHWARTZ

Northern Illinois University

Individual differences in cognition were studied in the form of the hypothesis that arousal, as indexed by personality measures of extraversion and neuroticism, affects the way in which verbal material is organized in memory. Subjects pretested on measures of these personality variables participated in either a paired-associates learning or a free-recall experiment. On the paired-associates task, subjects who were thought to be high on arousal made fewer errors when response terms were semantically similar than low arousal subjects. On the other hand, subjects thought low on arousal made fewer errors when response words were phonetically similar than high arousal subjects. On the free-recall task, low arousal subjects were found to cluster words together on the basis of semantic category at a higher rate than high arousal subjects. These results were taken to support the view that high arousal (as indexed by personality measures) leads to a focus on the physical aspects of verbal material, whereas low arousal leads to a memory organized around semantic aspects. The implications of these findings for other views of memory are discussed.

Psychologists have been aware of individual differences in cognitive functioning for some time. Recently, however, the technological (e.g., intelligence test) orientation of the past has given way to an interest in questions of a more theoretical nature (e.g., Hunt, Frost & Lunneborg, 1973). It is the purpose of the present paper to carry this work further by exploring some of the relationships between personality and memory as well as the implication of these relationships for a theory of cognition.

A personality theory with important implications for memory has been developed by Eysenck (1967). In his theory, the descriptive concepts of extraversion–introversion and neuroticism–stability are linked with the physiological constructs, arousal and activation, respectively. Introverts are thought to have higher cortical arousal levels than extraverts, whereas neurotics are characterized by higher levels of autonomic ac-

This research was supported by grants from the Northern Illinois University Dean's Fund. The author wishes to thank H. J. Eysenck for his comments on an earlier draft of this paper. Some of the research discussed here was presented at the annual meeting of the Psychonomic Society, Boston, November 1974.

Requests for reprints should be sent to Steven Schwartz, Division of Child Psychiatry University of Texas Medical Branch, Galveston, Texas 77550.

tivation than those falling at the stable end of the neuroticism scale.

Arousal, induced experimentally, has been related to memory by Kleinsmith and Kaplan (1963, 1964) who reported that arousing paired-associate items were harder to remember than nonarousing items when recall was tested immediately after acquisition but better recalled when the test was delayed 20 min to 1 wk. This finding was taken as support for the hypothesis that arousal protects a neural trace from interference (by rendering it inaccessible) until it is consolidated (Walker, 1958). Similar findings have been obtained when personality traits were used to reflect arousal (McLean, 1968). Unfortunately, a great deal of conflicting evidence (Archer & Margolin, 1970; Corteen, 1969; Hörmann & Todt, 1960; Maltzman, Kantor & Langdon, 1966; Schönpflug, 1966) suggests that the consolidation hypothesis is incorrect. In these experiments, arousal during acquisition was found to facilitate immediate as well as delayed recall.

Thus, although it appears that arousal during acquisition influences subsequent memory, the precise arousal–recall relationship is unclear. Since memory, in some experiments, improved from immediate to delayed recall, arousal could not have resulted in any permanent information loss. Rather, it seems plausible to assume that arousal affected the accessibility of stored information. The way in which arousal exerts such an effect is just beginning to be clarified. Recent research (Hörmann & Osterkamp, 1966; Hamilton, Hockey & Quinn, 1972; Schwartz, 1974) suggests that arousal influences the cues which are used to organize recall. Specifically, it appears that arousal orients memory toward the physical[1] characteristics of verbal material while adversely affecting memory for its semantic aspects (see also, Schwartz, 1973). Depending on the type of material, arousal may either facilitate or hinder memory, and contradictory experimental results are to be expected. The occasional reversal obtained with delay may be a function of arousal's dissipation with time.

Evidence in support of the view that arousal influences the way in which memory is organized has been obtained when the personality trait "anxiety" was used to index arousal (Zubrzycki & Borkowski, 1973; Mueller, 1974). Anxiety, however, may not be as clear-cut a measure of arousal as one would like (Saltz, 1970). The present experiments were designed to assess the hypothesis that arousal (indexed by measures of extraversion and neuroticism) focuses memory on physical cues while adversely affecting memory for semantic cues.

---

[1] The term "physical" is employed here to represent the visual and acoustic aspects of linguistic material in contrast to the semantic and syntactic aspects.

EXPERIMENT I

McLaughlin and Eysenck (1967) explored the relationship between personality and memory for paired-associates. On an easy task (neither the stimulus words nor the response words were similar to one another), arousal was curvilinearly related to performance. That is, if personality is conceived of in terms of an arousal continuum ranging from stable-extraverts (SE's), who are low on arousal, through stable-introverts (SI's) and neurotic-extraverts (NE's), who are intermediate, and ending with neurotic-introverts (NI's), who are high, the SI's and NE's performed best, and the SE's and NI's performed poorly. On a difficult task (low-stimulus/high-response similarity), the relationship between arousal and performance was linear. The low arousal SE's performed best, and the remaining groups performed more poorly. Although these results were interpreted as supporting a modified consolidation hypothesis, they are also consistent with the present view because response similarity on the hard task was varied along a "physical" dimension. That is, response members shared letters in common. If, as hypothesized, low arousal subjects concentrate on the semantic aspects of verbal material while high arousal subjects focus on physical aspects, then we would expect that only the latter group would be confused by physical similarity among the responses. (On the easy task, concentrating on one type of cue or the other is not differentially disturbing; thus, both SE's and NI's do about as well.) The present view predicts that if response similarity were along a semantic dimension, the linear relationship between arousal and memory would be reversed. That is, NI's would perform best and SE's poorly. This was the hypothesis of the first experiment.

Method

Lists. Unlike the McLaughlin and Eysenck experiment, the present study employed words rather than nonsense syllables. Two lists were constructed. On both lists, *stimulus* words were chosen that were both unrelated to one another semantically as well as phonetically. List 1 response words were all phonetically similar (billow, pillow, willow, etc.), while List 2 response words were all chosen from a single semantic category (spoon, fork, pot, etc.). Words in this latter list were chosen from the category members determined by Battig and Montague (1969).

Subjects and procedure. Forty-eight male and female introductory psychology students were chosen from among over 300 tested earlier with the Eysenck Personality Inventory (Eysenck & Eysenck, 1964). On the basis of their scores, subjects were assigned to one of the four personality groups. The mean extraversion score of those classified as NE's and SE's was 16.78, whereas the mean score for SI's and NI's on the extraversion scale was 8.66. On the neuroticism scale, NI's and NE's achieved a mean score of 15.10, whereas SI's and SE's achieved a mean of 5.00. Twelve subjects were assigned to each personality group. Half of each group learned List 1; half learned List 2. Testing continued until each subject learned the assigned list to a criterion of one errorless trial. The lists were presented by a memory drum to each subject individually, and errors were noted. The

STEVEN SCHWARTZ

words, typed in capitals, appeared at a 2:2-sec rate (2 sec for the stimulus word and 2 sec for both the stimulus and response words) with a 6-sec intertrial interval. Each list consisted of seven pairs and was presented in three different orders.

Results and Discussion

Males did not differ from females in any condition, so data from both sexes were grouped together. Figure 1 contains the results of the experiment in terms of the mean total number of errors made until the criterion was achieved. As predicted, the two types of lists were not learned equally well by the various personality groups. Specifically, the NI's performed best on the phonetically similar list. The triple interaction (list × neuroticism × extraversion) was significant $(F(1,40) = 12.32, p < .01)$. An *a posteriori* test on the mean error scores (Winer, 1962, pp. 309–313) indicated that four major differences contributed to this interaction. On the phonetically similar list, NI's made more errors than SE's $(p < .01)$, whereas the reverse was true on the semantically similar list $(p < .01)$. In addition, SE's made more errors on the semantically similar than on the phonetically similar list $(p < .05)$, whereas the opposite was true of NI subjects. There were no other meaningful differences obtained in this experiment with the exception of a main effect for lists $(F(1,40) = 5.33, p < .05)$. The semantically similar list was easier (in most cases) than the phonetically similar list.

Although the results of this experiment are consistent with the view that arousal, indexed by personality measures, influences the way in which memory is organized, a word should be said about a possible alternative explanation. That is, it may be that discriminating phonetically similar words from one another is easier than semantic differentiation and that these results, then, are actually in support of McLaughlin and Eysenck's (1967) hypothesis. The literature, however, does not support

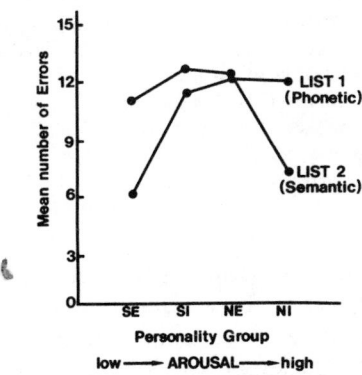

FIG. 1. Total number of errors for each personality group on each of the two lists. (Each point represents the mean number of errors until the criterion was achieved.)

such a contention. In almost every experiment dealing with such distinctions, semantic encoding seems no more difficult and leads to greater recall than phonemic encoding (see Mueller, 1974; Nelson & Brooks, 1974; Schwartz & Witherspoon, 1974). Moreover, the results of Expt I indicated that the semantic list was actually easier than the phonetically similar list. The results of Expt I, then, support the notion that high arousal subjects (NI's) who focus on the physical characteristics of verbal material are not adversely affected by semantic similarity, and low arousal subjects (SE's) who concentrate on the semantic characteristics are not adversely affected by phonetic similarity. This hypothesis implies that in a free-recall situation differences in the order of recall of semantically organized lists should be obtained as a function of personality. That is, semantic clustering should be observed in the free-recall of SE's, whereas NI's free-recall should be sequential (rote). This was the hypothesis of the second experiment.

EXPERIMENT II

Method

Subjects and lists. Twelve subjects from each of the four personality groups described in the first experiment served in the second experiment. Their scores on the EPI did not differ significantly from those reported in Expt I. Two lists were constructed so that each list contained 10 words from each of three categories:

List 1. Kitchen utensils, parts of the body, tools.
List 2. Sports, articles of clothing, vegetables.

These words were chosen from among the moderate frequency category members of the lists provided by Battig and Montague (1969).

Procedure. Each list was presented in two conditions. In the blocked condition, all words within a single category were presented contiguously, whereas in the pseudorandom condition, words from the various categories were mixed so that on only four occasions did two words from the same category follow one another. Words were presented via slides shown for 2.5 sec with a 1-sec intertrial interval. At the conclusion of a list, subjects were given 2 min to write as many words as they could recall on an answer sheet. Each list was presented to each subject four times (twice in the blocked order and twice in the pseudorandom order) for a total of eight list presentations. The sequence of list presentations was balanced as to list order (blocked or pseudorandom) and list type (List 1 or List 2). That is, half the subjects in each personality group studied List 1 followed by List 2, and half studied the blocked lists before the pseudorandom, whereas the remaining half studied the pseudorandom list first.

Results and Discussion

Free-recall was scored for the total number correct and the number of category repetitions relative to the maximum number of possible repetitions. (Other clustering scores were computed, but all yielded the same logical and statistical conclusions.)

Two 3-way analyses of variance (personality × list × order) were conducted (one using the total number of words recalled and the other using

STEVEN SCHWARTZ

clustering scores as the dependent variable). As the analyses indicated no significant effect for list type on either the number of words recalled ($F(1,33) = 2.10$, $p > .10$) or on clustering ($F(1,33) = 2.00$, $p > .10$), only the mean data across lists is reported in Table 1. The analysis employing total number of words recalled as the dependent variable found no significant differences for personality or for list order ($p > .10$ in both cases). This result indicates once again that experimenter imposed list organization need not necessarily result in increased recall (see also Hunt *et al.,* 1973). As might be expected, clustering was relatively high for all groups in the blocked condition. There was, however, a marked difference between groups in the pseudorandom condition. The interaction between list order and personality was significant ($F(3,33) = 3.12$, $p < .05$). An *a posteriori* test conducted on the mean clustering scores indicated that the locus of the interaction was a substantial decrease in clustering for the NI's in the pseudorandom condition relative to the blocked condition ($p < .05$). The remaining groups showed fairly small (nonsignificant) drops in clustering. As indicated in Table 1, difference scores calculated by subtracting, for each subject, the clustering score in the pseudorandom condition from the clustering score in the blocked condition reinforce this finding. In order to determine whether the NI's tended to recall the pseudorandom lists in the order in which they were presented, a score equivalent to the clustering score was calculated for rote memory (the number of original list repetitions relative to the maximum possible number of repetitions). For the blocked condition, this is identical to the score reported in Table 1, and although NI's did not differ significantly from the others, their score is in the predicted direction. In the pseudorandom condition, the rote clustering scores were .28, .35, .26, and .51 for the SE, SI, NE, and NI groups respectively. A test of planned comparisons (see Winer, 1962) indicated that only the NI group differed significantly from the others ($p < .01$) and that no other differences were significant. It appeared that

TABLE 1

MEAN RECALL AND CLUSTERING SCORES FOR THE FOUR PERSONALITY GROUPS

Personality group	Total words recalled		Clustering score		Difference[a]
	Blocked	Random	Blocked	Random	
Stable—Extraverts	21.41	22.00	.71	.63	−.08
Stable—Introverts	20.75	21.50	.71	.65	−.06
Neurotic—Extraverts	21.72	20.10	.77	.62	−.15
Neurotic—Introverts	19.85	21.20	.79	.48	−.31

[a] $p < .01$ for comparison of NI's with all other groups (Tukey "b" procedure, Winer, 1962).

the NI's tended to recall the pseudorandom lists in the order in which they were presented.

GENERAL DISCUSSION

The results of both experiments are consistent with the view that arousal, indexed by personality measures, influences the way in which memory is organized. Specifically, high arousal subjects focus on the physical aspects of verbal material, whereas low arousal subjects organize memory around semantic cues. These findings have implications for the way in which verbal memory is viewed by psychologists. Although few psychologists have trouble conceiving of a semantically organized verbal memory, some seem to doubt the idea of a memory organized along physical lines that lasts more than just a few seconds. There is good reason to believe, however, that memory for the physical aspects of verbal material lasts much longer than a few seconds. "S," a mnemonist studied by Luria (1968), relied almost exclusively on visual images and a "memory walk" method of memory retrieval. Furthermore, recent experiments conducted by Kirsner (1973), Kolers (1973), and Nelson and Brooks (1974) indicate that even non-mnemonists can retain for rather long periods fairly detailed information about the visual aspects of verbal material. The results of the present experiments serve to reinforce these findings.

The mechanism by which personality (arousal) exerts its effect on memory is unclear. From a neurophysiological point of view, the midbrain reticular activating system (generally considered the part of the brain primarily responsible for the control of arousal) has no known role in higher mental processes. Nevertheless, some writers (e.g., Kesner, 1973; Penfield & Roberts, 1959) have postulated some such role for the reticular activating system. Kesner (1973) suggested that arousal's effect is primarily to increase the degree of ongoing neural activation. In that case, arousal magnifies the neural events accompanying both correct perception and storage as well as those accompanying misperceptions and false memories. If one assumes that both presented and semantically related nonpresented items in memory have a "trace strength" (subject to random Gaussian fluctuations) greater than zero which is further incremented by arousal, then, assuming a fixed criterion for deciding whether or not an item was presented, arousal will increase the number of semantically related "false alarms" making memory based on semantic relationships ineffective. Perhaps, when a semantic strategy is rendered ineffective, one automatically turns to a physical strategy. Clearly, this line of reasoning is highly speculative, and discovering the neurological correlates of arousal's effect on memory must await further research.

STEVEN SCHWARTZ

REFERENCES

Archer, B. U., & Margolin, R. R. Arousal effects in intentional recall and forgetting. *Journal of Experimental Psychology*, 1970, **86**, 8–12.

Battig, W. F., & Montague, W. E. Category norms for verbal items in 56 categories: A replication and extension of the Connecticut category norms. *Journal of Experimental Psychology Monograph*, 1969, **80**, No. 3, Part 2.

Corteen, R. S. Skin conductance changes and word recall. *British Journal of Psychology*, 1969, **60**, 81–84.

Eysenck, H. J. *The biological basis of personality*. Springfield: C. C. Thomas, 1967.

Eysenck, H. J., & Eysenck, S. B. G. *Manual of the Eysenck personality inventory*. London: University of London Press, 1964.

Hamilton, P., Hockey, G. R. J., & Quinn, J. G. Information selection, arousal and memory. *British Journal of Psychology*, 1972, **63**, 181–189.

Hörmann, H., & Osterkamp, U. Uber den Einfluss von kontinuierlichem Larm auf die Organisation von Gedachnisinhalten. *Zeitschrift fur Angewandte Psychologie*, 1966, **13**, 31–38.

Hörmann, H., & Todt, E. Larm und lernen. *Zeitschrift fur Angewandte Psychologie*, 1960, **7**, 422–426.

Hunt, E., Frost, N., & Lunneborg, C. Individual differences in cognition: A new approach to intelligence. In G. H. Bower (Ed.), *The psychology of learning and motivation*. New York: Academic Press, 1973, Vol. 7.

Kesner, R. A neural system analysis of memory storage and retrieval. *Psychological Bulletin*, 1973, **80**, 177–203.

Kirsner, K. An analysis of the visual component in recognition memory for verbal stimuli. *Memory and Cognition*, 1973, **1**, 449–453.

Kleinsmith, L. J., & Kaplan, S. Paired-associate learning as a function of arousal and interpolated interval. *Journal of Experimental Psychology*, 1963, **65**, 190–193.

Kleinsmith, L. J., & Kaplan, S. Interaction of arousal and recall interval in nonsense syllable paried-associate learning. *Journal of Experimental Psychology*, 1964, **67**, 124–126.

Kolers, P. A. Remembering operations. *Memory and Cognition*, 1973, **1**, 347–355.

Luria, A. *The mind of a mnemonist*. New York: Basic Books, 1968.

Maltzman, I., Kantor, W., & Langdon, B. Immediate and delayed retention, arousal, and the orienting and defense reflexes. *Psychonomic Science*, 1966, **6**, 445–446.

McLaughlin, R. J., & Eysenck, H. J. Extroversion, neuroticism, and paired-associate learning. *Journal of Experimental Research in Personality*, 1967, **2**, 128–132.

McLean, P. D. Induced arousal and time of recall as determinants of paired-associate recall. *British Journal of Psychology*, 1969, **60**, 57–62.

Mueller, J. Anxiety in human learning and memory: Cue utilization. In M. Zuckerman and C. D. Spielberger (Eds.), *Emotions and anxiety: New concepts, methods and applications*. Washington, DC: Winston, 1974.

Nelson, D. L., & Brooks, D. H. Relative effectiveness of rhymes and synonyms as retrieval cues. *Journal of Experimental Psychology*, 1974, **102**, 277–283.

Penfield, W., & Roberts, L. *Speech and brain mechanisms*. Princeton: Princeton University Press, 1959.

Saltz, E. Manifest anxiety: Have we misread the data? *Psychological Review*, 1970, **77**, 568–573.

Schonpflug, W. Paarlernen, Behaltensdauer und Aktivierung. *Psychologische Forschung*, 1966, **29**, 132–148.

Schwartz, S. Arousal and recall: Effect of noise on two retrieval strategies. *Journal of Experimental Psychology*, 1974, **102**, 896–898.

Schwartz, S. Effects of arousal on two strategies of selective retrieval in short term memory. Paper presented at the annual meeting of the Midwestern Psychological Association, Chicago, May, 1973.

Schwartz, S., & Witherspoon, K. D. Decision processing in memory: Factors influencing the storage and retrieval of linguistic and form information. *Bulletin of the Psychonomic Society,* 1974, **4,** 127–129.

Taylor, J. A. A personality scale of manifest anxiety. *Journal of Abnormal and Social Psychology,* 1953, **48,** 285–290.

Walker, E. L. Action decrement and its relation to learning. *Psychological Review,* 1958, **65,** 129–142.

Winer, B. J. *Statistical principles in experimental design.* New York: McGraw–Hill, 1962.

Zubrzycki, C. R., & Borkowski, J. G. Effects of anxiety on storage and retrieval processes in short term memory. *Psychological Reports,* 1973, **33,** 315–320.

PART IX

COGNITION AND CREATIVITY

There has been much research and theorizing in recent years concerning differences between "divergent" and "convergent" thinking, on the hypothesis that the former was concerned with mental activities of a rather different character as compared with the latter. In particular, the hypothesis was formulated (Guilford, 1959; Getzels and Jackson, 1962) that "divergent" thinking was in some way related to originality and creativity. If this were true, one might have to say that tests of this kind measured an aspect of the "structure of the intellect", to use Guilford's phrase, different from that measured by orthodox IQ tests. The evidence for such a contention is at best inconclusive, and an alternative theory must at least be considered. This theory goes back to Spearman (1927) under whose aegis "divergent" thinking tests were first developed, and who demonstrated that tests of "fluency" (as he called them then) did indeed constitute a group factor within the general field of general intelligence. However, his explanation was quite different from that given by modern authors; he postulated that in so far as fluency test scores were not simply determined by general intelligence, they were a reflection of the extraverted or introverted personality of the subject, extraverts being more fluent, introverts less. This hypothesis is related to the impulsive nature of the extravert, uninhibited by dictates of having to make proposals which make sense, or which are not out of line with the rules of polite society. In more modern terms, we would make such a prediction on the basis of the wider basis for memory search which is associated with lower arousal, as explained in an earlier section. However we arrive at the deduction, it seems clear that we would expect differences in "fluency" or "divergent thinking" as between extraverts and introverts, with the former doing rather better. Several of the papers reprinted here have tested this hypothesis, and on the whole the evidence is very much in favour of the deduction.

Other problems which arise in the cognitive field relate to such problems as the relationship between achievement in cognitive tasks, such as school and university examinations, and personality; the question of mental speed in extraverts and introverts; and the interaction of these factors with age. Several reprinted articles take up these questions, and demonstrate that personality does indeed play an important part in cognitive tasks.

This relationship becomes particularly clear at the university level. Wankowski (1973) has followed up all incoming students at the University of Birmingham for a number of years, each of whom filled in a personality questionnaire on entry. He found a clear negative correlation between achievement and extraversion, and an equally clear one between achievement and neuroticism. The combination of E and N was positively lethal; only one in eight of the students so afflicted obtained a good honours degree, as opposed to one in three of introverted students (stable or unstable). Conversely, of the E and N students, one in three withdrew without obtaining a degree, while only one in five of stable introverts withdrew. Personality also determined choice of course. Stable people tended to congregate in the "practically" oriented courses and subjects of study, whilst those with neurotic tendencies predominated in "people oriented" areas of study. Introverts preferred theoretical and extraverts practical or "people oriented" areas. (Sociology was peopled *par excellence* by neurotic extraverts!) Findings such as these, taken together with the more experimental studies contained in this section, open up a fascinating and potentially important field much in need of further research.

REFERENCES

GETZELS, J. and JACKSON, P. W. *Creativity and intelligence: explorations with gifted students.* New York: Wiley, 1962.
GUILFORD, J. P. The structure of intellect. *American Psychologist*, 1959, *14*, 469–479.
SPEARMAN, C. *The abilities of man.* London: Macmillan, 1927.
WANKOWSKI, J. A. Temperament, motivation and academic achievement. Birmingham: University of Birmingham, Educational Survey and Counselling Unit, 1973.

From K. White (1968). Journal of Creative Behavior, *2*, 119–127, *by kind permission of the author and* The Creative Education Foundation

KINNARD WHITE

Anxiety, Extraversion-Introversion, and Divergent Thinking Ability*

RESEARCH
BASIS FOR STUDY

Considerable research interest recently has been focused on the relationship between personality factors and divergent thinking functions. The rationale for pursuing research in this area has been stated by Barron (1955), who argues that original responses occur with regularity among some persons while among others original responses are virtually nonexistent. If this is true, then it becomes possible for the researcher to focus his study on the relatively enduring underlying personal characteristics that may be expected to be related to the production of original responses.

Studies using "known groups" of adults, that is, groups of adults who are generally engaged in the performance of tasks that are judged to be creative in nature as opposed to groups of adults not generally engaged in the performance of these tasks, have reported general agreement in terms of the personality traits that are important to these sorts of tasks. Persons generally engaged in the performance of creative tasks have been typically described as being nonaggressive, sensitive, and somewhat asocial (Bloom, 1963; Drevdahl & Cattell, 1958; White, 1965). In terms of Eysenck's (1960) distinction between introversion and extraversion, these persons would generally be classified as introverts.

*This article provides psychological theories which support creativity-development principles such as deferred judgment. The research was supported by a grant from the University Research Council of the University of North Carolina, Chapel Hill, North Carolina.

Among persons not generally engaged in "creative work," but who are categorized as having "creative potential" on the basis of their scores on tests of divergent thinking ability, some research data suggest that we might expect relationships with personality that conflict with the above findings. Rivlin (1959) has reported that high school students who score high on divergent thinking tasks were rather sociable and generally evaluated themselves as being confident in their relationships with people. Cashdan and Welsh (1966) have also reported that, among talented high school students, those with high creative potential were not interpersonal recluses, but rather individuals who welcomed social contact; in addition, these students were self-assertive and independent. Further, the research by Smith (1961) has suggested that self-confidence was a primary factor in divergent thinking ability among educated adults. Also, studies conducted in England have shown quite clearly that cognitive measures which could be classified in the same category as the divergent thinking measures used in the United States are correlated with the personality type termed extraversion (Eysenck, 1960). Further work by Eysenck (1967) has clearly indicated that extraverts ought to perform better than introverts on tests requiring rapid adaptive changes. Hudson (1966) in a recent study conducted with English schoolboys has shown that students classified as divergent thinkers were more fluent, emotionally more outgoing, and more sociable than those classified as convergent thinkers. Fluency, emotional projection and sociability are all characteristics of extraverts.

HYPOTHESES   Analysis of this research indicated that a direct test of the relationship between extraversion-introversion and divergent thinking ability was needed. The research reported here was designed, therefore, to test hypotheses concerning the effects of this relatively broad personality dimension on measures of divergent thinking ability. In addition hypotheses were tested simultaneously concerning the effects of anxiety level and its interaction with extraversion-introversion on measures of divergent thinking ability. The rationale for testing the hypotheses concerning anxiety derives primarily from the early work of Spence (1956), which suggested that anxiety is a drive and furthermore that very strong drives or levels of anxiety can prevent adaptive changes in behavior. It follows from these hypotheses that persons with high levels of anxiety should score lower on tests requiring quick adaptive changes, or, in other words, on divergent thinking tasks, which certainly require this kind of adaptability.

The two major personality dimensions investigated, extraversion-introversion and anxiety, were viewed within the context of this research as being relatively broad descriptive categories that are general organizing influences on personality. Although research on the personality dimension extraversion-introversion has not received the attention from American researchers that it has from British researchers (Eysenck, 1960), the recent conceptualization of this dimension by Cattell and Scheier (1961) as a second-order personality factor derivable from previously established first-order traits measured by the *Sixteen Personality Factor Questionnaire* (*16 PF*) (Cattell & Eber, 1957) makes research on this dimension more feasible. The first-order traits of the *16 PF* which constitute this dimension are Factors A (warm, sociable), E (dominance), F (surgency), H (lack of shyness), and Q_2 (socially group dependent). These first-order personality factors appear to summarize a cluster of personality characteristics which the results of previous investigations have indicated should be related to divergent thinking ability. This dimension was used, therefore, to test the hypothesis that the personality dimension extraversion-introversion is related to performance on divergent thinking tasks.

Research focusing on the second personality dimension studied (anxiety-dynamic integration) has resulted in numerous conceptualizations of anxiety, but the one used in this study was that anxiety is a second-order personality factor composed of first-order factors assessed by the *16 PF*. The factors on the *16 PF* which contribute to this dimension are Factors C (low emotional stability), H (restrained), L (suspicious), O (apprehensive), Q_3 (poor self-sentiment), and Q_4 (tenseness). Again these elements of the anxiety dimension appear to summarize a cluster of personality traits which previous investigators have indicated are relevant to divergent thinking ability. This dimension was used, therefore, to test the hypothesis that the level of anxiety does affect performance on divergent thinking tasks.

METHOD
Subjects

Ss were two hundred male freshmen, one summer out of high school, who were enrolled at the University of North Carolina. Selection was made from classes in the Physical Education Department. Since all male freshmen are required to be in attendance in that department regardless of their health rating, this sample represents a cross-section of the freshman males at the university.

Independent Variables

The independent variables for this study were all derived from the *Sixteen Personality Factor Questionnaire* (*16 PF*), Form A (Cattell & Eber, 1957). This instrument yields measures on sixteen primary dimensions of personality. Factor analytic studies using the *16 PF* have resulted in the establishment of two major second-order factors, Anxiety (A_x), and Extraversion-Introversion (E-I). The A_x factor is designed to assess anxiety levels somewhat similarly to a consensus assessment by clinicians. This second-order factor has been shown to correlate in the .80's with the Taylor scale and from .40 to .50 with an anxiety checklist (Cattell & Scheier, 1961). Persons scoring high on this factor have been described as having higher tension, higher susceptibility to annoyance, less confidence in rational performance, lower self-sentiment, and less persistence in rewarding activities (Cattell & Scheier, 1961). The behavioral manifestations of the E-I, or Extraversion-Introversion, factor toward the extraversion end of the dimension are reported to be higher fluency on self characteristics, higher fluency on other people's behavior, more objects seen in unstructured drawings, preference for strange, and dramatic rather than familiar themes. Cattell (1965) describes the extravert as being a socially uninhibited, fluent, optimistic, person-oriented, not self-critical, individual.

These two second-order factors were derived as described in the Handbook (Cattell & Eber, 1957). The assessment was conducted within one month after Ss had entered the university. Testing was done in groups of about thirty.

Dependent Variables

Ss were assessed on two divergent thinking tasks which yielded three scores. The divergent thinking assessments were the *Alternate Uses* test (Wilson, *et al.*, 1960), which yields a measure of spontaneous verbal flexibility; and the *Consequences* test (Christensen, *et al.*, 1960), which yields measures of ideational fluency and originality. These measures derived from the *Alternate Uses* and the *Consequences* tests are classified by Guilford (1959) as flexibility—the divergent production of classes from semantic content; ideational fluency—the divergent production of semantic content; originality—the divergent production of transformations with semantic content. These tasks were scored in the manner suggested in the manual for the instruments.

The divergent thinking assessments were made about one week after Ss had sat for the personality assessment and were also conducted in groups of about thirty.

ANALYSIS OF
DATA

To assess the main effects of the A_x and E-I variables, as well as their interactions, on the measures of divergent thinking, the A_x and E-I scores were split at the norm mean (5.5; the means for these samples were $A_x = 5.3$; E-I = 5.5) to define two classifications of each variable. Ss with a score of 6 or above were considered high on the variable while Ss with a score of 5 or below were considered low. This procedure resulted in a two-way ($A_x \times$ E-I) classification.

Since both A_x and E-I are considered to be second-order factors which can be broken down into first-order factor components, correlations were calculated between each of the first-order factors of the 16 PF and the three assessments of divergent thinking. In this way relationships may be observed both between the first-order factors which contribute to A_x and E-I as well as between the other 16 PF factors and divergent thinking.

RESULTS

Table I at the end of the article presents the means and standard deviations on the divergent thinking tasks for the two A_x groups and the two E-I groups. Each of three assessments of divergent thinking ability was submitted to an analysis of variance, and the results for all three of the divergent thinking ability tasks were highly similar. In the cases of the significant main effects, the low A_x group scored higher on the flexibility task than the high A_x group; and the high E-I group scored higher on the flexibility task than the low E-I group.

The analysis of variance of scores on the ideational fluency task yielded significant main effects for A_x and E-I. Again, the low A_x group scored higher on the ideational fluency task than the high A_x group, and the high E-I group scored higher on the ideational fluency task than the low E-I group.

The analysis of variance of scores on the originality tasks also yielded significant main effects for A_x and E-I. Similar to the previous analyses, the low A_x scored higher on the originality task than the high A_x group; the high E-I group scored higher on the originality task than the low E-I group. Furthermore, the differentially high performance on the originality task by the low A_x/high E-I subgroup was the primary contributor to a significant interaction effect which had not shown up in the other two analyses.

The correlation matrix of divergent thinking scores and 16 PF scores is reported in Table 2 (at the end of the article). Of particular interest is the pattern and direction of the significant correlations between the three assessments of divergent thinking ability and the *16 PF* factors which contribute to the second-order factors of A_x and E-I. These correlations not only corroborate the findings in the analysis of variance, but in addition give some insight into the more important first-order personality factors involved. Both the number and size of the significant correlations reported in this table are relatively high for the type of relationships studied.

DISCUSSION   The results of this study indicate that persons with relatively low levels of anxiety perform significantly better on divergent thinking tasks than persons with high levels of anxiety. Similarly, all three assessments of divergent thinking ability had negative correlations to anxiety. This finding substantiates previous statements by Spence (1956), Cattell and Scheier (1961), Eysenck and Eysenck (1962), Getzels and Jackson (1962), and Ruebush (1963). Of all the factors of the *16 PF* contributing to the anxiety dimension, Factor H (restrained) and Factor O (apprehensive) were the highest and most consistently related to divergent thinking ability. Even the simple one-word description of these factors presented here suggests that this relationship is a meaningful one.

The relationships obtained between extraversion-introversion and divergent thinking ability conjunct with the findings reported by Cashdan and Welsh (1966) and by Rivlin (1959). Also the findings of this research follow logically from the hypotheses and data presented by Eysenck and Eysenck (1962), who have demonstrated that rigidity is highly related to introversion and neuroticism (anxiety). In fact, a factor analysis of rigidity as assessed by a questionnaire indicated that the variance of the rigidity scores could be accounted for primarily by introversion and neuroticism (anxiety). The notion of rigidity in mental processes clearly seems to be opposed to the ability to engage in divergent thinking tasks. That rigidity, introversion, and neuroticism are related has been further substantiated by the recent research of Watson (1967). He has demonstrated that neurotic-introverts were highly inflexible and had very low ability to utilize change responses in comparison with stable extraverts. It appears likely therefore that there is operating here a type of response set or style that is in some way mediated by the basic personality dimensions of anxiety and extraversion-introversion.

The correlations between the assessments of divergent thinking ability and the first-order *16 PF* factors that contribute to the second-order extraversion-introversion factor suggest some contradictions between the results of this study and studies using "known groups" of creative adults. Particularly outstanding are the significant positive correlations between factors H (lack of shyness), E (dominance), and Q_2 (socially group dependent). These same factors have been reported to have negative correlations to membership in groups judged to be engaged in creative activities (Cattell & Drevdahl, 1955; Drevdahl & Cattell, 1958; White, 1965).

Reversals such as these are difficult to explain, but among the possible reasons for them, the following are suggested as feasible avenues for further investigation. First, the influence which a given activity has on the person pursuing that activity is not well understood. Many sociologists feel that a person's work is quite important in shaping an individual's personality and style of life. It is currently unclear as to whether the differences in personality between people who are found in different occupational groups comes about because the individuals were attracted to the group as a result of certain personality attributes they possessed or whether they acquired certain personality attributes as a result of becoming associated with the group. Secondly, the notion of creativity is difficult if not impossible to define in such a way as to permit definitive research. In the type of study reported here, creativity as such was not being assessed. Rather some other characteristic of the individual was assessed, one which was assumed to be an index of his potential creativity. Yet when more ultimate criteria are used to assess creativity, questions concerning the basis for judging an act as being creative always arise. Perhaps persons found in "known groups" and persons assessed by the methods used in this study do, in fact, have different sorts of creative potential, or demonstrate their creativity in different ways.

Although some apparent contradictions currently exist, two conclusions appear to be in order. First, the problem which has been posed by this research clearly calls for conducting longitudinal studies to observe whether or not correlated changes do occur in personality and divergent thinking ability. Secondly, the results of the present study as well as inferential evidence from research previously cited clearly indicate that the personality dimensions of anxiety and extraversion-introversion should be taken into account in future studies of divergent thinking ability. The best evidence is that persons high on divergent thinking ability are not interpersonal recluses as some popular literature might lead one to believe, nor are they shy, apprehensive, and generally anxious.

TABLE 1   Means and Standard Deviations on Divergent Tasks for A_x and E-I Groups

| | High A_x | | | | Low A_x | | | |
| | High E-I | | Low E-I | | High E-I | | Low E-I | |
	X	SD	X	SD	X	SD	X	SD
Flexibility	19.12	5.52	17.48	5.20	22.50	4.85	18.30	6.18
Ideational Fluency	32.14	11.17	26.34	9.18	36.12	13.44	31.06	11.68
Originality	22.50	8.40	21.60	7.41	30.04	7.58	21.38	9.56

TABLE 2   Correlations Between 16 PF Factors and Scores on Divergent Thinking Tasks

16 PF Factors	Flexibility	Ideational Fluency	Originality
A ‡	10	10	10
C +	00	16*	04
E ‡	25**	04	29**
F‡	24**	21**	10
G	−05	24**	10
H + ‡	26**	25**	22**
I	13	−03	20**
L +	00	08	06
M	01	−23**	14*
N	−02	14*	13
O +	−15*	−19**	−12
Q_1	04	−22**	12
Q_2 ‡	−23**	−26**	−14*
Q_3 +	−02	−01	−05
Q_4 +	−07	−19**	−09

Note: Decimals have been omitted.
   + Primary factors in anxiety.
   ‡ Primary factors in extraversion-introversion.
   * $p < .05$
   ** $p < .01$

The Journal of Creative Behavior

REFERENCES BARRON, F. The disposition toward originality. *J. of Abn. & Soc. Psychol.* 1955, *51*, 478-485.

BLOOM, B. S. Report on creativity research at The University of Chicago. In C. W. Taylor & F. Barron (Eds.), *Scientific creativity.* New York: Wiley 1963. Pp. 251-264.

CASHDAN, S., & WELSH, G. S. Personality correlates of creative potential in talented high school students. *J. of Pers.,* 1966, *34,* 445-455.

CATTELL, R. B. *The scientific analysis of personality.* Baltimore: Penguin Books, 1965.

CATTELL, R. B., & DREVDAHL, J. E. A comparison of the personality profile (16 PF) of eminent researchers with that of eminent teachers and administrators and of the general population. *British J. of Psychol.,* 1955, *46,* 248-261.

CATTELL, R. B., & EBER, H. W. *Handbook for the sixteen personality factor questionnaire.* Champaign, Ill.: Institute for Personality and Ability Testing, 1957.

CATTELL, R. B., & SCHEIER, J. H. *The meaning and measurement of neuroticism and anxiety.* New York: Ronald, 1961.

CHRISTENSEN, P. R., MERRIFIELD, P. R., & GUILFORD, J. P. *Consequences.* Beverly Hills, Calif.: Sheridan Supply, 1960.

DREVDAHL, J. E., & CATTELL, R. B. Personality and creativity in artists and writers. *J. of Clinical Psychol.,* 1958, *74,* 107-111.

EYSENCK, H. J. *The structure of human personality.* (2nd ed.) London: Methuen, 1960.

EYSENCK, H. J. Intelligence assessment: A theoretical and experimental approach. *British J. of Educ. Psychol.,* 1967, *37,* 81-98.

EYSENCK, S. B. G., & EYSENCK, H. J. Rigidity as a function of introversion and neuroticism: A study of unmarried mothers. *International J. of Soc. Psychiatry,* 1962, *8,* 180-184.

GETZELS, J. W. & JACKSON, P. W. *Creativity and intelligence: explorations with gifted students.* New York: Wiley, 1962.

GUILFORD, J. P. The structure of intellect. *Amer. Psychol.,* 1959, *14,* 469-479.

HUDSON, L. *Contrary imaginations.* New York: Schocken, 1966.

RIVLIN, L. Creativity and the self-attitudes and sociability of high school students. *J. of Educ. Psychol.,* 1959, *50,* 147-152.

RUEBUSH, B. K. Anxiety. In H. W. Stevenson (Ed.), *Child psychology: The sixty-second yearbook of the National Society for the Study of Education,* Part I. Chicago: Univ. of Chicago Press, 1963. Pp. 460-516.

SMITH, W. J. The prediction of research competence and creativity from personal history. *J. of Appl. Psychol.,* 1961, *45,* 59-62.

SPENCE, K. W. *Behavior theory and conditioning.* New Haven: Yale University Press, 1956.

WATSON, D. L. Introversion, neuroticism, rigidity, and dogmatism. *J. of Cons. Psychol.,* 1967, *31,* 105.

WHITE, K. P. Personality characteristics of educational leaders: a comparison of administrators and researchers. *School Rev.,* 1965, *73,* 292-300.

WILSON, R. C., CHRISTENSEN, P. R., MERRIFIELD, P. R., & GUILFORD, J. P. *Alternate Uses.* Beverly Hills, Calif.: Sheridan Supply, 1960.

Kinnard White, Associate Professor, School of Education. Address: University of North Carolina, Chapel Hill, North Carolina 27514.

From W. J. Di Scipio (1971). British Journal of Psychology, *62*, 545–550, *by kind permission of the author and Cambridge University Press*

DIVERGENT THINKING:
A COMPLEX FUNCTION OF INTERACTING DIMENSIONS OF EXTRAVERSION–INTROVERSION AND NEUROTICISM–STABILITY*

By WILLIAM J. DI SCIPIO

Bronx State Hospital, New York, U.S.A.

Divergent thinking was measured by word fluency and word originality in a sample of 300 university students. After controlling for verbal intelligence, divergent thinking was found to be a complex function of extraversion–introversion and neuroticism–stability. Stable extraverts were significantly more fluent than stable introverts, but neurotic extraverts and introverts attained fluency scores approximating the mean of the extreme stable counterparts. The effect is explained in terms of Eysenck's arousal theory of personality types.

Introduction: A brief review of the literature

Research into the measurement of divergent thinking processes can be traced back to the early psychometric studies concerned with the faculty of 'imagination'. These studies demonstrated two distinct modes of expression: verbal fluency and originality. Verbal fluency defined a quantitative estimate of the rate of verbal output, while originality defined an estimate of the frequency of rare verbal responses with respect to a reference population. Reviews of the early work in this field may be found in Rogers (1953), Rim (1953), Eysenck (1960), Burt (1962, 1967) and Torrance (1967).

General intelligence, as defined by the early mental testers in Britain and America, was distinguished from the concept of 'imagination' in that general intelligence reflected the ability to reproduce information according to predetermined 'right' and 'wrong' test response criteria. Spearman (1927), however, held the view that tests of imagination scored for originality of response defined a specific cognitive factor which was only one of many others and might be employed in a wide battery of tests to yield a comprehensive estimate of the general intelligence factor g.

Hargreave's (1927) experimental studies of verbal fluency upheld Spearman's views and demonstrated that fluency, as measured by open-ended verbal tests, is a composite function of factors of general verbal ability, memory and motor speed of writing or speaking. Partial correlations among the fluency tests proved high enough to suggest that some further element remained to be accounted for (factor x) after removing the influence of the above factors. Hargreaves concluded that factor x was probably related to the absence of inhibitions, possibly a lack of self-criticism, thus attributing a conative explanation to verbal fluency.

Cattell (1934) placed greater emphasis upon the conative correlate of verbal fluency and renamed the tests of imagination 'Tests of Temperament'. In developing a battery of tests of perseveration and verbal fluency, Cattell found that a subtest of

---

* This paper formed part of a Ph.D. thesis by the author at the University of London, 1968.

WILLIAM J. DI SCIPIO

the latter factor, Speed of Cognitive Output (SCO), proved to be the best predictor of temperament. The test required the subject to list all the two-syllable words which he could think of in $2\frac{1}{2}$ min. The test correlated $0\cdot30$ ($n = 62$) with 'surgency', a personality trait denoting extraversion and measured by means of a self-rated questionnaire. The retest reliability of the SCO was $0\cdot57$ after one week.

The research to follow Cattell's lead continued to demonstrate the positive relationship of new verbal fluency tests to tests of temperament (Studman, 1935; Carroll, 1941; Notcutt, 1943; Gewirtz, 1948; Rim, 1954; Rogers, 1956; Hofstaetter *et al.*, 1957; Getzels & Jackson, 1962; Wallach & Kogan, 1965; Ramsey, 1966). Cattell's description of the surgency correlate of fluency as being one of sociability and the early replications of his findings led Eysenck (1960) to conclude that verbal fluency was related to extraversion, a personality type which incorporated traits of sociability and impulsivity.

Guilford (1950) introduced a new direction in the use of fluency and other divergent thinking tests by relating the abilities tapped by these tests to the abilities and patterns of character traits possessed by the 'creative' individual. The pattern of creative abilities was postulated to vary with the sphere of creative activity. Creative products varied with interests, attitudes and temperamental factors. Guilford's approach was useful, but only within the context of his factor structure of the intellect. Divergent thinking tests became loosely defined criteria of 'creativity', which did not account for the social acceptance of creative output for a given field.

Although Guilford's influence diverted further investigations from Cattell's and Eysenck's notion of fluency as a function of extraversion, the evidence continued to suggest that the individual who scored highly on fluency or 'creativity' tests tended to be impulsive, sociable, talkative and uninhibited, in addition to having a wide range of interests and preferring arts to sciences (Barron, 1953; Getzels & Jackson, 1962; Hudson, 1966; Bowers, 1967; Schaefer & Anastasi, 1968).

White (1968), in a recent paper, reports on the distinction between the personality correlates of creative behaviour as determined by known groups of creative individuals in contrast to creative individuals determined by high scores on divergent thinking tests. He suggests that personality correlates of divergent thinking tests are not *a priori* measures of creative ability as displayed by individuals who are judged by others as possessing 'creative talent'. White presents evidence for 200 male university freshmen which indicated that the extravert, as defined by Cattell's 16 PF, obtains higher scores on divergent test measures (flexibility, fluency and originality) than the introvert, with the relationship applying in the same order for stable *v.* neurotic personalities.

A contradictory note on the subject of personality correlates of divergent thinking is introduced by Rim (1953) in a study which attempted to establish a differential diagnostic criterion for hysterics (neurotic extraverts) and dysthymics (neurotic introverts). Rim did not find a significant difference between these clinical groups in verbal fluency.

It appears therefore that the only firm conclusion to be drawn from the literature at present is that divergent thinking varies as a function of personality typology in normal individuals. Several aspects of intellectual capacity and sex differences which may be relevant in this area have not been accounted for in the design of many

Divergent thinking

studies. The need for further research is therefore obvious. The work reported in this paper tests the hypothesis that divergent thinking, as measured by word fluency and word originality, is a function of personality variables of extraversion–introversion and neuroticism–stability when the influence of general verbal intelligence has been accounted for. Extraverts are predicted to be more fluent and original than introverts. Measures of the relationship of neuroticism–stability to divergent thinking are included in order to assess further possible interactions of personality types in modes of thinking.

METHOD

Description of the sample. A total of 100 male and 200 female students was tested at a large American university with a student population of 20,000. An approximate cross-sectional sample was obtained by setting age limits of 16–25 years (mean age = 19 yr.) and recruiting both voluntary students and others required to take experimental examinations as part of their introductory psychology courses. The students were tested by the same examiner in groups varying in size from six to 61. Testing atmosphere was similar to most other examinations familiar to the students in the university setting. The general purpose of the tests was described as experimental and in no way relevant to the students' university academic status. Twenty students volunteered to return for results and were retested for reliability estimates.

Description of the test measures. The assessment of general intellectual level was made by the Scholastic Aptitude Test – Verbal (SAT-V), which was administered approximately 4–6 months prior to admission by the university as a required entrance examination. The scores were available for 53 of the male and 134 of the female sample.

The experimental test session consisted of the following measures: (*a*) Eysenck Personality Inventory, Form A (EPI), a self-rated 57-item questionnaire designed to measure the independent dimensions of extraversion–introversion and neuroticism–stability; (*b*) Speed of Cognitive Output Test (SCO; Cattell, 1934), which requires the subject to list as many two-syllable words as he can think of, with the limitations that they not be objects in the room. Subjects were asked to circle the last word completed at a signal which was given at 30 sec. intervals. Verbal fluency scores were based upon the total number of words for a $2\frac{1}{2}$ min. period.

Word originality scores were obtained by assigning a score of one to each word used by a subject which did not appear in a reference sample of 100 subjects (33 male, 67 female) selected randomly from the full sample pool of 300 subjects.

Analysis of data. Dichotomous groups of introverts and extraverts were determined by dividing the total sample at the mean EPI score for extraversion–introversion. The same procedure was applied to form dichotomous neurotic and stable groupings. Mean verbal fluency and originality scores were computed for each independent sex and personality variable. In order to minimize loss of subjects in an attempt to maintain proportional cells for analysis of variance, three factorial designs were computed for each main effect and interaction of interest. An analysis of covariance employing the SAT-V as a single covariate was included in the design, although further loss of subjects whose SAT-V scores were not available was unavoidable. An additional covariance analysis was included which accounted for verbal fluency scores as a covariate when taking originality scores as the dependent variable.

RESULTS

There were no significant differences between males and females for either personality (EPI) or verbal intelligence (SAT-V) variables. The orthogonality of the E–I and N–S personality dimensions was upheld ($r = -0.17$, $n = 300$).

Word fluency. Table 1 presents means, S.D.s and numbers for the sample with SAT-V scores available for analysis. The results of the 2×2 analyses of variance for this sample contain two significant personality effects: extraverts are significantly more fluent than introverts ($F = 3.95$; d.f. = 1, 154; $P < 0.05$), and a significant

WILLIAM J. DI SCIPIO

interaction of extraversion–introversion and neuroticism–stability ($F = 8.94$; d.f. $= 1, 154$; $P < 0.003$). The interaction effect qualifies the main effect in that stable extraverts are significantly more fluent than stable introverts. The neurotic extravert is *less* fluent than the stable extravert and the neurotic introvert is *more* fluent than the stable introvert. Both neurotic groups approximate a mean fluency value lying between their stable counterparts. The covariance analyses, which covaried SAT-V scores, revealed that the above personality differences increased in level of significance ($F = 5.83$; d.f. $= 1, 153$; $P < 0.02$; and $F = 9.50$; d.f. $= 1, 153$; $P < 0.002$ respectively). Females were significantly more fluent than males ($F = 4.46$; d.f. $= 1, 280$; $P < 0.05$). Sex differences in fluency scores did not emerge as significant effects after covariance analysis.

Table 1. *Means and S.D.s of word fluency scores for personality dimensions summed over sexes*

	n	Mean	S.D.
Neurotic extraverts	45	25·49	7·65
Neurotic introverts	45	26·24	8·03
Stable extraverts	34	29·29	7·37
Stable introverts	34	22·59	7·94

Word originality. Word fluency and originality scores of the SCO correlated 0·67 ($n = 100$) for males and 0·61 ($n = 200$) for females. All analyses applied to the verbal fluency scores were repeated on originality scores. The single significant effect to emerge was that males were significantly more original than females ($F = 6.10$; d.f. $= 1, 280$; $P < 0.02$). This finding was upheld in covariance analyses when covarying both SAT-V scores and verbal-fluency scores ($F = 7.20$, d.f. $= 1, 181$, $P < 0.01$; $F = 12.32$, d.f. $= 1, 181$, $P < 0.001$).

Test–retest reliability coefficients were 0·92 for word fluency and 0·64 for word originality for 20 subjects tested at approximately one-week intervals.

DISCUSSION

The SCO test appears to be a better correlate of general verbal ability (SAT-V) for females ($r = 0.30$; $n = 134$) than for males ($r = 0.04$; $n = 53$) when scored for word fluency as well as for word originality ($r = 0.29$ and 0·03 respectively). After removing the influence of the fluency score from the originality score, there is less evidence of a sex difference for the relationship of originality to verbal intelligence ($r = 0.17$ and 0·08 respectively). The low positive correlation between word fluency and verbal intelligence for females is consistent with the findings first reported by Hargreaves (1927), but is now qualified by the sex difference in the present sample. The originality variable, however, shows very little relationship to intelligence for both sexes, which is in unqualified agreement with Hargreaves. A possible explanation of this finding may concern the operational criterion of word originality used in this study. Originality, as defined by unusual or rare two-syllable word production, does not involve attention to verbal meaning or verbal context and therefore does not tap vocabulary ability or general verbal reasoning. The word fluency measure,

Divergent thinking

however, is closely related to a general store of vocabulary and consequently this variable may be expected to correlate with the SAT-V test because of the shared variance both tests contain for vocabulary ability.

A further result which lends support to the independence of scores of fluency and originality within the same test is the significant sex differences found in opposite directions for each variable. Females are found to be more fluent than males. On the other hand, males are found to give more original responses than females. These sex differences are somewhat equivocal with respect to covariance analysis in that verbal IQ, the covariate, does not appear to be a linear function of word fluency for males, nor word originality for both sexes. The analysis of personality differences is therefore combined for both sexes because of the statistical advantage of increased sample size and the positive linear relationship between verbal IQ and word fluency for the full sample ($r = 0 \cdot 20$; $n = 300$).

The most salient finding to appear in this study is a qualification of the stated hypothesis when considering the interaction of the neuroticism–stability dimension. The hypothesis that divergent thinking as measured by word fluency and originality is higher for extraverts than introverts was upheld for word fluency but not originality. Neuroticism is found to decrease the fluency of extraverts and increase the fluency of introverts. Both neurotic groups of E and I approach the overall mean of the stable E and I groups. This finding explains why Rim (1953) was not able to find a significant word fluency difference between his two criterion groups of hysterics and dysthymics. Although both of Rim's clinical groups represent extremes in E and I, both are clinical conditions of high neuroticism.

A general *post hoc* formulation to account for the E–N interaction and based upon neurotic instability may be formulated in the following terms. Traits such as verbal fluency are manifested in extreme forms in opposite directions for introverts and extraverts, if both groups are stable or non-neurotic. Defining neuroticism or high anxiety as a disturbance in normal function, the mechanism which would normally maintain traits at upper and lower limits can no longer be assumed to function at these limits consistently. Consequently, the behaviour would regress toward the mean of the stable groups. In accordance with Eysenck's (1967) theory of arousal and personality, the mechanism which underlies the control of traits such as verbal fluency may be postulated as one of cortical inhibition versus excitation. In its most general form, this theory states that extraverts function with minimal levels of cortical inhibition of the central nervous sytem, while introverts function with maximal levels. The extravert would therefore respond behaviourally in a more impulsive and divergent manner than the introvert. Neuroticism introduces a weakening of higher cortical functioning and consequently would bring about an inability to maintain personality traits usually manifested by the E–I continuum in stable individuals. Predictions could no longer be made in relation to high and low verbal fluency, except that overall performance of neurotics at either end of the extraversion–introversion continuum would fall somewhere between the extremes of the stable groups.

The study suggests implications for clinical research in so far as divergent thinking tests may prove to be a useful diagnostic instrument in assessing the influence of neuroticism or high anxiety on spontaneous verbal output. Changes during the course of therapy might be monitored by assessing the rate at which the individual

WILLIAM J. DI SCIPIO

approaches a verbal fluency score appropriate to his sex, intellectual level and stable personality type.

I wish to thank Drs W. A. Winnick and G. A. Pierson, Queens College, New York, for administrative assistance, and Maria Di Scipio, R. N. and Dr M. M. Singh, Bronx State Hospital, New York, for reviewing the manuscript. The Ph.D. thesis was sponsored by Professor H. J. Eysenck, Institute of Psychiatry, London.

REFERENCES

BARRON, F. (1953). Complexity–simplicity as a personality dimension. *J. abnorm. soc. Psychol.* **48**, 163–172.

BOWERS, P. G. (1967). Effect of hypnosis and suggestions of reduced defensiveness on creativity test performance. *J. Personality* **35**, 311–322.

BURT, C. (1962). The psychology of creative ability. *Br. J. educ. Psychol.* **32**, 292–298.

BURT, C. (1967). Book review of *Contrary Imaginations* by Liam Hudson. *Br. J. Psychol.* **58**, 173–174.

CARROLL, J. B. (1941). A factor-analysis of verbal abilities. *Psychometrika* **6**, 279–308.

CATTELL, R. B. (1934). Temperament tests. II. Tests. *Br. J. Psychol.* **24**, 20–49.

EYSENCK, H. J. (1960). *The Structure of Human Personality.* London: Methuen.

EYSENCK, H. J. (1967). *The Biological Basis of Personality.* Springfield: Thomas.

GEWIRTZ, J. L. (1948). Studies in word-fluency. II. Its relation to eleven items of child behaviour. *J. genet. Psychol.* **72**, 177–184.

GETZELS, J. W. & JACKSON, P. W. (1962). *Creativity and Intelligence: Explorations with Gifted Students.* London: Wiley.

GUILFORD, J. P. (1950). Creativity. *Am. Psychol.* **5**, 444–454.

HARGREAVES, H. L. (1927). The faculty of imagination. *Br. J. Psychol. Monogr. Suppl.* **3**, 10.

HOFSTAETTER, P. R., O'CONNOR, J. P. & SUZIEDELIS, A. (1957). Sequences of restricted associative responses and their personality correlates. *J. gen. Psychol.* **57**, 219–227.

HUDSON, L. (1966). *Contrary Imaginations: a Psychological Study of the English Schoolboy.* London: Methuen.

NOTCUTT, B. (1943). Perseveration and fluency. *Br. J. Psychol.* **33**, 200–208.

RAMSAY, R. W. (1966). Speech patterns and personality. (Unpublished Ph.D. thesis, University of London.)

RIM, Y. (1953). Perseveration and fluency as measures of introversion–extraversion in abnormal subjects. (Unpublished Ph.D. thesis, University of London.)

RIM, Y. (1954). Perseveration and fluency as measures of introversion–extraversion in abnormal subjects. *J. Personality* **23**, 324–334.

ROGERS, C. A. (1953). The structure of verbal fluency. *Br. J. Psychol.* **44**, 368–380.

ROGERS, C. A. (1956). The orectic relations of verbal fluency. *Aust. J. Psychol.* **8**, 27–46.

SCHAEFER, C. E. & ANASTASI, A. (1968). A biographical inventory for identifying creativity in adolescent boys. *J. appl. Psychol.* **52**, 42–48.

SPEARMAN, C. (1927). *The Abilities of Man: their Nature and Measurement.* London: Macmillan.

STUDMAN, L. G. (1935). Studies in experimental psychiatry. V. 'W' and 'F' factors in relation to traits of personality. *J. ment. Sci.* **81**, 107–137.

TORRANCE, E. P. (1967). New types of items for measuring the creative thinking abilities. *International Workshop on Possibilities and Limitations of Educational Testing.* Berlin: Pädagogisches Zentrum.

WALLACH, M. A. & KOGAN, N. (1965). *Modes of Thinking in Young Children.* New York: Holt, Rinehart & Winston.

WHITE, K. (1968). Anxiety, extraversion–introversion, and divergent thinking ability. *J. creative Behav.* **2**, 119–127.

(*Manuscript received 23 June* 1970; *revised manuscript received 7 August* 1970)

From G. Leith (1972). British Journal of Educational Psychology, *42*, 240–247, *by kind permission of the author and Scottish Academic Press*

THE RELATIONSHIPS BETWEEN INTELLIGENCE, PERSONALITY AND CREATIVITY UNDER TWO CONDITIONS OF STRESS

By G. LEITH

(*Department of Research in Education, University of Utrecht*)

SUMMARY. The experiment set out to determine whether responses to creativity tests are influenced by the personality of the subjects and by the amount of stress imposed by different testing procedures. 106 children aged 9, 11 and 13 years were given an intelligence test and tests of extraversion and anxiety according to test manual directions and three verbal, creativity tests were given in a relaxed atmosphere to half of the children and in a moderately stressful manner to the remainder. The results indicate that the number and originality of responses is greater in the stressful condition and that there is a disordinal interaction of both extraversion and anxiety with stress.

INTRODUCTION

IN attempting to define and assess originality or creativity, investigators have claimed that conventional measures of ability fail to detect a wide area of cognitive capacity. This area is thought to be diagnostic of creative ability rather than conventional scholastic aptitude and to represent a sphere which has been overlooked by many educators and psychologists who give weight to intelligence as the major factor in school performance. The claim is that some children may be creative but relatively less able in intelligence tests, while some others have high IQs but score low on tests of creative ability as well as others who score high or low on both (Getzels and Jackson, 1962). The evidence for this position is, however, equivocal (Ripple and May, 1962 ; Butcher, 1968).

Wallach and Kogan (1965) surveyed the research on creativity and concluded that evidence for the existence of a unitary factor of creativity different from intelligence was not well founded. Their own study, however, did provide evidence of coherent clustering among creativity tests and of their independence from IQ. A feature of their design was the adoption of an individual, ' game ' approach to measurement. This was intended to overcome the mental-testing atmosphere of previous studies which had group administration, time limits, etc., and presumably invoked the same kinds of personal stress and set-to-respond as conventional tests.

In order to test the hypothesis that removal of a mental-testing atmosphere is an important aspect of measuring creativity, a group of 43 education students was given a number of tests, including the AH5 verbal scale, personality tests and a short set of verbal items similar to items from three of Wallach and Kogan's scales (Leith, 1971). The tests were simultaneously administered to a whole group but many steps were taken to bring about a relaxed atmosphere of responding. Thus, overt precautions to preserve anonymity, the manifest purpose of collecting data for group practical work, avoidance of anxiety-provoking cues and competitiveness, etc., contributed to an informal situation in which external threats were removed.

Findings from this small, pilot study were that : the three kinds of responses which were evoked (Associations, Uses, Similarities) were significantly inter-correlated (as high as 0·6) ; that verbal intelligence had no relationship with

G. Leith

these measures ; that extraversion (but not anxiety) was related to creativity scores. These results are consistent with Wallach and Kogan's and seem to endorse the need to avoid conventional group-test methods.

It would be unwise, however, to accept this conclusion without first making some attempt to find contrary evidence. Indeed, another hypothesis might be put forward that, since mild stress may facilitate ' arousal,' and since arousal is claimed to excite wider and more remote sets of associations, then the contrary view is tenable. This counter-hypothesis would assert that, if a test situation is mildly (but not severely) stressful, it will facilitate arousal, a state in which more remote associations than the conventional or stereotyped responses (which occur early in the repertoire) will be facilitated.

It is necessary, therefore, to manipulate experimental conditions to find when subjects respond under conditions of moderate stress and in stress-reduced situations :

(a) Whether relationships among creativity tests and between them and intelligence are different in the two situations ;

(b) Whether a difference in the number and originality of responses occurs.

The experiment was carried out with 106 boys and girls from three classes (3, 5 and 7) of a school in the area of Konstanz, in Germany. The children were aged 9, 11 and 13, respectively. Half of the children within each age group were randomly allocated to each treatment. One of these was similar to normal test administration, i.e., there were statements about testing the ability to carry out tasks, injunctions to " do your best," instructions to avoid delay, and so on. The other was conducted in a room having pleasant associations, e.g., the cookery room. In this case children were informed that they were helping in experimental work, that their individual scores would not earn or lose credit, that the purpose was to find how many different kinds of words children of their age knew in order to help educators to learn the words which were familiar to them. At the same time they were urged to do their best.

In the same session they completed a short personality questionnaire (Hallworth, 1962) followed by three kinds of open-ended response situations : Think of as many different things as you can like—; as many different ways in which you can use—; as many ways in which X is like Y. Three stimuli of each kind were presented. In the moderate stress (MS) condition a three-minute time limit was announced for each item and show of accurate timing was made. In the reduced stress (RS) conditions, the same three-minute span was unobtrusively applied. A week later, Raven's Standard Progressive Matrices was given, in the children's own classrooms, with standard instructions.

Three kinds of evidence were looked for in the responses :

(1) Evidence of relationships between six measures of creativity (each set of items being scored for number of responses and novelty) and between creativity and intelligence, and of differences in these correlations, between the treatments.

(2) Evidence that the MS and RS groups differ in number and novelty of responses.

(3) Evidence of interaction between personality characteristics (extraversion/ introversion and general anxiety) and treatments.

The first question relates to the possibility that certain relationships will emerge more strongly in one rather than the other experimental group. The second refers to the two hypotheses that a relaxed, game-like atmosphere

Effects of Stress Conditions

facilitates flexibility, fluency and novelty of responding or that mild stress induces arousal and hence the same properties of responding. The third anticipates that some kinds of individuals are more easily aroused or, alternatively, are 'freed' by the absence of external contraints, or even that what is facilitating for some may be inhibiting to others.

RESULTS

The six sets of scores were ranked within each treatment group and age level and Kendall's W (which assesses consistency of ranking in three or more ranks) was calculated (Siegel, 1956). The average rank order of the six measures was then correlated with the corresponding ranking of the children's intelligence test scores. Table 1 shows the relationships found.

TABLE 1

INTERCORRELATIONS BETWEEN SIX MEASURES OF CREATIVITY (ASSOCIATIONS, USES AND SIMILARITIES SCORED FOR FREQUENCY AND ORIGINALITY) AND INTELLIGENCE (RAVEN'S MATRICES).

Age Group	13 years		11 years		9 years	
Experimental Treatment	Moderate Stress	Reduced Stress	Moderate Stress	Reduced Stress	Moderate Stress	Reduced Stress
Creativity Tests	0·828*	0·471*	0·770*	0·614*	0·635*	0·491*
Intelligence and Creativity	0·303	–0·119	–0·326	0·327	0·172	·329

* $P < 001$.

Though the MS groups have slightly higher intercorrelations (W) than have RS groups, it must be emphasised that none of these differences is significant. On the other hand none of the correlations between creativity and intelligence is significant and, it should be noted, both negative and positive relationships are present. Since Raven's Standard Progressive Matrices test, though non-verbal, is highly saturated with 'g' and normally has substantial correlations with verbal tests, the zero level of correlation with the average ranks of creativity tests must be counted as an indication that the two measures are independent. In case the averaging of ranks of the six creativity measures had diminished or scattered links which might otherwise have been revealed, one of the measures was correlated with the average rank of all of them. The index of relationship found was as high as that of the original coefficient.

It can thus be affirmed that the three sets of stimulus materials elicited responses which are significantly intercorrelated in both the frequency and originality methods of scoring. At the same time, the creativity measures are not related to a measure of intelligence. A further point is that though there is a slightly higher relationship among creativity tests in all the MS groups than in the RS groups, the differences are quite small.

While the data presented above are sufficient to make the point that the evidence of clustering and of independence from intelligence obtains in both relaxed and stressed situations, a number of further points can be drawn out. In Table 2 the mean scores of all six measures are presented for each sub-group.

G. Leith

TABLE 2

MEAN CREATIVITY TEST SCORES (SD IN PARENTHESES) : CHILDREN RESPONDING UNDER TWO CONDITIONS OF STRESS.

Age Group	13		11		9	
Experimental Treatment	Moderate Stress	Reduced Stress	Moderate Stress	Reduced Stress	Moderate Stress	Reduced Stress
Associations :						
Frequency	42·9	36·4	33·8	30·9	26·9	18·1
	(12·9)	(6·1)	(8·5)	(5·9)	(7·6)	(3·5)
Originality...........	131·2	114·3	104·0	100·3	69·4	45·2
	(41·0)	(20·0)	(31·5)	(21·9)	(30·3)	(13·0)
Uses :						
Frequency	22·4	22·9	22·1	19·6	13·4	12·8
	(9·8)	(5·9)	(7·1)	(4·3)	(5·7)	(3·5)
Originality...........	72·4	64·3	60·1	55·2	36·2	31·4
	(29·9)	(23·8)	(26·3)	(16·8)	(25·0)	(14·1)
Similarities :						
Frequency	19·8	18·6	15·2	15·4	9·7	9·6
	(11·1)	(6·1)	(7·7)	(3·6)	(3·9)	(7·2)
Orginality	66·3	53·8	39·3	40·4	28·0	23·0
	(30·9)	(24·8)	(24·0)	(13·4)	(14·1)	(19·5)
N	11	12	15	15	25	28

Inspection of the data reveals two salient points. First, the overall averages of the MS groups are higher than those of the RS groups. Second, the variances of MS groups are greater (in many cases, significantly) than the corresponding RS groups' variances. The latter point explains why MS groups have slightly higher correlations than the RS groups. It also indicates the possibility of an interaction effect (which will be taken up later).

In spite of lack of homogeneity of variances, analyses (Walker and Lev, 1953) of all six measures were carried out by a method which adjusts for unequal numbers in cells, the test being robust and tolerant of departures from homogeneity of variance (Baker et al., 1966 ; Box, 1954). The probability levels may be doubled for a more conservative estimate of probability. In the case of the first two measures (Association—frequency and originality) the differences between treatments and between age groups were found to be significant. The remaining four showed significant age-level differences only. Tables 3 and 4 summarise the significant treatments analyses.

TABLE 3

ANALYSIS OF VARIANCE OF ASSOCIATIONS TEST SCORES (FREQUENCIES).

Source	df	ms	F	P
Treatments	1	55·21	16·38	·001
Ages	2	148·15	43·96	·001
Tr × A ..	2	4·42	1·31	
Error	100	3·37		
Total	105			

TABLE 4

ANALYSIS OF VARIANCE OF ASSOCIATIONS TEST SCORES (ORIGINALITY).

Source	df	ms	F	P
Treatments	1	334·50	7·51	·01
Ages	2	2239·86	50·32	·001
Tr × A ..	2	53·99	1·21	
Error	100	44·51		
Total	105			

It must be pointed out that, though non-significant, all the remaining treatments differences have the same direction as the above, viz., MS means, overall, are higher than RS means.

Effects of Stress Conditions

In order to gain further support for the interpretation in terms of arousal, it is necessary to show that those individuals who are particularly susceptible to arousal obtain higher scores than those who are less easily aroused. On theoretical grounds (Eysenck, 1970) introverts would be expected to be more readily roused than extraverts. Again, depending on the degree of stress, anxious individuals should more quickly show arousal—though a greater amount of stress may be expected to produce interference. To date, two analyses only have been made of scores on the Associations test, the number of responses measure. One of these analyses classified subjects, within sub-groups, into high and low (above and below the median scores) categories on the results of a test of general anxiety) H.B. Personality Inventory, in German translation). The other analysis made a similar grouping but according to level of extraversion/introversion from the same personality scale (Hallworth, 1962).

Mean scores for the two categorisations are given in Tables 5 and 6. The middle age group had a median extraversion score lower than that of the other two groups and it was dropped from the analysis.

TABLE 5

MEAN NUMBER OF RESPONSES OF ANXIOUS AND NON-ANXIOUS CHILDREN ON A TEST OF ASSOCIATIONS.

Age Group	Treatments			
	Moderate Stress		Reduced Stress	
	Anx.	Non-A.	Anx.	Non-A.
13	45·8	40·5	34·5	38·3
11	32·5	35·3	28·3	32·6
9	31·4	23·9	16·9	19·5

TABLE 6

MEAN NUMBER OF RESPONSES OF EXTRAVERTS AND INTROVERTS (CLASS 5 OMITTED) ON A TEST OF ASSOCIATIONS.

Age Group	Treatments			
	Moderate Stress		Reduced Stress	
	Extr.	Intr.	Extr.	Intr.
13	38·4	46·7	40·2	33·7
9	25·5	30·3	18·0	18·2

Tables 6 and 7 summarise the analyses of variance. In each test (of Association, frequency scores) the treatments difference is very highly significant as is the age levels difference. The effects of greatest interest, however, are the significant interactions of treatment conditions with anxiety and with extraversion/introversion.

TABLE 6

A/V ASSOCIATION (FREQUENCY) SCORES.

Source	df	ms	F	P
Treatments	1	126·75	19·56	·001
Anxiety....	1	·08	—	
Ages	2	282·23	43·55	·001
Tr × Anx.	1	46·75	7·22	·01
Tr × Age	2	8·60	1·32	
Anx. × Age	2	9·19	1·42	
Tr. × Anx. × Age	2	0·78		
Error	93	6·48		
Total	104*			

* One Subject 'lost.'

TABLE 7

A/V ASSOCIATION (FREQUENCY) SCORES.

Source	df	ms	F	P
Treatments	1	118·58	18·94	·001
Extraversion	1	5·78	—	
Ages	1	561·12	89·64	·001
Tr × E ...	1	47·04	7·51	·01
Tr × A ..	1	8·82	1·41	
E × A ...	1	1·28	—	
Tr × E × A..	1	13·01	2·08	
Error	67	6·26		
Total	74*			

* Class 5 omitted.

G. Leith

As was put forward in the 'arousal' hypothesis, anxious subjects in the MS treatment had higher scores than other sub-groups and the corresponding introvert sub-group was also highest in mean score. The interactions are shown graphically in Figures 1 and 2.

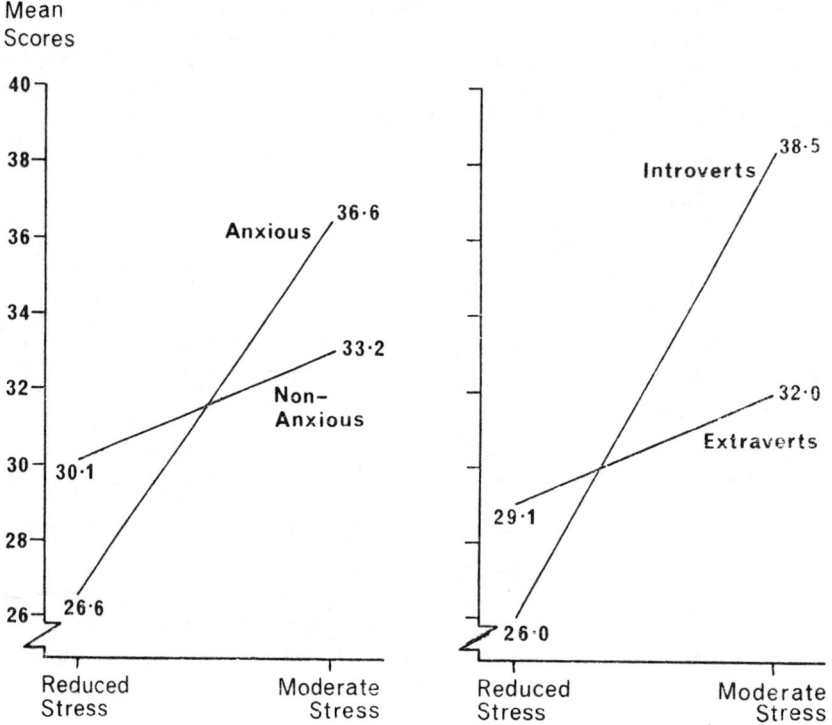

FIGURE 1

INTERACTION OF TREATMENTS AND
ANXIETY LEVELS.

FIGURE 2

INTERACTION OF TREATMENTS AND
AND EXTRAVERSION.

DISCUSSION AND CONCLUSIONS

The experiment was designed to obtain further evidence of the existence of a unitary trait which may be assessed by means of so-called 'creativity' tests and of its independence from general intelligence. At the same time, a particular hypothesis about the optimal conditions for assessing 'creativity' was tested. Wallach and Kogan's view, that their use of individual, untimed, gamelike situations, in which to obtain responses, is important, was first confirmed in a pilot study. In this preliminary investigation a modified procedure was adopted in which group testing was used in stress-reducing circumstances.

Effects of Stress Conditions

The present experiment took up the types of tests and procedures already validated and introduced an experimental contrast between stress-reduced and moderately stress-inducing test-procedures. The contrast was made in order to look for evidence disconfirming of the relaxation hypothesis and specifically to obtain evidence for an alternative view that moderate stress would facilitate arousal—thus inducing a wider range of available associations. On this view mild stress was considered likely to promote better performance on the part of introverts and anxious (i.e., above median) subjects. Also possible is the view that each situation might both help and hinder different kinds of individuals.

All of the hypotheses received confirmation. The creativity measures were significantly intercorrelated and were not significantly related to a measure of general intelligence. Slightly higher inter-relationships were found in the moderate stress condition but the differences were not marked. Stress tended to induce higher scores at all age levels than relaxed conditions, two of the differences being significant.

The hypotheses of interaction between treatments, introversion and anxiety have been verified in the two analyses so far carried out. Introverts and anxious subjects have been held to be more susceptible to arousal than extraverts and non-anxious. The findings, therefore, fit the account of arousal given by Hebb (1955). Since the interactions are disordinal (Lindquist, 1953 ; Lubin, 1961 ; though not according to the stricter rule suggested by Bracht, 1970), that is, in MS, while the introverts' mean is higher than the extraverts', in RS their ordinal position is reversed (extravert higher than introvert), the result is consistent with the pilot study's findings of a significant association between extraversion and creativity. In other words there may be some tendency for the responses of introverts to be *inhibited* in the relaxed condition (cf. Eysenck, 1970, pp. 439 ff).

The wider educational implications of these findings must necessarily be tentative and call for further information. If the conclusions set out above receive independent confirmation and elaboration, some hints about current policies and practices could be given. Thus, we could expect guidance about the need for differentiated teaching situations based on individual differences in cognitive style, personality and aptitudes other than general ability. Furthermore, we may be led to question some of the educational trends which foster views about optimal conditions for learning such as children should set their own pace of learning, giving directions is to be avoided, achievement stress must be eliminated, etc.—at least for some children.

REFERENCES

BAKER, B. O., HARDYCK, C. D., and PETRINOVICH L. F. (1966). Weak measurement *versus* strong statistics : an empirical critique of S. S. Stevens' proscriptions on statistics. *Educ. Psychol. Meas.* 26 291-309.

BRACHT, G. H. (1970). Experimental factors related to aptitude-treatment interactions. *Rev. educ. Res.* 40 627-645.

Box, G. E. P. (1954). Effects of inequality of variance and correlation between errors in the two-way classification. *Ann. math. Stat.* XXV 484-498.

BUTCHER, H. J. (1968). *Human Intelligence.* London : Methuen.

EYSENCK, H. T. (1970). *The Structure of Human Personality.* 3rd ed. London : Methuen.

GETZELS, J. W. and JACKSON P. W. (1962). *Creativity and Intelligence.* New York : John Wiley.

G. LEITH

HALLWORTH, H. J. (1962). *H.B. Personality Inventory.* School of Education, Birmingham University.

HEBB, D. O. (1955). Drives and the CNS (Conceptual Nervous System). *Psychol. Rev.,* 62, 243-254.

LEITH, G. O. M. (1971). A note on relationships between Intelligence, Creativity and Personality in a group of B.Ed. Students (unpubl.).

LINDQUIST, E. F. (1953). *Design and Analysis of Experiments in Psychology and Education.* New York : Houghton Mifflin.

LUBIN, A. (1961). The interpretation of significant interaction. *Educ. psychol. Meas.* 21, 807-817.

RIPPLE, R. E., and MAY, F. B. (1962). Caution in comparing creativity and IQ. *Psychol. Rep.,* 10, 229-230.

SIEGEL, S. (1956). *Nonparametric Statistics.* New York : McGraw Hill.

WALKER, H., and LEV, J. (1953). *Statistical Inference.* New York : Holt.

WALLACH, M. A., and KOGAN, M. (1965). *Modes of Thinking in Young Children.* New York : Holt, Rinehart and Winston.

(Manuscript received 23rd January, 1972)

From F. H. Farley (1966). British Journal of Social and Clinical Psychology, *5*, 306–309, *by kind permission of the author and Cambridge University Press*

Individual Differences in Solution Time in Error-Free Problem Solving

By F. H. FARLEY

Institute of Psychiatry, University of London

To investigate individual differences in the basic cognitive component of solution-time in errorless problem-solving, 30 subjects were given 21 Thurstone-type letter-series items to solve under stressed administration, and mean log speed scores of correct solutions were computed. Three groups of 10 subjects each were constructed on the basis of Maudsley Personality Inventory (MPI) extraversion scores, and their speed scores were compared. These groups were then reconstituted into three groups of 10 subjects each on the basis of MPI neuroticism (N) scores, and the speed scores of these groups were compared.

It was found that extraverts were significantly faster than introverts and ambiverts.

A curvilinear relationship between neuroticism and solution-time was suggested, with the mid N subjects performing significantly faster than the combined low N and high N subjects The low N and high N subjects did not differ significantly from each other.

The results could not be attributed to differences in age, verbal (vocabulary) intelligence, or sex.

The analysis of the separate determinants of performance in the solution of letter-series problems has isolated at least three basic components; speed of solution, accuracy and persistence (Furneaux, 1961). This analysis has been useful in elucidating the basic determinants of score in many intelligence and cognitive tests, as well as in the understanding of abnormal thought processes (Payne, 1961).

As it is no longer tenable to consider intelligence and cognition as independent of personality structure (Eysenck & White, 1964), then the basic determinants of speed, accuracy and persistence must also be considered in the light of individual personality differences.

The present paper reports an analysis of individual personality differences in the speed dimension of problem solving.

The essential requirements in the separate measurement of speed are that test items be easy, equal in difficulty, and only the speed of correct solutions be utilized in the score (Furneaux, 1952).

To meet these requirements, Furneaux (1955) has developed a test containing Thurstone-type letter-series items, with each item being timed separately, and only correct solutions being included in the speed-score. A relatively 'pure' error-free measure of speed is thus provided.

Eysenck's (1957, 1960) personality-behaviour theory has shown considerable heuristic and predictive value in the analysis of individual differences along dimensions of extraversion-introversion and neuroticism. Decrement in the time to achieve correct solutions over the course of a sixty problem, non-verbal intelligence test has been shown to be a function of extraversion with extraverts taking longer than

Individual Differences in Solution Time in Error-Free Problem Solving

introverts towards the end of the test (Eysenck, 1959*a*). Furneaux (1961) summarized an unpublished study on speed scores collected under conditions of change from non-stressed to stressed testing, yielding a stress-gain score, and reported that extraverted neurotics showed the greatest gain, and that introverted neurotics showed a decrement. Payne (1961) reviews evidence which suggests that neuroticism may bear a curvilinear relationship to speed over a number of speed tasks, and that extraverts tend to be faster than introverts. Eysenck & White (1964) and Lynn & Gordon (1961) have emphasized the likelihood of a curvilinear relationship between neuroticism and intelligence, and Lynn & Gordon have reported a study using a short version of the Raven's Matrices which supported this view.

Where speed is concerned, most measures employed have not been 'pure' error-free measures (Payne, 1961). The present study, therefore, utilizes the Nufferno speed test (Furneaux, 1955) which meets Furneaux's requirements outlined above. It consists of 21 letter-series problems. The first two problems and the last problem are not scored. The correct solution of each problem consists of identifying the recurring pattern in the sequence of letters, and writing down at the end of each item that letter which would appropriately continue the sequence. The test may be administered unstressed (covert timing, with no instructions to work rapidly), or stressed (overt timing, with instructions to work as rapidly as possible).

METHOD

Subjects

Thirty male and female domestic hospital staff, nurses, orderlies and university undergraduates served as subjects. The males (N = 16) did not differ significantly from the females (N = 14) in age.

Procedure

All subjects were administered the Nufferno test individually. In the same testing session they were also administered the Maudsley Personality Inventory (MPI) (Eysenck, 1959*b*), which yields scores on extraversion–introversion (E) and neuroticism (N). The experimenter did not know a subject's MPI scores at the time of administering the speed test. The stressed version of the Nufferno test was used.

The subjects were divided on the basis of their E scores into three groups of 10 subjects each. The low scoring group was labelled introvert, the middle group ambivert, and the high group extravert. There was no overlap in E scores between the extravert and ambivert groups, but two subjects having the same score had to be randomly assigned to the ambivert and introvert groups, one subject to each group.

The same subjects were then redivided on the basis of their N scores into three groups of 10 subjects each. These groups were labelled low N, mid N and high N. There was no overlap in N scores between the low N and mid N groups, but two subjects were randomly assigned between the mid N and high N groups.

As E and N are uncorrelated (Eysenck, 1959*b*) there was no reason to suspect that any differences in speed scores among the E groups could be due to differences in N, or that differences in speed scores among the N groups could be due to E. As a check, the N scores of the E groups were compared by analysis of variance, and the E scores of the N groups were likewise compared, but no significant differences were found.

RESULTS

The score for each subject was the mean log speed score of all problems correctly solved. The group means and standard deviations of the speed scores for the groups are: extraverts, $\bar{X} = 0.7824$, S.D. $= 0.1221$; ambiverts, $\bar{X} = 0.8752$, S.D. $= 0.1081$;

introverts, $\bar{X} = 0.9280$, s.d. $= 0.0173$. An analysis of variance was performed on these data which resulted in an F of 3.7062, $p < 0.05$ (2 and 27 d.f.). The analysis of variance was followed by Scheffé's test (Edwards, 1960) which demonstrated a significant difference between extraverts and ambiverts ($p < 0.05$), extraverts and introverts ($p < 0.001$), ambiverts + introverts versus extraverts ($p < 0.05$), but no significant differences in any of the remaining comparisons.

The group means and standard deviations of the speed scores for the N groups are: high N, $\bar{X} = 0.8740$, s.d. $= 0.0879$; mid N, $\bar{X} = 0.7792$, s.d. $= 0.1517$; low N, $\bar{X} = 0.9324$, s.d. $= 0.1096$. An analysis of variance was performed on these data resulting in an F of 4.1987, $p < 0.05$ (2 and 27 df). Scheffé's test following the analysis of variance showed the mid N to be significantly faster than the low N ($p < 0.05$), and also to be significantly faster ($p < 0.05$) than the low N and high N combined. None of the remaining comparisons were significant.

The number of problems correctly solved by the E groups were compared by analysis of variance, but no significant effect was found. This analysis was repeated on the N groups with the same result.

DISCUSSION

From the present data it would seem that when an error-free measure of solution time in problem solving is employed, extraverts are significantly faster than introverts. To check that the difference between the extraverts and introverts was not due to other factors, the age and verbal intelligence (Mill Hill Vocabulary Test, Raven, 1958) of the three E groups were compared by analysis of variance, but no significant effects were found. The mean log speed scores of the females (N = 14) were compared with those of the males (N = 16), but no significant difference was found ($t = 1.0936$). These results suggest that where the speed of arriving at correct solutions in human problem-solving is concerned, the personality of the problem-solver must be taken into consideration. Much of the 'error-variance' may be accounted for by at least the extraversion dimension.

The neuroticism dimension also bears a significant relationship to solution-time. The tendency towards a curvilinear relationship between neuroticism and speed is borne out by the significant superiority of the mid N over the combined low N and high N scores, and the lack of difference between the high and low N groups. These data clearly suggest a U-shaped relationship between neuroticism and stressed performance, as has been discussed by Jones (1961), Payne (1961) and others, but the restriction of sample size and the lack of a significant difference between the mid N and high N groups does not allow one to draw any more definite conclusion. As the present groups could not rightly be called extremes of neuroticism, it would be expected that the curvilinear relationship would become even more pronounced with larger, more extreme groups.

It is concluded that studies of the speed component of cognitive performance should take into account at least the personality dimensions of extraversion and neuroticism as sources of individual difference variance.

REFERENCES

EDWARDS, A. L. (1960). *Experimental Design in Psychological Research*, 2nd ed. New York: Holt, Rhinehart & Winston.

EYSENCK, H. J. (1957). *The Dynamics of Anxiety and Hysteria*. London: Routledge & Kegan Paul.

EYSENCK, H. J. (1959*a*). Personality and problem-solving. *Psychol. Rep.* **5**, 592.

EYSENCK, H. J. (1959*b*). *Manual of the Maudsley Personality Inventory*. London: University of London Press.

EYSENCK, H. J. (Ed.) (1960). *Experiments in Personality* (2 vols.). London: Routledge & Kegan Paul.

EYSENCK, H. J. & WHITE, P. O. (1964). Personality and the measurement of intelligence. *Brit. J. educ. Psychol.* **34**, 197–202.

FURNEAUX, W. D. (1952). Some speed, error and difficulty relationships within a problem-solving situation. *Nature*, **170**, 37–39.

FURNEAUX, W. D. (1955). The Nufferno Tests. *Bull. Nat. Found. educ. Res. England and Wales*, **6**, 32–36.

FURNEAUX, W. D. (1961). Intellectual abilities and problem-solving behaviour. In *Handbook of Abnormal Psychology* (ed. Eysenck, H. J.), pp. 167–192. New York: Basic Books.

JONES, H. G. (1961). Learning and abnormal behaviour. In *Handbook of Abnormal Psychology* (ed. Eysenck, H. J.), pp. 488–528. New York: Basic Books.

LYNN, R. & GORDON, I. E. (1961). The relation of neuroticism and extraversion to intelligence and educational attainment. *Brit. J. educ. Psychol.* **31**, 194–203.

PAYNE, R. W. (1961). Cognitive abnormalities. In *Handbook of Abnormal Psychology* (ed. Eysenck, H. J.), pp. 193–261. New York: Basic Books.

RAVEN, J. C. (1958). *The Mill Hill Vocabulary Scale*. London: H. K. Lewis.

Manuscript received 17 *September* 1965

From H. J. Eysenck and D. Cookson (1969). British Journal of Educational Psychology, *39*, 109–122, *by kind permission of the authors and Scottish Academic Press*

PERSONALITY IN PRIMARY SCHOOL CHILDREN:

1.—ABILITY AND ACHIEVEMENT.

BY H. J. EYSENCK

(*Institute of Psychiatry, London*)

AND D. COOKSON

(*Child Guidance Centre, Lichfield, Staffs.*)

SUMMARY. Scores of some 4,000 11-year-old boys and girls on the JEPI were analysed in relation to performance on scholastic and ability tests at the primary school leaving age. Analysis by correlation and analysis of variance methods revealed that extraverted boys and girls are scholastically superior to introverted ones, the regression being linear; that stable boys and girls did only marginally better than unstable ones, the regression being somewhat curvilinear; that interaction effects between N and E only occurred in conjunction with sex, unstable extraverted girls doing unexpectedly well, unstable extraverted boys unexpectedly poorly. Grammar school entrance proportions favoured extraverted and stable boys and girls, and disfavoured 'liars' on the L scale. Personality determined performance on ability/achievement tests more closely in the case of girls than of boys. The results suggest the importance of personality variables, particularly extraversion/introversion, in the attempt to predict scholastic success; it seems likely that introverts are 'late developers' as compared with extraverts, but in the absence of proper follow-up studies this conclusion remains speculative.

I.—INTRODUCTION.

THERE has been a resurgence of interest in recent years in the investigation of temperamental variables in relation to scholastic achievement. The discovery that intellectual ability is only one of the determinants of achievement is not of course all that recent, but the lack of suitable personality tests seemed to channel most research efforts into the cognitive field. The growth of dimensional theories of personality, together with the availability of inventories for the measurement of some at least of these dimensions, has changed the picture, and now we have quite a large series of studies comparing the intellectual status and the scholastic achievements of introverts and extraverts, or stable and unstable children and students. Cattell *et al.* (1966) have gone as far as to suggest that ability, temperament and motivation all contribute something like 25 per cent to the achievement variance, and such far-reaching claims are certainly worth investigating. However, such studies as have been reported have often seemed to give contradictory results; the same personality variable (e.g., extraversion) might correlate positively or negatively with achievement in different samples. Such contradictions lower one's faith in the validity of the findings, and require explanation.

One obvious hypothesis which would serve to integrate much of the evidence available is related to the concept of the 'late developer'; if introverts, say, develop more slowly than do extraverts, then superiority of achievement in extraverts during the first few years of schooling might turn into inferiority during later years. Evidence in favour of this hypothesis is in fact available, and comes out quite clearly even in such early pioneering studies as that of MacNitt (1930). This author studied 964 junior and high school pupils aged 13 and upwards, using a specially constructed introversion inventory; he analysed their average school marks in English, Mathematics Social Science, Physical Science and Foreign Languages and came to the following conclusion: " Those tending towards extraversion receive on the average higher marks than the introverts in Grades VII and VIII; slightly higher marks in Grades IX and X; and lower marks in Grades XI and XII. . . Those in the introverted group seem to increase their school marks on the average through the various grades, the extraverts' marks remaining on the average approximately the same . . . In general, there is a substantial relationship between introversion-extraversion and average school marks " (pp. 131-132). Taking Social Science as an example, we find correlations with introversion to be $-\cdot331$ in the youngest group, $-\cdot192$ in the middle group, and $+\cdot380$ in the oldest; for English the figures are $-\cdot379$, $-\cdot127$, and $+\cdot043$. Physical Science reaches a value of $+\cdot489$ for the oldest group, an interesting finding in virtue of Hudson's (1966) suggestion of a relationship between introverted personality traits and preference for science; in line with this possibility is the fact that achievement in foreign languages remains obstinately negative, with a value of $-\cdot494$ in the oldest group. Not too much should be made of these values, but they do suggest (1) a strong relationship, changing in time, between personality (specifically introversion-extraversion) and scholastic achievement, and (2) a differential direction of this relationship, with introversion predisposing pupils towards scientific achievement, and extraversion predisposing them towards linguistic achievement.

A similar inversion over time appears in the more recent work of S. B. G. Eysenck (1965), who correlated JEPI scores on extraversion with intelligence test scores; this correlation turned from positive at age 11 ($\cdot22$ for girls, $\cdot27$ for boys) to negative at age 14 for girls ($-\cdot25$) and at age 15 for boys ($-\cdot10$). Intelligence and achievement are of course two different concepts, but it should be remembered that intelligence tests in schools are often highly contaminated with knowledge, and are thus measures of Vernon's *v-ed* factor rather than of *g*. Other recent studies, mostly using either the Junior MPI or EPI, or else the Cattell scales, have also tended to find positive correlations between achievement and intelligence, on the one hand, and extraversion, on the other (Jones, 1960; Morrison *et al.*, 1965; Ridding, 1967; Rushton, 1966; Savage 1966); the children investigated were on the whole quite young. Thus, the evidence, while not unanimous, does seem to support the superiority of extraverted children in the primary school and at the beginning of the secondary school.

As regards the other main personality dimension studied in several researches, emotionality or neuroticism, the findings tend to suggest that among children high N scores are associated with poor performance (Butcher *et al.*, 1963; Callard and Goodfellow, 1962; Hallworth, 1961; Lunzer, 1960; Entwistle and Cunningham, 1968). These generalizations tend to break down when attention is turned to university students (Holmes, 1960; Furneaux, 1962; Lynn, 1959; Kelvin *et al.*, 1965); these tend to excel when high on introversion and on neuroticism. However, students are clearly a very unusual and highly selected sub-group, and should not necessarily be expected to show similar relations between personality and achievement to school children who tend to be quite unselected. Students must, by definition, have passed successfully through a long series of tests, weeding out those whose N component acted as a hindrance rather than as a motivational variable. In school children no such weeding-out process is likely to have taken place.

H. J. Eysenck and D. Cookson

In view of the considerable amount of agreement which has become apparent in the relation between personality and achievement, it may seem superfluous to carry out and report yet another study of a similar kind. There are several reasons for believing that such a study might produce useful results ; these reasons are related to certain weaknesses in design characteristic of several past studies. These may be briefly listed. (1) Boys and girls may show quite different regressions of achievement or ability on personality variables, yet very little attention has in fact been paid to this point. (The recent study of Entwistle and Cunningham, 1968, supports this argument, and emphasises the need for treating the sexes separately.) (2) Sampling has not always been very thorough ; usually just one or two schools have been used, although it is known that schools often differ profoundly from each other, and may give rise to quite different relationships in characteristics measured. (3) Statistical treatment has usually been very simple ; mostly product-moment correlation coefficients have been reported. The underlying assumption of linear regression may not be justified ; no tests for curvilinearity have been reported in most of the studies consulted. (4) The personality variables studied have usually been treated in isolation ; this is not justified unless it can be shown that no interaction is in fact taking place. Suppose that neurotic introverts and stable extraverts do particularly well on achievement tests ; simple tests against N or E separately will not disclose any significant correlations. There are too many examples of such interaction in the experimental literature (Eysenck, 1967) to allow us to dismiss this possibility as fanciful. Some form of zone analysis is clearly called for.

It is with these thoughts in mind that the experiment reported here was initiated ; the set-up and the analysis were dictated by the hope that more detailed study of such factors as sex or personality interaction might reveal interesting new facts additional to the expected positive correlation between achievement and extraversion, and the equally expected negative correlation between achievement and neuroticism. Our achievement variables contain, in addition to intelligence (verbal reasoning), the English and Mathematics papers of the 11+ examination and the success or failure of the pupil to gain access to a grammar school : this seemed of some interest in view of the prevailing lack of knowledge of the degree to which personality may influence selection. Reading ability is another achievement which is of obvious importance in connection with school work, and was consequently included.

II.—The study.

Subjects. All schools in Staffordshire with fourth-year junior children were asked to take part in the research. Of those that agreed to do so, 206 with about 6,000 fourth year children participated in all parts of the study and a further 55 with some 1,500 children participated to a more limited degree. In all about 77 per cent of all the 9,750 children in the age group were involved to some extent and all types of rural and urban areas within the county were well represented. At the time the research was done the children ranged in age from 10 years 9 months to 11 years 9 months, and all children in this age group from each school that took part were included.

General Procedure. The measuring techniques and instruments used in the research were investigated in a pilot study, but the carrying out of all parts of the main investigation, all scoring and all recording and dispatching of result was left entirely to the individual schools, each of which received a detailed manual of instructions and information.

Personality in Primary School Children—I

The data were collected during May, June and July, 1966, and the schools were allowed to administer the tests, etc., at any convenient times during this three months period, although certain stipulations were made regarding conditions of testing and the order in which various tests were to be carried out.

Main Measuring Techniques and Instruments.

The Junior Eysenck Personality Inventory. The most important measuring instrument for the purpose of the present analysis is the Junior Eysenck Personality Inventory (S. B. G. Eysenck, 1965), which was designed to measure the personality dimensions, neuroticism or emotionality and extraversion/introversion, and which also has a Lie Scale.

The children were asked to read the instructions on the test form, and additional oral explanations, mainly for the benefit of the duller children. were also given. They were not allowed to talk to each other about the questions, and no help was given with reading or in explaining the meanings of words or phrases. Teachers were asked to exclude those children who were unable to read the inventory.

The completed forms were checked to make sure no child had left out any item or had made some other error.

Abilities and Achievements. Already available were the results of two Moray House tests of verbal reasoning, one of Mathematics and one of English, taken six months earlier as part of the secondary selection procedure. For each test obtained marks are converted to ' quotients,' which are standard scores with a mean of 100 and a standard deviation of 15. It was also known whether or not a child had qualified for a grammar school place.

Reading level was measured by the Schonell Graded Word Reading Test (Schonell and Schonell, 1960) which is administered individually. Only the obtained score, which is the number of words correctly read, was used in the analysis, although it is usually converted to a Reading Age when the test is used by schools.

*Personality Ratings.** The four personality traits for which the teachers made ratings were: Emotional Stability, Perseverance, Sociability and Impulsiveness. For each trait there were five scale categories, ranging from 1 (highest) to 5 (lowest), and each category was accompanied by a description of children's behaviour or attributes considered most relevant to that level. The teachers were given the rough proportions of children expected in different categories, with a view to obtaining approximately normal distributions. Every child was rated on one trait before any child was rated on the next.

*Family Background.** Information on size of family and ordinal position in the family was obtained from the children. The classification of occupations used (Central Advisory Council for Education, 1954) is based on the Registrar-General's classification into social classes and has five categories, ranging from professional and magerial occuaptions (1) to unskilled occupations (5). Teachers were asked to find out from each child the occupation of his father or guardian.

Teachers rated the degree of interest in their child's progress shown by parents on a four-point scale from 1 (highest level of interest) to 4 (lowest). With each scale category was a description of parental attitudes considered appropriate at that level.

* These variables will be analysed and discussed in later papers.

H. J. Eysenck and D. Cookson

Summary of Main Variables.

Junior EPI	Extraversion (E)
	Neuroticism (N)
	Lie Scale (L)
Abilities and Achievements	Verbal Reasoning (Tests 70 and 71)
	Mathematics
	English
	Reading
	Grammar School pass/fail
Personality Ratings	Emotional Stability
	Perseverance
	Sociability
	Impulsiveness
Family Background	Size of family
	Ordinal position in family
	Occupational Classification
	Parental interest in child's progress.

Method of analysis.

On the basis of the distributions of N, E and L scores, a sample was selected for the purpose of an analysis of variance. As a first step all children with L scores over 8 were excluded. An attempt was then made to divide the two distributions (E and N) into thirds, in such a manner that a maximum number of cases should be included in each of the resulting 9 groups, for both sexes. The two sets of scores finally adopted were as follows: Low N, 0–11. Average N, 12–17. High N, 18–24. Low E, 0–15. Average E, 16–18. High E, 19–24. In this way we obtained, for the two sexes separately, 9 groups of children showing all possible combinations of low, average or high N, and low, average or high E. The number of cases in each of the 2×9 cells was 160, as a minimum, up to 182, as a maximum; the actual number used varied according to the availability of the achievement scores for the particular children involved. Thus the total number in a given analysis was never smaller than 2,880, and never larger than 3,276. In any particular analysis the number of children in each cell was of course kept constant. The reason for the marked variation in numbers was of course that if one child failed to complete his English test say, then 17 other children had to be dropped from the analysis in order to keep numbers in the cells equal. While these analyses of variance constitute the main part of our results, correlational analyses were also carried out on rather larger numbers in order to obtain data from non-selected groups; the analysis of variance group is of course highly selected, although preserving in its main features the characteristics of the total population.

III.—Results.

Verbal Reasoning. Two tests of verbal reasoning were given, VR 70 and VR 71; both were very similar and both are relatively orthodox measures of verbal intelligence. For the purpose of simplicity we shall refer to the scores on these tests as measures of intelligence, without wishing to beg any of the many questions raised by this term. An analysis of variance was carried out on the data from VR 70; these, it will be remembered, formed a $2 \times 3 \times 3$ design, with 2 sex groups, 3E groups and 3 N groups. The means for these various groups are given in Table 1. Sex, as expected, produces significant differences (girls higher) at better than the ·01 level of probability. E produces even more significant differences (p < ·001), with the more extraverted having higher scores ; this effect seems to be linear. N produces effects which are barely significant (p < ·05) ; the most stable having slightly higher scores than the other two groups. None of the interactions are significant ; thus the main effects can be evaluated without regard for possible cross-influences.

TABLE 1

SCORES ON VR 70.

	Male				Female			
	N —	A	N+	All	N —	A	N+	All
I	92·98	91·43	92·19	92·20	94·64	90·98	94·94	93·52
A	96·55	92·60	94·09	94·41	98·20	95·43	95·80	96·48
E	97·73	99·05	92·92	96·57	101·54	99·34	100·18	100·35
All	95·75	94·36	93·07	94·39	98·13	95·25	96·98	96·78

I=introverts. A=ambiverts, E=extraverts. N—=stable. A=average.
N+=emotionally unstable.

Results for VR 71 are shown in Table 2. Sex again plays a very significant part (p < ·001), as does E (p < ·001), but N is not significant. However, the N × E interaction is significant (p < ·05). as is the S × N × E interaction (p < ·01). The sex and E differences go in the same direction as before, i.e., girls and extraverts are superior. The significant interactions appear to originate with the emotional extravert groups ; for the girls, this group is the second highest (score 103·90), while for the boys this group is near the bottom (score 95·48). A similar difference actually appears in VR 70 also (100·18 as compared with 92·92), but is below the level of significance. This group occupies the position of psychopaths and prospective criminals in Eysenck's scheme (1964, 1967) and it seems possible that for boys (whose criminal propensities are well known to be much higher than those of girls) this combination of personality traits is more lethal, and interferes more with the massed practice involved in traditional intelligence tests (Eysenck, 1959), than in girls. However, before seeking too earnestly for an explanation of the finding it might perhaps be wise to replicate the findings itself ; the failure of the interactions to achieve significance in the VR 70 study suggests caution in accepting the results as necessarily genuine. Some support is given by the significant sex × E interaction found by Entwistle and Cunningham (1968) in their work with 13-year-old school children.

TABLE 2

SCORES ON VR 71.

	Male				Female			
	N —	A	N+	All	N —	A	N+	All
I	95·80	94·45	95·09	95·11	98·78	94·25	98·31	97·11
A	99·35	95·46	103·15	99·32	101·96	99·64	98·68	100·09
E	101·21	102·26	95·48	99·65	105·44	103·84	103·90	104·39
All	98·79	97·39	97·90	98·03	102·06	99·24	100·30	100·53

H. J. Eysenck and D. Cookson

Mathematics. The results of the mathematics examination fail to show any difference between the sexes ; the often documented superiority of males in dealing with figures apparently just makes good their inferiority in the verbal reasoning tests. (This explanation can be tested by looking at the English marks of the two sexes, where the girls should be very superior according to this hypothesis.) No differences are apparent, either, for N as a main effect, but E is again involved in producing marked differences in achievement (p < ·001) N×E×S and S×N×E interactions are both significant at the p < ·01 level. The detailed results are given in Table 3.

TABLE 3

Scores on Mathematics Test.

	Male				Female			
	N −	A	N+	All	N −	A	M+	All
I	91·08	90·79	91·70	91·19	92·93	87·88	92·76	91·22
A	96·28	91·81	100·11	96·06	95·81	94·46	93·59	94·62
E	98·52	99·32	92·96	96·93	99·85	98·36	97·60	98·60
All	95·29	93·98	94·92	94·73	96·20	93·60	94·65	94·81

The interaction effects are again mainly due to the extraverted, emotional children ; the girls in this group do well, the boys poorly, compared to their colleagues in the other groups. It may be surmised that this result is either due to lower intelligence in the male sub-group, or else to the reactive inhibition produced in the examination-taking situation when confronted with massed practice on relatively monotonous material.

English. The results for this test are given in Table 4 ; as far as sex is concerned they bear out our expectation that girls would be very superior to boys (p < ·001). The other results are identical with those found in the Mathematics paper ; N is significant, E highly significant (p < ·001), and the N×E and S×N×E interactions are significant at the ·01 level. Extraverts do better than ambiverts or introverts, and the interaction seems largely due to the emotional/extravert group, with the girls having good scores and the boys bad ones.

TABLE 4

Scores on English Test.

	Male				Female			
	N −	A	N+	All	N −	A	N+	All
I	90·85	90·63	92·23	91·23	95·71	92·48	96·67	94·95
A	95·71	91·76	100·89	96·12	98·44	97·78	95·87	97·36
E	97·53	99·21	92·49	96·41	103·42	101·28	100·62	101·77
All	94·70	93·87	95·20	94·59	99·19	97·18	97·72	98·03

Personality in Primary School Children—I

Reading. The reading test score again shows the familiar pattern, with girls superior (p < ·001) and extraverts superior (p < ·001) ; N shows a significant main effect (p < ·05) and a very significant interaction with E (p < ·001.) The detailed results are shown in Table 5. The N main effect would appear to be a curvilinear one, with N+ and N − groups having higher scores than A (average) groups. This effect is in fact universal in all our tests, although it is not usually significant ; inspection of the VR tests and the Mathematics and English will demonstrate this general tendency quite clearly. It would be idle to speculate at this point about the possible reasons for this curvilinear trend which in any case, while statistically significant over such a large number of children, is effectively very weak and of little practical importance.

TABLE 5

SCORES ON READING TEST.

	Male				Female			
	N −	A	N+	All	N −	A	N+	All
I	54·29	54·70	61·01	56·67	58·77	59 42	63·16	60·45
A	66·15	59·75	62·17	62·69	65·94	64·15	63·53	64·54
E	67·08	66·56	66·87	66·84	71·38	70·09	70·57	70·68
All	62·51	60·34	63·35	62·07	65·37	64·55	65·76	65·23

Grammar School Entrants : Proportions. Table 6 lists the proportions of grammar school entrants for the different personality configurations. Both E and N are highly significant (p < ·001), while sex and all interactions are non-significant. Extraversion is a favourable sign for grammar school selection (particularly among the girls, it would appear) and neuroticism/emotionality is an unfavourable sign (again the differences are somewhat larger among the girls than among the boys.) The differences are not only statistically significant, but they are clearly of practical importance ; the low E—high N girls send 9 per cent to the grammar school, the high E—low N girls 25 per cent. It would be idle to deny the importance in this connection of personality traits, even though some of the variance is presumably mediated through the connection between E and ability/achievement.

TABLE 6

PROPORTIONS OF GRAMMAR SCHOOL ENTRANTS IN DIFFERENT GROUPS.

	Male				Female			
	N −	A	N+	All	N −	A	N+	All
I	·1538	·1264	·1593	·1465	·2198	·0934	·0934	·1355
A	·1758	·1209	·1264	·1410	·2198	·1319	·1209	·1575
E	·2088	·1593	·1923	·1868	·2527	·2637	·2308	·2491
All	·1795	·1355	·1593	·1581	·2308	·1630	·1484	·1808

H. J. Eysenck and D. Cookson

Correlational analysis. Product-moment correlations were computed between variables discussed above, for altogether 2,162 girls and 1,869 boys. The correlations are given in Table 7 ; values for boys are set out below the leading diagonal of the matrix, values for girls above. The values in the two halves are reassuringly similar, showing that conclusions can with confidence be drawn from them, and that what is true of boys is equally true of girls. With numbers as large as these, correlations in excess of ·04 would be statistically significant, although of course not much psychological importance would be attributed to such very low coefficients.

TABLE 7

INTERCORRELATIONS OF SELECTED TESTS.

		1	2	3	4	5	6	7	8	9	10
1	Age		·06	—·03	—·04	·06	·05	—·05	—·03	—·05	—·01
2	E	·07		—·21	—·03	·22	·19	·18	·19	·19	·07
3	N	—·03	—·19		—·29	—·06	—·11	—·11	·11	—·10	—·09
4	L	—·06	—·03	—·28		—·17	—·15	—·15	—·13	—·15	—·08
5	Reading	·06	·23	—·06	—·16		·77	·74	·70	·76	·48
6	VR 70 ..	—·05	·19	—·11	—·15	·77		·94	·88	·85	·68
7	VR 71 .	—·05	·19	—·11	—·14	·74	·94		·90	·84	·69
8	Maths...	—·04	·20	—·11	—·12	·70	·87	·89		·78	·64
9	English	—·04	·19	—·10	—·15	·81	·90	·89	·82		·61
10	Grammar school .	—·01	·08	—·09	—·07	·48	·67	·68	·63	·65	

(Boys lower part, girls upper part of matrix.)

Age has been included in the table for the sake of interest, although of course the variance was very small. Nevertheless, there is a slight positive correlation with E and a slight negative one for N, both in line with the general age trend as set out in the Manual of the JEPI. Age also shows a very slight positive relationship with reading, but an even slighter negative one with intelligence and achievement tests ; these are replicated from one group to the other, and must therefore be considered significant statistically. However, the practical importance of these slight values is almost certainly nil, and we will disregard them.

Extraversion, as expected from the analyses of variance, shows positive correlations with the intelligence and achievement tests, ranging from ·23 to ·19 for the boys, and from ·22 to ·19 for the girls. Neuroticism gives smaller but still highly significant correlations with intelligence and achievement tests, ranging from —·06 to —·11 for the boys, and from —·06 to —·11 for the girls. The L scale, interestingly enough, also correlates very significantly with intelligence and achievement tests, values ranging from —·12 to —·16 for the boys, and from —·13 to —·17 for the girls. L does not correlate significantly with E, but does correlate significantly with N (—·28 and —·29 respectively for boys and girls) ; hence one variable could be used as a suppressor variable for the other. Even without doing this, it is clear that the contributions of N and L are additive.

The reading, verbal reasoning, Mathematics and English tests all correlate quite highly together and obviously form the nucleus of a ' scholastic aptitude ' factor ; all these tests show almost identical relationships with E, N and L. The correlation between VR 70 and VR 71 is of course artificially high because it is

Personality in Primary School Children—I

more of the nature of a reliability coefficient. Grammar school entrance is positively correlated with the scores on this scholastic aptitude factor, but the correlations are much lower than those between the tests ; they range from ·48 to ·69, thus leaving over half the variance to be attributed to non-scholastic factors. Personality features appear to play some part in this ; entrants are more likely to be extraverted (·08 and ·07 respectively, for boys and girls) and non-neurotic (−·09 for both sexes). In addition low scores on the L scale seem to be regarded with favour ; correlations of −·07 and −·08 are found. These correlations are not very high, suggesting that personality as measured contributes only something like 3 per cent to the selection process. This, however, is probably an underestimate ; when the figures are corrected for attenuation, as perhaps they ought to be for this purpose, the figure would become somewhat more respectable. Even then, of course, we cannot correct for chance factors in the selection process which probably assume quite a considerable importance, together with home influences and other causes not subject to measurement in this experiment. We would estimate that of the child-contributed variance to the entrance selection procedure, personality factors measured by the JEPI contribute something like 5 per cent to 10 per cent. Such estimates are of course difficult to justify without much more knowledge of all the factors active in the selection process, but they may serve as a base-line on which future research can improve.

Psychological significance. The statistical significance of many of the data reported should not blind us to the fact that with such large numbers of children even quite small differences appear significant, and that, even though these differences appear equally with boys and girls, and are hence replicable, yet their psychological and practical importance may be small. What is required is some yardstick to assess the general importance of observed differences, rather than a measure of statistical significance. A difference in IQ of one point may significantly discriminate between two very large groups, but would be dismissed as unimportant. Where does psychological importance begin, and how can it be indexed ? The most obvious index would seem to be some adaptation or other of the method of standard scores, i.e., an indication of the strength of the observed difference in terms of the total variance. In Table 8 we have set out, for boys and girls separately, the ratio of observed differences between extraverts and introverts on various tests to the standard deviation of these tests. It will be seen that for boys this ratio is never below one-third, and exceeds one-half in the case of the reading test ; for girls the ratio is in all cases but one in excess of one-half. Thus, if we consider the SD of IQ to be 15, the differences between extraverted and introverted boys would amount to something like 6 points, that between extraverted and introverted girls to something like 8 points. These differences are certainly not unimportant from the psychological point of view, and are larger than the sex differences usually reported, and considered of some interest.

TABLE 8

Ratio of Observed Differences to SDs of Tests for Extraverts *v.* Introverts.

	Boys	Girls
VR 70	·34	·52
VR 71	·33	·52
Mathematics	·40	·50
English	·38	·47
Reading	·55	·55

H. J. Eysenck and D. Cookson

It is clear that for girls the ratios given in Table 8 are larger than they are for boys. No explanation is offered for this phenomenon, which in any case may not be replicated in future research; until such replication is reported not too much importance should be attached to this difference. Entwistle and Cunningham (1968) have reported tentatively a similar suggestion.

IV.—DISCUSSION.

To what extent may our sample be regarded as representative? With respect to verbal intelligence and achievement in Mathematics and English our 1,869 boys and 2,162 girls are not far removed from the national average of 100; the figures are given below in Table 9. There is a slight inferiority, but it is too small to give much concern.

TABLE 9

MEAN SCORES ON VR 70, MATHS AND ENGLISH PAPERS.

	Boys	Girls
VR 70...............	98·25	98·35
Maths.	98·19	98·20
English	97·75	97·62
(N)	(1,869)	(2,162)

With respect to personality we would perhaps expect considerable agreement between the figures from this sample and the standardization data on extraversion; the actual figures bear this out. Boys score on the average 17·42, girls 17·42; this compares with standardization figures of 17·69 and 17·32 respectively. Variances too are almost identical. In so far as the standardisation sample may be regarded as a proper national sample, so far can we regard our present group as representative. With respect to L we would of course expect our present sample to have lower scores, because high scores were in fact excluded; the means for our group are 3·86 and 3·86 compared with standardization means of 4·79 and 5·49. Variances are slightly lower, but it is the drop in means which is important and relevant. Concurrent with this drop in L scores, and not unexpected because of the usual negative correlation between L and N, is a rise in N scores. For our group the means are 12·70 and 12·63; these figures should be compared with the standardization means of 11·10 and 11·83. Variances are slightly reduced, but the important and relevant figure is the difference in means. Our sample is obviously not representative, containing fewer 'liars' (high L scorers) and more 'neurotics' (high N scores). This slight failure to be representative is the price we have to pay for excluding potentially invalid inventories with high lie scores; it is impossible to be sure whether our choice was or was not a reasonable one. In any case the deviation from proper sampling norms is only a marginal one; it is unlikely that any of our main conclusions has been much affected by it.

These conclusions may be listed as follows:

(1) Extraverted boys and girls do better scholastically and on verbal reasoning tests than do introverted boys and girls; the relation is linear on the whole, and may be expressed by a product moment correlation coefficient of ·20 or thereabouts.

(2) Emotional boys and girls do only slightly less well than do stable ones, and the significance of N as a main effect is marginal. The relation is curvilinear, with high N and low N children doing better than those with average N.

(3) Interaction effects between E and N seem to be related to sex; emotional extraverts do well in the female group, but badly in the male group. This result is partly in line with the findings of Entwistle and Cunningham (1968).

(4) Sex differences are apparent in the English paper, but neither in VR nor in Mathematics; the superiority of the girls in English is equalled by their superiority in Reading.

(5) Grammar school entrance proportions favour extraverted and stable boys and girls; instability is actually a worse prognosticator for girls than for boys.

(6) E scores determine performance of girls more closely than performance of boys.

(7) 'Liars' on the L scale tend to be rejected from grammar school entrance; this would of course lower the observed relation between low N scores and acceptance, because of the known negative correlation between N and L. The figures might be more impressive had not very high 'liars' been excluded from the analysis.

These findings present us with some difficult and complex questions. To what extent can we find answers to the casual question implicit in much of what we have said—does intelligence 'cause' extraverted behaviour, or does extraversion 'cause' children to do well in school? We do not believe that our data enable us to answer this type of question, and indeed we are not certain that the question is a meaningful one as phrased. Further research of a more detailed and experimental kind is obviously called for. It is more easily possible to partial out intelligence scores from the personality-achievement correlations, but we have not done this because of doubts about the VR tests being even reasonably pure measures of Burt's " innate mental ability "; their very high correlations with the achievement tests suggest that scholastic achievement makes such a large contribution to VR scores as to make the task of partial correlation analysis of doubtful value. An exception to this general rule is presented by the grammar school entrance data; here clearly we must try and estimate the influence of personality variables when the influence of abliity/achievement is held constant, without however wishing to argue necessarily that the causal sequence goes along this direction. An analysis was undertaken, but will not be reported in detail; it revealed in essence that for most groups the admission rate was governed by ability/achievement, but that introverted boys (but not girls) were accepted more frequently than their VR scores would suggest, and that neurotic boys were selected more frequently, and neurotic girls less frequently, than would be expected on the basis of their VR scores. We do not find it easy to explain these findings. We will come back to these points in a later paper.

Our findings challenge comparison with the Entwistle and Cunningham (1968) paper, which is the only one of those quoted which based its findings on a really adequate number of cases. Working with a sample of 1,472 girls and 1,523 boys aged 13, these authors found a significant, negative, linear correlation between N and school achievement ($r = -\cdot16$); our own figure is slightly lower and there is a suggestion of curvilinearity in the analysis of variance. Possibly the differences are due to the differences in age of the two samples; possibly the curvilinearity is an artefact of the special selection process used to find equal-sized groups for our analysis of variance. In any case there is agreement on the detrimental effect of N school children, as far as school achievement is concerned. Entwistle and Cunningham failed to find a correlation between school achievement and E " because a distinct sex difference produces an overall non-linear relationship. Extraverted girls and introverted boys tend to be

H. J. Eysenck and D. Cookson

more successful in school work than children with the opposite personality characteristics." We did find a very significant relationship approximating the value of r= ·2 between E and school achievement for both sexes ; according to our hypothesis of the introvert ' late developer,' this difference between the two investigations would be explained by the age difference between the two samples. Had a 15-year-old sample been tested we would have predicted an actual inversion of our results, with introverts superior to extraverts. There may of course be a sex difference in the point of cross-over from E-superiority to I-superiority ; Entwistle and Cunningham's data suggest that this point may occur earlier for boys than for girls (but see S. B. G. Eysenck, 1965). Our data agree with Entwistle and Cunningham in suggesting that extraversion is a more positive influence towards school achievement in girls than in boys, although our data emphasise an E×N interaction which does not appear in their data in ours, of the emotional girls it is the extraverted one that does *best*, while of the emotional boys it is the extraverted one that does *worst*. There is no overall curvilinear regression of school achievement on E, for boys and girls together, or for each sex separately, as in their Fig. 2. This interaction effect (N×E) may also be a function of age, disappearing as the children get older.

It is clear that Entwistle and Cunningham are right when they say that we are dealing with " complex inter-relationships about which we still know all too little." The reason why the problem is a difficult one is clearly related to the differential influence of age and sex on personality and achievement ; this makes essential use of very large groups of children, and the coverage of different ages. The present study may serve as an introduction to the analysis of 11-year-old children, while the Entwistle and Cunningham one serves the same purpose for 13-year-old children. A study of 15-year-olds would give us an even better perspective, but of course all this would still only be cross-sectional ; what is most urgently needed is a good follow-up study, on large numbers of children, taking into account school achievement and intelligence, as well as personality and home background. The advantage we now have is simply that we can frame more clear-cut hypotheses than was possible a few years ago ; we are certainly still very far from having any firm answers to our questions.

Some hypotheses have already been suggested by Entwistle and Cunningham, and by us in a previous section ; here we wish merely to point out that the testing of such hypotheses demands a much more analytic approach than has been customary. Eysenck's attempt to make use of the Yerkes-Dodson law in relating achievement in school to N demands for its verification some measure of the *difficulty level* of the school work involved, as this is a crucial parameter of the law in question ; what is more, this difficulty level may differ from school to school, or even from class to class, and will almost certainly differ from pupil to pupil. Without measuring these aspects of difficulty level no proper assessment of the value of the theory is possible. Again, motivation is an important variable which is frequently neglected, although it plays a crucial role in the complex of hypotheses which we are considering (Eysenck, 1964) ; it might with advantage be measured along the lines suggested by Entwistle (1968). Possibly some of the observed differences between extraverts and introverts, and their relation to age, reflect differences in response to social motivation; this may be stronger in the primary school, to give way gradually to intrinsic scholastic motivation. This shift in turn may occur earlier in England than in the U.S.A., where schools are reputed to present a ' softer ' option than in England ; this may account for the later cross-over between achievement and extraversion in the work of MacNitt (1930) than in that of Eysenck (1965)

Personality in Primary School Children—I

Some attempt to measure this variable of ' formal work ' will have to be made if we wish to test adequately any of the theories which suggest themselves. Complexity in the data does not preclude scientific analysis, but it does demand corresponding complexity of analysis, theory and measurement.

ACKNOWLEDGEMENTS.—We are most grateful to the many primary school teachers in Staffordshire who supplied the bulk of the research data ; for such whole-hearted co-operation, often involving much effort and many hours of work, they deserve every praise. We are also grateful to the Staffordshire County Council Education Committee for permission to carry out the research and to numerous members of the Health and Education Departments for valuable advice and indispensable assistance. The Maudsley and Bethlem Research Fund gave support to the study.

V.—REFERENCES.

BUTCHER, H. J., AINSWORTH, M. E., and NESBITT, J. E. (1963). Personality factors and school achievement—a comparison of British and American children. *Brit. J. Educ. Psychol.*, 33, 276-286.

CALLARD, M. P., and GOODFELLOW, C. L. (1962). Three experiments using the Junior Maudsley Personality Inventory. Neuroticism and Extraversion in school boys as measured by JEPI, *Brit. J. Educ. Psychol.*, 32, 241-251.

CATTELL, R. B., SEALY, A. P., and SWENEY, A. P. (1966). What can personality and motivation source trait measurements add to the prediction of school achievement ? *Brit. J. Educ. Psychol.*, 36, 280-295.

CENTRAL ADVISORY COUNCIL FOR EDUCATION (1954). *Early Leaving : A Report of the Central Advisory Council for Education.* London : H.M.S.O.

ENTWISTLE, N. J. (1968). Academic motivation of school attainment. *Brit. J. Educ. Psychol.*, 38, 181-188.

ENTWISTLE, N. J., and CUNNINGHAM, S. (1968). Neuroticism and school attainment—a linear relationship ? *Brit. J. Educ. Psychol.*, 38, 123-132.

EYSENCK, H. J. (1959). Personality and problem solving. *Psychol. Rep.* 5, 592.

EYSENCK, H. J. (Ed.) (1964). *Experiments in Motivation.* Oxford : Pergamon Press.

EYSENCK, H. J. (1964). *Crime and Personality.* London : Routledge and Kegan Paul.

EYSENCK, H. J. (1967). *The Biological Basis of Personality.* Springfield : C. C. Thomas.

EYSENCK, S. B. G. (1965). *Manual of the Junior Eysenck Personality Inventory.* London : Univ. of London Press.

FURNEAUX, W. D. (1962). The psychologist and the university. *Universities Quart.*, 17, 33-47.

HALLWORTH, H. J. (1961). Anxiety in secondary school children. *Brit. J. Educ. Psychol.*, 31, 281-291.

HOLMES, F. J. (1960). Predicting academic success in a general college curriculum. *I.P.A.T. Information Bull.*, No. 4.

HUDSON, J. (1966). *Contrary Imaginations.* London : Methuen.

JONES, H. GWYNNE (1960). Relationship between personality and scholastic attainment. *Bull. Brit. Psychol., Soc.*, 40, 42.

KELVIN, R., LUCAS, C., and OJHA, A. (1965). The relationship between personality. mental health and academic performance in university students. *Brit. J. Soc. Clin. Psychol.*, 4, 244-253.

LUNZER, E. A. (1960). Aggressive and withdrawing children in the normal school. *Brit. J. Educ. Psychol.*, 30, 119-123.

LYNN, R. (1959). Two personality characteristics related to academic achievement. *Brit. J. Educ. Psychol.*, 29, 213-217.

MACNITT, R. D. (1930). *Introversion and Extraversion in the High School.* Boston : R. G. Badger, The Gorham Press.

MORRISON, A., MACINTYRE, D., and SUTHERLAND, J. (1965). Teachers' personality ratings of pupils in Scottish primary schools. *Brit. J. Educ. Psychol.*, 35, 306-319.

RIDDING, L. W. (1967). An investigation of the personality measures associated with over and under achievement in English and arithmetic. *Brit. J. Educ. Psychol.*, 37, 397-398.

RUSHTON, J. (1966). The relationship between personality characteristic and scholastic success in 11-year-old children. *Brit. J. Educ. Psychol.*, 36, 178-184.

SAVAGE, R. D. (1966). Personality factors and academic attainment in junior school children. *Brit. J. Educ. Psychol.*, 35, 91-92.

SCHONELL, F. T., and SCHONELL, F. E. (1960). *Diagnostic and Attainment Testing.* London : Oliver and Boyd.

(*Manuscript received 26th October, 1968*)

From G. M. Seddon (1975). British Journal of Psychology, *66*, 493–500, *by kind permission of the author and Cambridge University Press*

THE EFFECTS OF CHRONOLOGICAL
AGE ON THE RELATIONSHIP OF INTELLIGENCE AND
ACADEMIC ACHIEVEMENT WITH EXTRAVERSION
AND NEUROTICISM

BY G. M. SEDDON

University of East Anglia, Norwich

This study examines the possibility that the relationships of intelligence and academic achievement with both extraversion and neuroticism may vary with chronological age. A sample of 741 students in the 15–19 age group worked through a battery of four tests, two of which were tests of intelligence and two tests of achievement in chemistry. The nature of the relationships between performance on these tests and measures of extraversion, neuroticism and chronological age were then expressed as multiple regression equations. The results showed a consistently different pattern of significant relationships for both extraversion and neuroticism with the achievement tests on the one hand and with the intelligence tests on the other. Only the performance on the two achievement tests depended upon an interaction between extraversion and chronological age. There were no such interactions involving neuroticism and chronological age.

The possible existence of interactions involving chronological age in determining the relationships of both intelligence and academic achievement with extraversion and neuroticism has been indicated by a number of previous studies. For example, some results reported by Eysenck (1965) for students in the age range 11–16 suggest that the correlations of intelligence with both extraversion and neuroticism change from zero to negative over the age of 13. However, the correlations with the older students were obtained on such small numbers of students that no definitive conclusions can be drawn. There are also numerous studies in which different tests of academic achievement have been administered to different students over the age range 5–18 +, and which report the correlations of achievement with both extraversion and neuroticism as varying between −0·3 and +0·3 (Entwistle, 1972). In reviewing these experiments in some detail Entwistle concludes that the correlations may well vary systematically with age. In the case of extraversion he suggests that the relationships might change from positive to negative as age increases. Furthermore he feels that the change in sign could occur between the ages 12 and 15. Anthony (1973) has offered a tentative explanation of such an effect based upon the observed inverted-U type regression of extraversion on chronological age, in which the maximum of the curve appears to be somewhere in the age-range 12–15. For relationships with neuroticism the existence of any trend is less easily discerned than it is in the case of extraversion. However, Entwistle suggests that correlations might increase as chronological age increases.

Interesting though these changing relationships are, most of the experiments are insufficient in themselves to establish definitively the interactions involving age. In particular, there appear to be no studies in which the same achievement tests were administered to students of different ages. As a result the effects of changing chronological age are superimposed on the effects of changing the nature of the tests used as dependent variables. It is obvious, therefore, that no unequivocal conclusions can

G. M. SEDDON

be drawn from such a set of experiments. Moreover, there may be no need to invoke an interaction with chronological age, because it can be shown that the observed changes in the correlation coefficients may well be due entirely to very small concomitant changes in the nature of the test.

Thus if two tests, X and Y measure different aspects of academic achievement, the extent to which the two tests are different, may be reflected in the extent to which the correlation coefficient, r_{XY}, differs from unity. If P now represents one of the two personality tests, the correlation coefficients, r_{XP} and r_{YP}, may differ from each other considerably when r_{XY} differs from unity. Moreover, there is a mathematical relationship which describes by how much r_{YP} may differ from r_{XP} for particular values of r_{XY} and r_{XP} (Stanley & Wang, 1969; Glass & Collins, 1970). The limits of r_{YP} are:

$$r_{XP} \cdot r_{XY} \pm \sqrt{[(1 - r^2_{XP})(1 - r^2_{XY})]}. \tag{1}$$

Equation (1) may then be used to calculate the limits of r_{YP} for any combination of r_{XP} and r_{XY}. Now, as mentioned previously, the correlation coefficients between different tests of academic achievement and each of these personality variables usually range between -0.3 and $+0.3$. Also the correlation coefficients, r_{XY}, between different achievement tests tend to be positive and cover the whole range from 0.1 to say, 0.9. Hence, by substituting these values in equation (1), it is easily demonstrated that for each one of the various combinations of values for r_{XP} and r_{XY}, r_{YP} can range from being positive to being negative. Furthermore when r_{XY} is as high as 0.8, r_{YP} can be expected to be anywhere in the range -0.3 to $+0.3$. Thus as a result of making quite small differences between tests X and Y, r_{XP} and r_{YP} may be made to differ in a manner which corresponds exactly to the manner in which the correlations of academic achievement with these personality variables are found to vary over all the previous experiments. Therefore, it is reasonable to conclude that the observed changes in these latter relationships could well be due solely to changes in the nature of the tests of academic achievement.

However, this argument is not being presented in an attempt to deny the existence of interactions with chronological age. It is presented merely to emphasize that evidence from previous experiments in which students of different ages have worked through different tests, cannot be interpreted unequivocally in terms of interactions involving chronological age. A more clear-cut demonstration of an interaction involving chronological age has been reported by Leith & Davis (1972) in a study concerned with investigating the relationship between neuroticism and the amount learned from a self-instructional programme by 12 and 13 year olds. Leith & Davis observed a main effect corresponding to a significant inverted-U relationship, which was modified, on increasing the chronological age of the students, by the maximum of the curve moving towards higher levels of neuroticism.

In conclusion, there is as yet very little evidence which demonstrates unequivocally that the nature of the relationships of intelligence and academic achievement, with both extraversion and neuroticism varies with chronological age. The present experiment was therefore intended to produce results which allow more definitive conclusions to be drawn.

Effects of chronological age

Table 1. *Distribution of the subjects among the different age groups and types of academic institution*

Age group (years)	Schools	Colleges of education	Universities
15	97	0	0
16	247	0	0
17	178	0	12
18	11	0	141
19+	0	21	34
All groups	533	21	187

METHOD

The basic plan was to administer a variety of tests of intelligence and academic achievement to a group of students covering a range of ages and to investigate the nature of the relationships between performance on these tests with measures of extraversion, neuroticism, and chronological age. The relationships which were of particular interest were whether the regression of intelligence or academic achievement on each of extraversion and neuroticism is rectilinear or curvilinear, and whether there are significant interactions for each of these personality traits with chronological age.

Subjects

It is of course impracticable to attempt to administer the same tests of intelligence or academic achievement over the whole age range, 5–18 plus. It was therefore decided to concentrate on the 15–18 plus age range, where it is less difficult to devise tests which are suitable for use with all the students involved. In fact, all the subjects were students of chemistry in either secondary or tertiary institutions. The 25 secondary schools involved included comprehensive, grammar and public schools, drawn mainly from the Midlands. Each school was preparing the student for either 'O' or 'A' level chemistry examinations. From the higher education sector two colleges of education and three universities allowed all the first-year chemistry students who were potential candidates for honours degrees to participate. The number and distribution of the students among the different age groups and different types of institution are summarized in Table 1.

Tests

It was decided to use four tests as dependent variables. Two of them were to be tests of intelligence, whereas the other two were to be tests of achievement in chemistry. The intelligence tests were further subdivided into verbal and non-verbal intelligence, and the two achievement tests were also to cover different subject matter areas. In one case the test was to cover a very general area of subject matter and in the other a very specific area.

In choosing or constructing such intelligence and achievement tests, it is important, for the purpose of the present experiment, that they should be able to discriminate between students within each age group and between students over the whole age range. An ideal intelligence test here is AH5 (Heim, 1956) because each of the two parts (i.e. verbal and non-verbal) is specifically designed to discriminate well among students such as those in the sample. In the case of the achievement tests the students in the present sample could be considered to be at four distinct stages or standards of chemical achievement, i.e. fifth form, first-year sixth form, second-year sixth form and first year university or college of education. It follows that so far as content is concerned, the tests must sample a wide variety of topics including some which would normally be considered suitable for inclusion in examinations set at any of these levels. In the case of the test of general background knowledge one test was found to be suitable. It was 'High School Chemistry' 1965 (Part II) published by the American Chemical Society – National Science Teachers Association Cooperative Examinations Committee. As required, the items corresponding to each age group covered a wide range of subject matter. The test of specific background knowledge in chemistry was constructed specially for the experiment and was concerned with

G. M. Seddon

Table 2. *Means and standard deviations of the various tests for the different age groups*

Group		Age (years)	Verbal intelligence	Non-verbal intelligence	General background knowledge	Specific background knowledge	Extra-version	Neuroticism
15-year-olds	Mean	15·4	15·5	20·1	14·7	14·8	15·5	11·4
($n = 97$)	s.d.	0·25	3·9	5·0	6·5	9·1	3·8	4·0
16-year-olds	Mean	16·4	17·2	21·0	18·5	20·5	14·3	11·3
($n = 247$)	s.d.	0·29	4·1	4·6	6·1	9·9	4·0	4·0
17-year-olds	Mean	17·4	17·5	20·8	21·1	20·6	14·7	11·5
($n = 190$)	s.d.	0·27	3·8	4·8	6·7	10·5	3·8	4·4
18-year-olds	Mean	18·9	18·1	21·8	26·4	23·6	14·0	11·9
($n = 207$)	s.d.	1·5	4·1	4·3	6·0	10·9	4·1	4·3
All age groups	Mean	17·2	17·3	21·0	20·8	20·7	14·3	11·6
$n = 741$	s.d.	1·4	4·1	4·7	7·4	10·6	4·0	4·2

a very restricted set of objectives. Very briefly, these objectives required the student firstly to identify graphs showing the correct trends in the magnitudes of various physical properties of binary compounds in certain parts of the Periodic Table of the Elements, and secondly to identify diagrams showing the three-dimensional structures which could be adopted by these substances in the solid state.

The Eysenck Personality Inventory (Eysenck & Eysenck, 1964) was chosen to measure both extraversion and neuroticism, even though, strictly speaking, it has been validated only with subjects comparable to the older students in the present sample. However, an investigation into the suitability of these two scales for 15 and 16-year-olds (Seddon, 1969) indicated that they are still quite acceptable for the present purpose.

Procedure

In each institution the intelligence and personality tests were administered in the same week, EPI always being done first, and the students took the two achievement tests some time later (i.e. 6–10 weeks). All of the testing in the various institutions was carried out in the same six-month period at the end of the calendar year.

Results

Table 2 gives the means and standard deviations obtained by the various age groupings on each of the six tests.

A suitable method of analysis is multiple regression analysis, based upon an equation which relates scores, X_A, on each criterion task to the measures of extraversion, X_E, neuroticism, X_N, and chronological age, X_{CA}, in such a way that the nature of the terms included in this equation should be able to simulate the various curvilinear and interaction effects under investigation. The existence of each effect can then be investigated by testing the significance of the corresponding terms. In the event of the various curvilinear effects not appearing to be significant, it is obviously important to know whether the relationship is in fact rectilinear or just not significant at all. It was therefore decided to include terms corresponding to rectilinear effects as well as terms corresponding to curvilinear effects.

The actual form of the terms corresponding to rectilinear effects is standard and requires no further description. The terms corresponding to curvilinear effects must allow the complete curves to reach either a maximum – in accordance with the Yerkes–Dodson law, for example – or a minimum. The most convenient terms for this

Effects of chronological age

Table 3. *Results of the stepwise multiple regression analyses*

Variable	β-weights (× 10²)						
	(1) Verbal intelligence						
CA*	11	11	11	11	11	−09	−17
E	—	−04	−05	−24	−24	−34	−36
N	—	—	−07	−07	−11	−11	−17
E²	—	—	—	20	20	24	23
N²	—	—	—	—	04	04	04
CA × E	—	—	—	—	—	13	19
CA × N	—	—	—	—	—	—	15
R (× 10²)	11	12	14	14	14	15	16
P	—	—	—	—	—	—	—
	(2) Non verbal intelligence						
CA*	06	05	05	05	05	−08	−01
E	—	−05	−05	−14	−15	−26	−25
N	—	—	−04	−03	−20	−20	−18
E²	—	—	—	09	10	14	14
N²	—	—	—	—	17	17	18
CA × E	—	—	—	—	—	15	13
CA × N	—	—	—	—	—	—	−06
R (× 10²)	06	07	08	08	09	11	11
P	—	—	—	—	—	—	—
	(3) General background knowledge						
CA*	40	39	39	40	40	04	13
E	—	−17	−18	−11	−11	−42	−41
N	—	—	−11	−11	−11	−13	−10
E²	—	—	—	−07	−07	04	05
N²	—	—	—	—	00	02	02
CA × E	—	—	—	—	—	42	39
CA × N	—	—	—	—	—	—	−07
R (× 10²)	40	43	45	45	45	47	47
P	1 %	1 %	1 %	—	—	1 %	—
	(4) Specific background knowledge						
CA*	16	15	15	16	16	−13	−29
E	—	−13	−14	05	06	−19	−21
N	—	—	−11	−11	09	08	02
E²	—	—	—	−20	−21	−12	−13
N²	—	—	—	—	−20	−20	−20
CA × E	—	—	—	—	—	34	40
CA × N	—	—	—	—	—	—	14
R (× 10²)	16	20	23	23	24	27	27
P	—	1 %	1 %	—	—	1 %	—

* Ages are measured to the nearest quarter of a year

purpose are second order in the appropriate independent variables, e.g. X^2_E and X^2_N, with the sign and magnitude of the β-weights or partial regression weights indicating the direction and extent of curvature respectively. Finally the interactions are investigated by means of terms involving cross-products of raw-scores, e.g. $X_{CA}.X_E$ and $X_{CA}.X_N$. Hence the final multiple regression equation corresponds to equation (2):

$$\hat{X}_A = b_1.X_{CA} + b_2.X_E + b_3.X_N + b_4.X^2_E + b_5.X^2_N + b_6.X_{CA}.X_E + b_7.X_{CA}.X_N + \text{const.} \tag{2}$$

G. M. Seddon

Table 4. *Summary of the variables which turned out to be*
significant at the 1 per cent level

Terms concerned with	Dependent variables			
	Verbal intelligence	Non-verbal intelligence	General background knowledge	Specific background knowledge
Extraversion	—	—	$E\,(-)$ $CA \times E\,(+)$	$E\,(-)$ $CA \times E\,(+)$
Neuroticism	—	—	$N\,(-)$	$N\,(-)$

The results of the multiple regression analysis for each of the four criterion variables are shown in Table 3, which for each dependent variable presents a whole series of multiple regression equations gradually building up to the final equation by the addition of a new term on moving from one equation to the next. In this matrix format the β-weights and values of multiple-R for any one equation in this stepwise procedure are presented in one column, and the independent variables themselves are given, in the order in which they were introduced, down the left-hand column of the matrix. The significance of each term is assessed by testing whether or not the predictability is significantly improved after adding that particular term (McNemar, 1969, p. 321). In cases where terms are significant at the 0·01 level, this fact is indicated at the foot of the appropriate column in Table 3.

A brief overall summary of the results is given in Table 4, where for each dependent variable the terms found to be significant in the multiple regression analysis are listed together with a plus or minus sign according to whether the sign of the respective β-weight is positive or negative.

DISCUSSION

Table 2 shows that for each of the tests used as dependent variables, all four age groups have substantial and comparable standard deviations. The mean scores for each age group also increase fairly steadily over the whole age range. The four dependent variables are therefore regarded as giving adequate discrimination of the students within and over the different age groups.

Table 4 shows that there were no significant interactions involving chronological age and either extraversion or neuroticism in determining the relationships with either of the two intelligence tests. However, in the case of the two achievement tests there are significant interactions which operate so as to increase the partial relationship between achievement and extraversion as chronological age increases. In contrast to the experiment of Leith & Davis (1972), the present experiment does not reveal the existence of an interaction between neuroticism and chronological age. However, neither does it reveal the existence of a curvilinear relationship between performance and neuroticism, and it is possible that both these differences between the present results and those of Leith & Davis are due to other effects— e.g. the different age range of the students.

In considering the changing pattern of significant terms for the various tests it will be noted that the two achievement tests have identical sets of significant terms in the

Effects of chronological age

multiple regression equations, and that the two intelligence tests have no significant terms in theirs. It will be noted also that the terms which are significant for the achievement tests involve both extraversion and neuroticism. The results are therefore in agreement with the hypothesis that the relationships of the dependent variables with both extraversion and neuroticism change with the nature of the dependent variable. However, it is evident that neither the differences between the two types of intelligence test nor the differences between the two types of achievement test were sufficiently great to give rise to significantly different relationships for the two types of intelligence test on the one hand or the two types of achievement test on the other.

In conclusion it is important to emphasise that all the findings of this study refer only to students within the age range 15–18 + and within very restricted levels of ability. It is therefore quite possible that for both intelligence and academic achievement, different results will be obtained for students belonging to different age and ability ranges. It is also necessary to recognize that, as students progress through these different levels of the educational system, they are required to survive a sequence of selection procedures which considerably reduce the number of students transferring from the pre-'O'-level classes to the sixth forms at the age of 16 or so, and from the sixth forms to the universities and colleges of education at the age of 17/18. As a result, in the present study the changes in the age groups are confounded with concomitant changes in other traits and abilities which may be important in determining a student's performance on tests of achievement or intelligence. It must be acknowledged, therefore, that the results do not necessarily refer directly to the intrinsic effects of chronological age. The results describe effects which may be only incidentally related to chronological age, and which may be observed only in groups of students taken from sectors of the educational system where there is a similar succession of selection procedures as age increases.

Nevertheless, bearing these limitations in mind, the study has demonstrated that for students, as they are presently found at each age level within these particular sectors of the British educational system, there is one subject-matter area where the relationship between academic achievement and extraversion changes as chronological age increases. However, there appear to be no such changes in the relationship between achievement in the same subject matter area and neuroticism or in the relationship between intelligence and either extraversion or neuroticism.

REFERENCES

ANTHONY, W. S. (1973). The development of extraversion, of ability and of the relation between them. *Br. J. educ. Psychol.* **43**, 223–227.

ENTWISTLE, N. J. (1972). Personality and academic attainment. *Br. J. educ. Psychol.* **42**, 137–151.

EYSENCK, H. J. & EYSENCK, S. B. G. (1964). *Manual of the Eysenck Personality Inventory*. London: University of London Press.

EYSENCK, S. B. G. (1965). *Manual of the Junior Eysenck Personality Inventory*. London: University of London Press.

GLASS, G. V. & COLLINS, J. R. (1970). Geometric proof of the restriction on the possible values of r_{XY} when r_{XZ} and r_{YZ} are fixed. *Educ. psychol. Measur.* **30**, 37–39.

HEIM, A. W. (1956). *AH5 Group Test of High-Grade Intelligence*. Slough: National Foundation For Educational Research.

G. M. SEDDON

LEITH, G. O. M. & DAVIS, T. N. (1972). Age changes in the relationship between neuroticism and achievement. *Res. Educ.* **8**, 61–70.

McNEMAR, Q. (1969). *Psychological Statistics*, 4th ed. New York: Wiley.

SEDDON, G. M. (1969). Some information on the use of the Eysenck Personality Inventory in the 15–19 age range. (Unpublished report, University of East Anglia.)

STANLEY, J. C. & WANG, M. D. (1969). Restrictions of the possible values of r_{12} given r_{13} and r_{23} *Educ. psychol. Measur.* **29**, 579–581.

(Manuscript received 28 June 1974; revised manuscript received 8 January 1975)

From W. Revelle, P. Amaral and S. Turriff (1976). Science, *192*, 149–150, *by kind permission of the authors and the American Association for the Advancement of Science*

Introversion/Extroversion, Time Stress, and Caffeine: Effect on Verbal Performance

Abstract. Time pressure and caffeine differentially affected the performance of introverts on verbal ability tests similar to the Graduate Record Examination. With time pressure and 200 milligrams of caffeine, the performance of introverts fell by 0.63 standard deviation, but extroverts by 0.44 standard deviation.

A classic, although widely challenged, finding in human and animal performance is that efficiency of performance is a curvilinear function of the stress induced by the task. Both high and low levels of stress are thought to be associated with inefficient performance, and moderate levels lead to optimum performance (*1*). Many anecdotal examples can be found of performance decrements under high stress, usually that associated with military combat or natural disasters (*2*), but it is difficult to find clear examples of decrements in performance for normal levels of stress (*3, 4*). Such decrements are usually open to the criticism that they occurred as a result of increases in distracting stimuli or because of contradictory task demands (*5*). The stress induced by taking an examination is usually assumed to be too little to lead to inefficient performance although performance on tests has occasionally been claimed to demonstrate curvilinear effects (*3, 6*). If performance on tests is curvilinearly related to stress, and if some individuals are more susceptible to this stress than others, then changes in the testing situation that lead to slight increases in stress should be beneficial for some individuals and harmful to others. In correlational terms, susceptibility to stress should be positively related to performance for low levels of stress, unrelated at moderate levels, and negatively related at high levels. We have found this to be the case.

We predicted that introverted individuals should be more susceptible to performance decrements under moderate levels of stress than should extroverted individuals. We expected that, with moderate increases in stress, introverts would decline in efficiency (and hence in performance) and extroverts would improve. That is, we expected the correlation between the introversion-extroversion dimension and performance to increase as stress was increased. This prediction derived from a theory of the behavioral and physiological differences between introverts and extroverts (*7*). In brief, this theory states that when variations in the environmental level of stimulation are controlled, introversion is positively correlated with cortical activation or arousal (*7*). Many of the behavioral correlates of introversion and ex-

troversion reflect this differential arousal (*7, 8*). Other behaviors associated with introversion and extroversion are believed to be caused by homeostatic attempts to increase arousal (for example, by seeking stimulation) by underaroused extroverts and to decrease arousal (for example, by avoiding stimulation) by over-aroused introverts (*9*). When proper controls are applied, psychophysiological studies of the differences between introverts and extroverts tend to substantiate this theory (*7–9*), although there is considerable question as to the unidimensionality of the introversion-extroversion construct (*10*).

We gave verbal ability tests under conditions presumed to differ in their arousing properties. The results are consistent with our predictions and indicate that the personality dimension of introversion-extroversion is related to test performance in a complex manner, and that certain testing conditions favor one end of the dimension while other conditions favor the opposing end.

We administered three equivalent tests of verbal ability (*11*) under three separate conditions to each of 101 undergraduate students. The forms and conditions were randomized for each subject (*12*). On one night the subjects were instructed to solve all 60 problems and to

spend as much time as necessary. On another night, the subjects were allowed to spend only 10 minutes on the test, were told to work as quickly as possible, and were given two placebo pills which they were told contained 200 mg of either caffeine or lactose. The same procedure was followed on the third night, except that the pills actually contained 200 mg of caffeine (*13*). Subjects had been instructed not to consume any caffeine or other drugs for 6 hours preceeding each condition. They filled out the Eysenck Personality Inventory Form A (*14*) while waiting for the "caffeine" to take effect.

The correlations between number correct [corrected for guessing (*15*)] and the introversion-extroversion dimension were −.29 in the relaxed condition, −.18 under time pressure with placebos, and +.12 under time pressure with caffeine. Although the change in correlation from the relaxed to placebo conditions was not statistically significant, the change from placebo to caffeine conditions was (*t*-test of the difference between dependent correlations, $t = 3.38$, d.f. = 98, $P < .005$).

The distribution of introversion-extroversion scores can be divided into three groups, introverts, ambiverts, and extroverts (*14*) (Fig. 1). To allow for comparisons between scores achieved in different lengths of time, we converted all scores to standard scores. Scores from the relaxed condition were standardized separately, but means and variances from the two timed conditions were pooled before the scores were standardized. The appropriate correction for guessing (number correct − ¼ number incorrect) was applied to the scores before they were standardized (*16*).

The interaction between introversion-extroversion and situational stress (Fig. 1) is statistically significant (unweighted means analysis of variance, $F = 4.92$, d.f. = 4, 196, $P < .005$) (*17, 18*). In the two timed conditions, total performance can be separated into two components: speed (the number of problems attempted) and accuracy (the ratio of the number of problems correct to the number of problems attempted). The correlation between the introversion-extroversion dimension and speed did not increase significantly. For accuracy, however, there was a significant change in the correlation (from −.31 with placebos to +.02 with caffeine: $t = 3.15$, $P < .005$). For the grouped data, this indicated a decrease in accuracy from .69 to .63 for the introverts and an increase in accuracy from .60 to .64 for the extroverts. This implies that the locus of the effect is not merely a response style of trading off

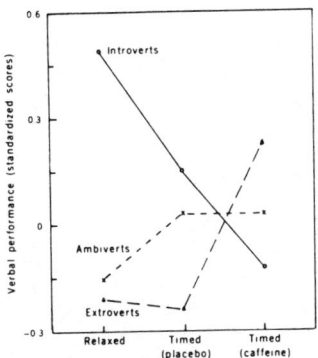

Fig. 1. Standardized performance scores (mean = 0, S.D. = 1) on practice verbal Graduate Record Examinations as function of introversion-extroversion, time pressure, and caffeine. The relaxed condition was standardized separately; the timed conditions were standardized together.

speed for accuracy on the part of the introverts.

Before we generalize from these results, several limitations should be considered. (i) The relaxed condition allowed the subjects as much time as they required to complete the test. This is more generous than even normal "power" (untimed) instructions. (ii) The timed conditions were shorter than normally allowed on standard ability tests. (iii) The performance shift from relaxed to time stress is a relative shift (scores were standardized within condition); almost all subjects solved more problems in the power condition. In the timed conditions, however, the shift is absolute rather than relative; when treated with caffeine, introverts correctly answered fewer problems and extroverts more problems. (iv) Differences in performance in the relaxed condition could be a result of differences in arousal (our hypothesis) or represent different levels of involvement in the task. If introverts are assumed to be relatively more interested in intellectual problems, they might be expected to do better when allowed unlimited time. In the timed conditions, however, this explanation is less convincing. In the same testing session some subjects were administered placebo and others caffeine—a condition that diminishes the likelihood of differential susceptibility of introverts and extroverts to possible expectations of the experimenter.

Our effects are interactive ones and not main effects. Caffeine-induced stress neither raises nor lowers average performance but rather increases the performance for some individuals and decreases it for others. Similarly, across the two drug conditions, there was no net superiority for either introverts or extroverts. These findings suggest a paradigm for studying the effects on performance of stressors in conjunction with dimensions of personality. Specifically, this methodology overcomes many of the objections raised to previous studies of the curvilinear relationship between stress and performance (5).

WILLIAM REVELLE
PHYLLIS AMARAL
SUSAN TURRIFF

Department of Psychology,
Northwestern University,
Evanston, Illinois 60201

References and Notes

1. R. M. Yerkes and J. D. Dodson, *J. Comp. Neurol. Psychol.* **18**, 459 (1908); P. L. Broadhurst, *Acta Psychol.* **16**, 321 (1959); E. Duffy, *Activation and Behavior* (Wiley, New York, 1962).
2. R. B. Malmo, *On Emotions, Needs, and Our Archaic Brain* (Holt, Reinhart, and Winston, New York, 1962).
3. J. E. Hokanson and M. Burgess, *J. Abnorm. Soc. Psychol.* **68**, 698 (1964); R. T. Wilkinson, S. El-Beheri, C. C. Gieseking, *Psychophysiology* **9**, 529 (1972).
4. P. Patkai, *Int. J. Psychiatry Med.* **5**, 575 (1974).
5. R. Näätänen, in *Attention and Performance IV*, S. Kornblum, Ed. (Academic Press, New York, 1973), pp. 155–174.
6. J. W. Atkinson and J. O. Raynor, Eds., *Motivation and Achievement* (Winston, Washington, D.C., 1974); C. D. Spielberger and I. G. Saronson, Eds., *Stress and Anxiety* (Halsted, New York, 1975); E. Gaudry and C. D. Spielberger, Eds., *Anxiety and Educational Achievement* (Wiley, New York, 1971).
7. H. J. Eysenck, *Biological Basis of Personality* (Thomas, Springfield, Ill., 1967); J. A. Gray, in *Multivariate Analysis and Psychological Theory*, J. R. Royce. Ed. (Academic Press, New York. 1973).
8. G. S. Claridge. *Personality and Arousal* (Pergamon, Oxford, 1967); M. G. H. Coles, A. Gale, P. Kline, *Psychophysiology* **8**, 54 (1971); A. Crider and R. Lunn, *J. Exp. Res. Pers.* **5**, 145 (1971); R. B. Sloane, P. O. Davidson, R. W. Payne, *Arch. Gen. Psychiatry* **13**, 19 (1965).
9. H. J. Eysenck, in *Emotions—Their Parameters and Measurement*, L. Levi, Ed. (Raven, New York, 1975), pp. 439–467; F. Farley and S. V. J. Farley, *Consult. Psychol.* **31**, 215 (1967).
10. J. P. Guilford, *Psychol. Bull.* **82**, 802 (1975).
11. G. R. Gruber and E. C. Gruber, *Graduate Record Examination Aptitude Test: A Complete Review for the Verbal and Math Parts of the Test* (Simon & Schuster, New York, 1973). The first 60 questions (20 each of analogies, antonyms, and sentence completions) of practice tests 2, 3, and 4 were used.
12. There were no noticeable relationships between performance and the sequence of either the conditions or the tests. All sessions began at approximately 7 p.m. to control for possible diurnal effects [M. J. F. Blake, *Nature (London)* **215**, 896 (1967)].
13. Actually 400 mg of caffeine citrate was administered. This contained 200 mg of caffeine which is roughly equivalent to one and one-half to two cups of coffee [J. F. Greden, *Am. J. Psychiatry* **131**, 1089 (1974)].
14. H. J. Eysenck and S. B. Eysenck, *Eysenck Personality Inventory* (Educational and Industrial Testing Service, San Diego, 1964). The scores defining each group were 2 to 9 (introverts, $N = 27$), 10 to 15 (ambiverts, $N = 45$), and 16 to 21 (extroverts, $N = 29$). The mean extroversion score was 12.5 (S.D. = 4.5).
15. The correlations with number right (uncorrected) were $-.28$, $-.13$, and $+.14$.
16. The means before standardization were 37.3, 21.1, and 21.9 (S.D. = 8.6, 8.5, and 9.0) for the relaxed, placebo, and caffeine conditions, respectively.
17. Similar analyses were done with the neuroticism scale from the Eysenck Personality Inventory, but there were no significant effects.
18. A preliminary study with 60 subjects and 100 mg of caffeine had similar results. Introverts ($N = 18$) fell from $+0.25$ to -0.36 sigma units, while extroverts ($N = 11$) rose from $+0.01$ to $+0.22$. Ambiverts ($N = 31$) rose slightly from -0.2 to -0.16.
19. We thank J. Barry and L. Gourley for assistance in collecting the data for the pilot study and L. G. Humphreys, M. Humphreys, and two anonymous reviewers for helpful comments on an earlier draft of this paper.

30 January 1976

PART X

SOCIAL BEHAVIOUR

There are many links between the physiology of arousal, through the personality trait of extraversion–introversion, and social behaviour. The most direct is probably through the arousing effect of social interaction; such factors as the simple presence of people, gazing at others, talking to them, or interacting with them in other ways have been shown to produce powerful arousing effects. Zajonc (1965) has surveyed a large number of studies on social facilitation which integrate very well with the major lessons imposed by work on learning and memory. It will be remembered that according to the inverted-U relationship between arousal and performance, easy tasks are facilitated by arousal, difficult ones made harder. Zajonc reviews studies in which learning and performance are studied under non-social conditions (i.e. without anyone present), and under social conditions (i.e. with other persons present). As early as 1924, Allport postulated that "the sights and sounds of others doing the same thing" augmented ongoing responses; this augmentation, however, was proposed to occur only for overt motor responses. "Intellectual or implicit responses of thought are hampered rather than facilitated by the presence of others," he thought. This might be thought of as an early adumbration of the application of the Yerkes–Dodson Law to the effects of social stimulation. Later work was more specific.

Zajonc sums up several later investigations by stating that "it would appear that the emission of well-learned responses is facilitated by the presence of spectators, while the acquisition of new responses is impaired. To put the statement in conventional psychological language, performance is facilitated and learning is impaired by the presence of spectators". He goes on to refine this statement by having recourse to a theoretical statement rather like Spence's general theory; if the dominant responses in a situation are the correct ones, social facilitation will occur. If the dominant responses are incorrect, social arousal will strengthen these incorrect responses, and thus make learning more difficult. These experiments all deal simply with the presence of specta-

tors, i.e. with other people who take no active part in the experiment. Other studies have dealt with the participation of others in a variety of tasks.

Zajonc (1965) also summarizes a series of well-known studies by Allport and Dashiell using the co-action paradigm, i.e. situations in which the subject acts either in the presence of others also active in the same task, or else not so active. Allport's subjects worked either in separate cubicles or sitting around a common table, and many different tasks were studied; the outcome of his work, and that of others, could again be fitted comfortably into a general theoretical statement such as that contained in the previous paragraph. Zajonc continues his survey with a consideration of work on animals, but this is too far removed from our present interest to be summarized, although he suggest that it too fits well into a general theoretical statement of the Spence type. We may thus say that social interaction has an arousing effect on learning and performance, that this effect is in line with work previously surveyed on the effects of arousal, and that it would seem to follow that under-aroused, extraverted people should be more likely to seek out personal contacts than would overaroused, introverted people. Thus the trait of sociability, which is central to most conceptualizations of extraversion, can be seen as a direct consequence of arousal differences between extraverts and introverts.

Work done since Zajonc's thesis was put forward has tended to support his views (e.g. Zajonc and Sales, 1966; Carment, 1970a, 1970b; Matlin and Zajonc, 1969; Martens, 1969a, 1969b; Hunt and Hillery, 1973; Cottrell, Rittle and Wack, 1967; Innes and Young, 1975; Geen, 1973, 1974; Desportes, 1976). However, certain theoretical criticisms have been made of the hypothesis that it is the mere presence of an audience which produces these effects. While some investigators are in agreement (e.g. Chapman, 1973, 1974), most have argued that what is required is that the subject should experience apprehension over being evaluated by the audience (e.g., Cottrell et al., 1968; Henchy and Glass, 1968; Sasfy and Okum,

1974). As Cottrell (1968, 1972) puts it, the presence of others would therefore appear to be a stimulus which elicits a learned drive associated with anxiety over being judged. This line of argument is consistent with traditional explanations of social facilitation in lower animals, most of which emphasize some aspect of the *behaviour* of conspecifics and not their mere physical presence. Weiss and Miller (1971) have discussed these theoretical points at some length, also raising the question of incentive motivation, i.e. whether the secondary drive in the social motivation situation could also be based on primary appetitive states (e.g., expectation of praise rather than criticism). A discussion of these issues would take us too far outside our topic; from the point of view of arousal produced by association with people the question of whether it is the mere presence, or expectations associated with their presence, which is causal is of secondary importance. The addition of some r_g-s_g mechanism to the "mere presence" paradigm would not invalidate arguments about introvert–extravert differences (and might indeed strengthen them). In any case, there are several papers in which social interaction effects have been linked with introversion–extraversion; the most important of these have been reprinted in Eysenck's (1971) set of *Readings in Extraversion–Introversion*. Unfortunately, the majority of papers taking up the crucial study of the interaction of personality and social facilitation have used anxiety as the personality variable preferred (Berkey and Hoppe, 1972; Cox, 1966, 1968; Ganzer, 1968; Pederson, 1970). We have already discussed the difficulties in interpretation raised by the choice of a variable which is in fact a mixture of E and N; it is difficult if not impossible to relate observed effects to one or the other of the two component traits of anxiety.

This is not the only link between arousal, at the one end of the chain, and social behaviour, at the other. Sensation-seeking at the sensory level clearly and directly leads to sensation-seeking at the social level; the attraction of the bright lights and loud music of the town for extraverted youths is well known, and may lead them into temptation which ultimately may result in criminal conduct. Perhaps even more important may be differences in strength of conditioning, depending on level of arousal; Eysenck (1976a) has suggested that, particularly in the presence of high N, the ready conditionability of introverts may lead to neurotic breakdown, and the poor conditionability of extraverts to criminal behaviour. There is much evidence to support this hypothesis (Eysenck, 1976b). There are many other types of social behaviour which can be looked at along these lines; only a few have been singled out for discussion in the reprinted papers which follow.

Quite generally, we would maintain that personality interacts with social situations in a manner which makes it impossible to make predictions from the situation alone, without taking into account personality. As an example, consider the work of Di Loreto (1971), who studied the effects of behaviour therapy on certain types of phobic disorders. He used three types of therapy, each represented by two experienced therapists (in order to eliminate or control variance due to therapist's personality): Wolpe's desensitization treatment, Ellis' rational–emotional therapy, and Rogers' client-centred therapy. All the patients involved were tested and divided into extraverted and introverted; Di Loreto postulated and found that the Ellis type of therapy was much more effective with introverts, the Rogerian type of therapy with extraverts (there were no differences with respect to Wolpe's method). These results suggest that no prediction can be made on the basis of specifying method of treatment alone; prediction only becomes possible when the personality of the patient is measured and used as part of the forecasting formula. This is not an isolated finding, of course; quite universally throughout this book we have found that personality and treatment interact, and prediction of outcome is only possible when both are taken into account. If this is true of experimental laboratory studies, it is equally true of social situations and experiments. General, experimental and social psychology need the concepts of personality theory as much as personality theory needs the concepts of general psychology and physiology; the relation is symbiotic.

It may be appropriate here to go back to an argument stated implicitly in the first section, namely that of the genetic basis of extraversion–introversion, and the relationship between sociability and impulsiveness. How is it possible for behaviour to be determined genetically? Surely only physiological–anatomical structures can be determined in such a manner? We are now in a position to suggest a plausible chain of causation. We begin with genetically determined differences in ARAS reactivity, causing in turn different arousability in the cortex, and hence mean differences in arousal level between extraverts, ambiverts, and introverts. Given that intermediate degrees of arousal are pleasant, and hence produce adient responses, while very low and very high degrees of arousal are unpleasant, and hence produce abient responses, extraverts will seek out situations which are productive of high arousal, while introverts will avoid such situations; we have reviewed much evidence of an experimental kind to that effect. Now we have seen that interaction with other people can be conceptualized as arousing; it would seem to follow, *ceteris paribus*, that extraverts would seek out other people, interact with them, and thus derive a certain amount of arousal which they experience as positively reinforcing; this in turn would lead to a continuation of this habit.

Introverts, conversely, would experience degrees of arousal in excess of the optimum level on interacting with other people, and would hence tend to be negatively reinforced by social contact, and consequently avoid it. Thus sociability would be a good measure of extraversion, provided other things were indeed equal, which of course they only too often are not—hence the failure of observed correlations to be perfect. Social contacts may produce negative reinforcement for other reasons than too high arousal level; a person may be rejected for reasons of dullness, age, race, ugliness, deformity, or any of a dozen other reasons. He would thus learn to avoid negative reinforcement, and become introverted in his behaviour, although genetically possibly extraverted. This general model is of course testable; it would require seeking out subjects who on experimental testing give results which differ drastically from their questionnaire responses, i.e. the non-concordant subjects. The theory makes a universal statement about invariance; where invariance fails, the theory suggests the intrusion of other factors which, in order to make the theory scientific, must be specifiable and testable. Little seems to have been done along these lines, but results of such research might be of considerable interest.

Impulsiveness would be conceptualized as a lack of constraint; this constraint, in turn, would be considered the outcome of life experiencing leading to conditioning favouring inhibition. Conditioning, in this case, would be considered a function of arousal, higher arousal leading to stronger conditioning, and hence to greater inhibition, i.e. to less impulsive behaviour. In this way we can account for the genetic link between sociability and impulsiveness, through arousal. The environmental link is somewhat more problematical, and only a rather speculative suggestion can be made. Social interaction means establishing contacts with other people, and inhibitions of all sorts may make this process difficult—it seems reasonable to assume that impulsive people, little bothered about rejection and other possible consequences of their action, are more likely to make social contacts than people made shy through inhibitions of one kind or another. Again this hypothesis is testable, and if true would put some flesh on the bare bones of the original genetic study reprinted in part I. It is unfortunate that so little direct evidence is available on these important points; the reason is probably that these problems have not engaged the interest of personality theorists mostly unconcerned with the elaboration of genetic determinants and the resulting paradigms alike. Work on criminality (Eysenck, 1976a, 1976b) and sexual behaviour (Eysenck, 1976c) suggests that these theoretical considerations may be along the right lines.

REFERENCES

ALLPORT, F. H. *Social psychology*. Boston: Houghton Mifflin, 1924.

BERKEY, A. S. and HOPPE, R. A. The combined effect of audience and anxiety on paired-associates learning. *Psychonomic Science*, 1972, *29*, 351–353.

CARMENT, D. W. Rate of simple motor responding as a function of coaction, competition and sex of the participants. *Psychonomic Science*, 1970a, *19*, 340–341.

CARMENT, D. W. Rate of simple motor responding as a function of differential outcomes and the actual and implied presence of a coactor. *Psychonomic Science*, 1970b, *20*, 115–116.

CHAPMAN, A. J. Social facilitation of laughter in children. *Journal of Experimental Social Psychology*, 1973, *9*, 528–541.

CHAPMAN, A. J. An electromyographic study of social facilitation: a test of the "mere presence" hypothesis. *British Journal of Psychology*, 1974, *65*, 123–128.

COTTRELL, N. B. Performance in the presence of other human beings: mere presence, audience, and affiliation effects. In: R. A. Simmel, G. Hoppe and A. Milton (Eds.), *Social Facilitation and Imitative Behavior*. Boston: Allyn and Bacon. 1968.

COTTRELL, N. B. Social facilitation. In: C. G. McClintock (Ed.), *Experimental social psychology*. New York: Holt, Rinehart, and Winston, 1972.

COTTRELL, N. B., RITTLE, R. H., and WACK, D. L. The presence of an audience and list type (competitional or noncompetitional) as joint determinants of performance in paired-associate learning. *Journal of Personality*, 1967, *35*, 423–434.

COTTRELL, N. B., WACK, D. L., SEKERAK, G. J., and RITTLE, R. H. Social facilitation of dominant responses by the presence of an audience and the mere presence of others. *Journal of Personality and Social Psychology*, 1968, *9*, 245–250.

COX, F. N. Some effects of test anxiety and presence or absence of other persons on boys' performance on a repetitive motor task. *Journal of Experimental Child Psychology*, 1966, *3*, 100–112.

COX, F. N. Some relationships between test anxiety presence or absence of male persons and boys' performance on a repetitive motor task. *Journal of Experimental and Child Psychology*, 1968, *5*, 1–12.

DAVIDSON, P. O. and KELLEY, W. R. Social facilitation and coping with stress. *British Journal of Social and Clinical Psychology*, 1973, *12*, 130–136.

DESPORTES, J. P. Les effets de la présence de l'expérimentateur dans les sciences du comportement. Paris: Editions du Centre National de la Recherche Scientifique, 1976.

DI LORETO, A. O. *Comparative psychotherapy: an experimental analysis*. New York: Aldine-Atherton, 1971.

EYSENCK. H. J. (Ed.) *Readings in extraversion–introversion* (3 vols.). London: Staples, 1971.

EYSENCK, H. J. *Crime and personality* (3rd Edition). London: Routledge and Kegan Paul, 1976a.

EYSENCK, H. J. Psychopathy, personality and genetics. In: R. D. Hare and D. Schalling (Eds.) *Psychopathic behaviour*. London: John Wiley and Sons, 1976b.

EYSENCK, H. J. *Sex and personality*. London: Open Books, 1976c.

GANZER, V. J. Effects of audience presence and test anxiety on learning and retention in a serial learning situation. *Journal of Personality and Social Psychology*, 1968, *8*, 194–199.

GEEN, R. G. Effects of being observed in short and long-term recall. *Journal of Experimental Psychology*, 1973, *100*, 395–398.

GEEN, R. G. Effects of evaluation apprehension on memory over intervals of varying length. *Journal of Experimental Psychology*, 1974, *102*, 908–910.

HENCHY, T. and GLASS, D. C. Evaluation apprehension and the social facilitation of dominant and subordinate responses. *Journal of Personality and Social Psychology*, 1968, *10*, 446–454.

HUNT, P. J. and HILLERY, J. M. Social facilitation in a co-action setting: an examination of the effects over learning trials. *Journal of Experimental Social Psychology*, 1973, *9*, 563–571.

INNES, J. M. and YOUNG, R. F. The effect of presence of an audience, evaluation apprehension and objective self-awareness on learning. *Journal of Experimental Social Psychology*, 1975, *11*, 35–52.

MARTENS, R. Effect of an audience on learning and performance of a complex motor skill. *Journal of Personality and Social Psychology*, 1969a, *12*, 252–260.

MARTENS, R. Palmar sweating and the presence of an audience. *Journal of Experimental Social Psychology*, 1969b, *5*, 371–374.

MATLIN, M. V. and ZAJONC, R. B. Social facilitation of word associations. *Journal of Personality and Social Psychology*, 1969, *10*, 435–460.

PEDERSON, A. M. Effects of test anxiety and coacting groups on learning and performance. *Perceptual and Motor Skills*, 1970, *30*, 55–62.

SASFY, J. and OKUM, M. Form of evaluation and audience expertness as joint determinants of audience effects. *Journal of Experimental Social Psychology*, 1974, *10*, 461–467.

WEISS, R. G. and MILLER, F. G. The drive theory of social facilitation. *Psychological Review*, 1971, *78*, 44–57.

ZAJONC, R. B. Social facilitation. *Science*, 1965, *149*, 269–274.

ZAJONC, R. B. and SALES, S. M. Social facilitation of dominant and subordinate responses. *Journal of Experimental Social Psychology*, 1966, *2*, 160–168.

From F. J. Vingoe and S. R. Antonoff (1968). Journal of Counseling Psychology, *15,* 91–93, *by kind permission of the authors and The American Psychological Association*

Personality Characteristics of Good Judges of Others[1]

FRANK J. VINGOE AND STEVEN R. ANTONOFF

Colorado State University

This paper explored the personality characteristics of good and poor judges of others. Ss took the Eysenck Personality Inventory (EPI) and the California Personality Inventory (CPI) and rated themselves and their peers on the EPI variable of Extraversion and the 5 CPI variables of Dominance, Sociability, Self-Acceptance, Responsibility, and Psychological-Mindedness. Good raters were differentiated from poor raters on the basis of the discrepancy between the peer rating on each variable and the rating derived from the ratee's actual test score. The 11 best judges were compared to the 10 poorest judges. Results indicated that good judges minimize their worries and complaints, are well-adjusted, introverted, self-controlled, tolerant, and tend to "fake good."

There have been a number of reports on the characteristics of good judges. Taft (1955, 1956) has reported on investigations in this general area. In his review of the literature, Taft (1955) noted that "there is evidence that judgments are more accurate when J and S are similar in cultural backgrounds, also in age and sex . . . [p. 6]." He indicated that the ability "to judge others on analytic modes correlates positively with emotional adjustment; presumably the more psychologically significant aspect of this correlation is that poor judges tend to be poorly adjusted and, therefore, probably more likely to allow personal biases to affect their judgments [p. 14]."

Using a group of 40 subjects undergoing a "living-in" assessment program, Taft (1956) found the good judge of others to be,

a serious, organized and reasonable person who apparently relies upon the use of his intelligence and conservatism in meeting successfully the hazards of life. On the other hand, the poor judge is socially oriented but not socially adjusted. Support for this picture is offered by the subject's own check on the adjective list. The good judges prefer to use terms that indicate achievement orientation at the expense of social relations, e.g., industrious, logical, painstaking, reserved and retiring. The poor judges preferred adjectives almost all of which reveal social organization, e.g., noisy, show-off, egotistical, emotional, affectionate, clever—but also careless [p. 26].

In summary, Taft's (1955, 1956) work suggests that some of the more important factors

involved in judging others are the frame of reference used in making the judgment, position of the judge on the adjustment–maladjustment continuum, and the position of the judge on the introversion–extraversion continuum. However, a recent study (Eysenck & Eysenck, 1964) found no relationship between the position of judges on the Neuroticism and Extraversion scales of the Eysenck Personality Inventory (EPI; Eysenck & Eysenck, 1963) and the excellence of their judgments of others on the Extraversion scale.

In the present study the attempt was made to differentiate good from poor judges of others on the basis of their respective personality characteristics. The major assumption made was that freshmen of the same age and sex who lived together in the same dormitory would be in an optimum position to judge each other.

Judgmental ability was measured by the difference between the peer rating on each of six personality variables and the rating derived from the ratee's actual test score on each of these variables.

The following specific hypotheses were made:

1. Good judges are significantly less neurotic than poor judges.

2. Good judges are significantly less extraverted than poor judges.

3. Good judges score significantly higher on the California Psychological · Inventory (CPI) scales of (*a*) Well-Being, (*b*) Tolerance, and (*c*) Intellectual Efficiency.

The predictions made in Hypothesis 3 are based on the correlation of EPI Neuroticism with the CPI scales (Vingoe, 1966). The three CPI scales of Well-Being, Tolerance, and Intellectual Efficiency were the three most highly

[1] A modified version of a paper presented at the meeting of the Colorado-Wyoming Academy of Science, April 1967.

Notes and Comments

correlated with neuroticism. Thus, it was hypothesized that there are five personality variables—EPI Neuroticism and Extraversion and CPI Well-Being, Tolerance, and Intellectual Efficiency—which differentiate good from poor judges of others.

PROCEDURE

The Ss were 66 18-year-old freshmen women living in the same dormitory. The following instruments were administered: (a) Self-Rating Booklet, (b) the CPI (Gough, 1964), (c) EPI, and (d) the Peer-Rating Booklet. Both the Self-Rating and the Peer-Rating booklets were based upon material developed by Goldberg and Rorer (1963). The horizontal graphic rating scale used for the peer ratings was based on Guilford (1959). The Ss rated themselves and their peers on five CPI variables—Dominance, Sociability, Self-Acceptance, Responsibility, and Psychological-Mindedness and on the EPI variable of Extraversion. Since Ferguson (1949) indicated a significant relationship between accuracy in rating and acquaintance with ratee, acquaintanceship ratings were also obtained in the present study. All ratings were made on a seven-point scale. Each S was also asked what she thought she would get (on the average) if the other girls on her wing were to rate her on the six personality variables (estimated mean peer rating). The Ss rated those who lived in the same wing of their dormitory. Only the ratings made which were associated with a high degree of acquaintance of the ratee (Ratings 6 and 7) were used in the data analysis. However, all 66 Ss were known well or fairly well by at least one other S.

Discrepancy scores for each of the six variables were determined for each rater between her rating of each S on each of the traits indicated above and the ratings derived from the ratee's actual test scores. Since both peer ratings and self-ratings were made on a seven-point scale, the EPI and CPI percentile scores were transformed into a

seven-point rating scale to facilitate calculations. The test score percentiles were divided into seven categories. The categories were based on the distribution of the normal curve and included the same percentage of cases. The ratings were determined by percentile scores as follows: Rating 1, 2nd–15th; Rating 2, 16th–29th; Rating 3, 30th–43rd; Rating 4, 44th–57th; Rating 5, 58th–71st; Rating 6, 72nd–85th; and Rating 7, 86th–99th. The individual discrepancy scores were then summed for the six variables to obtain a total discrepancy score (total judgmental ability score). Only the total judgmental ability score is reported in this article.

From the original group of 66 Ss, the 11 with the lowest total discrepancy scores (good raters; 2 Ss obtained the same score) and the 10 with the highest total discrepancy scores (poor raters) were compared in terms of differences between each of the CPI and EPI variables.

RESULTS

The significance of the difference between means was computed by t test, and the results are presented in Table 1. As predicted, good raters showed significantly different scores on the CPI variables of Well-Being and Tolerance and the EPI variables of Extraversion and Neuroticism. More specifically, good raters were significantly less neurotic at the 5% level and significantly less extraverted at the 2.5% level. In addition, good raters scored significantly higher on Well-Being at the 5% level and were significantly more tolerant at the 2.5% level. Thus, Hypotheses 1, 2, 3a, and 3b were supported. Although the trend of the data was suggestive, support was not found for Hypothesis 3c; that is, good raters tended to be more intellectually efficient, but the difference between good and poor raters on this variable did not reach significance. It was also found that good and poor raters were differentiated by CPI Self-Control and EPI Lie scale at the .02 and .01 levels, respectively. In summary, the results indicate that good judges minimize their worries and complaints, are tolerant, introverted, and relatively well-adjusted. In addition, good judges are more self-controlled and tend to "fake good" as measured by the EPI Lie scale.

DISCUSSION

The ability to accurately judge others on certain defined personality characteristics is an asset in a number of occupations in which evaluation and selection are important tasks. If one can distinguish good from poor judges of others on the basis of judges' personality characteristics, a major step forward will have been made. In the present investigation, good raters

TABLE 1
Factors Differentiating Good and Poor Raters of Others

Variable	Good raters[a]		Poor raters[b]		t	p
	M	SD	M	SD		
Neuroticism	9.1	4.25	12.3	3.38	1.85	.05
Extraversion	10.8	4.13	14.8	4.12	2.10	.025
Well-Being	36.3	3.62	31.4	4.71	2.03	.05
Tolerance	23.3	4.90	20.1	3.38	2.10	.025
Intellectual Efficiency	38.8	7.97	35.9	8.20	1.04	ns
Lie	2.9	1.07	1.8	0.31	3.28	.01[c]
Self-Control	28.7	3.55	21.9	5.27	2.77	.02[c]

[a] N = 11.
[b] N = 10.
[c] Two-tailed test.

Notes and Comments

were differentiated from poor raters on six personality variables. However, the importance of the particular criterion used in the measure of judgmental ability should be borne in mind. Taft (1956) used two separate criteria: (a) mean staff ratings and (b) median peer ratings on the personality traits. In a study involving the judging of acquaintances and strangers, Taft (1966) used a Q-sort technique in which the judge sorted statements as he felt the subject would sort them.

In the present study, ratings on each of the personality variables derived from the ratee's actual test scores on these variables were used as the criteria for judgmental ability. However, the derivation of the ratings from test score percentiles was somewhat arbitrary, and establishing the reliability of this procedure was not practicable. Although self-ratings were available and their test-retest reliability adequate, it was felt that the subject's test scores would be less distorted. In general, the results of this study support Taft's (1956) conclusions. Although Taft suggested that some of the characteristics found to differentiate good and poor judges in his sample of advanced graduate students might not differentiate subjects from another sample, the results of the present study using college freshmen verified his results, in that good judges were found to be relatively well-adjusted, self-controlled, and introverted.

REFERENCES

EYSENCK, H. J., & EYSENCK, S. B. G. *Manual for the Eysenck Personality Inventory*. San Diego: Educational Testing Service, 1963.

EYSENCK, S. B. G., & EYSENCK, H. J. The personality of judges as a factor in the validity of their judgments of extraversion-introversion. *British Journal of Social and Clinical Psychology*, 1964, **3**, 141–144.

FERGUSON, L. W. The value of acquaintance ratings in criterion research. *Personnel Psychology*, 1949, **2**, 93–102.

GOLDBERG, L. R., & RORER, L. G. An intensive study of sociometric measures. Unpublished manuscript, Oregon Research Institute, 1963.

GOUGH, H. G. *Manual for the California Psychological Inventory*. Palo Alto: Consulting Psychologists Press, 1964.

GUILFORD, J. P. *Personality*. New York. McGraw-Hill, 1959.

TAFT, R. The ability to judge peopde. *Psychological Bulletin*, 1955, **52**, 1–23.

TAFT, R. Some characteristics of good judges of others. *British Journal of Psychology*, 1956, **47**, 19–29.

TAFT, R. Accuracy of empathic judgments of acquaintances and strangers. *Journal of Personality and Social Psychology*, 1966, **3**, 600–604.

VINGOE, F. J. A note of the validity of the California Psychological Inventory. Unpublished manuscript, Colorado State University, 1966.

(Received May 12, 1967)

From R. W. Ramsay (1966). Journal of Personality and Social Psychology, *4*, 116–118, *by kind permission of the author and The American Psychological Association*

PERSONALITY AND SPEECH [1]

R. W. RAMSAY

Institute of Psychiatry, Maudsley Hospital, London

Recordings were made of Ss reading, conversing, describing TAT pictures, and making up stories about TAT pictures. Measurements were made from the recordings of the lengths of sound and lengths of silence in speech. It was found that there is a highly significant difference in lengths of sound and silence between tasks; the tasks requiring higher cognitive activity having longer silences. Ss were divided on the basis of the personality continua of extraversion and neuroticism, and almost a quarter of the inter-S variance could be accounted for in terms of extraversion. The extraverts use longer sounds and shorter silence than the introverts. No consistent effects due to neuroticism were found.

Most of the psychological studies of speech have concentrated on content—what is said rather than how it is said; in fact, as Mahl (1959, p. 105) points out, the standard text in the psychology of speech and communication (Miller, 1951) barely mentions what Mahl calls nonlexical aspects of speech. Chapple (1939, 1940) pioneered the work of trying to measure the noncontent aspects of speech—how long a person speaks and how long he is silent—during interpersonal interaction. He and others, notably Goldman-Eisler, Hargreaves, Mahl, Matarazzo, Saslow, and Starkweather, have extended the early work so that a small body of information has been built up in this area. Starkweather (1964) summarizes most of the relevant literature.

The research approach in this field encounters two problems. The first is the technical difficulty of measuring speech, and a separate paper (Ramsay, in press) attempts to deal with this. There is also the problem of trying to measure the complex interaction of many variables. Many studies have used interpersonal interaction as their test situation—two people conversing, or psychiatric patients in psychotherapy. These are highly complex situations, and it is therefore not surprising that the results of some of the studies are equivocal and difficult to interpret. Rosenthal (1964) gives ample evidence of the confounding interaction effects due to the experimenter. Before trying to measure complex problems of interpersonal interaction, levels of anxiety, differences in tasks, differences in situation, etc., it may be profitable to investigate the more basic aspects of how and why people differ in their speech patterns, that is, to try to account

for the large intersubject variance in terms of personality.

Eysenck (1957), showing a preference for dealing with a few broad variables in his dimensional approach to personality, has concentrated his interest on four factors: intelligence, extraversion-introversion (E-I), neuroticism (N), and psychoticism. Because of the particular factor-analytic technique used, these dimensions are orthogonal to each other, and it is possible to investigate personality differences along the two dimensions of E-I and N, and assume a random distribution of intelligence and psychotic tendency.

Speech has been shown to consist of short bursts of sound interspersed with silence. If the extravert is more expansive and expressive in his movements (Davis, 1948; Rachman, 1961), this should be reflected in his less reserved and introspective speech patterns. The present study investigates the correlates of speech patterns with differences in personality along the dimensions of E-I and N. No detailed hypotheses from Eysenck's theories were formulated, and the approach was more exploratory than hypothetico deductive.

METHOD

The subjects were 23 volunteer first-year teacher-training college students, female, with an average age of 18.5 years. Before the speech-testing session the subjects were required to fill in an Eysenck Personality Inventory (Eysenck & Eysenck, 1964) to establish their position on the dimensions of E-I and N, and they also filled in the Mill Hill Vocabulary Scale (Raven, 1948) to give a rough measure of verbal intelligence.

The verbal tasks were:

1. An initial unrecorded reading task to get the subjects used to the microphone, and to allow the subjects to habituate to some extent to the testing

[1] This study was supported by a scholarship from the Canada Council.

BRIEF ARTICLES

situation. This also gave the experimenter a chance to get a volume-level setting for the subject.

2. Reading a short passage of prose (average time taken for reading approximately 1 minute).

3. Reading a short passage of direct speech (average time taken approximately 3 minutes).

4. A 10-minute conversation with the experimenter on the subject of teaching as a career.

5. A description of the pictures on four Thematic Apperception Test (TAT) cards. No time limit.

6. Four stories made up about the same TAT cards used previously. No time limit.

In the 10-minute conversation the experimenter only spoke if the subject was silent for 3 seconds or more. This was done in an effort to minimize the interaction effects of the experimenter, as Goldman-Eisler (1961a) has found that in discussion pauses are no longer than 3 seconds and that 99% are less than 2 seconds.

The complete operation for continuous speech duration measurement consisted of recording a subject's verbalizations by means of a throat microphone onto magnetic tape at a constant volume. The taped verbalizations were then passed at a constant volume through a relay into a recording device which registered the time the relay was closed (speech), and the time the relay was open (silence), correct to .01 second.

RESULTS

The data consisted of mean lengths of speech, mean lengths of silence, and a ratio of total time of speech over total time of silence. The lengths of sound and silence are treated separately as they appear to be two different processes (average r over all tasks = $-.346$, $df = 21$). The mean scores for sound and silence were not normally distributed but positively skewed, so a log transformation was used for the statistical analysis.

As a check on the reliability of the results, the data for the reading tasks were correlated.

The correlation obtained was .746. Similarly the picture description and story correlation was .743.

As preliminary correlations between E-I scores and lengths of sound were significant (average $r = .407$, $df = 21$, $p = .05$), analyses of variance were done on the data. Of the 23 subjects in the sample, 16 were selected to fall into the four quadrants of stable introvert (SI), stable extravert (SE), neurotic introvert (NI), and neurotic extravert (NE). The analyses were of the split-plot design with two levels for extraversion, two levels for neuroticism ($n = 4$ at each level), and four repeated measures for each subject. The repeated measures were for Tasks, 2, 3, 5, and 6; Task 4 (conversation) is confounded by interaction with the experimenter and so was dealt with separately. The results for Task 4 were similar to the other results but at a lower level of significance.

The results of the analyses of variance are summarized in Table 1. Extraverts and introverts differed significantly in the lengths of sound and silence; extraverts produce longer bursts of sound than introverts, and shorter periods of silence between sounds. The ratio of total sound to total silence shows even more clearly the effect due to E-I; extraverts have a high ratio, indicating that they spend more time in speech and less time in silence. There is also a highly significant difference between tasks. To test this difference between tasks further, the two reading tasks were combined, and the picture and story tasks were combined, as these tasks seemed logically to be similar. Tasks 2 and 3 were then compared with Tasks 5 and 6, using Scheffé's (1953) test for multiple comparisons. There was a highly significant difference between the reading and picture tasks in sound and silence (F sound = 354.1, $p = .001$; F silence = 304.4, $p = .001$).

TABLE 1

RESULTS OF ANALYSES OF VARIANCE ON LENGTHS OF SOUND, SILENCE, AND SOUND/SILENCE RATIO

Source	Sound			Silence			Sound/silence ratio		
	df	MS	F	df	MS	F	df	MS	F
Extraversion (A)	1	83,197	5.95*	1	63,372	5.30*	1	3,922,679	12.13*
Neuroticism (B)	1	20,454	—	1	31,228	—	1	260,660	—
A × B	1	22,443	—	1	6,680	—	1	66,850	—
Error (a)	12	13,989		12	11,968		12	323,478	
Tasks (C)	3	542,318	108.82**	3	691,212	86.44**	3	36,575,940	154.85**
A × C	3	3,203	—	3	89	—	3	765,946	3.24
B × C	3	15,097	3.03	3	30,493	3.81	3	107,027	—
A × B × C	3	3,918	—	3	7,863	—	3	140,250	—
Error (b)	36	4,983		36	7,996		36	236,208	

Note.—Significance levels based on conservative test suggested by Greenhouse and Geisser (1959).
* $p = .05$.
** $p = .001$.

BRIEF ARTICLES

An analysis of variance on the results of the verbal intelligence test results showed no significant difference between groups.

DISCUSSION

The results in general agree with those found by other investigators. The distribution of sounds and silences follow a reversed J curve, with most being of short duration. This study has shown that the personality variable of E-I plays an appreciable part in speech. As was stated in the introduction, no definite predictions could be made concerning the effects of N, and the results showed some slight tendency for N to interact with E-I on length of sound. These results are difficult to explain and therefore, until further experimentation in this area has been done, it seems preferable to leave the effects of N an open question.

Returning to the E-I dimension, the lengths of sound produced by an individual correlate significantly with this dimension. If a correction is made for attenuation, it is found that almost one quarter of the variance can be accounted for by this factor alone. The introvert gives short bursts of speech and long pauses, the extravert long bursts of speech and short pauses. Goldman-Eisler (1961b) has stated that pauses are used for higher cognitive activity, and she has shown that there is an appreciable difference in length of pauses between two tasks, one requiring little thought and the other requiring a great deal of thought. The results of this study confirm her findings: Reading, which is a well-learned habit for most people and so requires little thought, has short silences; picture description and story telling require more thought and the silences are longer.

REFERENCES

CHAPPLE, E. D. Quantitative analysis of the interaction of individuals. *Proceedings of the National Academy of Sciences*, 1939, **25**, 58–67.

CHAPPLE, E. D. Personality differences as described by invariant properties of individuals in interaction. *Proceedings of the National Academy of Sciences*, 1940, **26**, 10–16.

DAVIS, D. R. *Pilot error: Some laboratory experiments*. London: His Majesty's Printing Office, 1948.

EYSENCK, H. J. *The dimensions of anxiety and hysteria*. London: Routledge & Kegan Paul, 1957.

EYSENCK, H. J., & EYSENCK, S. B. G. *The Eysenck Personality Inventory*. London: University of London Press, 1964.

GOLDMAN-EISLER, F. The distribution of pause duration in speech. *Language and Speech*, 1961, **4**, 232–237. (a)

GOLDMAN-EISLER, F. The significance of change in the rate of articulation. *Language and Speech*, 1961, **4**, 171–174. (b)

GREENHOUSE, S. W., & GEISSER, S. On methods in the analysis of profile data. *Psychometrika*, 1959, **24**, 95–112.

MAHL, G. F. Exploring emotional states by content analysis. In I. Pool (Ed.), *Trends in content analysis*. Illinois: University of Illinois Press, 1959. Pp. 89–130.

MILLER, G. A. *Language and communication*. New York: McGraw-Hill, 1951.

RACHMAN, S. J. Psychomotor behaviour and personality. Unpublished doctoral dissertation, University of London, 1961.

RAMSAY, R. W. The measurement of duration of speech. *Language and Speech*, in press.

RAVEN, J. C. *The Mill Hill Vocabulary Scale: Form 1 Senior*. London: H. K. Lewis, 1948.

ROSENTHAL, R. The effect of the experimenter on the results of psychological research. In B. A. Maher (Ed.), *Progress in experimental personality research*. Vol. 1. London: Academic Press, 1964. Pp. 80–114.

SCHEFFÉ, H. A method of judging all contrasts in the analysis of variance. *Biometrika*, 1953, **40**, 87–104.

STARKWEATHER, J. A. Variations in vocal behavior. In D. McK. Rioch & E. A. Weinstein (Eds.), *Disorders of communication*. Baltimore: Williams & Wilkins, 1964.

(Received August 16, 1965)

From H. B. Gibson and M. E. Corcoran (1975). British Journal of Psychology, *66*, 513–520, *by kind permission of the authors and Cambridge University Press*

PERSONALITY AND DIFFERENTIAL SUSCEPTIBILITY TO HYPNOSIS: FURTHER REPLICATION AND SEX DIFFERENCES

BY H. B. GIBSON AND M. E. CORCORAN

The Hatfield Polytechnic, Hatfield, Hertfordshire

Following the study of Gibson & Curran (1974), a further sample of 45 subjects was tested on the Eysenck Personality Inventory (EPI) and a slightly modified form of the Stanford Hypnotic Susceptibility Scale (SHSS) in precisely the same way. The results in this second sample were broadly the same as those obtained in the earlier study. Combining the two samples, it was found that the sex variable provided some interesting contrasts. The power of the lie scale of the EPI to predict hypnotic susceptibility observed earlier was found to be a significant effect only for males. While there was no significant difference between the sexes in terms of the means and s.D.s of the extraversion (E) and neuroticism (N) scales, when the interaction of these scales was studied males and females differed significantly. The population from the two studies ($n = 88$) was analysed by means of polar coordinates in the manner suggested by Eysenck (1966) with regard to the E and N scales. Eysenck's prediction as to hypnotic susceptibility was strikingly confirmed. These data are briefly discussed in terms of alternative approaches to hypnosis from the 'state' and the 'non-state' viewpoints.

A recent study (Gibson & Curran, 1974) was designed to replicate work on the personality correlates of differential hypnotic susceptibility which had been done at the Maudsley (Furneaux & Gibson, 1961) and at Stanford (Hilgard & Bentler, 1963). In brief, the Maudsley study, using the Maudsley Personality Inventory (MPI), had shown that subjects who scored high on the lie scale tended to be insusceptible to hypnosis; moreover, 'stable extraverts' (SE) and 'neurotic introverts' (NI) tended to be the most susceptible, and 'neurotic extraverts' (NE) and 'stable introverts' (SI) the least susceptible. The Stanford study produced results which were not only statistically significant but were diametrically opposed in direction.

The 1974 study of Gibson & Curran used the more modern personality test, the Eysenck Personality Inventory (EPI), and more sophisticated means of measuring hypnotic susceptibility (Curran & Gibson, 1974). The results supported the earlier Maudsley study but were based on a rather limited number of subjects ($n = 43$). The present study reports further work replicating the 1974 study exactly, with an independent sample of 45 subjects. It is reasoned that only by testing independent samples will the controversy eventually be resolved and some insight be gained into the extremely puzzling interaction between personality variables which account for differential susceptibility to hypnosis. This work is important not only in the field of hypnotic research, but because of its implications for the whole methodology of assessing personality by means of written questionnaires.

METHOD

Subjects

The subjects were 45 students comprising the majority of two later years' intake on the degree course in psychology which supplied the subjects for the earlier 1974 study. All were volunteers, and no pressure to participate was used, in contrast to the Stanford study.

H. B. Gibson and M. E. Corcoran

Table 1. *Basic data of samples 1 and 2 compared*

	Sample 1		Sample 2	
	Mean	S.D.	Mean	S.D.
SHSS	4·91	3·23	4·82	3·40
Lie	2·91	2·03	3·27	2·50
Extraversion	26·60	9·57	25·93	7·13
Neuroticism	23·98	8·15	23·80	9·31

Materials and procedure

These were identical with the earlier study. A full account of the procedural details is now published elsewhere (Curran & Gibson, 1974) with the factorial structure of the Stanford Hypnotic Susceptibility Scale (SHSS) as found.

RESULTS

Between sample comparisons

The basic data of the two samples in terms of the means and S.D.s of the four scales used are shown in Table 1. None of the differences between the two samples is statistically significant; in fact they are closely similar on all scales.

Lie scale and hypnotic susceptibility

In sample 1, as reported by Gibson & Curran (1974), both the L scale and the SHSS were dichotomized at their medians and shown to be negatively related. The relationship is shown below and compared with the same treatment applied to sample 2, the SHSS being dichotomized at $\leqslant 4$.

	Sample 1		
		− L	+
	+	13	9
SHSS			
	−	7	14

$r_t = -0.40$, n.s.

	Sample 2		
		− L	+
	+	13	6
SHSS			
	−	11	15

$r_t = -0.40$, n.s.

The relationship between the two scales in terms of r_t is precisely the same for these two independent samples dichotomized at their respective medians. In fact, as the L scores for sample 2 were slightly higher than for sample 1 (as shown in Table 1) the median was 1 point higher.

Extraversion, neuroticism and susceptibility

In the 1974 study following the method employed at Stanford by Hilgard & Bentler (1963), the cases in the SE and NI quadrants were pooled and compared with the pooled NE and SI quadrants with respect to hypnotic susceptibility. This treatment was also applied to the data of sample 2 and the results are compared below:

	Sample 1	
	− SHSS	+
SE and NI	9	17
NE and SI	12	5

$r_t = 0.54$, $\chi^2 = 3.98$, $P < 0.05$

	Sample 2	
	− SHSS	+
	9	10
	17	9

$r_t = 0.26$, n.s.

483

Susceptibility to hypnosis

Table 2. *Basic data of the two sexes compared*

	Males		Females	
	Mean	S.D.	Mean	S.D.
SHSS	3·89	2·63	5·62	3·08
Lie	3·45	2·55	2·88	2·06
Extraversion	25·03	7·71	27·18	8·82
Neuroticism	22·11	9·51	25·06	7·60

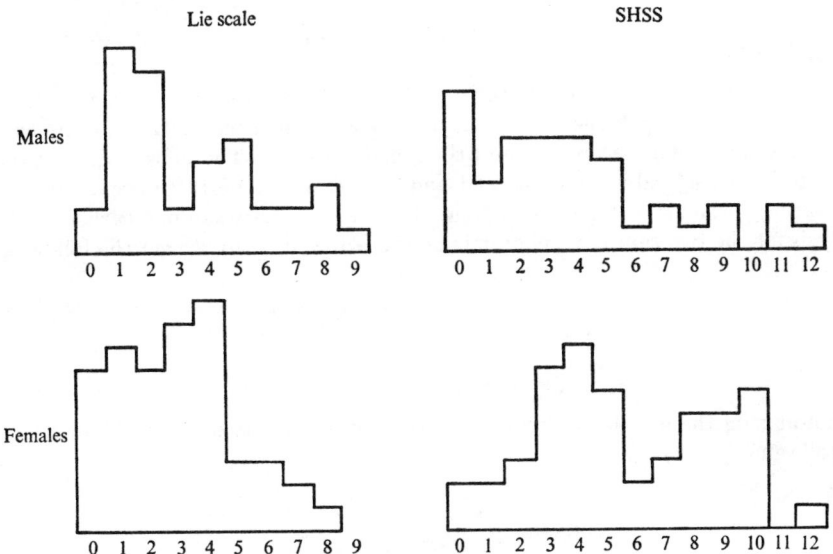

Fig. 1. Histograms of score distributions of males and females on the Lie scale and SHSS.

As shown above, the interaction in sample 2 is the same as in sample 1, although it does not reach statistical significance. In further analyses of the data in order to examine any possible differences between the two samples which might account for a lowered interaction, it was found that they differed with regard to their proportional sex composition.

Between sexes comparisons

The sex composition of the two samples was as follows:

	Sample 1	Sample 2
Males	16	22
Females	27	33

The basic data of the two sexes in terms of the means and S.D.s of all the scales are shown in Table 2.

Lie scale, hypnotic susceptibility and sex

From Table 2 it might be concluded that there was little difference between the sexes on the L scale or the SHSS. A very different picture is presented if we study

H. B. Gibson and M. E. Corcoran

Table 3. *Interaction between extraversion and neuroticism with respect to sex, with mean L score in parenthesis*

	Males	Females	Total
Stable extraverts	9 (2·44)	15 (2·73)	24
Neurotic extraverts	9 (2·89)	13 (2·77)	22
Stable introverts	15 (4·73)	5 (3·80)	20
Neurotic introverts	5 (2·40)	17 (2·82)	22
Total	38	50	88

$\chi^2 = 12\cdot35$ with 3 d.f.; $P < 0\cdot01$.

the actual histograms of scores as shown in Fig. 1. Whereas the mean L score of males is shown to be slightly higher than that of females, if their modal L scores are compared, the male modal score is 1 and the female one is 4. The male L distribution tends to be considerably more skewed and a median cut of 19/19 occurs at $\leqslant 2$. Comparing the male L scores with their SHSS scores (as was done earlier in this analysis for the two samples dichotomizing the SHSS at $\leqslant 5$), we get the following:

		− L	+
	+	11	2
SHSS			
	−	8	17

$r_t = -0\cdot76, \chi^2 = 7\cdot48, P < 0\cdot01$

Dichotomizing the female L scores at the same median cuts on both scales, we get the following:

		− L	+
	+	12	16
SHSS			
	−	10	12

$r_t = 0\cdot04$, n.s.

Thus in contrast to the significant power of the L scale to predict hypnotic susceptibility among the males, the L scale has no such power among the females. Several exploratory cutting points were also tried in the female distributions (including their own group median) but no relationship could be found.

Comparisons with extraversion and neuroticism

The E and N scores shown in Table 2 imply that there is no difference between the sexes on these two scales. However, if we examine the *interaction* between the two scales as in Table 3, a significant difference is apparent. The whole population has been divided as equally as possible into four quadrants and among the more extraverted half of the population sex has little bearing on the distribution. Among the more introverted half, however, sex makes a very significant difference; male introverts are predominantly on the stable side and female introverts on the neurotic side.

The mean L scores of each quadrant are shown in parenthesis and it can be seen that for both males and females the highest mean L score is in the SI quadrant. The statistical significance of this was tested by dichotomizing the L scale as before, and on a 2 × 2 table comparing the L scores in the SI quadrant with those in all other quadrants pooled. For the males the difference is significant ($\chi^2 = 3\cdot96$; $P < 0\cdot05$).

Susceptibility to hypnosis

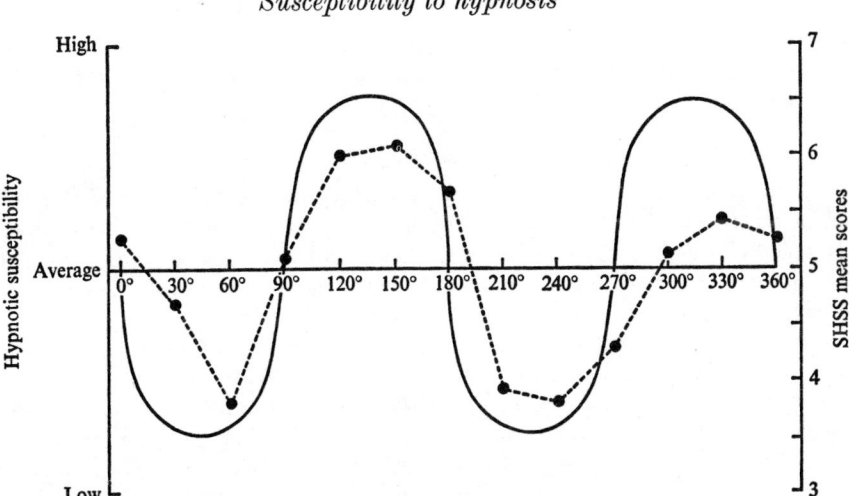

Fig. 2. Polar coordinates of the SHSS related to E and N, superimposed on the curve predicted by Eysenck (1966).

The interaction between E, N and SHSS is shown below for males and females separately.

	Males		Females	
	− SHSS +		− SHSS +	
SE and NI	7	7	12	20
NE and SI	18	6	10	8
	$r_t = 0.41$, n.s.		$r_t = 0.28$, n.s.	

The interaction of the two EPI scales with hypnotic susceptibility is thus seen to be in the same direction for both sexes, although the difference between the sexes with regard to the interaction of E with N has been shown to be significant in Table 3. If both sexes are considered in one population of 88 subjects, we get the following interaction:

	−	SHSS +
SE and NI	19	27
NE and SI	28	14

$$r_t = 0.39, \chi^2 = 4.70, P < 0.05$$

Analysis by polar coordinates

Analysis by means of dichotomizing scales invariably leads to considerable error variance in the outcome. An alternative form of analysis has been suggested by Eysenck (1966) with regard to relating E and N scores to hypnotic susceptibility. Eysenck suggested the use of polar coordinates and his actual figure has been reproduced in Fig. 2 (Fig. 8, Eysenck, 1966). Superimposed on Eysenck's theoretical curve, which he predicted would represent the relationship between suggestibility scores and the polar coordinates of E and N, are the actual data found in this study. These points were arrived at by dividing the scatter-plot on the E and N axes into 12 30° segments. Each point represents the mean of the SHSS scores lying 30° ± each of the radial cutting lines. By this method of determining the curve each individual contributes to two means and a smoother curve is obtained. It will be observed that the curve thus empirically determined conforms extremely well to the wave form which Eysenck predicted.

DISCUSSION

This study set out to do the limited task of replicating the study of Gibson & Curran (1974) with a second sample of subjects. As a total population of 88 subjects was thereby tested, certain interesting interactions with sex were discovered by serendipity, and hence a broader discussion of the significance of these results seems warranted.

Most of the major theorists in the field of hypnotic research take one of two alternative approaches. This difference is sometimes referred to in terms of the 'state' and 'non-state' viewpoints of hypnosis (Coe, 1973). The first approach treats hypnosis as a presumed altered state of awareness or 'trance' (e.g. Hilgard, 1965) as it is also considered in the traditional Pavlovian work (e.g. Pavlov, 1923). The second approach does not consider such an assumption necessary and tends to view hypnosis more in terms of the subject's goal-directed strivings and role-playing skills (e.g. Sarbin & Coe, 1972). All theorists are agreed, however, that there exists a real and reliable inter-subject difference in susceptibility. The former approach can be extended to suggesting that there are reliable personality differences, perhaps having a physiological basis, underlying differential susceptibility. The latter approach would lead us to place more importance on situational variables and explain differential susceptibility more in terms of the 'will' of the subject.

The work that has been reported here can be seen from either approach. No very strong association between personality parameters as measured by the EPI, and hypnotic susceptibility as measured by the SHSS, has been demonstrated, but at least the type of association has been shown to be *reliable* by the similar results coming from three independent studies. The unexpected power of the L scale to predict susceptibility in male subjects tends to support the argument that susceptibility is *situational* rather than a function of enduring personality parameters. Work on L scales shows that they may measure situational variables; subjects will 'fake good' or 'fake bad' according to the circumstances in which the test is administered (e.g. Salas, 1968). However, the whole of the association cannot be explained as an artifact of the L scale, for it is manifest with females also, and the L scale does not predict hypnotic susceptibility for them.

It is pertinent at this juncture to discuss why the L scale should be different both in distribution (see Fig. 1) and implication for the two sexes. Males are generally less well-behaved than females and society recognizes this difference, e.g. in the grossly different rates of delinquency among males and females. This difference is certainly reflected in children's lie scale data where males score fairly consistently lower than females (Gibson, 1964; S. B. G. Eysenck *et al.*, 1966). One might have expected the male students in this study to have a lower L scale distribution than the female students; instead, the males have a lower mode but a higher mean due to the more pronounced skew of their distribution. It is suggested that those males in the upper part of the distribution are exhibiting a tendency to resist experimental investigation of their personality parameters, and that this defensive trait is manifest in the

Susceptibility to hypnosis

hypnosis situation. Higher L scores for females may be closer to objective self-report and thus have less implication of defensiveness which might imply resistance to hypnotic induction. The 'high liars' have not been excluded from the analysis as in the Maudsley study, and it may be seen that because they are rather more frequent in the NI quadrant, this enhances the observed effects, at least for males. It is no more meaningful to state that 'high liars tend to represent themselves as stable introverts' than it is to state that 'stable introverts tend to give high lie scores'. One cannot determine which is the more meaningful statement.

In the manual of the EPI it is stated that 'Correlations with sex are not large, because items giving large sex differences were eliminated during the construction of the inventory' (Eysenck & Eysenck, 1964, p. 18). This may be so, but the present study has shown a significant difference between the sexes with regard to the *interaction* of E and N. It will be of interest to see if other researchers using the EPI find the same sex difference if they use the same method of interaction analysis rather than just reporting means and s.d.s.

If the data on the L scale in relation to hypnotic susceptibility, for males, lends some support to the situational, 'non-state' view of hypnosis, the study as a whole cannot be said to do so. It must be acknowledged that Eysenck (1966) has had his prediction strikingly confirmed by the data shown in Fig. 2. All the detailed qualifications of L scale differences, of sex differences and various interactions do not override the lawful relations between E and N with regard to hypnotic susceptibility which are apparent when we study a large enough population. If Eysenck's theory is sound (Eysenck, 1967) then there is an underlying biological basis for the parameters of E and N and this would be in harmony with a 'state' theory of hypnosis.

It must be admitted regretfully that these additional data bring us no nearer the resolution of the conflict between the Maudsley and the Stanford studies referred to earlier. Re-reading the latter study we find that 87 per cent of their subjects were males, a feature which makes their finding of a *positive* association between high L scoring and hypnotic susceptibility even more surprising in the light of the findings of the present study, and which calls for independent testing in other laboratories.

REFERENCES

COE, W. C. (1973). Experimental designs and the state–nonstate issue in hypnosis. *Am. J. clin. Hypnosis* **16**, 118–128.

CURRAN, J. D. & GIBSON, H. B. (1974). Critique of the Stanford Hypnotic Susceptibility Scale: British usage and factorial structure. *Percept. mot. Skills* **39**, 695–704.

EYSENCK, H. J. (1966). Personality and experimental psychology. *Bull. Br. psychol. Soc.* **19**, no. 62, 1–28.

EYSENCK, H. J. (1967). *The Biological Basis of Behaviour*. Springfield, Ill.: Thomas.

EYSENCK, H. J. & EYSENCK, S. B. G. (1964). *Manual of the Eysenck Personality Inventory*. London: University of London Press.

EYSENCK, S. B. G., SYED, I. A. & EYSENCK, H. J. (1966). Desirability response set in children. *Br. J. educ. Psychol.* **36**, 87–90.

FURNEAUX, W. D. & GIBSON, H. B. (1961). The Maudsley Personality Inventory as a predictor of susceptibility to hypnosis. *Int. J. clin. exp. Hypnosis* **9**, 167–177.

GIBSON, H. B. (1964). A lie scale for the Junior Maudsley Personality Inventory. *Br. J. educ. Psychol.* **34**, 120–124.

GIBSON, H. B. & CURRAN, J. D. (1974). Hypnotic susceptibility and personality: a replication study. *Br. J. Psychol.* **65**, 283–291.

H. B. Gibson and M. E. Corcoran

Hilgard, E. R. (1965). *Hypnotic Susceptibility*. New York: Harcourt, Brace & World.

Hilgard, E. R. & Bentler, P. M. (1963). Predicting hypnotizability from the Maudsley Personality Inventory. *Br. J. Psychol.* **54**, 63–69.

Pavlov, I. P. (1923). The identity of inhibition with sleep and hypnosis. *Sci. Mon.* **17**, 603–608.

Salas, R. G. (1968). Fakeability of responses on the Eysenck Personality Inventory. *Aust. J. Psychol.* **20**, 55–57.

Sarbin, T. R. & Coe, W. C. (1972). *Hypnosis: a Social Psychological Analysis of Influence Communication*. New York: Holt, Rinehart & Winston.

(*Manuscript received 5 February* 1975; *revised manuscript received 19 March* 1975)

From H. J. Eysenck (1971). British Journal of Psychiatry, *118*, 593–608, *by kind permission of the author and the Royal Medico-Psychological Association*

Personality and Sexual Adjustment

By H. J. EYSENCK*

INTRODUCTION

In view of the considerable importance attached to sexual adjustment by many psychologists and psychiatrists, it is disappointing that very little work seems in fact to have been done in this field. There are, it is true, surveys of 'normal' sexual behaviour, such as those associated with Kinsey, but these are characterized on the whole by the serious limitation of using entirely descriptive statistics; these are useful in a limited sense, but are not very informative. The value of a mean of $2 \cdot 34$ for the number of times that members of a given sample indulge in intercourse during the week is doubtful when it is realized that some members of the sample have intercourse once or twice a year, while others have it several times a night; even if one could take the unaided recall of such events very seriously, and even if the rate for a given person were less fluctuating than it probably is, nevertheless when variances are as large as these means have little meaning or relevance. Clearly the important question centres on quite a different problem, namely that of personality traits and other factors giving rise to these very marked individual differences in sexual behaviour and adjustment. Kinsey and his followers have concentrated on the factors of social class and age, perhaps because these are relatively easy to ascertain; it is not so easy to ascertain the psychological factors involved, as many critics of Kinsey's work have pointed out. Nor have psychiatrists, in spite of their professional interest in this field, been more forthcoming; apart from isolated statements about the lower fertility of psychotics, the loss of libido in depression, its excess in manic states, and the

widespread sexual troubles of neurotics, little serious and detailed work appears to have been done to relate personality traits, or even descriptive diagnostic labels, to specific types of sexual behaviour. Psychologists have been equally remiss; apart from a few undistinguished and not very meaningful studies reviewed by the writer (Eysenck, 1971) little use has been made of the well-established research methodologies and psychometric tests available to them for use in such a situation.

The only apparent exceptions to this general rule are two studies both of which are based on the writer's general theory of personality description in terms of E (extraversion) and N (neuroticism); this theory enables us to make fairly specific deductions regarding behaviour and attitudes in the sexual field (Eysenck, 1967; Eysenck and Eysenck, 1969). Both these studies (Giese and Schmidt, 1968; Eysenck, 1971) make very similar deductions, and as these are also relevant to the study here to be described they may with advantage be summarized here in brief. As far as E is concerned, these deductions are based on the postulated greater cortical arousal of introverts, leading (a) to lower sensory thresholds and (b) to better and quicker formation of conditional responses; there is ample experimental support for these two points (Eysenck, 1967). According to theory, extraverts, having higher sensory thresholds, would seek for stronger sensory stimulation ('sensation-seeking behaviour'); being less easy to condition, they would form the conditioned responses necessary for 'socialization' less readily, and would therefore be less likely to behave in a socially approved manner. The theory is of course much more complex than this but even in this brief statement will suffice to mediate the following predictions: 1. Extraverts will have intercourse *earlier* than introverts. 2. Extraverts will have intercourse

* I am indebted to Miss Maureen Castle and Mr. Maurice Yaffe for help in collecting the data here analysed.

The assistance of the Maudsley and Bethlem Royal Research Fund is acknowledged.

more frequently than introverts. 3. Extraverts will have intercourse with *more different partners*. 4. Extraverts will have intercourse in *more diverse positions* than introverts. 5. Extraverts will indulge in more *varied* sexual behaviour outside intercourse. 6. Extraverts will indulge in longer pre-coital love play than introverts. These predictions are made with some confidence because they represent fairly direct deductions from psychological theory, based on large numbers of laboratory investigations of sensory thresholds, conditioning, alternation and other types of behaviour of introverts and extraverts; such predictions can of course still be disconfirmed, but at least the expectations are clear-cut and follow from theory.

With respect to N, predictions are less clear, and are therefore made with less confidence. On the whole one would perhaps expect high N scorers, who are theoretically characterized by a labile and overactive autonomic system, and are thus susceptible to fear and anxiety to a degree which may make them less likely to indulge in sexual behaviour, to worry about sex, to be disgusted by sex, and to have fewer contacts with sexual partners; this would be particularly true of unmarried subjects, because of the well-known difficulties in social relations of high N scores (Eysenck and Eysenck, 1969). There being no reason to assume that high N scorers would have less sexual drive than low N scorers, one might assume also that the reduction in direct outlets postulated above might lead to substitute outlets being adopted; masturbation, pornography and prostitution suggest themselves in this context. These predictions are more speculative than those concerned with E, and are not offered in any spirit of confidence, but they may be useful in outlining the field of study. The general predictions made are perhaps supported by the frequent observation of a direct connection between neurotic pathology and sexual difficulties, but in dealing with non-pathological samples such considerations may carry little weight.

A third general trait of personality has been investigated in the present study, namely the so-called 'psychoticism' dimension (P for short). This variable and its measurement have been discussed by H. J. Eysenck and S. B. G. Eysenck (1968), and by S. G. B. Eysenck and H. J. Eysenck (1968, 1969a, 1969b); essentially this factor purports to describe the personality underlying psychoses of all types (approximating perhaps to some degree the 'psychotic triad' of the MMPI). Traits such as hostile, impersonal, cruel, play a large part in this factor; details of the items included in the questionnaire are given in the papers quoted above. Prediction is difficult, as very little is in fact known about this factor. The lack of personal involvement, the lack of human feeling, and the cruelty/hostility feelings which play such a large part in this factor suggest that normal sexual relations would not be likely to be associated with high P scoring, and that instead we might find relations reduced to a more starkly biological level. Again, it should be stressed that this is not a firm prediction, but a surmise based on the psychological content of the factor in question; disconfirmation of such speculative predictions would not be unexpected.

Giese and Schmidt (1968), using a very short scale for the measurement of E and N, administered questionnaires regarding their sexual conduct to over 6,000 German students, both male and female; most of these were unmarried. It would not of course be possible to quote in extenso the results of their study, which has been published in book form; some relevant facts are reproduced in Table I. It will be seen that extraverts masturbate less, pet to orgasm more, have coitus more frequently, have coitus earlier, adopt more different positions in coitus, indulge in longer pre-coital love play, and practise fellatio and cunnilingus more frequently. It should be added that on some of these items differences are much greater for men than for women; this is expected on the grounds that in our society it is men who set the pace in sexual relationships, so that their personality is expressed more clearly in the procedures adopted. High N scorers (male) masturbate more frequently, have greater desire for coitus, and claim to have spontaneous erections more frequently; females have less frequent orgasm and stronger menstrual pains. No questions were asked regarding P, and consequently no results are available. (In this

BY H. J. EYSENCK

Table only unmarried students are included. Groups were subdivided according to their extraversion score into introverts (E_1), ambiverts (E_2), and extraverts (E_3). There were more men than women in this sample.)

Eysenck (1971), using a personality inventory measuring P, E and N, tested 423 male and 379 female unmarried university students with a 19 item scale of sexual behaviour, ranging from kissing to 'soixante-neuf'; factor analysis of this scale resulted in three meaningful factors identified as *petting*, *intercourse*, and *perversion*. (The term 'perversion' is here used to refer to cunnilingus, fellatio, and unusual positions for sexual intercourse; this use is somewhat arbitrary, but is adopted for ease of reference.) N was correlated negatively with all three factors; high N scorers did less petting, had less intercourse and took less part in perverted practices. E was correlated positively with all three factors, but particularly factors 1 and 2; correlations with 3 were very small. P, on the other hand, had correlations with factor 3, and hardly at all with 1 and 2; in other words, perverted behaviour was related to P rather than to E. These correlations, in so far as comparisons can be made, are similar to those reported by Giese and Schmidt (1968),

and bear out on the whole the set of predictions made on the basis of the writer's theory. It should be noted, however, that all the facts summarized so far deal with sexual *activities*, which are often circumscribed by external restrictions and opportunities; of equal interest would be possible differences in *attitudes* towards sex of persons differing in respect of E, N or P. It is the purpose of this paper to report such a study; predictions are of course similar to those already discussed.

DESIGN OF RESEARCH

The sample used in this research was the same as that described in connection with the previous study (Eysenck, 1971); it consisted of 423 unmarried male students and 379 unmarried female students. These had been administered the P, E and N inventory and the 19-question sexual questionnaire mentioned above; details about administration and structure of sample are given in the previous paper. In addition all subjects filled in a Sexual Attitudes Inventory, consisting of almost 100 questions; this is reproduced as Appendix A of this paper. A number of the questions were taken from, or adapted from, the Sex Inventory of Thorne

TABLE I

	Males: (percents shown in italics)			Females:		
	E_1	E_2	E_3	E_1	E_2	E_3
(1) Masturbation at present	*86*	*80*	*72*	*47*	*43*	*39*
(2) Petting: at 17	*16*	*28*	*40*	*15*	*19*	*24*
Petting: at 19	*31*	*48*	*56*	*30*	*44*	*47*
Petting: at present age	*57*	*72*	*78*	*62*	*71*	*76*
(3) Coitus: at 17	*5*	*13*	*21*	*4*	*4*	*8*
Coitus: at 19	*15*	*31*	*45*	*12*	*20*	*29*
Coitus: at present age	*47*	*70*	*77*	*42*	*57*	*71*
(4) Median frequency of coitus per month (sexually active students only)	*3·0*	*3·7*	*5·5*	*3·1*	*4·5*	*7·5*
(5) Number of coitus partners in last 12 months; unmarried students only 1	*75*	*64*	*46*	*72*	*77*	*60*
2–3	*18*	*25*	*30*	*25*	*17*	*23*
4+	*7*	*12*	*25*	*4*	*6*	*17*
(6) Long pre-coital sex play	*21*	*25*	*28*	*21*	*16*	*18*
(7) Cunnilingus	*52*	*62*	*64*	*58*	*69*	*69*
(8) Fellatio	*53*	*60*	*69*	*53*	*59*	*61*
(9) More than 3 different coital positions	*10*	*16*	*26*	*12*	*18*	*13*
(10) Experience of orgasm nearly always	—	—	—	*17*	*32*	*29*

Sexual activities of introverts (E_1), ambiverts (E_2) and extraverts (E_3). From Giese and Schmidt (1968).

(1966); others were specifically written to investigate certain theoretical expectations and predictions. Also given in the Appendix are the overall percentages of 'Yes' answers of the male and female students to those questions, in so far as the questions can be answered by a simple 'Yes' or 'No'; these figures will be referred to again in connection with our discussion of sex differences. Several questions had to be changed in dealing with men and women; only the male set is given in the Appendix. Question 76, for example, is reworded in the passive sense for women: 'I get very excited when men touch my breasts.' These changes will be very obvious in each case, and do not require more detailed documentation.

Subjects were divided into groups for the purpose of analysis, taking each of the three personality dimensions in turn. Those high on a given factor are referred to as P+, or N+, or E+; those low on a given factor are referred to as P−, or N−, or E−. Subjects average on a given factor are referred to as P=, or N=, or E=. The numbers in these groups are as equal as possible, but as scores on the inventory scales rise by unit steps it was not always possible to prevent group sizes from becoming dissimilar. Table II shows the actual numbers in each group, for men and women separately.

Most comparisons in this article will be made in terms of percentage 'yes' answers, and in view of the large number of these it would be impossible to give significance levels in each case. Table III gives the S.E._p values for N = 400 and for N = 120, for different levels of p (p is the proportion of 'yes' answers, or the proportion of 'no' answers, whichever is the smaller). By and large, differences of 12 per cent will be significant for the N = 120 value, i.e. for comparisons between the personality groups, and differences of 6 per cent will be significant for the N = 400 values i.e., for comparisons between the sexes; these values will be smaller for lower values of p. More important perhaps is the consideration that in each case where personality values are concerned there are three groups, so that if there is a monotonic relation this adds considerably to the significance of the observed differences. It would of course have been possible to have carried out analyses of variance for each comparison, but the results would have been prohibitively voluminous to print, and in any case only apply to single comparisons, not to large sets given below. Furthermore, we are concerned, not so much with individual values but rather with groups of items measuring certain factors; congruence in these comparisons again validates conclusions which might not be significant for single questions.

TABLE II

	Male	Female
P +	110	87
P =	138	142
P −	175	150
Total	423	379
E +	125	121
E =	156	133
E −	142	125
Total	423	379
N +	139	116
N =	135	137
N −	149	126
Total	423	379

Number of subjects in different groups.

TABLE III

P =	N = 400	N = 120
5%	1·0897	1·9896
10%	1·5	2·7386
15%	1·7854	3·2596
20%	2·0000	3·6515
25%	2·1651	3·9528
30%	2·2913	4·1833
35%	2·3848	4·3541
40%	2·4495	4·4721
45%	2·4875	4·5415
50%	2·5	4·5644

Size of S.E._p for different values of P and N.

RESULTS

The relationships existing between the individual questions and the personality factors P, E and N are given in detail in Table IV, V

BY H. J. EYSENCK

and VI. Each Table lists, for men and women separately, the percentage of 'Yes' answers given to each question by high, average and low scorers on the P scale (Table IV), the E scale (Table V), and the N scale (Table VI). In addition, each Table lists the correlations between each question and the personality variable in question, again separately for men and women. These two ways of setting out the

TABLE IV

	\+	P_M =	−	r_p	\+	P_F =	−	r_p
1.	35	36	42	−·06	44	61	67	−·17
2.	27	47	58	−·17	64	85	85	−·26
3.	21	15	25	−·05	37	44	45	−·14
4.	29	38	48	−·13	53	58	65	−·10
5.	11	18	18	−·10	6	25	33	−·30
6.	1	7	5	−·06	3	15	16	−·15
7.	51	49	43	·09	49	48	36	+·13
8.	5	6	9	−·04	15	23	23	−·11
9.	59	53	53	·08	55	48	39	+·09
10.	65	59	59	·05	43	41	31	+·07
11.	32	19	26	·09	16	6	5	+·22
12.	5	6	5	·00	7	6	4	−·01
13.	47	49	35	·12	24	8	8	+·22
14.	66	60	65	·04	75	77	71	+·04
15.	14	6	11	·06	3	6	5	−·06
16.	6	1	3	·10	5	2	1	+·08
17.	29	36	39	−·08	41	39	43	−·00
18.	13	14	11	·01	21	18	29	−·06
19.	12	14	8	·06	16	18	15	−·01
20.	55	51	45	·07	28	27	23	+·04
21.	38	43	46	−·08	40	32	37	+·01
22.	45	39	34	·10	25	27	18	+·07
23.	32	36	38	−·01	25	29	23	+·03
24.	2	2	2	−·02	7	4	11	−·03
25.	30	28	29	−·02	40	43	40	−·00
26.	73	69	63	·10	92	70	64	+·23
27.	20	14	13	·10	22	9	11	+·14
28.	36	25	25	·11	26	14	16	+·11
29.	22	17	19	·01	33	27	21	+·13
30.	17	15	15	·02	18	6	7	+·15
31.	67	68	76	−·04	85	77	81	+·03
32.	24	23	22	·02	15	15	7	+·04
33.	76	59	66	·06	32	35	27	+·10
34.	33	32	26	·07	31	25	20	+·09
35.	15	10	13	·04	8	7	6	+·10
36.	5	2	3	·12	3	6	4	+·04
37.	51	48	58	−·12	48	49	46	−·02
38.	95	96	93	·03	100	96	97	+·09
39.	90	86	89	−·00	69	72	66	−·01
40.	52	38	43	·07	48	31	31	+·15
41.	91	81	82	·09	66	53	43	+·19
42.	7	6	9	−·02	6	25	27	−·23
43.	68	51	61	·04	30	30	21	+·08
44.	11	19	23	−·17	43	73	69	−·29

TABLE IV (*cont.*)

	\+	P_M =	−	r_p	\+	P_F =	−	r_p
45.	5	4	9	−·08	13	37	35	−·25
46.	32	22	22	·14	7	2	3	+·08
47.	61	62	60	·02	15	8	5	+·20
48.	21	16	17	−·01	24	27	27	−·02
49.	8	5	8	−·03	11	15	12	−·06
50.	35	34	29	·08	32	27	23	+·07
51.	27	20	27	−·02	16	15	13	+·05
52.	13	4	5	·21	5	0	1	+·22
53.	29	20	25	·08	23	16	9	+·18
54.	61	72	65	−·00	80	76	83	−·07
55.	5	1	1	·10	5	2	3	+·04
56.	15	9	12	−·01	7	6	5	+·06
57.	23	25	29	−·05	22	21	27	−·08
58.	25	20	26	−·01	14	14	18	−·04
59.	93	90	94	−·03	86	78	74	+·10
60.	30	17	21	·05	16	13	11	+·06
61.	85	82	85	·03	78	62	61	+·14
62.	7	10	15	−·04	33	40	51	−·12
63.	24	13	13	·08	20	22	19	+·06
64.	55	61	55	·03	56	58	45	+·03
65.	32	26	23	·09	28	15	15	+·13
66.	9	7	10	−·03	8	4	13	−·04
67.	37	34	31	·07	29	25	18	+·16
68.	91	87	88	·01	79	65	55	+·19
69.	8	3	3	·08	20	20	24	−·08
70.	62	42	34	·25	10	8	5	+·09
71.	56	55	46	·11	44	42	42	+·09
72.	75	68	64	·10	55	57	50	+·04
73.	30	23	12	·21	23	14	3	+·18
74.	5	6	5	−·06	6	11	9	−·06
75.	79	67	75	·01	59	59	51	+·06
76.	58	52	61	−·06	45	51	39	+·03
77.	39	38	22	·16	23	11	11	+·17
78.	72	78	73	−·02	74	70	68	+·08
79.	82	75	65	·18	53	34	26	+·32
80.	43	45	27	·20	60	42	27	+·23
81.	62	63	63	·02	21	8	5	+·27
82.	39	45	41	·01	11	8	7	+·13
83.	49	36	40	·12	16	13	9	+·12
84.	69	58	53	·18	41	30	28	+·15
85.	58	64	64	−·01	47	36	21	+·24
86.	59	53	46	·12	55	43	47	+·07
87.	5	4	9	−·02	3	14	17	−·14
88.	33	33	31	−·01	31	27	22	+·00
89.	19	7	5	·23	2	2	1	+·12
90.	9	5	6	·11	1	5	3	−·06
91.	72	62	57	·16	57	35	33	+·22
92.	87	82	73	·20	52	33	31	+·20
93.	82	75	73	·09	57	37	33	+·25
94.	74	64	51	·21	7	3	3	+·18

Percentage of 'yes' answers for P+, P= and P− scores for 94 items of inventory; also correlations between P and each item. Data are given separately for men and women.

PERSONALITY AND SEXUAL ADJUSTMENT

TABLE V

	E_M				E_F			
	+	=	−	r_E	+	=	−	r_E
1.	31	38	45	−·12	50	63	64	−·15
2.	42	54	49	−·08	77	86	78	−·09
3.	17	23	22	−·05	40	50	39	−·07
4.	42	42	37	−·09	58	66	54	·03
5.	14	13	20	−·04	21	23	27	−·08
6.	3	3	6	−·03	8	14	16	−·06
7.	45	49	42	·03	54	44	33	·18
8.	6	7	8	−·04	23	20	21	−·01
9.	63	55	46	·13	56	45	38	·15
10.	58	60	64	−·06	36	42	34	·02
11.	16	24	34	−·18	8	4	12	−·13
12.	5	7	4	−·00	5	4	8	−·09
13.	51	40	39	·09	14	11	11	·04
14.	67	62	63	·05	75	74	74	−·01
15.	7	6	17	−·17	4	5	6	−·18
16.	2	1	6	−·07	1	2	4	−·09
17.	42	35	30	·07	50	43	31	·14
18.	14	12	12	·00	20	20	30	−·12
19.	7	9	16	−·17	14	15	19	−·11
20.	40	47	62	−·19	23	28	26	−·05
21.	48	40	42	·00	31	40	37	−·03
22.	33	36	47	−·11	17	20	32	−·17
23.	23	33	49	−·27	12	18	46	−·36
24.	2	1	3	−·01	4	10	7	−·06
25.	25	33	27	·00	48	35	42	−·00
26.	77	65	62	·06	80	71	68	·16
27.	14	15	15	·00	12	11	14	·00
28.	22	28	33	−·08	14	15	24	−·15
29.	17	19	22	−·05	30	28	20	·08
30.	15	15	18	−·03	11	5	12	−·04
31.	84	76	54	·29	93	86	62	·40
32.	13	23	31	−·18	12	11	14	−·05
33.	71	64	65	·05	37	32	25	·12
34.	23	28	37	−·09	22	23	29	−·07
35.	3	13	19	−·19	6	5	10	−·12
36.	2	2	7	−·12	3	7	3	−·02
37.	50	52	56	−·07	43	54	45	−·07
38.	93	96	94	−·03	98	95	98	·01
39.	90	85	89	·02	76	67	64	·12
40.	42	46	43	−·05	37	38	29	·08
41.	87	82	83	·01	58	53	45	·16
42.	6	8	8	−·09	15	22	27	−·13
43.	57	60	63	−·03	32	28	20	·18
44.	11	20	23	−·19	53	70	70	−·19
45.	3	4	11	−·14	21	35	35	−·14
46.	28	26	20	·13	5	2	4	·03
47.	56	63	62	·00	8	7	10	−·04
48.	11	20	21	−·11	29	25	26	·00
49.	7	7	7	·02	10	16	13	−·03
50.	32	38	25	·08	32	28	20	·11
51.	10	22	41	−·29	9	10	25	−·27
52.	6	4	8	−·07	1	2	2	−·07
53.	20	31	20	·03	12	14	18	−·03
54.	83	70	47	·28	87	86	66	·27
55.	0	1	5	−·15	3	2	4	−·10
56.	2	8	25	−·34	1	4	12	−·26

TABLE V (cont.)

	E_M				E_F			
	+	=	−	r_E	+	=	−	r_E
57.	15	27	35	−·17	17	20	33	−·13
58.	17	23	30	−·11	8	14	24	−·24
59.	96	96	86	·11	86	80	70	·21
60.	14	21	30	−·15	15	9	16	−·05
61.	91	79	84	·01	69	64	62	·05
62.	10	12	12	·01	39	44	45	−·03
63.	8	19	19	−·14	15	21	25	−·09
64.	62	58	53	·07	64	46	48	·14
65.	22	28	29	−·03	13	15	26	−·15
66.	6	7	13	−·15	3	5	16	−·23
67.	37	33	31	·06	26	27	15	·08
68.	91	93	81	·13	71	62	60	·10
69.	2	4	7	−·15	15	20	30	−·20
70.	52	44	37	·14	13	5	3	·06
71.	54	54	47	·02	47	45	35	·08
72.	70	68	66	·05	57	57	47	·08
73.	23	21	17	·04	14	12	10	−·02
74.	6	4	6	−·00	9	9	10	−·09
75.	70	74	77	−·05	60	58	49	·11
76.	55	58	58	−·04	51	44	40	·07
77.	48	30	19	·22	19	11	12	·09
78.	71	76	75	−·04	72	71	67	·02
79.	76	71	72	·03	41	34	30	·14
80.	34	37	40	−·04	50	35	35	·04
81.	58	65	65	−·03	10	10	9	·00
82.	40	42	43	−·01	12	8	6	·12
83.	42	33	49	−·04	11	14	10	−·02
84.	66	58	52	·11	33	34	29	·07
85.	68	66	54	·12	38	31	29	·09
86.	59	49	48	·05	51	50	40	·09
87.	3	6	9	−·09	14	11	14	−·07
88.	34	30	32	·01	25	32	20	·04
89.	10	10	8	·07	4	1	2	·04
90.	5	6	9	−·02	6	3	2	·01
91.	73	59	58	·08	44	38	36	·10
92.	88	79	73	·14	41	32	38	·06
93.	82	78	68	·15	41	41	38	·06
94.	75	63	47	·21	6	3	2	·09

Percentage of 'yes' answers for E+, E= and E− scores for 94 items of inventory; also correlations between E and each item. Data are given separately for men and women.

information are complementary; the percentages show clearly whether the regressions are linear, a point assumed in calculating meaningful product-moment correlations, while the correlations give a single figure to indicate the strength of the observed relationship, as well as its direction. These three Tables constitute the basic data of this study. In addition, a factor analysis was carried out on the intercorrelations

BY H. J. EYSENCK

TABLE VI

	N_M +	=	−	r_N	N_F +	=	−	r_N
1.	43	36	36	·10	60	61	56	·03
2.	50	50	46	·07	79	82	79	−·05
3.	28	19	16	·11	47	44	39	·06
4.	25	41	53	−·27	49	53	77	−·30
5.	17	19	13	·01	20	28	22	−·05
6.	3	4	6	−·12	6	15	16	−·17
7.	57	47	34	·25	53	37	42	·12
8.	8	7	5	·05	25	20	20	−·02
9.	59	58	48	·07	48	44	47	·02
10.	64	61	57	·09	42	39	31	·14
11.	37	22	16	·25	13	9	2	·20
12.	5	6	5	·04	8	7	2	·09
13.	45	44	41	·02	11	13	11	·00
14.	64	61	66	−·07	71	73	79	−·05
15.	18	5	7	·15	8	4	3	·10
16.	6	2	1	·11	4	2	1	·05
17.	28	36	42	−·16	25	45	52	−·24
18.	14	16	7	·08	25	26	18	·07
19.	14	10	8	·11	24	15	10	·15
20.	70	47	34	·31	35	29	13	·24
21.	39	41	49	−·08	30	36	41	−·13
22.	53	37	26	·29	34	26	10	·28
23.	42	36	30	·12	27	28	22	·04
24.	4	1	1	·09	9	7	6	·04
25.	38	32	17	·20	55	39	30	·23
26.	59	66	77	−·11	79	73	67	·11
27.	22	11	11	·16	19	10	10	·11
28.	40	29	15	·25	29	15	10	·21
29.	29	20	9	·24	35	27	16	·23
30.	23	14	10	·17	14	7	7	·09
31.	64	73	76	−·12	79	77	85	−·05
32.	35	22	11	·26	23	7	6	·19
33.	73	64	62	·14	38	27	29	·03
34.	39	33	18	·18	39	22	14	·27
35.	24	11	2	·33	12	7	2	·18
36.	6	2	2	·14	6	4	3	·05
37.	55	49	54	·04	49	48	45	·02
38.	95	95	94	·01	97	96	98	·02
39.	91	88	85	·08	60	71	75	−·15
40.	48	41	41	·11	41	35	29	·08
41.	90	85	77	·18	56	50	49	·05
42.	7	9	6	·01	15	27	21	−·07
43.	65	61	54	·15	34	23	24	·05
44.	19	21	15	·05	72	61	63	·04
45.	8	7	4	·07	28	34	29	−·03
46.	27	21	24	·04	4	2	4	·01
47.	65	64	54	·08	13	7	5	·13
48.	30	17	7	·27	48	21	12	·33
49.	9	9	3	·14	16	13	10	·03
50.	42	30	26	·18	34	25	22	·14
51.	41	16	17	·30	23	15	6	·21
52.	14	2	2	·27	3	1	0	·08
53.	33	24	16	·16	23	15	7	·19
54.	53	68	77	−·21	72	80	87	−·14
55.	4	1	0	·18	4	3	2	·04
56.	20	7	9	·22	8	6	3	·11

TABLE VI (cont.)

	N_M +	=	−	r_N	N_F +	=	−	r_N
57.	35	23	20	·15	34	23	13	·15
58.	32	22	17	·23	22	15	10	·11
59.	88	95	94	−·07	78	77	80	·02
60.	44	16	7	·42	28	11	2	·32
61.	81	84	87	−·07	66	66	63	·09
62.	9	13	13	−·08	44	43	41	−·06
63.	30	11	6	·34	39	15	9	·33
64.	60	59	52	·06	53	53	52	−·02
65.	36	27	17	·19	29	16	10	·20
66.	16	4	6	·18	10	9	5	·05
67.	30	39	32	·01	30	20	20	·06
68.	85	90	91	−·10	72	60	63	·05
69.	6	4	3	·08	27	19	20	·04
70.	47	42	43	·05	8	7	7	−·05
71.	53	53	49	·02	45	42	40	·03
72.	74	63	67	·03	60	49	53	·05
73.	25	21	15	·18	16	15	5	·12
74.	4	7	4	·09	9	9	10	−·03
75.	77	71	73	·06	57	55	55	·02
76.	54	63	55	·05	52	44	40	·05
77.	35	33	29	·02	14	16	12	·02
78.	75	72	76	−·01	72	72	67	·05
79.	71	71	76	−·06	41	36	28	·12
80.	50	36	26	·21	53	39	29	·18
81.	65	67	57	·10	12	9	8	·05
82.	47	46	33	·16	11	7	8	·09
83.	50	41	33	·14	16	9	11	·07
84.	60	56	60	·01	36	31	29	·06
85.	63	61	63	−·01	41	28	29	·12
86.	53	49	52	·02	58	46	39	·10
87.	11	4	3	·11	9	16	13	−·06
88.	33	32	30	·02	28	24	26	−·04
89.	9	8	10	·05	2	2	2	·01
90.	10	4	5	·09	3	5	2	·01
91.	68	62	59	·05	45	37	36	·08
92.	83	79	77	·09	41	36	33	·02
93.	77	76	75	·00	49	38	34	·10
94.	61	59	64	·05	3	4	4	·10

Percentage of 'yes' answers for N+, N= and N− scores for 94 items of inventory; also correlations between N and each item. Data are given separately for men and women.

between the items, for men and women separately; the fourteen factors which emerged will not be here discussed in detail, as this would take us beyond the confines of our concern with personality factors determining sexual adjustment; occasional mention will be made of these factors in our discussion when this seems helpful. The nature of the factors may be surmised from the labels given them.

The data given in Tables IV, V and VI

clearly require considerable effort to work through for the reader, and for his convenience an attempt has been made in this section to interpret these numerous figures and discuss their import. Inevitably, certain subjective elements will enter into such an interpretation, and the reader will wish to refer back to the primary data in order to make his own decisions about the accuracy and adequacy of the interpretation offered. Discussion will be arranged in such a way that each personality factor is taken in turn; brief mention will be made of the main factor loadings on the relevant sex factors, and then a summary will be given of the individual items loading significantly (above ·1) on the personality factor in question.

The first personality factor to be discussed is P. This presents an interesting combination of promiscuity, pre-marital sex and curiosity with hostility and lack of satisfaction; the picture is of a 'lady killer' who has little love or kindness towards his victims, and who is on the whole dissatisfied with his sex life. None of the loadings of P on these sex factors are very large (·3, with pre-marital sex, is the highest, followed by ·25 for promiscuity), but they form a meaningful pattern, and show congruence for the two sexes.

The highest loading individual items refer to lack of concern with virginity (items 5 and 26), liking for impersonal sex (2 and 13), pre-marital sex (42 and 45), libertinism (44 and 79), liking for pornography (47, 81 and 84), liking for prostitution instead of marriage (85, 89), dislike of sexual censorship (91, 92, 93, 94), promiscuity (77), voyeurism (83), and strong sexual excitement (52, 3, 6, 7, 33, 37, 41, 46, 53, 82). These items indicate an intense preoccupation with sex in its biological aspect; other items indicate the morbid and indeed pathological aspect of the high P scorer's attitude. He considers himself deprived sexually (11) and dissatisfied with his sex life (4, 22), in spite of the fact that he has had more sexual experience than the low P scorer; he feels hostility to his sex partner (73, 80), is troubled by perverted thoughts (28, 29), and has homosexual leanings (16, 30, 36, 40). Taking one's pleasures where one finds them (70) has clearly not brought him much happiness;

the libertinism is marred by a pathological streak which may justify the clinical connotations of the 'P' label.

The high E scorer is also characterized by the promiscuity factor, but in him it is allied most prominently with lack of nervousness and with satisfaction. The highest loadings are with lack of nervousness (·35) and with promiscuity (·27); here apparently we have a happy philanderer, who derives satisfaction from his sexual behaviour. The individual items having the highest loadings emphasize the extravert's social facility with the opposite sex (23, 31, 56, 51, 54, 58, 66, 17), his liking for sexual activity (59, 69, 9, 18, 19, 32, 41, 55), his contentment with his sexual life (11, 15, 20, 22) and his lack of worry about it (60, 63). He too is easily excited sexually, (7, 33, 39, 43, 46) and endorses pre-marital sex (26, 42, 45); he too is promiscuous (77, 44), but he lacks the pathological element of the high P scorer (28, 35), and his liking for pornography is very slight (84, 85, 91, 92, 93, 94). Homosexuality (36) is no problem to him, and offers no attraction.

High N scorers show a different combination of excitement and approval for pre-marital sex with the other factors: they are characterized by low satisfaction and high guilt feelings. Loadings are highest on guilt (·30), and lack of satisfaction (·25); excitement loads more highly for the men (·20). Individual items emphasize the same features; particularly prominent are the lack of satisfaction derived from sex (4, 20, 22), the guilt feelings associated with a strong conscience (48, 25), the worry about sexual activities (60, 63), the problem of controlling sexual thoughts (35, 7, 28, 29), and the fears and difficulties associated with contacts with the opposite sex (56, 17, 54, 56, 31). Blame is attached to the inhibiting influence of the parents (34), religion (49) and 'bad experiences' (27). Sexual behaviour is seen as both troublesome (21, 19, 66) and disgusting (11), and the high N scorer stresses his inability to contact members of the other sex (15, 23); in spite of all this he has strong sexual drives (33, 41, 43, 50, 52) which he finds it difficult to control (32, 53). Homosexuality is a problem (16, 36, 40). There is some evidence of liking for pornography (83, 85, 93, 94), but much less so than in the high P scorer; it almost seems a substitute for the unattainable sexual contacts with real life partners. Lastly, there is a tendency to be hostile to the sex partner (80, 73), but again the context suggests a different interpretation to the hostility of the high P scorer; here the hostility may spring from the failure to acquire a sex partner in the first place!

Taking an overall view, one might say that, as expected, high P and N scorers show a distinctly pathological pattern of sexual reactions. Both are characterized by strong sexual drives (the former less so than the latter), but whereas the high P scorer 'acts out' his libidinous, promiscuous and perverse desires, the high N scorer does not; instead he is beset by a whole set of inhibitions, worries, and guilt feelings which effectively prevent him from consummating his desires. Yet both groups are dissatisfied with their patterns of sexual performance, although presumably for different reasons; this dissatisfaction constitutes the strongest evidence for the hypothesis that both are to some degree 'pathological'. (It would clearly not be adequate to justify this term on the grounds of either statistical infrequency of occurrence, or of moral and ethical undesirability of the conduct in question; it is because both groups are so dissatisfied with their behaviour that one may justly infer that it is not appropriate.) Both groups are similar in that they view their sex partners with some hostility, like pornography, and have homosexual leanings; yet as already pointed out, the different setting in which these items occur suggests different interpretations of the motivation involved, at least for the first two points.

As regards the E factor, the evidence would seem to suggest that here we have two nonpathological ways of sexual adjustment, the extraverted and the introverted, which are opposed in a very meaningful manner. The extravert endorses the 'permissive', promiscuous approach to sex, with frequent change of sex partner and much 'healthy appetite' for frequent sexual contacts. The introvert endorses the orthodox Christian approach with fidelity, stress on virginity, and less purely biological factors as the prime contents. Taken to their extremes, these approaches become the 'liber-

tine' and the 'puritan' respectively, but if not taken to excess they are probably both viable modes of adjustment. The extravert seems more satisfied with his way of life, and is of course better able to contact members of the opposite sex, but this may be an artefact of the particular sample taken; at 20, unmarried youngsters quite naturally have some difficulties in living up to introverted ideals. At 40, the happily married introvert may show better adjustment than the extravert suffering from the 'seven year itch'. This is of course merely speculation, but it may serve to emphasize the restrictions imposed on interpretation by the specific nature of the sample studied.*

*The data presented in Tables IV, V and VI enable us to say something about the consistency of the personality-attitude relations between sexes, and also about the similarity or dissimilarity of attitudes held by different personality types. Given in these Tables are six columns (r_P, r_E, and r_N, each replicated for males and females) which report the correlations of each of the 94 items with P, E and N. These six columns were themselves correlated, in the hope that the results would throw some light on the two problems mentioned above. First consider the male-female correlations within personality type, i.e. P_M vs. $P_F = \cdot 69$; E_M vs. $E_F = \cdot 80$; N_M vs. $N_F = \cdot 77$. These demonstrate that personality scale–attitude item correlations which are high for one sex are also high for the other; there is clearly a considerable amount of consistency here, particularly for the E scale, slightly less so for the N scale, and least of all for the P scale. This is not unexpected, as the P scale is the least reliable and has had much less experimental work associated with it than the other two scales. When we turn from these intra-scale correlations to inter-scale correlations, we find results which may be set out in the form of a small Table:

	P × E	P × N	E × N
Male vs. male: ..	·28	·23	− ·61
Female vs. female: ..	·39	·38	− ·25
Male vs. female: ..	·22	·33	− ·39
Female vs. male: ..	·32	·14	− ·44

Clearly the sexual attitudes of high P scorers are a little like those of high E scorers, and also a little like those of high N scorers; the degree of similarity does not amount to more than about 8 per cent or 9 per cent of the variance. High E scorers are somewhat more markedly unlike high N scorers; the degree of dissimilarity amount to something like 17 per cent of the variance. The within-sex comparisons are no different on the whole from the between-sex comparisons, and all are in good agreement with each other. The between-scale correlations are clearly lower than the within-scale correlations, demonstrating that our results are consistent across sex. On the whole these figures are very encouraging; they suggest that different personality types do indeed have different attitudes towards sex, regardless of the sex of the respondent.

Having thus briefly discussed the sexual attitudes associated with P, E and N, it may be worth while to devote a few sentences to a discussion of the observed differences between male and female attitudes, as set out in numerical form in the Appendix. (In assessing percentage differences, it is of course essential to bear in mind the different S.E.s at different levels of p, as set out in Table III.) Overwhelmingly outstanding among items giving marked differences between the sexes are items relating to pornography (47, 81, 84, 91, 92, 93), orgies (44, 94), voyeurism (83, 62) and prostitution (85), closely followed by impersonal sex (2, 13). Sexual excitement is close behind (33, 41, 43, 46, 82, 3, 39); in all this of course males have higher rates of endorsement than females. Pre-marital sex is also favoured more by the males (45, 70, 79, 42), as is promiscuity (77). But contentment in their sex life is more marked among women (4, 20, 11, 22), perhaps unexpectedly. Masturbation is more a male pastime (10, 8), and men are also less prudish in general (18, 68, 69, 59), and feel less guilt (25). Most of these differences are not unexpected, although one should not overinterpret them; some of the replies may represent little but widely held views unthinkingly endorsed. The only unexpected feature of the study is the apparent satisfaction of the women with their sex lives; it used to be thought that the 'permissive' society favoured men, as did the Victorian era. Possibly the clue lies in the greater sex drive apparent in the men, and the difficulties which this strong drive must give rise to when confronted with the stark reality that over half the women in our sample were still virgins and apparently intent on holding on to this status. In this sellers' market, women clearly have the upper hand, and may enjoy this status; again the nature of our sample may be responsible for a finding which is not likely to be duplicated for older men and women. There is an interesting finding in Schofield's book (1968), in which he showed that female adolescents who had had intercourse were not very attractive on the whole, while male adolescents who had had intercourse were; the explanation presumably is again in terms of the sellers' market—men must be attractive

to get a girl, but a girl who is attractive does not need to trade her virginity for male attention. Specific research devoted to a clarification of these relations might be of considerable interest.

RESULTS: SEXUAL PATHOLOGY

Two questions in the inventory related to sexual reactions which might be considered medically pathological, although use of this term is of course somewhat arbitrary in this context. The questions relating to male subjects were numbers 95 and 96, as shown in the Appendix; they are concerned with impotence and ejaculatio praecox respectively. For the women, these two questions referred instead to frigidity (from a = never to f = always) and orgasm during intercourse (from a = very often to f = never). The actual wording of the possible answers (a to f) was identical to that of the male questions. The wording of the female questions was: Have you ever suffered from frigidity? and Do you usually have orgasm during intercourse? These questions are only meaningful for respondents who have in fact had intercourse, and were only answered by them; in consequence they could not be included in the factor analysis, and results are discussed separately in this section.

The distributions of replies, as expected, are very asymmetrical, and in order to make possible the use of t tests an attempt was made to divide the distribution at a point which would give as nearly as possible groups of equal size; this aim was not accomplished with any very great success, due to the piling up of data in certain categories. Nevertheless, the results are suitable for statistical treatment. The male results will be discussed first, followed by the female results. In each case, the P, E and N scores of the groups which showed or did not show the pathological behaviour in question were calculated and compared, significance of differences being assessed by means of the t technique.

(1) *Male impotence.* The great majority of men gave answer (a), i.e. 'never', to this question (n = 164); consequently all other answers were grouped together to form the 'pathological' group (n = 120). Mean scores on P, E and N

are shown in Table VII; it will be seen that impotent men are somewhat (non-significantly) higher on P, more introverted, and significantly (p < ·05) higher on N.

(2) *Ejaculatio Praecox.* A majority of men gave answers (e) and (f), i.e. never or hardly ever (n = 152); consequently all other answers were grouped together to form the 'pathological' group (n = 132). Mean scores on P, E and N are shown in Table VII; it will be seen that men suffering somewhat from ejaculatio praecox are slightly (non-significantly) lower on P, slightly more introverted, and significantly higher on N.

(3) *Female frigidity,* The great majority of women gave answer (b), i.e. once or twice; this was grouped with answers (c) to (f) to constitute the 'pathological' group, with those answering 'never' (a) constituting the non-pathological group. Mean scores on the personality dimensions are given in Table VII; frigid women (using this term somewhat inaccurately for our 'pathological' group) are somewhat more introverted, but not significantly so, and score higher on N, but also not significantly so. Numbers are only 49 in the non-pathological group, and 122 in the pathological group; had the numbers been as large as those in the male groups, these differences might have reached significance. Clearly repetition of the study with larger numbers is called for.

(4) *Orgasm.* Many women gave answer (a), i.e. 'very often' or (b), i.e. 'often'; these were combined to form the non-pathological group (n = 83). The other answers were combined

to form the 'pathological' group (n = 86). Neither P nor E seem to be related to orgasm frequency; N, however, differentiates the two groups at the ·05 level of statistical significance. Higher N scores go with lower orgasm frequency.

The results of this analysis are not unexpected; it is found that sexual pathology as defined here is associated with neuroticism (significantly in three cases out of four, and almost significantly in the fourth case). Introverts show slightly greater pathology, but these differences never reach significance. High P scorers do not differ significantly from low P scorers, and may in fact have slightly less pathology as regards these indices of behaviour.

It is doubtful if the behaviours called 'pathological' really deserve this name, in view of the frequency with which they occur in this normal group, and it seemed of some interest to study the personality correlates of the much smaller more extreme groups giving more definitely pathological reactions. Five males admitting to having suffered from impotence often, more often than not, or always; they showed a markedly elevated P score of 7·00, which is significantly higher than average. The E score of this group fell to 11·9, and the N score rose to 12·8; these changes are in line with expectation, but not significant in view of the very small size of the sample. Six women admitted to frigidity often, more often than not, or always. Their P scores went up to 4·58, and their N score reached the very high value of 17·83; the latter value is significant beyond the 1 per cent level, but the former is not significantly different from average. The other

TABLE VII

		P	E	N
1. Male Impotence:	Non-pathological	4·37	13·09	10·58
	Pathological	4·82	12·65	11·84
2. Ejaculatio Praecox:	Non-pathological	4·62	13·04	10·54
	Pathological	4·48	12·70	11·70
3. Frigidity:	Non-pathological	3·00	12·59	12·05
	Pathological	2·80	11·58	13·41
4. Orgasm:	Non-pathological	3·06	11·87	12·29
	Pathological	2·77	11·84	13·75

Mean P, E and N scores of students pathological and non-pathological, with respect to four sexual disorders.

extreme groups do not add anything of interest to the data already presented. It is interesting that in spite of the small size of the sample of frigid women, the greater degree of pathology involved has now made the relation with N significant. We may conclude, therefore, that all four types of sexual pathology are related to N, but that P is only involved significantly with high frequency of impotence.

General Discussion

There would be little point in repeating the many detailed findings which this study has given rise to, or in summarizing the various conclusions. Discussion will be confined to two main points: (1) the problems of sampling and (2) the problem of veridical report. The correlations here established between sexual attitudes and personality variables are meaningful only in so far as they can be considered to transcend the particular sample on which they were established. Correlations are not as subject to sampling distortions as are population parameters such as means, but nevertheless some evidence is required to show that our sample is not so highly selected with respect to relevant variables as to make the conclusions of doubtful generality. Eysenck (1971) has shown that the sample is very similar to unselected population samples of similar age with respect to percentage of men and women with experience of coitus, and also with respect to the scores on P, E and N. In other words, our sample is representative of the population of unmarried adolescents of 18 to 22 years of age with respect to the two main variables we are concerned with, i.e. sexual experience and personality; it seems unlikely that our data are entirely idiosyncratic and unrepresentative. No doubt some distortion of sampling has taken place through the act of volunteering and other associated factors, but these are probably not so serious as to invalidate the results.

As regards veridical reports, we have two lines of argument. The first relates to internal evidence; thus, duplicated items gave very highly correlated results, which suggests that items were not filled in randomly or with intention to deceive. The large number of comments written on the questionnaire returned suggested that respondents took the task very seriously. Most important, meaningful factors are not likely to arise from an analysis of correlations between items which were not in fact completed with some degree of honesty. Furthermore, the higher correlations between sexual behaviour patterns and personality in males are unlikely to have arisen from faked data.

More convincing perhaps are various bits of external evidence. If the relations established in this paper are real, then it should be possible to find evidence in the literature of factual consequences of these relations. Eysenck (1971) has argued, for instance, that if extraverts are in fact more promiscuous, then V.D. patients and unmarried mothers should be particularly extraverted; Eysenck (1961) and Wells (1969) have found evidence in favour of these predictions. Sex differences in line with our results have been discovered in an experimental investigation by Sigurt *et al.* (1970). Psychiatrists have repeatedly found a relation between neurosis and sexual pathology; our data are very much in line with these suggestions. Ultimately, of course, there can be no absolute proof for the veridical nature of the answers given, but such evidence as has been quoted makes it unlikely that the data seriously misrepresent the truth. After all, respondents were assured of anonymity and had no motivation to tell lies; furthermore, much concentrated work was required to fill in the various questionnaires properly and post them back to the author, and few people would be likely to undertake all this just in order to mislead.

It might also be pointed out that other writers, using different methods, have reported results which, where comparable, were similar to ours. Mention has already been made of the work of Giese and Schmidt; we might also mention the interviewing studies of Schofield (1968), and of Bynner (1969), which also resulted in congruent results. There is thus beginning to build up a set of findings linking personality factors with sexual attitudes and behaviours which seems to hang together and be reproducible from study to study, even when different methods of information gathering and different samples, of different nationality, are involved. Finally, it should be noted that these results are for the most part in excellent agreement with prediction from theory; respondents could hardly have known these theories, or filled in their inventories in such a way as to support prediction!

If we can accept that the results are along the right lines, even though of course requiring replication, and relevant only to unmarried adolescents of between 18 and 22, then we can frame certain general conclusions. Sexual attitudes and behaviours seem to coalesce around two main and relatively independent factors: sexual pathology and sexual libido. Both these factors denote continua; pathology may be present to varying degree, and libidinal strength may vary from little to great. High N scorers are clearly most likely to suffer from sexual pathology; this emerges, for both men and women, from both the factor analysis and also from the separate analysis of frigidity, orgasm frequency, impotence and ejaculatio praecox. High P scorers, while also slightly prone to pathology, are particularly high on libido. Extraverts are somewhat higher on libido than introverts, and somewhat less pathological, but we have argued that this pathological association with introversion may be found only in this particular age range. As pointed out before, both the high N and the high P attitudes are probably undesirable; healthy and acceptable reactions, although entirely different, are those of extraverts and introverts, adopting respectively the hedonistic and the stoic philosophies (or the permissive and the Victorian point of view, if these terms be preferred). These are of course only the bold outlines of the picture; much of the finer detail has been disclosed in the body of this paper. If more questions are raised than answered, this should be blamed on the relative neglect of this whole field by psychologists and psychiatrists alike; it seems odd that 70 years after Freud insisted so dramatically on the importance of the study of sexual impulses so little should be known about this vital topic.

Summary

Some 800 unmarried male and female students were administered a personality inventory measuring psychoticism, extraversion and neuroticism, as well as a 98 item questionnaire of sexual attitudes. Factor analysis showed that some 15 factors were sufficient to account for the attitudes sampled; most of these were similar for the two sexes. High- and low-scorers on the three personality variables were compared for their responses to the attitude items, and numerous highly significant differences were found; similarly, male and female students' responses were compared. Personality scores were found to be correlated with some of the sex attitude factors. In general, high N scorers showed the greatest degree of pathology, followed by high P scorers; extraverts showed an absence of pathology. P scorers showed strong libidinal desires. These and many other findings are considered in the context of the writer's personality theory which had provided certain tentative predictions about the sexual attitudes and behaviour of different personality types.

References

BYNNER, J. M. (1969). 'The association between adolescent behaviour and attitudes as revealed by a new social attitude inventory'. London: Univ. of London, unpublished Ph.D. thesis.

EYSENCK, H. J. (1967). *The Biological Basis of Personality.* Springfield, Ill. C. C. Thomas.

—— (1971). *Personality and Sexual Behaviour.* To appear.

—— and EYSENCK, S. B. G. (1968). 'A factorial study of psychoticism as a dimension of personality.' *Multivariate Behav. Res.*, Special Issue, 15–31.

—— —— (1969). *The Structure and Measurement of Personality.* London: Routledge and Kegan Paul.

EYSENCK, S. B. G. (1961). 'Personality and gain assessment in childbirth of married and unmarried mothers.' *J. ment. Sci.*, 417–30.

EYSENCK, S. B. G., and EYSENCK, H. J. (1968). 'The measurement of psychoticism: a study of factor stability and reliability.' *Brit. J. soc. clin. Psychol.*, 7, 286–94.

—— —— (1969a). '"Psychoticism" in children: a new personality variable.' *Res. in Educ.*, 1, 21–37.

—— —— (1969b). 'Scores on three personality variables as a function of age, sex, and social class.' *Brit. J. soc. clin. Psychol.*, 8, 69–76.

GIESE, H., and SCHMIDT, A. (1968). *Studenten Sexualität.* Hamburg: Rowohlt.

SCHOFIELD, M. (1968). *The Sexual Behaviour of Young People.* London: Pelican Books.

SIGURT, V., SCHMIDT, G., RHEINFELD, S., and WEIDEMANN-SUTOR, I. (1970). 'Psycho-sexual stimulation: sex differences.' *J. Sex Res.*, 6, 10–24.

PERSONALITY AND SEXUAL ADJUSTMENT

THORNE, F. C. (1966). 'The sex inventory.' *J. clin. Psychol.*, Monogr. Suppl. No. 21.

WELLS, B. W. P. (1969). 'Personality characteristics of V.D. patients.' *Brit. J. soc. clin. Psychol.*, 8, 246–52.

APPENDIX

INVENTORY OF ATTITUDES TO SEX

This questionnaire is anonymous, to encourage truthful answers

Read each statement carefully, then underline the 'yes' or the 'no' answer, depending on your views. If you just cannot decide, underline the '?' reply. Please answer *every* question. There are no right or wrong answers. Don't think too long over each question; try to give an immediate answer which represents your *feelings* on each issue. Some questions are similar to others; there are good reasons for getting at the same attitude in slightly different ways.

		Percentage 'YES' Answers	
		Male:	Female:
1.	The opposite sex will respect you more if you are not too familiar with them.	38	59
2.	Sex without love ('impersonal sex') is highly unsatisfactory.	49	80
3.	Conditions have to be just right to get me excited sexually.	21	43
4.	All in all I am satisfied with my sex life.	40	60
5.	Virginity is a girl's most valuable possession.	16	24
6.	I think only rarely about sex.	4	13
7.	Sometimes it has been a problem to control my sex feelings.	46	44
8.	Masturbation is unhealthy.	7	21
9.	If I loved a person I could do anything with them.	55	46
10.	I get pleasant feelings from touching my sexual parts.	61	37
11.	I have been deprived sexually.	25	8
12.	It is disgusting to see animals having sex relations in the street.	5	6
13.	I do not need to respect a woman, or love her, in order to enjoy petting and/or intercourse with her.	43	12
14.	It is alright for children to see their parents naked.	64	74
15.	I am rather sexually unattractive.	10	5
16.	Frankly, I prefer people of my own sex.	3	2
17.	Sex contacts have never been a problem to me.	35	41
18.	It is disturbing to see necking in public.	12	23
19.	Sexual feelings are sometimes unpleasant to me.	11	16

		Percentage 'YES' Answers	
		Male:	Female:
20.	Something is lacking in my sex life.	50	26
21.	My sex behaviour has never caused me any trouble.	43	36
22.	My love life has been disappointing.	39	23
23.	I never had many dates.	36	26
24.	I consciously try to keep sex thoughts out of my mind.	2	7
25.	I have felt guilty about sex experiences.	29	41
26.	It wouldn't bother me if the person I married were not a virgin.	68	73
27.	I had some bad sex experiences when I was young.	15	13
28.	Perverted thoughts have sometimes bothered me.	28	18
29.	At times I have been afraid of myself for what I might do sexually.	19	26
30.	I have had conflicts about my sex feelings towards a person of my own sex.	16	9
31.	I have many friends of the opposite sex.	71	80
32.	I have strong sex feelings but when I get a chance I can't seem to express myself.	23	12
33.	It doesn't take much to get me excited sexually.	66	31
34.	My parents' influence has inhibited me sexually.	30	25
35.	Thoughts about sex disturb me more than they should.	12	7
36.	People of my own sex frequently attract me.	4	4
37.	There are some things I wouldn't want to do with anyone.	53	47
38.	Children should be taught about sex.	94	97
39.	I could get sexually excited at any time of the day or night.	88	69
40.	I understand homosexuals.	44	35
41.	I think about sex almost every day.	84	52
42.	One should not experiment with sex before marriage.	7	21
43.	I get sexually excited very easily.	60	27
44.	The thought of a sex orgy is disgusting to me.	18	65
45.	It is better not to have sex relations until you are married.	6	31
46.	I find the thought of a coloured sex partner particularly exciting.	24	3

BY H. J. EYSENCK

		Percentage 'YES' Answers	
		Male:	Female:

		Percentage 'YES' Answers	
		Male:	Female:

47. I like to look at sexy pictures. .. — Male: 61, Female: 8
48. My conscience bothers me too much. .. .. — Male: 18, Female: 26
49. My religious beliefs are against sex. .. .. — Male: 7, Female: 13
50. Sometimes sexual feelings over-power me. .. .. .. — Male: 32, Female: 27
51. I feel nervous with the opposite sex. .. .. — Male: 25, Female: 15
52. Sex thoughts drive me almost crazy. .. .. — Male: 6, Female: 2
53. When I get excited I can think of nothing else but satisfaction. — Male: 24, Female: 15
54. I feel at ease with people of the opposite sex. .. .. .. — Male: 66, Female: 80
55. I don't like to be kissed. .. — Male: 2, Female: 3
56. It is hard to talk with people of the opposite sex. .. .. — Male: 12, Female: 6
57. I didn't learn the facts of life until I was quite old. .. .. — Male: 26, Female: 23
58. I feel more comfortable when I am with my own sex. .. .. — Male: 24, Female: 16
59. I enjoy petting. .. .. — Male: 92, Female: 78
60. I worry a lot about sex. .. — Male: 22, Female: 13
61. The Pill should be universally available. .. .. .. — Male: 84, Female: 65
62. Seeing a person nude doesn't interest me. .. .. .. — Male: 11, Female: 43
63. Sometimes thinking about sex makes me very nervous. .. — Male: 16, Female: 20
64. Women who get raped are often partly responsible themselves... — Male: 57, Female: 53
65. Perverted thoughts have some-times bothered me. .. .. — Male: 26, Female: 18
66. I am embarrassed to talk about sex. .. .. — Male: 9, Female: 8
67. Young people should learn about sex through their own experience. .. .. .. — Male: 34, Female: 23
68. Sometimes the woman should be sexually aggressive. .. .. — Male: 88, Female: 64
69. Sex jokes disgust me. .. .. — Male: 4, Female: 22
70. I believe in taking my pleasures where I find them. .. .. — Male: 44, Female: 7
71. A person should learn about sex gradually by experimenting with it. .. .. — Male: 52, Female: 42
72. Young people should be allowed out at night without being too closely checked. .. .. — Male: 68, Female: 54
73. Did you ever feel like humiliat-ing your sex partner? .. .. — Male: 20, Female: 12
74. I would particularly protect my children from contacts with sex. — Male: 5, Female: 9

75. Self-relief is not dangerous so long as it is done in a healthy way. .. .. — Male: 74, Female: 56
76. I get very excited when touching a woman's breasts. .. .. — Male: 57, Female: 45
77. I have been involved with more than one sex affair at the same time. .. .. — Male: 32, Female: 14
78. Homosexuality is normal for some people. .. .. .. — Male: 74, Female: 70
79. It is alright to seduce a person who is old enough to know what he or she is doing. .. .. — Male: 73, Female: 35
80. Do you ever feel hostile to your sex partner? .. .. .. — Male: 37, Female: 40
81. I like to look at pictures of nudes. .. .. — Male: 63, Female: 10
82. Buttocks excite me. .. .. — Male: 42, Female: 8
83. If you had the chance to see people making love, without being seen, would you take it? — Male: 41, Female: 12
84. Pornographic writings should be freely allowed to be pub-lished. .. .. — Male: 59, Female: 32
85. Prostitution should be legally permitted. .. .. .. — Male: 62, Female: 32
86. Decisions about abortion should be the concern of no one but the woman concerned. .. — Male: 52, Female: 47
87. There are too many immoral plays on TV. .. .. .. — Male: 6, Female: 13
88. The dual standard of morality is natural, and should be con-tinued. .. .. — Male: 32, Female: 26
89. We should do away with mar-riage entirely. .. .. .. — Male: 9, Female: 2
90. Men marry to have intercourse; women have intercourse for the sake of marriage. .. .. — Male: 7, Female: 3
91. There should be no censorship, on sexual grounds, of plays and films. .. .. — Male: 63, Female: 39

Please underline the correct answer

92. If you were invited to see a 'blue' film, would you: .. — Male: 80, Female: 37
(a) Accept   (b) Refuse
93. If you were offered a highly pornographic book, would you: — Male: 76, Female: 40
(a) Accept it   (b) Reject it
94. If you were invited to take part in an orgy, would you: .. — Male: 61, Female: 4
(a) Take part   (b) Refuse

95. Given availability of a partner, would you prefer to have intercourse:
   (a) Never
   (b) Once a month
   (c) Once a week
   (d) Twice a week
   (e) 3–5 times a week
   (f) Every day
   (g) More than once a day

96. Have you ever suffered from impotence:
   (a) Never
   (d) Often
   (b) Once or twice
   (c) Several times
   (e) More often than not
   (f) Always

97. Have you ever suffered from ejaculatio praecox (premature ejaculation)?
   (a) Very often
   (b) Often
   (c) Middling
   (d) Not very often
   (e) Hardly ever
   (f) Never

98. At what age did you have your first intercourse . . . .

H. J. Eysenck, Ph.D., *Professor of Psychology, Institute of Psychiatry, De Crespigny Park, Denmark Hill, London, S.E.5*

(*Received 3 June 1970*)

505

From J. F. Allsopp and M. P. Feldman (1974). Social Behavior and Personality, *2*, 184–190, *by kind permission of the authors and the Society for Personality Research Inc.*

EXTRAVERSION, NEUROTICISM, PSYCHOTICISM AND ANTISOCIAL BEHAVIOR IN SCHOOLGIRLS

JOHN F. ALLSOPP*
and
M. PHILIP FELDMAN
University of Birmingham

Four groups of Ss, ranging from 11 and 12 year-olds to 14 and 15 year-olds, were tested on the Junior P.Q., a new measure of E, N and P in children, and on an anonymous self-report questionnaire of antisocial behavior (ASB). An objective measure of school naughtiness (Na) was also available. The results followed similar trends in each group and showed that ASB is positively related to E, N and P, and Na to E and P. It is concluded that Eysenck's theory of antisocial behavior is capable of predictions concerning the range of misbehavior engaged in by secondary school girls.

Studies designed to test the theory proposed by Eysenck (1964, 1970), that criminality is causally related to the continuous orthogonal personality dimensions of extraversion (E) and neuroticism (N), have generally considered E and N scores independently, and compared a group of institutionalized offenders with a control group of non-institutionalized non-offenders. Such studies have consistently shown that adult male prisoners are significantly higher than normal control groups on N, but in general no such differences have emerged on E (Bartholomew, 1959; Field, 1959; Fitch, 1962; Eysenck and Eysenck, 1970, 1971b). Similar findings have been reported by Little (1963) for boys in borstal. Recently, however, Burgess (1972) has described three studies in which independent E and N scale comparisons provided similar results, but in each of which a quadrant analysis showed the prisoners to be significantly over-represented in the high E high N quadrant. Adult female prisoners have been found much higher on N and higher on E than control Ss (Bartholomew, 1963; Eysenck, 1964; Eysenck and Eysenck, 1964), and borstal girls have been shown to be extremely high on both N and E (Price, 1968). However, Hoghughi and Forrest (1970) have described a number of studies in which samples of approved school boys of various ages were found to score significantly higher on N, but significantly lower on E, than corresponding standardization samples.

On the other hand, studies using a self-report questionnaire measure of antisocial behavior (ASB), based on the work of Gibson (1967), and constructed by the second author of the present study, have

*Now at Institute of Psychiatry, University of London.

suggested that delinquent behavior in boys of this age is related to extraversion. Allsopp (1968), having found no significant E difference between early teenage remand school and secondary school boys, showed that when the Ss were divided into high and low ASB scorers the former group was significantly higher on the E scale. Further, with two male and two female samples of fourth form secondary school children, Saxby *et al.* (1970) found a significant linear relationship between ASB score and levels of E. The question arises as to which studies have provided a valid relationship between delinquency and extraversion. The studies using the ASB questionnaire indicate that it provides a valid measure of a continuous dimension of antisocial behavior and, while appreciating that more precise information needs to be obtained, the authors suggest that the most likely explanation for the negative findings with respect to E obtained from the other studies with male Ss is that proposed by Eysenck and Eysenck (1970), namely, that certain questions on the E scale produce different interpretations and answers in institutionalized populations.

The studies with the ASB questionnaire suggest that Eysenck's theory may be applicable to a far wider range of behavior than adult criminality. The present study was an attempt to investigate whether the theory can be used to predict the relationships between the personality and antisocial behavior of ordinary school girls. The ASB questionnaire was expanded in an attempt to cover the complete range of misdemeanours committed by secondary school girls. There was also available an objective measure of school naughtiness (Na). Following the prediction of Eysenck (1964, 1970) of a relationship between criminality and the E and N personality dimensions on the basis of their mutual connection with conditioning, it was hypothesized that ASB and Na are positively related to both E and N. Eysenck (1970) has extended his theory to include the prediction that psychoticism (P) is related to certain types of adult criminality, and two studies which have used a P scale (Eysenck and Eysenck, 1970, 1971b) have shown that prisoners are clearly higher than controls on this dimension. The similarity of many of the ASB questionnaire items to criminal acts appeared sufficient reason to follow Eysenck's (1970) prediction, and hypothesize a positive relationship between ASB and P, but it did not seem appropriate to predict the existence of such a relationship for school misbehavior.

METHOD

SUBJECTS

The Ss were members of the first four year groups of a Warley secondary girls school, ranging in age from 11 to 12 years old to 14 to 15 years old. The E was a teacher at the school. It was possible to test virtually all the girls on the school roll and, when Jamaican and Indian Ss, for whom the results were analyzed separately (Allsopp, 1972), were excluded, there were available for analysis questionnaire responses from 54, 45, 50 and 48 Ss in the four groups taken in ascending order of age.

SOCIAL BEHAVIOR AND PERSONALITY

QUESTIONNAIRES

The E, N and P personality dimensions were measured with the Junior P.Q., a new inventory designed for use with children (Eysenck and Eysenck, 1973). The ASB questionnaire[1] along with details of its development has been described in detail elsewhere (Allsopp, 1972). It consisted of the 28 items of the original questionnaire to which were added another 20 items chosen following detailed discussion with small groups in oral English lessons on the range of misbehavior engaged in by girls of their age. The items range from very mild acts (*e.g.*, making a noise in class or whilst moving about the school) to serious offences (*e.g.*, breaking into private property to steal something). The questionnaire asked the Ss not to include their name as the answers would be "private and confidential" and, on the basis of this, "please be honest when you tick each item". The Ss were required to indicate whether they had undertaken the acts "never", "once or twice", or "three or more times". The questionnaire was scored by giving two points for a "three or more times" response, and one point for a "once or twice" response. There was also available a measure of school naughtiness (Na) consisting of the total number of marks lost for bad behavior over two full terms, one either side of the time of testing.

RESULTS

Table 1 shows the correlations for ASB and Na with each of E, N and P. For ASB, all correlations with the personality variables are

TABLE 1: CORRELATIONS OF ASB AND Na WITH EACH OF E, N AND P

| | | ASB | | | Na | |
	E	N	P	E	N	P
Year 1	0.13	0.15	0.22	0.34*	−0.21	−0.05
Year 2	0.13	0.24	0.34*	0.12	0.06	0.39*
Year 3	0.11	0.32*	0.61*	0.02	0.22	0.54*
Year 4	0.30*	0.21	0.40*	0.36*	0.02	−0.06

*$p < 0.05$.

positive, although the values only reach significance with E in the fourth year group, with N in the third year group, and with P in the oldest three age groups. For Na, the youngest and oldest groups show a significant correlation with E and a virtually zero correlation with P, while the middle two age groups show a clearly positive and highly significant correlation with P and only a low correlation with E. None of the correlations between Na and N is significant.

In order to determine the possible effects of interactions between the personality variables in determining ASB and Na scores, the Ss were divided within each age group into ENP octant groups by dichotomizing about the mean on E and N, and about the median on P. Analysis of variance on both ASB and Na scores within these

---

[1] Copies of the questionnaire may be obtained from the authors.

octant groups indicated no interactions between the personality variables and age, and so the S groups were combined for the purpose of further analysis. For ASB, significant effects were shown to exist for E (1% level), N (5% level), P (0.1% level), and the E × N interaction (5% level). For Na significant effects were shown for only E (5% level) and P (0.1% level). When this combined group of Ss is considered the trends suggested by the correlation data of Table 1, that is, that ASB is positively related to each of E, N and P, and Na to both E and P, are all significant. Inspection of Table 2 showing mean ASB scores for the four EN quadrants suggests that the E × N interaction effect can be accounted for by the relationship with E and N being due to low E low N quadrant Ss scoring abnormally low on ASB.

TABLE 2: MEAN ASB SCORES FOR EN QUADRANTS FOR ALL SUBJECTS COMBINED

High E High N	High E Low N	Low E High N	Low E Low N
18.22	17.94	16.73	9.16

The data were analyzed in one further way. Within each age group the Ss were divided into four subgroups according to whether they had scored in the upper or lower level, as defined above, on all three, two, one, or none of the E, N and P scales. The mean ASB and Na scores for these subgroups are plotted in Fig. 1. To test the significance of the relationships suggested by Fig. 1, an analysis of variance was

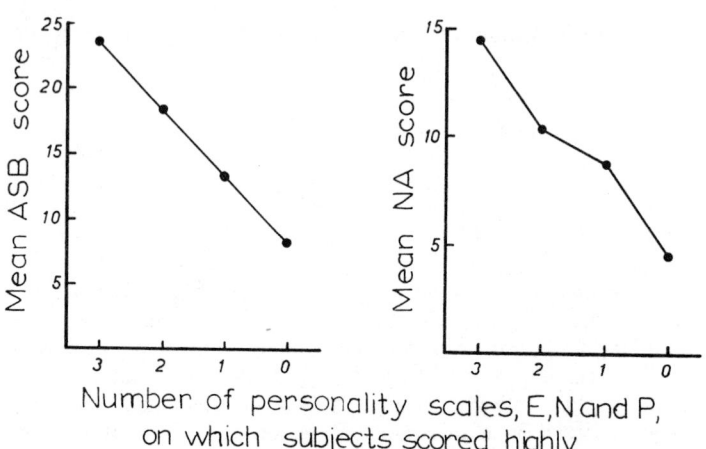

FIG. 1: *Mean ASB and Na scores for all subjects combined in upper level on three, two, one, or none of the personality scales E, N and P.*

undertaken on both ASB and Na scores divided into the four subgroups. In both cases the Years × Subgroups interaction was quite insignificant but the difference between the groups highly significant ($p < 0.001$).

DISCUSSION AND CONCLUSIONS

The correlations between ASB and Na for the four year groups, in ascending order of age, were: 0.35, 0.57, 0.44, and 0.44. Considering that many of the ASB items are concerned with misbehavior far more serious than that for which children would be disciplined in school, these values, all of which reach 5% significance, would appear sufficiently high to argue for the validity of the ASB questionnaire responses. While we do not imply that some Ss do not distort their reports, or that most Ss provide a perfectly accurate self-report, it is suggested that the ASB questionnaire provides a reasonably accurate measure of a S's position on a continuous dimension of antisocial behavior.

The hypotheses that E and N are related to ASB are supported. When the various age groups are considered separately, the results reach significance for only one group in each case. However, all results are in the hypothesized direction, suggesting that with larger samples satisfactory levels of significance would have been obtained with each independent group. The hypothesis that P is positively related to ASB is also supported. For each year group and for all groups combined this relationship is stronger than that for either E or N with ASB and fails to reach significance only for the youngest group of girls.

When the Ss are combined, the hypothesis that E is related to Na is supported, although this relationship only reaches significance for the youngest and oldest groups considered independently. The girls in the middle two age groups do, however, show a strong relationship between Na and P. The explanation of this latter finding perhaps lies in the type of misbehavior that Na measures, for the second and third year girls were by far the most difficult to discipline in the school, and so here the Na scores reflect more serious misdemeanors. The hypothesized relation between Na and N is not supported by the present data. This could be due to children who score high on N being too anxious to misbehave in school where detection by a teacher is both virtually certain and instantaneous. It is interesting in this connection that the group of girls new to the school, to whom the argument would be especially expected to apply, actually provide a negative correlation approaching significance between Na and N. If the explanation proposed is correct this tendency will work against that predicted by Eysenck, so that more precise categorizations of types of school misbehavior will be needed before adequate predictions on the basis of Eysenck's theory can be made in this connection.

The only significant interaction effect is that between E and N in determining ASB score. The data shown in Table 2 suggest that for girls in this age range both E and N are predictive of antisocial behavior, but that the combination of a high E and high N score is not, as suggested by Burgess (1972) for adult criminality, the crucial factor. In the absence of further information no reliable conclusion can be drawn as to the implication of this finding. It is possible that different interactions between E and N operate in determining varying types of delinquent behavior in different populations, and that the effect found here occurs when considering the milder types of antisocial behavior indulged in to some degree by virtually all school children.

In relation to both ASB and Na, all interactions of E and N with P are quite insignificant, the highest F ratio only slightly exceeding unity. In general the results support the findings of a study by Eysenck and Eysenck (1971a) who obtained a "criminal propensity" score by considering the 40 items of their 80-item inventory which showed most discrimination between prisoner and control groups. They argued that, assuming criminals to be higher on all three of the P, E and N scales, and hence to come from one octant of the three dimensional space, the reliability of this combined score would be increased. As this was not found to be so, they concluded that "P, E and N are partly independent and additive, rather than combinational and multiplicative, factors in predisposition to criminal activity" (Eysenck and Eysenck, 1971a, p. 58). With the possible exception of an interaction effect existing between E and N in determining ASB score, and of N not predicting Na scores, the results of the present study fit in well with this conclusion. Figure 1 shows clearly the additive effect of the E, N and P dimensions. There is a clear monotonic relationship for both ASB and Na with the number of personality scales on which the Ss score highly, and, especially for the former measure of misbehavior, the relationship is virtually linear. On each measure the Ss in the high ENP octant scored on average about three times as high as those in the low ENP octant.

The present study has shown that general antisocial behavior of secondary school girls is positively related to the E, N and P personality dimensions. The conclusions to be drawn with respect to school misbehavior are less clear. It appears that the milder types of school naughtiness are related to E and the more serious types to P. It has been tentatively suggested that the hypothesis that N is related to misbehavior in school was not upheld as the effect predicted by Eysenck's theory is confounded by children high on N being too anxious to misbehave in the presence of a teacher where detection is virtually inevitable. In general the results suggest that the personality variables have an independent and additive effect in predicting the degree of misbehavior in girls of this age. These findings provide strong support for the generality of the theory explaining antisocial behavior presented by Eysenck (1964, 1970). The theory is clearly capable of predictions concerning much wider categories of antisocial behavior than serious crimes committed by a small proportion of the population. Further studies, using similar measures to those adopted here, are needed to test the theory's predictions with regard to the continuum of delinquency in the general population.

ACKNOWLEDGEMENTS

We are indebted to the Colonial Research Fund for the support of this investigation. We would like to thank Miss O. M. Bartlett, Headmistress of Shireland Girls School, Warley, for her willing co-operation in providing subjects, and Professor P. L. Broadhurst, Professor H. J.

SOCIAL BEHAVIOR AND PERSONALITY

Eysenck, Dr Sybil B. G. Eysenck, Dr D. W. Fulker and Mr T. W. Teasdale for advice given at various stages of the study.

REFERENCES

Allsopp, J. F. 1968: Extraversion, neuroticism, sensation-seeking and antisocial behavior in remands and controls as measured by self-report. Unpublished undergraduate dissertation, University of Birmingham, Department of Psychology.

Allsopp, J. F. 1972: The effect of extraversion, neuroticism, and psychoticism on measures of antisocial behavior in secondary school girls. Unpublished M.Sc. thesis, University of Birmingham.

Bartholomew, A. A. 1959: Extraversion-introversion and neuroticism in first offenders and recidivists. *British Journal of Delinquency, 10:* 120-9.

Bartholomew, A. A. 1963: Some comparative Australian data for the Maudsley Personality Inventory. *Australian Journal of Psychology, 15:* 46-51.

Burgess, P. K. 1972: Eysenck's theory of criminality: A new approach. *British Journal of Criminology, 12:* 74-82.

Eysenck, H. J. 1964: *Crime and Personality.* Routledge & Kegan Paul, London.

Eysenck, H. J. 1970: *Crime and Personality,* 2nd edn. Paladin, London.

Eysenck, H. J.; Eysenck, S. B. G. 1964: *Manual of the Eysenck Personality Inventory.* University Press, London.

Eysenck, H. J.; Eysenck, S. B. G. 1970: Crime and personality: An empirical study of the three-factor theory. *British Journal of Criminology, 10:* 225-39.

Eysenck, H. J.; Eysenck, S. B. G. 1971a: Crime and personality: Item analysis of questionnaire responses. *British Journal of Criminology, 11:* 49-62.

Eysenck, S. B. G.; Eysenck, H. J. 1971b: A comparative study of criminals and matched controls on three dimensions of personality. *British Journal of Social and Clinical Psychology, 10:* 362-6.

Eysenck, S. B. G.; Eysenck, H. J. 1973: Test re-test reliabilities of a new personality questionnaire for children. *British Journal of Educational Psychology, 43:* 126-30.

Field, J. G. 1959: The personalities of criminals. Paper presented at the Annual Conference of the British Psychological Society, Cambridge. April, 1959.

Fitch, J. H. 1962: Two personality variables and their distribution in a criminal population: An empirical study. *British Journal of Social and Clinical Psychology, 1:* 161-7.

Gibson, H. B. 1967: Self-reported delinquency among schoolboys and their attitudes to the police. *British Journal of Social and Clinical Psychology, 6:* 168-73.

Hoghughi, M. S.; Forrest, A. R. 1970: Eysenck's theory of criminality. An examination with approved school boys. *British Journal of Criminology, 10:* 240-54.

Little, A. 1963: Professor Eysenck's theory of crime: An empirical test on adolescent offenders. *British Journal of Criminology, 4:* 152-63.

Price, J. B. 1968: Some results of the Maudsley Personality Inventory from a sample of girls in borstal. *British Journal of Criminology, 8:* 383-401.

Saxby, P. J.; Norris, A. J.; Feldman, M. P. 1970: Questionnaire studies of self-reported anti-social behaviour and extraversion in adolescents. Unpublished paper, University of Birmingham, Department of Psychology.

JOHN ALLSOPP, PH.D.,
Department of Psychology,
Institute of Psychiatry,
De Crespigny Park,
Denmark Hill, London SE5 8AF,
England.

Reprints of this paper are available from Dr Allsopp.